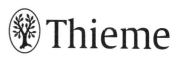

Functional Reconstructive Nasal Surgery

2nd Edition

Egbert H. Huizing, MD, PhD
Professor Emeritus and Former Chairman
Department of Otorhinolaryngology
University Medical Center Utrecht
The Netherlands

John A.M. de Groot, MD, PhD
Formerly Assistant Professor
Department of Otorhinolaryngology
University Medical Center Utrecht
The Netherlands

869 illustrations

Thieme
Stuttgart • New York • Delhi • Rio de Janeiro

Library of Congress Cataloging-in-Publication Data
is available from the publisher.

© 2015 by Georg Thieme Verlag KG

Thieme Publishers Stuttgart
Rüdigerstrasse 14, 70469 Stuttgart, Germany
+49 [0]711 8931 421, customerservice@thieme.de

Thieme Publishers New York
333 Seventh Avenue, New York, NY 10001 USA
+1 800 782 3488, customerservice@thieme.com

Thieme Publishers Delhi
A-12, Second Floor, Sector-2, Noida-201301
Uttar Pradesh, India
+91 120 45 566 00, customerservice@thieme.in

Thieme Publishers Rio, Thieme Publicações Ltda.
Argentina Building 16th floor, Ala A, 228 Praia do Botafogo
Rio de Janeiro 22250-040 Brazil
+55 21 3736-3631

Cover design: Thieme Publishing Group
Typesetting by Thomson Digital, India

Printed in Germany at Aprinta Druck, Wemding   5 4 3 2 1

ISBN 978-3-13-129412-8

Also available as an e-book:
eISBN 978-3-13-164122-9

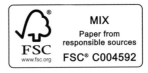

Contents

Contents

Preface

It is rewarding that our book has been used and appreciated in so many teaching clinics in Europe, the United States, Asia, and South America. We were also pleased to witness publication of the first edition in Italian, Turkish, and Chinese—and even some illegal copies!

Some time ago, Mr. Stephan Konnry from Thieme Publishers Stuttgart persuaded us to bring out a second and revised edition of our book. This posed a problem, as we both resigned from the practice of Rhinology and Rhinosurgery several years ago. We felt that this made us unable to update a book like ours. Fortunately, many of our younger colleagues currently teaching in functional reconstructive nasal surgery were willing to update the various chapters without impairing the concept of the book. We are extremely grateful to all of our contributors for their loyalty and help.

Apart from the main contributors, we gratefully acknowledge the remarks given by Dr. René Poublon (Rotterdam) and Dr. Koen Ingels (Nijmegen).

Finally, we would like to thank our editors Mr. Stephan Konnry and Dr. Vicki Gregory (Cambridge, UK) as well as Ms. Nidhi Chopra, Mr. Immanuel Jäger, and Dr. Michael Wachinger for their support.

We hope that this second edition will be received as well as the first one.

Egbert H. Huizing, MD, PhD
John A.M. de Groot, MD, PhD

Contributors

Ronald L.A.W. Bleys, MD, PhD
Professor of Clinical Anatomy
University Medical Center Utrecht
Utrecht, The Netherlands

Peter A.R. Clement, MD, PhD
Emeritus Professor of Otorhinolaryngology
Free University Brussels (V.U.B.)
Ixelles, Belgium

Peter W. Hellings, MD, PhD
Professor of Otorhinolaryngology
University Hospitals Leuven
Leuven, Belgium

Eugene B. Kern, MD, PhD
Emeritus Professor of Rhinology
   and Facial Plastic Surgery
Mayo Clinic Medical School
   Rochester, Minnesota;
Emeritus George M. and Edna B. Endicott
   Professor of Medicine
Mayo Foundation for Medical Education
   and Research;
Professor of Otorhinolaryngology
State University of New York
   Buffalo, New York

Jörg Lindemann, MD, PhD
Professor of Otorhinolaryngology
Department of Otorhinolaryngology
   and Head & Neck Surgery
University Hospital Ulm
Ulm, Germany

Adriaan F. van Olphen, MD, PhD
Formerly Assistant Professor of Otorhinolaryngology
University Medical Center Utrecht
Utrecht, The Netherlands

Wolfgang Pirsig, MD, PhD
Emeritus Professor of Otorhinolaryngology
University of Ulm
Ulm, Germany

Marc O. Scheithauer, MD, PhD
Professor of Otorhinolaryngology
Department of Otorhinolaryngology
   and Head & Neck Surgery
University Hospital Ulm
Ulm, Germany

Abel-Jan Tasman, MD, PhD
Privat-Dozent of Otorhinolaryngology
Kantonsspital St. Gallen
St. Gallen, Switzerland

Chapter 1

Basics

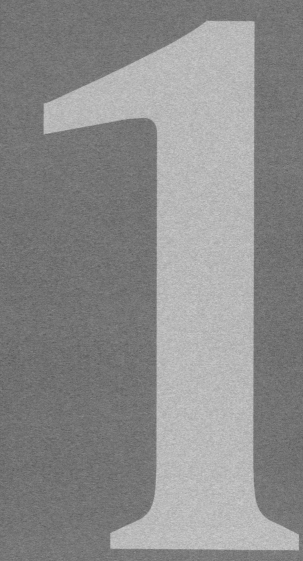

1 Basics

1.1 Surgical Anatomy

1.1.1 Face

Orientation

Both in diagnosis and surgery, the following terms should be used for orientation (▶ Fig. 1.1):
- Cranial (or superior)
- Caudal (or inferior)
- Dorsal (or posterior)
- Ventral (or anterior)

These definitions are to be preferred above others as they are universal and do not change with body position. In the American literature, the term "cephalic" is often used for "cranial."

Proportions

The human face shows considerable variations in size, form, and proportions. The primary factors involved are race, gender, and age; the secondary factors are growth and trauma. It is therefore difficult to distinguish between normal and abnormal. It is even more difficult— and, in principle, impossible—to define "the beautiful face." The concept of beauty has not been consistent throughout history, and various human civilizations have aspired to different ideals. Even within the same culture, these ideals have changed over time.

The Western Standard

Our ideas about facial proportions originate in the work of the artists Leonardo da Vinci (1452–1519) and Albrecht Dürer (1471–1528). According to their concept of harmony, the human face may be divided into three equal horizontal and five equal vertical parts (▶ Fig. 1.2 and ▶ Fig. 1.3). It may be helpful to draw horizontal, verti- cal, and base lines on photographs of the patient when analyzing facial proportions and the relationship of the external nose with other parts of the face. Other than as an aid to partitioning, however, the Leonardo–Dürer con- cept should not be used. First, the concept is not applica- ble to all races; second, age and gender play a dominant role; and finally, the concept of beauty is highly subjec- tive. In our opinion, the primary responsibility of a nasal surgeon is to recreate a nose with normal function and normal form. Enhancement of beauty is of secondary importance.

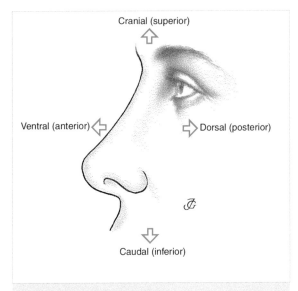

Fig. 1.1 Topographic terminology to be used in nasal surgery.

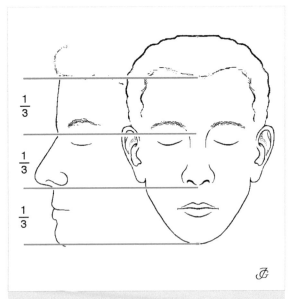

Fig. 1.2 Horizontal division of the face into three equal sections.

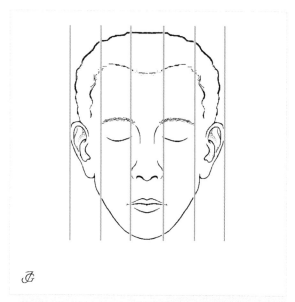

Fig. 1.3 Vertical division of the face into five equal sections.

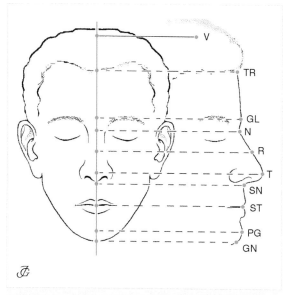

Fig. 1.4 The most important midline points of the face and the nose.
GL = glabella; GN= gnathion; N = nasion; PG = pogonion; R = rhinion; SN= subnasale; ST = stomion; T = tip; TR = trichion; V = vertex.

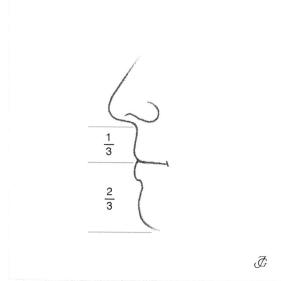

Fig. 1.5 The height of the upper lip is about half the distance from the gnathion to the stomion.

Horizontal Division

The face is made up of three equal sections: hairline–nasion = nasion–subnasale = subnasale–pogonion (► Fig. 1.2 and ► Fig. 1.4). The height of the external nose is equal to that of the forehead and to that of the lower face. This division can be greatly influenced by hair growth, hairstyle, and spectacles.

The lower part of the face can be divided into two parts: the upper lip (one-third) and lower lip with chin (two-thirds) (► Fig. 1.5).

Vertical Division

The face can be divided into five equal sections: the nasal section, two eye sections, and two lateral sections (► Fig. 1.3).

Lobular Base Division

When looked at caudally, the nasal lobule forms a triangle. The height and base of this triangle differ according to race, gender, and age (see ► Fig. 1.17). In the Caucasian race, the distance from the lobular base to the upper corner of the nostril (the length of the columella) is about twice as long as the length of the tip (► Fig. 1.6).

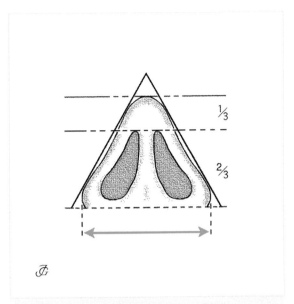

Fig. 1.6 Triangular shape of the lobule. In the Caucasian nose, the distance from the lobular base to the upper corner of the nostril is about twice as long as the length of the tip.

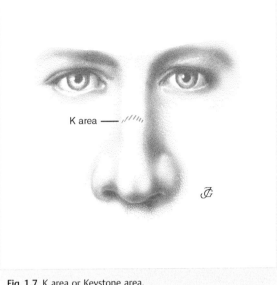

Fig. 1.7 K area or Keystone area.

Points

When analyzing the face, several anthropometric points may be used. Some of these are on the skull (bony landmarks), while others are on the skin (clinical points). The following points are important in nasal analysis.

Midline Points (▶ Fig. 1.4)

- *Vertex (clinical)*: highest point of the head when it is oriented in the Frankfort horizontal plane
- *Trichion (clinical)*: midpoint of the frontal hairline
- *Glabella (clinical and bony)*: midline elevation above the nasal root at the level of the eyebrows
- *Nasion (clinical and bony)*: midpoint of the frontonasal sutures; deepest point at the transition between the forehead and the nose
- *Rhinion (clinical and bony)*: most caudal point of the internasal suture
- *Tip (pronasale; clinical)*: most prominent point of the lobule
- *Subnasale (clinical)*: midpoint of the nasolabial angle overlying the anterior nasal spine
- *Stomion (clinical)*: imaginary point at the crossing of the vertical facial midline and the horizontal labial fissure between the lips
- *Pogonion (clinical and bony)*: most ventral midpoint of the chin
- *Gnathion (clinical and bony)*: midpoint of the caudal margin of the chin

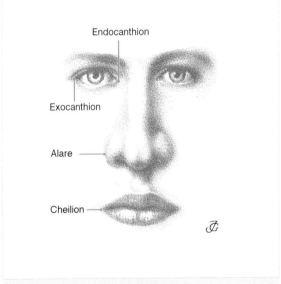

Fig. 1.8 The most important paranasal points.

Keystone or K Area (Clinical)

The keystone or K area is the region where the nasal bones, triangular cartilages, and cartilaginous septum unite. (see ▶ Fig. 1.7) The term was coined by Cottle to emphasize that the nasal vault resembles a Gothic arch closed by a keystone.

Paranasal Points (▶ Fig. 1.8)

- *Nasal canthus (medial canthus, endocanthion; clinical)*: inner commissure of the eye fissure
- *Temporal canthus (lateral canthus, exocanthion; clinical)*: outer commissure of the eye fissure

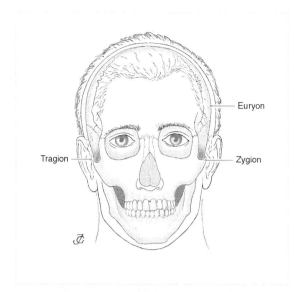

Fig. 1.9 The most important lateral points.

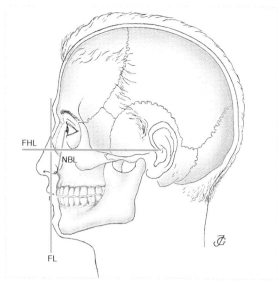

Fig. 1.10 Frankfort horizontal line (FHL), facial line (FL), and nasal base line (NBL).

- *Alare (clinical)*: most lateral point of the alar curvature; used to measure the lobular width
- *Cheilion (clinical)*: the point located at each labial commissure

Lateral Points (▶ Fig. 1.9)

- *Euryon (clinical and bony)*: most prominent lateral point on each side of the skull
- *Zygion (clinical and bony)*: most lateral point of the zygomatic arch
- *Tragion (clinical)*: notch on the upper margin of the tragus

Lines

The most important lines on the head are the Frankfort horizontal line (FHL) and the facial line (FL). They are used both anthropometrically and clinically. A third line that is helpful in surgery is the nasal base line (NBL) (▶ Fig. 1.10).

Frankfort Horizontal Line

The FHL is the line on the skull from the inferior orbital margin to the upper margin of the external bony ear canal (tragion). In clinical practice, the line between the inferior orbital margin and the upper border of the tragus is used. The FHL should be horizontal when side-view photographs are taken.

Facial Line

The FL is the line from the glabella to the pogonion. It serves as the baseline for calculating the nasofrontal and the nasolabial angles. The FL helps to analyze and define the dimensions of the nasal pyramid in relation to the midface, forehead, and chin.

Nasal Base Line

NBL is a slightly oblique line on the skin at the nasal base from the medial canthus to the alar-facial groove. The prominence (*projection, salience*) of the bony and cartilaginous pyramid and the lobule is measured from this line. In performing lateral osteotomies and wedge resections, the NBL is used as a line of reference.

Angles

The following text describes the most important angles in nasal analysis.

Nasofrontal Angle

The nasofrontal angle is the angle between the FL and the line over the dorsum of the bony pyramid (▶ Fig. 1.11a). Its magnitude depends on race and age. In Caucasian adults, it measures about 150°. In Asians and blacks, it is larger. The magnitude of the nasofrontal angle has no relation to nasal function. From an aesthetic point of view, a large variation is generally acceptable, reflecting ethnic differences.

Nasolabial Angle

The nasolabial angle is the angle between the base of the columella (subnasale) and the upper lip (▶ Fig. 1.11b). In Caucasian males, this angle measures 80 to 90°, in females 90 to 110°. In Asians and blacks, it is usually larger.

The nasolabial angle is, to a certain extent, related to nasal function. The smaller this angle, the more vertical the inspiratory airstream that enters the nose and the higher in the nasal cavity the air will reach. Also, aesthetically, the nasolabial angle is considered more important than the nasofrontal angle.

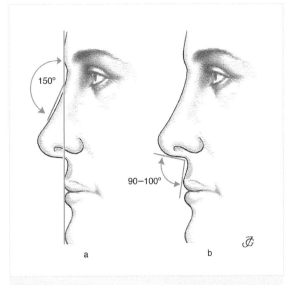

Fig. 1.11 (a) Nasofrontal angle. (b) Nasolabial angle.

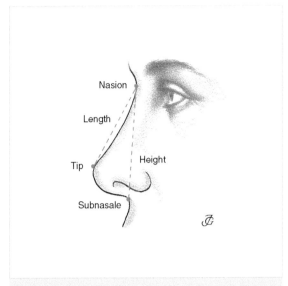

Fig. 1.12 Height and length of the nose.

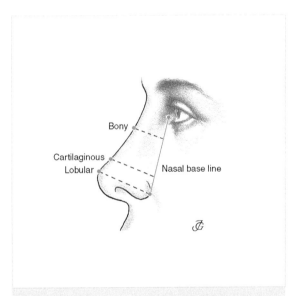

Fig. 1.13 Prominence of the bony pyramid, cartilaginous pyramid, and lobule.

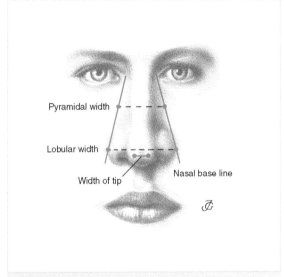

Fig. 1.14 Width of the pyramid, lobule, and tip.

Dimensions

- *Height of pyramid*: distance between nasion and subnasale (columellar base) (▶ Fig. 1.12)
- *Length of pyramid*: distance between nasion and tip (▶ Fig. 1.12)
- *Prominence (projection, salience)*: ventral projection of the pyramid measured from the NBL (▶ Fig. 1.13)
- *Bony prominence*: distance between the NBL and most prominent part of the bony dorsum

- *Cartilaginous prominence*: distance between the most prominent part of the cartilaginous dorsum and the NBL
- *Lobular (tip) prominence*: distance between the tip and the NBL at the alar-facial groove
- *Width of pyramid*: horizontal dimension of the base of the pyramid and of the tip (▶ Fig. 1.14)
- *Pyramidal width*: distance at the base of the bony cartilaginous pyramid between the left and right NBL

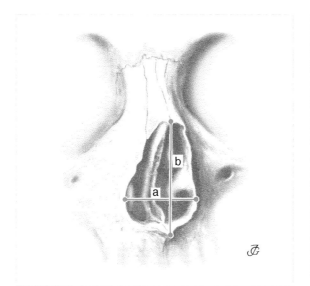

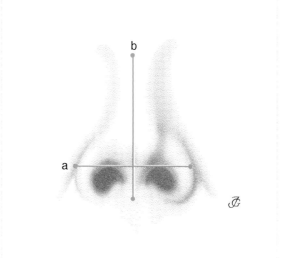

Fig. 1.15 Anatomical nasal index.
Width of piriform aperture (a) × 100
Length of piriform aperture (b)
Normal values:
- Leptorrhine (Caucasian): < 46.9
- Platyrrhine (black): 47.0–50.9
- Chamaerrhine (e.g., Asian): 51.0–57.9
(After Knuszmann 1988.)

Fig. 1.16 Clinical nasal index.
Width of piriform aperture (a) × 100
Height of pyramid (b)
Normal values:
- Leptorrhine (Caucasian): 55.0–69.9
- Platyrrhine (black): 70.0–84.9
- Chamaerrhine (e.g., Asian): 85.0–99.9
- Hyperchamaerrhine (black): > 100.0

- *Lobular width*: distance between the lateral walls of left and right alar cartilages
- *Width of tip*: distance between the two domes

Nasal Indices

The following anatomical and clinical indices may be useful in nasal surgery:
- Nasal index (anatomical and clinical)
- Lobular (tip) index
- Projection index

The way they are measured is illustrated in ▶ Fig. 1.15, ▶ Fig. 1.16, ▶ Fig. 1.17, and ▶ Fig. 1.18. Determining nasal indices may be helpful in analyzing nasal abnormalities and assessing the results of surgery (e.g., in shortening the nose, increasing the projection of the tip or the cartilaginous dorsum, and narrowing the lobule).

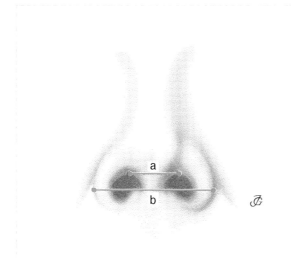

Fig. 1.17 Lobular (tip) index.
Width of tip at ventral border of nares (a) × 100
Maximum width of lobule (b)
This index is normally about 70. It is smaller in the platyrrhine, black, and growth-disturbed nose. It is greater in patients with excessive prominence of the nasal pyramid.

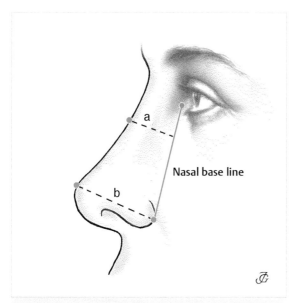

Fig. 1.18 Projection index.

Projection of dorsum (a) × 100

Projection of lobule (b)

(a) Projection from the nasal base line of the bony dorsum at the nasion.

(b) Projection from the nasal base line of the lobule at the level of the tip.

The projection index is usually 55–65. Its clinical value is limited.

1.1.2 External Nose (External Pyramid)

The external nose consists of four major parts (▶ Fig. 1.19):
1. Bony pyramid
2. Cartilaginous pyramid
3. Lobule
4. Soft-tissue areas

The bony pyramid, cartilaginous pyramid, and lobule comprise about one-third of the external nose. Together they form an integrated anatomical–physiological entity. This is the result of the rigid fixation of the cartilaginous vault to the lower margin of the bony pyramid (underlap of 1.0 to 1.5 mm; ▶ Fig. 1.20, and also ▶ Fig. 1.34 and ▶ Fig. 1.93) and the junctions between the lobule and the cartilaginous pyramid, in particular the connection (and overlap) between the lateral crus of the lobular cartilage and the lower margin of the triangular cartilage (▶ Fig. 1.20). At four different areas, the pyramid consists of soft tissue, allowing a certain amount of mobility (▶ Fig. 1.19 and ▶ Fig. 1.30).

The external nasal pyramid is covered (from the outside to the inside) by skin, subcutaneous connective fatty tissue, and muscle fibers. The thickness and extent of these various layers show considerable individual variation.

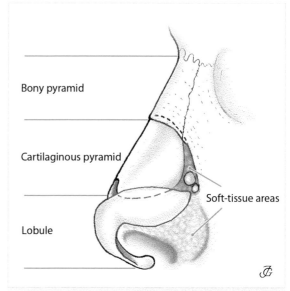

Fig. 1.19 The four major parts of the external nose: bony pyramid, cartilaginous pyramid, lobule, and soft-tissue areas.

Bony Pyramid

The bony pyramid (or bony vault) is the bony part of the external nose that projects above and anterior to both NBLs. Its upper midpoint is the depth of the nasofrontal angle or nasion. Its lowest point is the rhinion or K area.

The bony pyramid consists of the nasal bones, the nasal part of the frontal bone including the nasal spine (spina nasalis ossis frontalis), and the two frontal processes of the maxilla (▶ Fig. 1.21).

The *nasal bones* are small, oblong, and quadrangular. They are thicker and narrower cranially and thinner and wider caudally. They are attached to each other in the midline by slightly serrated borders that form the internasal suture. Cranially, they unite with the nasal part of the frontal bone to form the frontonasal suture. About halfway down the sloping side of the pyramid, their lateral margins meet the frontal process of the maxilla at the frontomaxillary suture. Their inside (dorsal) surface is smooth and forms part of the anterior wall of the nasal cavity. It has an oblong groove, the ethmoidal sulcus, for the anterior branch of the ethmoidal nerve. The nasal bones often show small perforations (nasal foramina) through which blood vessels penetrate.

- The *frontal processes of the maxillae* are situated between the nasal and lacrimal bones and make up the dorsal part of the bony vault. They are thicker than the adjacent caudal parts of the maxillae. Lateral osteotomies are usually carried out in this part of the bony vault.
- The *piriform aperture* is the anterior nasal aperture as seen in a skull (▶ Fig. 1.21). It is bounded by the nasal bones and the maxillae.

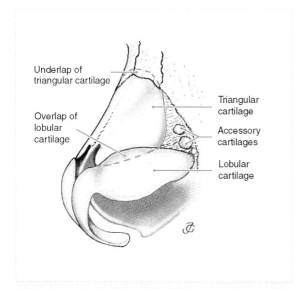

Fig. 1.20 Bony pyramid, cartilaginous pyramid, lobule, and soft-tissue areas.

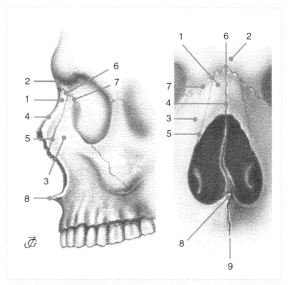

Fig. 1.21 Bony pyramid.
1 = nasal bone; 2 = frontal bone (nasal part); 3 = frontal process of maxilla; 4 = internasal suture; 5 = nasomaxillary suture; 6 = frontonasal suture; 7 = frontomaxillary suture; 8 = anterior nasal spine; 9 = intermaxillary suture.

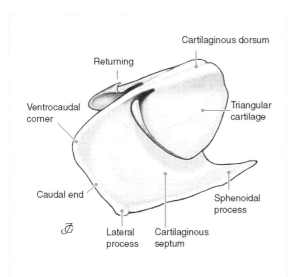

Fig. 1.22 Septolateral cartilage with reflection of the medial part of the caudal margin of the triangular cartilage.

Cartilaginous Pyramid

The cartilaginous pyramid or vault is made up by the septolateral cartilage and the two lateral membranous areas with one to three accessory cartilages (▶ Fig. 1.20).

The septolateral cartilage (▶ Fig. 1.22) consists of:
- The cartilaginous septum (cartilago septi nasi) that rests on the premaxilla including its anterior nasal spine, dividing the internal nose into two cavities, and
- The two triangular cartilages that form the greater part of the dorsal and lateral walls of the cartilaginous vault

The attachment of the cartilaginous vault to the bony pyramid is rigid. The upper margin of both triangular cartilages underlap the lower margin of the nasal bones by 1 to 2 mm over a distance of 5 to 10 mm (▶ Fig. 1.20). See also ▶ Fig. 1.93 and ▶ Fig. 1.94; page 38. The area where the nasal bones, the septal cartilage, and the two triangular cartilages unite is commonly called the keystone or K area (see ▶ Fig. 1.7).

The cartilaginous vault is a T-shaped construction. Its angle gradually diminishes from about 15° at the lower margin of the triangular cartilage to almost 90° at the K area (▶ Fig. 1.23). See also ▶ Fig. 1.95 and ▶ Fig. 1.96; page 39. In this way, a funnel-type construction is created that plays an important role in breathing and conditioning of the inspired air (see page 51).

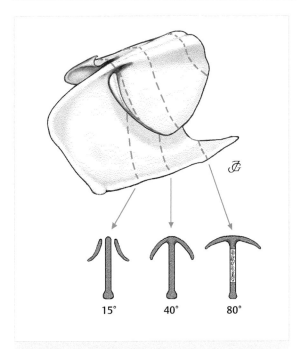

Fig. 1.23 Cross sections through the septolateral cartilage at the valve area, posterior to the valve, and at the K area.

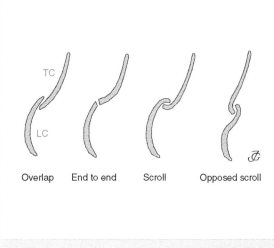

Fig. 1.24 Most common relationships between the triangular cartilage (TC) and the lobular cartilage (LC).

The *septal cartilage (cartilaginous septum)* rests with its base on a bony pedestal consisting (from ventral to dorsal) of the anterior nasal spine, the anterior part of the nasal crest of the maxilla (often referred to as the premaxilla), and the vomer. Caudally, it has a free, somewhat mobile end that is connected to the columella by the membranous septum. Dorsally, it is united with the perpendicular plate of the ethmoid bone. Ventrally, it is continuous with the two triangular (or upper lateral) cartilages. Together they make the cartilaginous vault and dorsum. See also ▶ Fig. 1.67, ▶ Fig. 1.68, ▶ Fig. 1.69, and ▶ Fig. 1.70; page 30 and page 31.

The *triangular cartilages (upper lateral cartilages)* are continuous with each other and with the septal cartilage. Together they constitute the cartilaginous vault. Cranially, their margins are underlying, and firmly fixed to, the caudal margin of the nasal bones. Medially, the triangular cartilage is lined by mucosa. It covers the inside of the cartilaginous part of the internal nasal cavity. Dorsally, it is connected with the lateral soft-tissue or "hinge" area (see ▶ Fig. 1.20). Ventrally, it is continuous with the septum in its upper two-thirds, while in its lower third, a small cleft with loose connective tissue is found between its medial margin and the septum (medial soft-tissue area or paraseptal cleft). The length of this cleft is variable and related to the length of the nose

The caudal margin of the triangular cartilage is free and protrudes into the vestibule. Its lateral side is covered by skin (the "cul de sac"). The medial third of the caudal margin is usually rotated upward 160 to 180°. This is called returning, scrolling, or curling (see ▶ Fig. 1.22).

The caudal margin of the triangular cartilage moves inward and outward with respiration (valve function). These movements are possible because of its relatively loose fixation to the medial and lateral soft-tissue areas (the cleft and the hinge areas, respectively). The reflection of the medial part of the lower margin, on the other hand, increases its rigidity and thus counteracts an easy collapse of the lateral nasal wall on inspiration.

The relationship between the triangular cartilage and the lateral crus of the lobular cartilage shows large variations. The most common relationship is a certain overlap of the caudal margin of the triangular cartilage by the cranial margin of the lateral crus of the lobular cartilage. Other relationships that may be found are: "end-to-end," "scroll," and "opposed scroll" (Dion 1978) (▶ Fig. 1.24). In the dense connective tissue that connects the lateral crus to the triangular cartilage, several sesamoid cartilages can be found. They provide both mobility and stability, allowing the intercartilaginous area to act more or less as a joint (see also ▶ Fig. 1.95, ▶ Fig. 1.96, and ▶ Fig. 1.97; page 39).

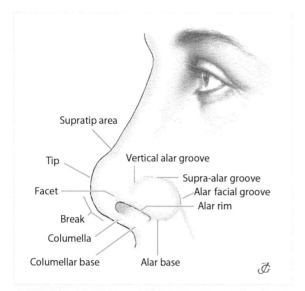

Fig. 1.25 Lateral view of the lobule with its major anatomical–clinical structures.

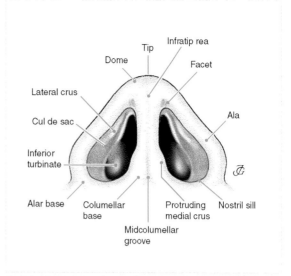

Fig. 1.26 Base view of the lobule with its main structures.

Nomenclature of Triangular Cartilage

Nomina Anatomica (NA): cartilago nasi lateralis (lateral nasal cartilage)
North America: upper lateral cartilage (ULC)
Germany: Seitenknorpel
France: cartilage laterale
This book: triangular cartilage (TC)

Lobule

The lobule is the mobile lower third of the external nasal pyramid. It is made up of two lobular cartilages, muscle fibers, subcutaneous connective and fatty tissue, and a relatively thick skin with sebaceous glands. The major structures of the lobule are illustrated in ▶ Fig. 1.25 and ▶ Fig. 1.26.

Tip

The *tip (apex nasi)* consists of the two domes, the interdomal connective tissue fibers, and the overlying skin.
- *Supratip area*: a slight depression just cranial to the tip ("the dip before the tip")
- *Tip-defining point*: most prominent area of the dome of the lobular cartilage; the tip is made up of the two tip-defining points
- *Infratip area*: part of the lobule anterior (ventral) to the nostrils and the columella

Alae

The alae are the mobile lateral walls of the lobule that are made up of the lateral crura of the lobular cartilage and the overlying muscles and skin.

- *Alar rim*: caudal margin of the ala; together with the columella and the nostril sill, it forms the nostril (ostium externum or naris)
- *Alar base (alar foot)*: area of attachment of the ala to the face
- *Facet*: flat area at the ventrocaudal part of the ala corresponding to the caudal lobular notch (see ▶ Fig. 1.30)
- *Vertical alar groove*: vertical groove or depression of the ala just medial to the dome
- *Supra-alar groove or crease*: horizontal groove just above the cranial margin of the lateral crus
- *Alar-facial groove*: fold at the alar base between the ala and face

Columella

The columella is the midline structure running from the upper part of the lobule to the upper lip, consisting of the medial crura of the lobular cartilage. The columella is more or less broadened due to the lateral (outward) curvature of the end of the medial crura.
- *Columellar break*: slight bend of the lower margin of the columella at the level of the upper (ventral) margin of the nostril
- *Midcolumellar groove*: vertical groove in the skin between the medial crura

Nostril (Naris, Ostium Externum)

The orifices of the lobule are usually called the nostrils or nares. They are bounded by the columella, lower alar rim, and the nostril sill.
- *Nostril sill*: inferior (dorsal) rim of the nostril

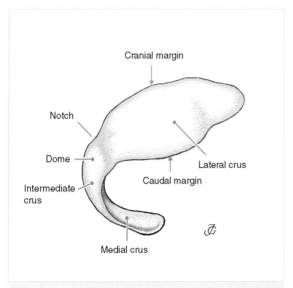

Fig. 1.27 Left lobular cartilage with its anatomical parts.

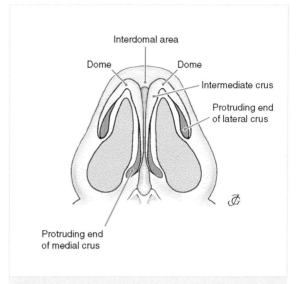

Fig. 1.28 Lobular cartilages in relation to the tip, alae, and columella.

Vestibule

The vestibule is the skin-covered cavity between the nostril and the valve area. Its upper part, lateral to the protruding caudal margin of the triangular cartilage, is a blind-ending pouch commonly called the cul de sac. The caudal part of the vestibule bears hairs (vibrissae) that help protect the entrance of the respiratory tract against insects, etc.

Nomenclature of Lobular Cartilage

Nomina Anatomica (NA): cartilago alaris major (greater alar cartilage)
North American: lower lateral cartilage; alar cartilage
German: Flügelknorpel
This book: lobular cartilage

Lobular Cartilages

The lobular cartilages are horseshoe-shaped cartilages that support the structured anatomy of the whole lobule. They determine the position and form of the tip, the alae, and the columella as well as the configuration of the nares and vestibules.

The lobular cartilage can be divided into three or four parts (▶ Fig. 1.27):
• Medial crus
• Intermediate part (not always identifiable)
• Dome
• Lateral crus

Medial Crus

The medial crus is the slightly bent medial part of the lobular cartilage. It supports the columella, nares, and tip. Its length and width vary greatly. As the medial crura run into the columella, they become closely associated and form a support for the septal cartilage. Their free ends protrude slightly into the vestibules, broadening the columellar base (▶ Fig. 1.28). The space between the medial crura is filled with loose connective tissue. There are no crossing fibers between the two crura. See also ▶ Fig. 1.101 and ▶ Fig. 1.102; page 41.

Intermediate Part

The intermediate part may be defined as the transitional segment between the medial crus and the dome. It cannot always be clearly identified as a separate part of the lobular cartilage. Many authors therefore do not recognize it as a separate structure.

Dome

The dome is the strongly bent part of the lobular cartilage between the medial and lateral crura. Its curvature varies greatly from 80° (ballooning type) to 10° (narrow type). Its cranial border is often notched. The two domes together make the nasal tip. It has been suggested that the two domes are connected by a bundle of midline crossing fibers, an interdomal ligament, or Pitanguy ligament. In a histological study (Zhai et al 1995), we were unable to confirm the presence of horizontal, midline-crossing fibers, and certainly not a ligament (see ▶ Fig. 1.98, ▶ Fig. 1.99, and ▶ Fig. 1.100).

Although a true ligament characterized by highly organized fiber directions is not present, the connecting

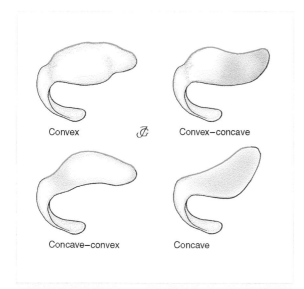

Fig. 1.29 Most common shapes of the lateral crus of the lobular cartilage.

Convex Convex–concave

Concave–convex Concave

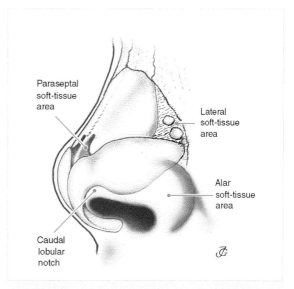

Fig. 1.30 The four soft-tissue areas.

Paraseptal soft-tissue area

Lateral soft-tissue area

Alar soft-tissue area

Caudal lobular notch

tissue between the domes and adjacent intermediate parts of the lobular cartilages is biomechanically important.

Lateral Crus

The lateral crus is the lateral extension of the lobular cartilage supporting the ala. Its shape may be convex, convex–concave, concave–convex, concave, or flat (▶ Fig. 1.29). The convex type is the most frequent. Its length (mediolateral dimension) varies from 16 to 30 mm, its maximal height (craniocaudal dimension) from 6 to 16 mm. The distance of its caudal margin to the alar rim increases in the ventrodorsal direction.

Soft-Tissue Areas

The external nasal pyramid has four soft-tissue areas. Unfortunately, there is considerable confusion about their terminology in the literature. We suggest using the following nomenclature (▶ Fig. 1.30):
- Paraseptal cleft or paraseptal soft-tissue area
- Lateral soft-tissue area or hinge area
- Caudal lobular notch
- Alar soft-tissue area

The *paraseptal cleft (paraseptal soft-tissue area)* is a narrow triangular opening between the cartilaginous septum and the lower third of the medial margin of the triangular cartilage, filled with loose connective tissue. It allows the outward and inward movement of the lower part of the triangular cartilage during respiration.

The *lateral soft-tissue area (hinge area)* is a more or less triangular soft-tissue area between the lateral margin of the triangular cartilage and the lateral wall of the piriform aperture. It consists of relatively dense connective tissue fibers with two to three accessory cartilages. It allows

outward and inward movements of the triangular cartilages (and valve) and alae. It is therefore also called the hinge area.

The *caudal lobular notch* is found medially at the lower margin of the lateral crus. It does not seem to have any special functional significance. It deserves special attention and needs to be carefully preserved during lobular surgery.

The *alar soft-tissue area* is the most dorsal and caudal part of the ala inferior to the lateral crus of the lobular cartilage. The ala is not completely occupied by the lobular cartilage.

Skin and Connective, Muscular, and Fatty Tissues Overlying the External Nose

The external nasal pyramid is covered from outside to inside by:
- An epidermis of varying thickness and a dermis with sebaceous glands and hair follicles
- A connective tissue layer of varying thickness containing the vascular and nerve supply, and a variable amount of fatty tissue
- A muscle layer
- A thin, loose connective tissue layer permitting gliding movements of the overlying tissues
- A periosteal or perichondrial layer that is attached to the bone or cartilage

Nowadays, some authors like to speak of a superficial musculoaponeurotic system (SMAS), consisting of a superficial fatty layer, a fibromuscular layer, a deep fatty layer, a longitudinal fibrous layer, and an intercrural ligament (Letourneau and Daniel 1988). However, we prefer to reserve the term SMAS for a connective tissue layer containing a variable number of muscle fibers that extends cranially from the platysma, covers the parotid

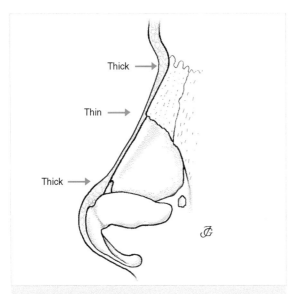

Fig. 1.31 Thickness of the skin and subcutaneous tissues overlying the external pyramid.

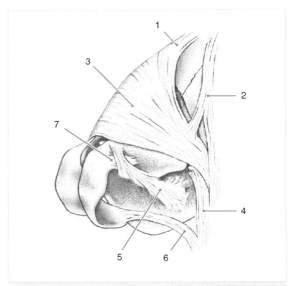

Fig. 1.32 The seven most important nasal muscles superimposed on a 3D computerized reconstruction (artist's impression) of the bony and cartilaginous structures in a 45-year-old male (from Bruintjes et al 1996).
1 = procerus muscle; 2 = levator labii alaeque nasi muscle; 3 = transverse part of nasalis muscle; 4 = alar part of nasalis muscle; 5 = dilator naris muscle (m. dilatator naris); 6 = depressor septi muscle; 7 = apicis nasi muscle.

gland and facial nerve branches, and stops at the level of the zygomatic arch. Anteriorly, the SMAS is continuous with the orbicularis oculi and zygomaticus major muscles. Because this layer is in the same level as the facial muscles, it can best be regarded as the vestige of the facial muscle layer in a region where such muscles are not needed anymore (i.e., the parotid region). Indeed, in primates, the cranial border of the platysma runs as high as the zygomatic arch (Jost and Levet 1984). Therefore, we do not follow the distinction between the various layers as described by Letourneau and Daniel (1988); moreover these layers show considerable differences in the various parts of the external nasal pyramid. See also ▶ Fig. 1.95, ▶ Fig. 1.96, and ▶ Fig. 1.97; page 39.

The *bony pyramid* is covered in its upper part by relatively thick skin with a considerable amount of subcutaneous connective tissue and muscle fibers (procerus). In its lower part, the nasal bones are covered by a rather thin skin, a thin layer of loose connective tissue, and some transverse muscle fibers (transverse part of nasalis) (▶ Fig. 1.31).

The loose subcutaneous layer allows movement of the skin over the bone while offering protection against trauma and pain from pressure. This is illustrated by patients in whom this layer has not been preserved during surgery; they often complain of tenderness in this region.

The *cartilaginous pyramid* is covered by a somewhat thicker layer of soft tissue. The skin has a larger number of sebaceous glands and hair follicles. The muscle fiber layer is also thicker. See also ▶ Fig. 1.95 and ▶ Fig. 1.96; page 39.

The *lobule* has a thick covering consisting of epidermis, dermis with hair follicles and numerous sebaceous glands, fat, connective tissue with the vascular supply, lymph vessels and nerves, muscle fibers, and areolar tissue.

The thickness and quality of the skin depend on a great number of factors, including gender, age, and climatological influences. The subcutaneous connective tissue layer is relatively thick, especially between the cartilages. A variable amount of fatty tissue can be found in the midline just above the interdomal area and laterally. See also ▶ Fig. 1.104 and ▶ Fig. 1.105; page 41.

Four different muscles can be distinguished. The fibers run from the lobular cartilage into the skin, adding to the rigidity of the lateral lobular wall or ala. As a result, the lobular skin is not freely movable over the lobular cartilage.

Musculature

The external nasal pyramid is almost completely covered by a thin layer of musculature. There is no consensus on the number of muscles that can be distinguished and no agreement on their names.

Terminologia Anatomica (1998) recognizes five nasal muscles. Most anatomical and rhinosurgical textbooks, however, mention seven or nine.

All nasal muscles have a mimic function. Some of them also play a role in breathing and provide stability for the lateral nasal wall. In this section we follow the work of Bruintjes et al (1996), who recognized seven different nasal muscles (▶ Fig. 1.32).

- The *procerus muscle* is an unpaired layer of muscle fibers. These originate in the nasofrontal suture area, fan in a caudal direction (hence the alternative name, pyramidalis), and insert in the skin over the bony pyramid. These muscle fibers produce transverse wrinkling of the skin at the root of the nose. Some fibers may reach as low as the ala and thus may assist in elevating the ala and dilating the nostril.

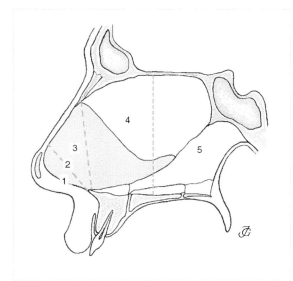

Fig. 1.33 The five areas of the internal nose according to Cottle (1961): Area 1 = level of nostril; Area 2 = valve area; Area 3 = region underneath the cartilaginous vault ("the attic"); Area 4 = region of the heads and anterior parts of the inferior and middle turbinate; Area 5 = region of the posterior parts of the inferior and middle turbinates.

- The *levator labii superioris alaeque nasi muscle* arises from the frontal process of the maxilla. It has a small medial part that inserts into the perichondrium of the lateral crus. It can thus act as a dilatator of the nostril and elevator of the lateral lobular wall.
- The *nasalis muscle (transverse part)* originates in the maxilla above the canine tooth and the skin over the nasolabial fold. It runs to the midline of the nasal dorsum. It acts as a stabilizer of the lateral nasal wall. See also ▶ Fig. 1.99 and ▶ Fig. 1.100; page 41.
- The *nasalis muscle (alar part)* also originates in the maxilla but at a point somewhat more medial than the transverse part. It inserts at the lateral and lower margin of the ala. These fibers may draw the ala laterally and dilate the valve area. This muscle is the most important stabilizer of the lateral nasal wall.
- The *dilator naris* arises from the lateral crus and superimposing alar skin and inserts into the skin of the nasolabial groove. However, not all authors accept this view. The muscle acts together with the alar part of the nasalis muscle as alar abductors and openers of the nostril.
- The *depressor septi muscle* originates in the maxilla above the incisor tooth, together with the fibers of the alar part of the nasal muscle, and inserts in the medial crus. It pulls the membranous septum down, widening the nostril.
- The *apicis nasi muscle* is a very small muscle lying on the lower medial part of the lateral crus. Its function is a matter of debate.

1.1.3 Internal Nose

Anatomically, embryologically, and physiologically we distinguish:
- Two nasal cavities (two noses)
- Three nasal passages on both sides: the lower, middle, and upper meatus
- Three nasal openings on both sides: the nostril (external ostium, naris), the valve area (internal ostium), and the choana

Anatomical–Physiological Subdivision of the Nasal Organ

Over the years, several systems have been suggested to divide the different parts of the nose on the basis of anatomical, physiological, and/or pathological differences.

External versus Internal Nose

The oldest subdivision is the distinction between the external and the internal nose: the external nose, specific to humans, is the prominent bony, cartilaginous and soft-tissue pyramid in the middle of the face; while the internal nose, with its mucosa, turbinates, and septum, is the nasal organ proper.

Five-Area Division of Cottle

For the purpose of diagnosis and documentation, as well as to correlate pathology with symptomatology, Cottle (1961) proposed to divide the internal nasal cavity into five areas (▶ Fig. 1.33).
- *Area 1*: nostril (external ostium, naris), formed by the alar rim, the lateral border of the columella, and the floor of the vestibule
- *Area 2*: the nasal valve area (internal ostium, isthmus)
- *Area 3*: the area underneath the cartilaginous vault (also called the "attic")
- *Area 4*: the anterior half of the nasal cavity, including the heads of the turbinates and the infundibulum or ostiomeatal complex
- *Area 5*: the posterior half of the nasal cavity, including the tails of the turbinates

This five-area division was adopted by several authors including ourselves. In several German textbooks (Masing 1977, Ey 1984, Rettinger 1988), however, the denomination "area 3" was given to a different region (the premaxillary area) than in the Cottle system. This has diminished the value of the five-area division.

Five-Structure Division of Bachmann–Mlynski

Bachman (1982), and more recently Mlynski et al (2001), have divided the nose on the basis of its inspiratory function into five different structural elements: the vestibulum, the isthmus, the anterior cavity, the area of the turbinates, and the posterior cavity, choanae, and epipharynx.

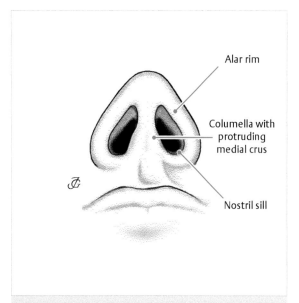

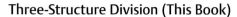

Fig. 1.34 Structures bounding the nostril.

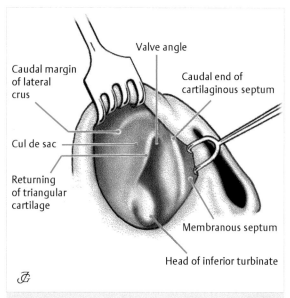

Fig. 1.35 Vestibule and valve area with its various structures.

Three-Structure Division (This Book)

In this book we suggest a subdivision into three anatomical–physiological parts (Huizing 2003) (see also ▶ Fig. 1.119):
- The *anterior segment* or upstream area, consisting of the nostril, vestibule, and valve area
- The *middle segment* or functional area proper, consisting of the mucosa-lined nasal cavity with the turbinates, septum, and sinus ostia
- The *posterior segment* or downstream area, with the tails of the turbinates, anterior wall of the sphenoid, and choanae

Nostril (Naris, External Ostium)

The nostril is formed by the alar rim, the lateral border of the columella with the protruding end of the medial crura, and the nostril sill (▶ Fig. 1.34). In a normal adult Caucasian nose, the nostril has an ovaloid form with a slightly oblique axis. In newborns and young children, it is almost round. It gradually changes to the adult ovaloid aperture during school age and puberty.

In the noses of blacks and Asians, the nares are also more round. In some types of noses of blacks, the external ostium may have an almost horizontal axis. These racial and age variations are also expressed in the magnitude of the lobular index.

Vestibule

The vestibule is the skin-covered inner part of the lobule (▶ Fig. 1.35). The following structures are of clinical and surgical significance (see also ▶ Fig. 1.95, ▶ Fig. 1.96, and ▶ Fig. 1.104):

- Medially:
  - The columella with the medial crus of the lobular cartilage
  - The membranous septum (the membrane that connects the medial crura of the lobular cartilage to the lower edge of the septal cartilage) and its covering skin
  - The skin covering the caudal end of the septal cartilage
- Internal ostium or laterally:
  - The inside of the ala with the lateral crus and its more or less protruding end
  - The cul de sac or infundibulum, a shallow pouch bounded laterally by the cranial part of the lateral crus and medially by the caudal part of the triangular cartilage

Valve Area (Internal Ostium)

The valve area is a more or less triangular or teardrop-shaped area that gives access to the internal nasal cavity (▶ Fig. 1.36). Its original name was ostium internum (Zuckerkandl 1882) or isthmus nasi. Later, it was considered a "valvular device controlling the inflow of air" (Mink 1902, 1920). Nowadays, we call it the valve area (Kern e.g., 1978). As the narrowest region of the internal nose, it causes the greatest resistance to breathing. The valve area is bounded:
- Medially by:
  - The cartilaginous septum
  - The premaxillary wing
- Laterally by:
  - The lower margin of the triangular cartilage or limen nasi
  - The fibrofatty tissue area
  - The head of the inferior turbinate
- Caudally by:
  - The skin-covered floor of the piriform aperture

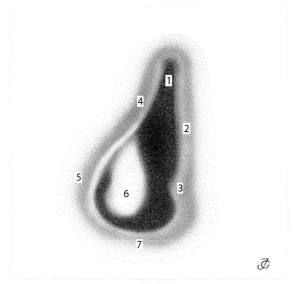

Fig. 1.36 Nasal valve area.
1 = valve angle; 2 = cartilaginous septum; 3 = ventrolateral process of the cartilaginous septum and premaxillary wing; 4 = caudal margin of the triangular cartilage (limen nasi); 5 = fibrofatty tissue area; 6 = head of the inferior turbinate; 7 = nasal floor.

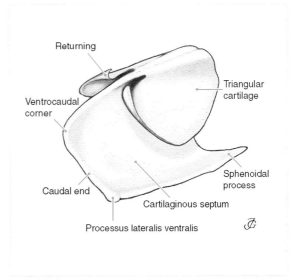

Fig. 1.37 Septolateral cartilage consisting of the cartilaginous septum and the two triangular cartilages.

The medial wall of the valve area is rigid, whereas the lateral wall is mobile. On inspiration, it moves inward due to the negative pressure caused by the inspiratory airflow. On expiration, it moves outward. The inward movement is counteracted by the mass and stiffness of the triangular and lobular cartilages, soft-tissue areas, and the connecting fibers and musculature (see also ▶ Fig. 1.95, ▶ Fig. 1.96, and ▶ Fig. 1.97; page 39).

Terminology of the Valve Area

- *Valve area*: narrowest area (area 2) of the internal nose
- *Valve*: the moving part of the lateral wall of the valve area (i.e., the caudal margin of the triangular cartilage)
- *Valve angle*: the angle between the caudal margin of the triangular cartilage and the septum
- *Ostium internum*: old name for the valve area; this name was introduced by anatomists (Zuckerkandl 1883) in the 19th century in contrast to "ostium externum" (naris, nostril)
- *Isthmus*: narrowest area of the nasal cavity (valve area)
- *Limen nasi*: lower margin of the triangular cartilage (valve)

External Nasal Valve

Recently, some authors (e.g., Riechelmann et al 2010) suggest the presence of another valvular structure, the *external nasal valve*. They attribute a valvular function to the relative narrowing of the nasal vestibule that is caused by the slightly protruding caudal margin of the lateral crus (sometimes named the vestibular fold) and the protruding caudal end of the medial crus. Cottle 1955 named these protrusions "baffles" and pointed out that they add to nasal resistance and influence airstream. Cole 2003 recognized four components of the nasal valve. It is well known that pathology of the lateral crus or the medial crus may, indeed, lead to inspiratory breathing obstruction. This condition is usually called alar collapse. We doubt if the term *external nasal valve* is justified to describe the function of these two vestibular airway resistors that only indirectly affect the functioning of the much more important (internal) nasal valve.

Septum

The nasal septum consists of: (1) the cartilaginous septum; (2) the perpendicular plate of the ethmoid bone; (3) the vomer; and (4) the septal framework.

Cartilaginous Septum

The cartilaginous septum is part of the septolateral cartilage. The following structures are of special clinical and surgical interest (▶ Fig. 1.37):
- The free caudal end
- The processus lateralis ventralis: a broadening of its caudal margin in the area where the cartilage is connected to the premaxilla
- The ventrocaudal corner (anterior–inferior corner)
- The sphenoidal process (posterior process): a posterior extension of the cartilaginous septum between the perpendicular plate and the vomer; see also ▶ Fig. 1.67, ▶ Fig. 1.68, ▶ Fig. 1.69, and ▶ Fig. 1.70; page 30 and page 31.

Perpendicular Plate of the Ethmoid Bone (Lamina Perpendicularis)

The perpendicular plate of the ethmoid bone is a more or less quadrangular, thin, bony plate. Its upper border is ventrally attached to the posterior surface of the nasal spine of the frontal bone (frontoethmoidal suture). More

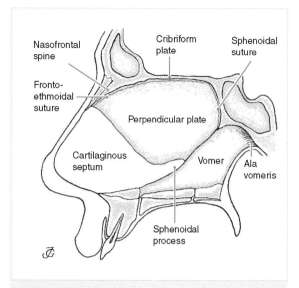

Fig. 1.38 Perpendicular plate of the ethmoid bone and the vomer.

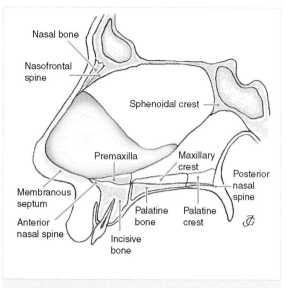

Fig. 1.39 Septal framework.

posteriorly, it is united to the inferior surface of the cribriform plate (▶ Fig. 1.38). The posterior margin unites with the sphenoidal crest (sphenoidal suture). The caudal margin is attached to the anterior border of the vomer. The ventral margin unites with the cartilaginous septum. This part often has two cortical layers with spongiotic bone marrow in between. On rare occasions, a bulla may be present (see also ▶ Fig. 1.73 and ▶ Fig. 1.74).

Vomer

The vomer is an unpaired, oblong, quadrangular bone resembling a plowshare. Its cranial margin is broad and split into two lateral leaves (alae vomeris). These are attached to the sphenoid bone. Its posterior margin forms the medial wall of the choanae. Its inferior margin, which is sharp and serrated, is connected to the nasal crests of the maxilla and palatine bone. The anterior (to some extent also cranial) margin is somewhat thickened. It has a groove in which the inferior margin of the perpendicular plate and the cartilaginous septum are fixed.

Septal Framework

The septal framework holding the septum consists of eight different anatomical structures (▶ Fig. 1.39):
- Caudally:
  - Anterior nasal spine (spina nasalis anterior)
  - Premaxilla with the premaxillary table and the premaxillary wings
  - Maxillary crest (crista nasalis maxillae)
  - Palatine crest (Crista nasalis ossis palatini)
  - Membranous septum (septum membranaceum)
- Ventrally:
  - Bony ridge at the dorsal side of the nasal bones
- Cranially:
  - Bony ridge at the junction of the cribriform plates

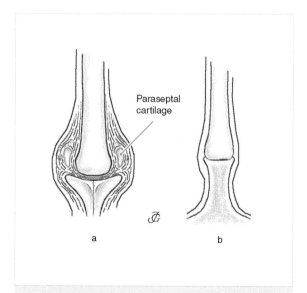

Fig. 1.40 Chondropremaxillary complex (a) and the chondro-maxillary junction (b).

- Dorsally:
  - Sphenoidal crest (crista sphenoidalis), a bony ridge at the junction of the two sphenoidal sinuses

Junctions between the Septum and its Framework

Precise knowledge of the connections between the various parts of the septum is of the utmost importance in septal surgery. In particular, the junctions between the cartilaginous septum and the anterior nasal spine and the premaxilla are of great importance. Detailed information is presented in ▶ Fig. 1.39, ▶ Fig. 1.40, ▶ Fig. 1.41, and ▶ Fig. 1.42 (and also

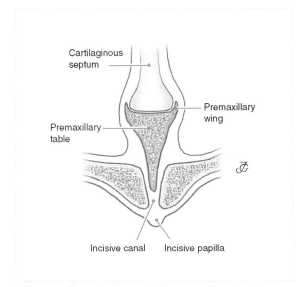

Fig. 1.41 Premaxilla and premaxillary wings.

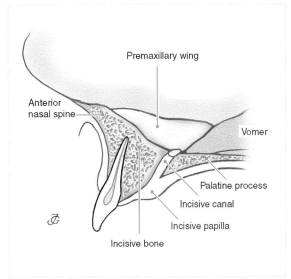

Fig. 1.42 Premaxilla and incisive canal.

in ▸ Fig. 1.67, ▸ Fig. 1.68, ▸ Fig. 1.69, ▸ Fig. 1.70, ▸ Fig. 1.71, ▸ Fig. 1.72, ▸ Fig. 1.73, and ▸ Fig. 1.74).

Incisive Bone

Although the terminology of ▸ Fig. 1.39, ▸ Fig. 1.40, ▸ Fig. 1.41, and ▸ Fig. 1.42 is common in clinical practice, it is different from that found in major anatomical textbooks. The existence of an incisive bone (os incisivum) is indisputable since it has centers of ossification that are distinct from those of the main maxillary mass. The fusion of the incisive bone with the maxillary bone takes place well before birth and does not leave a trace on its facial aspect. On the palatine side, however, a suture (the incisive suture), running from the incisive fossa in the anterolateral direction, is visible at birth. This suture may persist for several decades.

The incisive bone might therefore be described as the part of the maxilla anterior to the incisive fossa and incisive canals. It may be considered the same bone as the premaxilla, which is a separate bone in most vertebrates. In anatomical textbooks, the structure referred to as the premaxilla in ▸ Fig. 1.39, ▸ Fig. 1.40, ▸ Fig. 1.41, and ▸ Fig. 1.42 is described as the most anterior part of the nasal crest of the maxilla, and is also known as the incisor crest. It is the highest part of the nasal crest. It projects ventrally, together with its contralateral fellow, as the anterior nasal spine, and flattens superiorly to form the premaxillary table and wings (▸ Fig. 1.40a and ▸ Fig. 1.41).

Turbinates and Turbinate-Like Structures

In each nasal cavity, six to eight turbinates and turbinate-like structures can be distinguished (▸ Fig. 1.43 and ▸ Fig. 1.44).

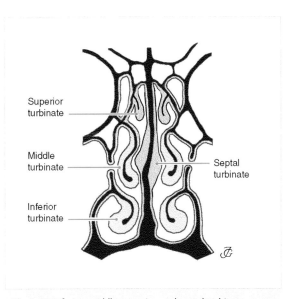

Fig. 1.43 Inferior, middle, superior, and septal turbinate.

On the lateral nasal wall we find:
1. The inferior turbinate (concha nasalis inferior)
2. The middle turbinate (concha nasalis media)
3. The superior turbinate (concha nasalis superior)
4. The agger nasi, and in some cases
5. The supreme turbinate (concha nasalis suprema)

On the medial nasal wall we find:
1. The septal turbinate (also known as tuberculum septi, intumescentia septi, and Kiesselbach ridge), and in some cases several
2. Posterior septal ridges or folds

(See also ▸ Fig. 1.87).

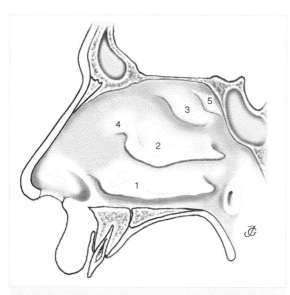

Fig. 1.44 Lateral nasal wall with inferior turbinate (1), middle turbinate (2) superior turbinate (3), agger nasi (4), and supreme turbinate (5).

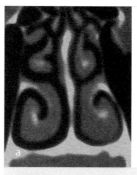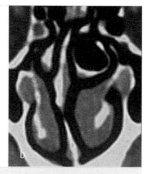

Fig. 1.45 a, b CT scans of the inferior turbinate demonstrating the large variation of the angle between the turbinate bone and the bony lateral nasal wall. (a) Large angle, almost 90 degrees. (b) Small and asymmetric angles; the asymmetry suggests that apart from genetic factors, postnatally developed pathology may play a role.

Hippocrates called the turbinates "sleeves." Casserius (1610) gave them their present name. (He wrote: "[...] the use of the turbinate bones is to break the force of the entering air and warm it and cleanse it.")

Turbinates

The turbinates should be considered separate structures with a similar, but not completely identical, function. Their bony skeleton may be lamellar, spongy, or bullous.

- The *lamellar type* is the most common, especially in the inferior turbinate. Its architecture may differ in the way the bony lamella protrudes into the nasal cavity.
- The *spongy type* is frequently seen in the inferior and middle turbinates and also in the bony septum underlying the septal turbinate.
- The *bullous type* is present in the middle turbinate in about 25% of the population. It is a very rare finding in the inferior turbinate.

The cavernous parenchymal tissue is by far the most developed in the inferior turbinate. It is also relatively thick at the medial and posterior part of the middle turbinate. It is negligible in the superior turbinate. These variations illustrate the functional differences of the turbinates and their parts.

The mucosal lining of the various turbinates also shows certain differences in the number of cilia-bearing cells and glands.

Because of their extensive submucosal capillary bed and the abundance of serous and mucous glands, the mucosal surface greatly contributes to the humidification, warming, and cleansing of inspired air. This is made possible by the thick mass of cavernous tissue in between the submucosa and the bony skeleton. The conchal parenchyma is made up of arterioles, venules, and an extensive capillary bed embedded in loose connective tissue. Congestion and decongestion of the cavernous plexus is regulated by a complex autonomic nerve system that is influenced by a number of endogenous and exogenous factors (see page 25).

The *inferior turbinate* is the largest of the four lateral turbinates. It is an independent bone which is attached to the maxilla. As in mammals, it may therefore be called the "maxilloturbinale." For clinical and surgical purposes we distinguish a turbinate head, body, and tail. These three parts differ in terms of function and pathology.

The bony skeleton consists of a solid or spongiotic lamella extending from the lateral bony nasal wall into the nasal cavity (see page 37 and ▶ Fig. 1.88). The angle between the turbinate bone and the bony lateral nasal wall may vary considerably, from about 20 to 90° (▶ Fig. 1.45). These differences may contribute to inferior turbinate pathology. They should therefore be taken into account in planning turbinate surgery. The mucosa of the inferior turbinate is thicker than in the upper part of the nasal cavity. The cavernous parenchyma of the inferior turbinate is much more massive than that of other turbinates. In the congestive state, it may increase its volume three to four times compared with its decongested state, thereby almost completely blocking the inferior nasal passage (see also page 37, ▶ Fig. 1.87, ▶ Fig. 1.90, and ▶ Fig. 1.91).

The *middle turbinate* is part of the ethmoid bone. This explains why its skeleton may be more or less pneumatized. It is comparable to the ethmoidoturbinale I in mammals. The bony skeleton (▶ Fig. 1.46) may be of the lamellar, spongy (concha spongiosa), or bullous type (concha bullosa).

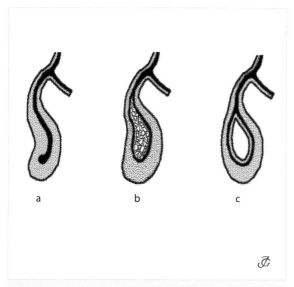

Fig. 1.46 a–c Middle turbinate. (a) Plate or lamellar type.
(b) Cancellous or spongy type. (c) Bullous type.

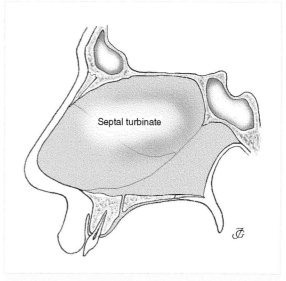

Fig. 1.47 Septal turbinate, lateral view.

- The *lamellar type* is characterized by a curved bony plate extending from the lamina papyracea. This plate divides the ethmoid bone into an anterior and posterior part. Its free end may be more or less straight, curved inward, or curved outward.
- The *spongy type* is less common. The bony skeleton is made up of two cortical layers and spongiotic bone with bone marrow in between. As a result, the turbinate may be relatively thick, which may play a role in pathology.
- The *bullous type* is a common variation found in about 25% of normal individuals. The skeleton consists of an ovaloid ethmoidal cell with thin walls. Its inside is lined with mucosa, and it usually drains through an ostium into the infundibulum. A concha bullosa may have a considerable size and may be multichambered. As a result, it may be in permanent contact with the septum and/or obstruct the infundibulum. Although a normal variation, a concha bullosa may thus play a role in nasal and sinus pathology.

The cavernous parenchyma of the middle turbinate is less voluminous than that of the inferior turbinate. It is thinnest at its head and thicker in the middle part and tail. It varies from 1 mm in the decongested state to 2 to 3 mm in the congested state. The mucosa of the middle turbinate is of moderate thickness and has numerous glands.

The *superior turbinate* is also part of the ethmoid bone. It is comparable with the ethmoidoturbinale II in mammals. It has little or no functional and pathological significance. It is a rudimentary structure consisting of a ridge at the cranioposterior wall of the nasal cavity of about 2 cm in length with some cavernous tissue and a relatively thin mucosa (see ▶ Fig. 1.87 and page 37).

The *supreme turbinate* is the remains of the ethmoidoturbinale III in mammals. In humans it is only present in about one-third of individuals.

Turbinate-Like Structures

The *septal turbinates* present themselves as local thickenings or ridges of the septal mucosa. Considering their histology and location, these mounds and plicae should be considered turbinates as they play a role in regulating and conditioning inspired air.

- *The tuberculum septi anterior (intumescentia septi),* the most conspicuous septal turbinate, lies opposite the head of the middle turbinate. It was described by Morgagni (1706), and later by Zuckerkandl (1892). Its height is 1 to 2 cm, its length about 2 cm (▶ Fig. 1.43 and ▶ Fig. 1.47). See also ▶ Fig. 1.87 and ▶ Fig. 1.92; page 37. The underlying perpendicular plate in this area is usually of the spongy type.
- *Septal ridges (plicae septi, tuberculum septi posterior):* Two or three narrow mucosal ridges or folds may be seen running downward on the lower (vomeral) part of the bony septum. Their course is parallel to the course of the inspiratory airstream. They are more common in children than in adults.
- The *agger nasi* is a mound or ridgelike elevation at the lateral nasal wall anterior to the head of the middle turbinate. Because of its location and structure it is to be considered a (rudimentary) turbinate.

Mucoperichondrium, Mucoperiosteum

The mucoperichondrium and mucoperiosteum consist of the following structures: (1) the mucous membrane with ciliated and nonciliated cells, goblet cells, and basal cells; (2) a basement membrane; (3) a lamina propria with seromucous glands; and (4) the perichondrium or periosteum. See also ▶ Fig. 1.75 and page 33.

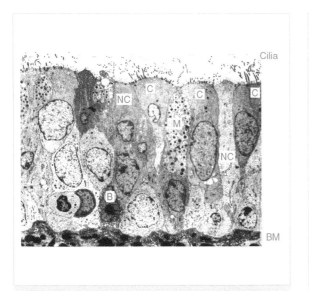

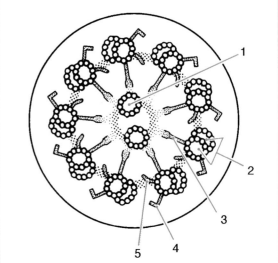

Fig. 1.48 Nasal mucosa (TEM) (from Schuil, Thesis Utrecht 1994).
B = basal cell; BM = basement membrane; C = ciliated columnar cell; M = mucus-producing goblet cell; NC = nonciliated columnar cell.

Fig. 1.49 Schematic representation of a cilium.
1 = central microtubule; 2 = peripheral doublet of microtubule; 3 = radial spoke; 4 = outer dynein arm; 5 = inner dynein arm.

Mucous Membrane

The nasal cavity is lined by a membrane that is composed of four different types of cells: ciliated columnar cells, nonciliated columnar cells, secretory cells or goblet cells, and basal cells (▶ Fig. 1.48).

The *ciliated columnar cells* are long slender cells. They are covered by 300 to 400 microvilli as well as some 100 to 250 cilia that are in constant movement (▶ Fig. 1.49). The cilia are embedded in a layer of thin fluid and covered by a layer of thicker mucus. This superficial blanket of mucus is transported over the thinner fluid layer in a posterior direction by the ciliary beat movement, the so-called mucociliary transport (MCT). This system is one of the most important defense mechanisms of the upper respiratory tract (Cilia page 60).

The *nonciliated columnar cells* are similar in size to the ciliated cells. They are only provided with microvilli that increase their functional surface area.

The *secretory cells or goblet cells* are covered by microvilli and filled with granules. The number of granules in the cytoplasm gradually increases with time. These granules distend the cell (hence the name goblet), which finally leads to a discharge of secretions through its upper surface (called apocrine secretion). The goblet cells produce the more viscous component of the mucus.

According to the studies of Tos and collaborators (1982), the number of goblet cells varies from about 5,700/mm² on the septum to 6,000/mm² in the sinuses, 8,000/mm² on the middle turbinate, and 11,000/mm² on the inferior turbinate. Their density is higher in children than in adults. In the nasal cavity, their density slightly increases from anterior to posterior. In general, the number of goblet cells is higher in areas where the mucosa is not in contact with air currents, for example the lateral wall of the inferior turbinate. (Experimental) breathing obstruction has been found to cause an increase of goblet cells.

The *basal cells* are short and rest on the basement membrane. They do not reach the epithelial surface and are probably replacement cells.

Basement Membrane

The basement membrane consists of a thin continuous layer with a thicker layer of collagen fibers underneath. This membrane separates the epithelial cells from the submucosa or lamina propria.

Lamina Propria (Submucosa)

In the submucosa, three layers can be recognized:
- A superficial layer of fenestrated capillaries
- A layer of mixed tubuloalveolar glands
- A zone of venous plexuses of various thickness that rests on the perichondrium or periosteum and may develop into a thick mass of cavernous tissue in the various turbinates

Seromucous Glands

The nasal mucosa is provided with a large number of glands that produce the more liquid superficial layer of mucus.

There are two types:

1. The anterior glands (altogether some 20 to 30) with relatively long ducts that open into the vestibule.
2. The small seromucous glands that are present in the whole mucosa. Their total number amounts to some 16,000. In contrast to the goblet cells, their density slightly decreases from anterior to posterior. Their numbers are somewhat higher on the septum than on the inferior and middle turbinates (Tos 1982).

Perichondrium, Periosteum

The perichondrium and periosteum consist of several layers of connective tissue fibers running parallel to the cartilage or bone. Small blood vessels and nerves run between the fibers of its outer layers (see ▶ Fig. 1.75).

Mucous Layer

The mucous layer is composed of two sheets:

- A lower layer of thin fluid, the periciliary or sol layer, which surrounds the cilia
- An upper gel layer with a higher viscosity

The mucous blanket adds water and warmth to the inspired air and captures particles in its upper layer (pollutants, micro-organisms, allergens, etc.). Its thickness varies between 0.5 and 1.0 mm. The mucus is produced by the goblet cells and seromucous glands.

Cilia

Phylogenetically, cilia are among the oldest biological structures. They can even be found on the surface of protozoa. The length of a respiratory cilium is 5 to 7 mm. It consists of an axoneme and a surrounding cell membrane. It has a basal body and a basal root fixed into the epithelium. The axoneme is made up of two central single microtubules and nine pairs of peripheral microtubules with outer and inner dynein arms (▶ Fig. 1.49). These arms are missing in patients with primary (genetic) ciliary akinesia.

Vomeronasal Organ (Organ of Jacobson)

The vomeronasal organ is a small canal and pouch lined with chemosensory cells, located in the deep layers of the septal perichondrium at the base of the anterior septum (▶ Fig. 1.50). For details see also ▶ Fig. 1.78, ▶ Fig. 1.79, and ▶ Fig. 1.80; page 34. It is considered a vestige of an earlier phylogenetic accessory olfactory organ. Its dimensions vary considerably (length: 3 to 12 mm; volume: 2.0 to 34.10⁻⁴ mL). It develops from the medial wall of the olfactory placode and detects chemical signals, especially

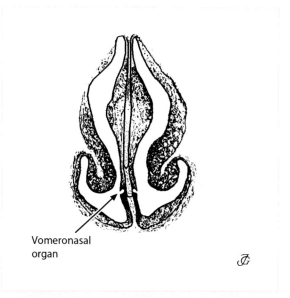

Fig. 1.50 Vomeronasal organ (organ of Jacobson), consisting of a short duct and a small pouch lined with high columnar epithelium located in the perichondrium of the base of the anterior part of the cartilaginous septum.

odors with a sexual or territorial significance called pheromones. The vomeronasal organ is found in all mammals, and recent clinical and cadaveric studies have shown it to be present in about 80% of human adults. No differences between males and females have been observed. In septal surgery, the vomeronasal organ should be respected. This means that the mucoperichondrium should be elevated underneath the deepest perichondrial fibers using a blunt elevator.

1.1.4 Vasculature of the Nose

The nasal structures receive their blood supply from the external as well as the internal carotid system (ECS and ICS; ▶ Fig. 1.51). See ▶ Fig. 10.56 for more details.

The anterior septum, the ethmoid bone, and the major part of the external pyramid receive their blood from the internal carotid system through branches of the ophthalmic artery.

The turbinates, inferior part of the septum, palate, the paranasal area, upper lip, vestibule, columella, and lower lip are supplied by the external carotid system through two of its main branches, the maxillary and the facial arteries.

Knowledge of the differences between the basins of the two systems is of utmost importance in managing nasal blood loss. Serious recurrent epistaxis from the lower half of the nasal cavity may be treated by clipping the maxillary artery or by ligation of the external carotid artery (ECA). Bleeding from the cranial part of the nasal cavity requires coagulation or clipping of the anterior and/or

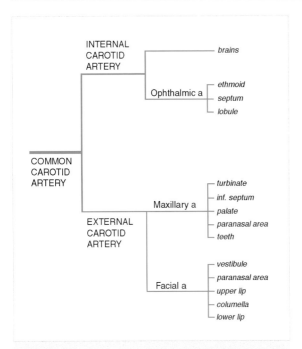

Fig. 1.51 The vascular supply of the internal and external nose is derived from both the internal and the external carotid system.

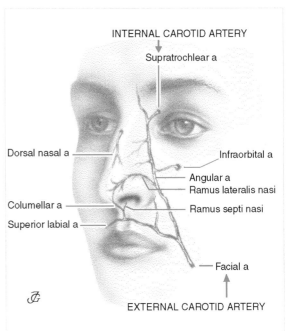

Fig. 1.52 Vascularization of the external nasal pyramid by a network of anastomoses between the internal and external carotid system.

posterior ethmoidal artery. This may be done either endonasally or through a paranasal, transorbital approach.

Vasculature of the External Nasal Pyramid

The blood supply of the external nasal pyramid is very variable and usually asymmetric. The nasal pyramid receives its blood supply mainly from the facial artery (ECS). In addition, the nasal dorsum is partially supplied by the ICS through the dorsal nasal artery, a terminal branch of the ophthalmic artery that leaves the orbit below the trochlea, and by the external nasal branch of the anterior ethmoidal artery, which emerges between the nasal bone and the triangular cartilage (▶ Fig. 1.52).

The facial artery branches into the superior labial artery at the corner of the mouth. This artery courses along the labial margin between the mucous membrane and the orbicularis oris muscle, and communicates with its contralateral fellow. It gives rise to an alar branch and, in the midline, to the columellar artery that supplies the columella and the lobular tip. The columellar artery also sends a branch to the nasal septum. Therefore, in the Terminologia Anatomica, the columellar artery is called the nasal septal branch.

By the side of the nose at the level of the ala, the facial artery branches into the lateral nasal branch, which supplies the dorsum and ala of the nose. The part of the facial artery distal to the lateral nasal branch is called the angular artery. The angular artery proceeds alongside the margin of the nose to the medial angle of the eye. It has several side branches towards the nasal dorsum and the cheek, and usually communicates with a medial branch of the infraorbital artery.

Facial artery branches to the external nasal pyramid may anastomose broadly with each other, their fellows from the opposite side, and the dorsal nasal artery.

Vasculature of the Septum

The septum receives its blood supply through five different arteries which originate both in the ICS as well as in the ECS (▶ Fig. 1.53):

- *Superior–anterior*: anterior ethmoidal artery (ophthalmic artery–internal carotid artery [ICA])
- *Superior–posterior*: posterior ethmoidal artery (ophthalmic artery–ICA)
- *Inferior–anterior*: superior labial artery (facial artery–external carotid artery [ECA]) and greater palatine artery (maxillary artery–ECA)
- *Inferior–posterior*: sphenopalatine artery (maxillary artery–ECA)

As illustrated in ▶ Fig. 1.53, there is a wide overlap between these five providers. This explains why, in some cases, it is so difficult to deal with epistaxis.

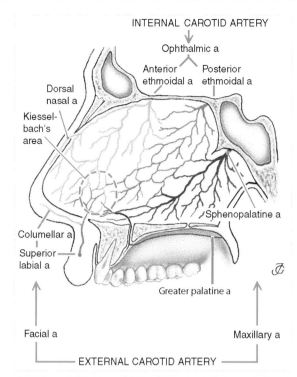

Fig. 1.53 Vascularization of the septum. Anastomoses between the internal (ethmoidal arteries) and external (superior labial and sphenopalatine arteries) carotid system.

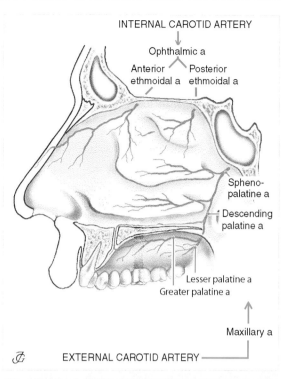

Fig. 1.54 Vascularization of the lateral nasal wall. Anastomoses between the internal (ethmoidal arteries) and external (sphenopalatine artery) carotid system.

The well-known locus Kiesselbach is a vulnerable area on the anterior septum where the terminal vessels of the various arteries meet and anastomose.

Vasculature of the Lateral Wall and Turbinates

The lateral nasal wall and the turbinates are supplied in a similar way to the septum (▶ Fig. 1.54).
- *Anterior ethmoidal artery*: lateral wall area 3, 4; head of turbinates; anterior ethmoidal cells
- *Posterior ethmoidal artery*: lateral wall area 4, 5; superior turbinate; posterior ethmoidal cells
- *Sphenopalatine artery*: lateral wall area 5; turbinates; nasal floor
- *Superior labial artery*: vestibule

Resistance and Capacitance Vessels

The nasal mucosa has a very complex and characteristic vasculature. Two types of vessels may be distinguished: a rich capillary network in the subepithelial zone and around the seromucous glands, and a cavernous venous plexus deep in the lamina propria. The capillaries are named the resistance vessels; the plexus of venous sinusoids, the capacitance vessels. The latter are so well developed that they resemble erectile tissue. They may contract and distend. When congested, they cause swelling of the mucosa and increased

nasal resistance. They are particularly found in the anterior half of the inferior turbinates and the anterior part of the septum.

1.1.5 Nerve Supply of the Nose

The nasal structures have an intricate nerve supply involving four different systems (▶ Table 1.1):
- Somatosensory system
- Somatomotor system
- Sympathetic system (visceromotor)
- Parasympathetic system (visceromotor)

Table 1.1 The four nervous systems of the nose, their neurotransmitters and effects

System	Neurotransmitters	Effects
Somatosensory	SP, NKA, CGRP, etc.	Sensibility skin and mucosa
Somatomotor	ACh	Musculature
Sympathetic	NA, NPY, etc.	Vasoconstriction Quality of secretion
Parasympathetic	ACh, VIP, PHI, etc.	Vasodilation Stimulation of secretion

Abbreviations: Ach, acetylcholine; CGRP, calcitonin gene–related peptide; NA, noradrenaline; NKA, neurokinin A; NPY, neuropeptide Y; PHI, peptide histidine isoleucine amide; SP, substance P; VIP, vasoactive intestinal peptide

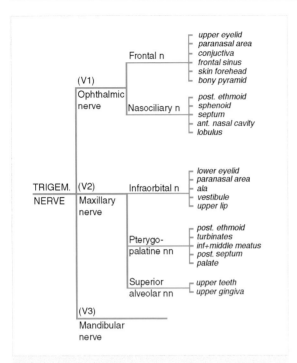

Fig. 1.55 Schematic diagram of internal and external nasal innervation.

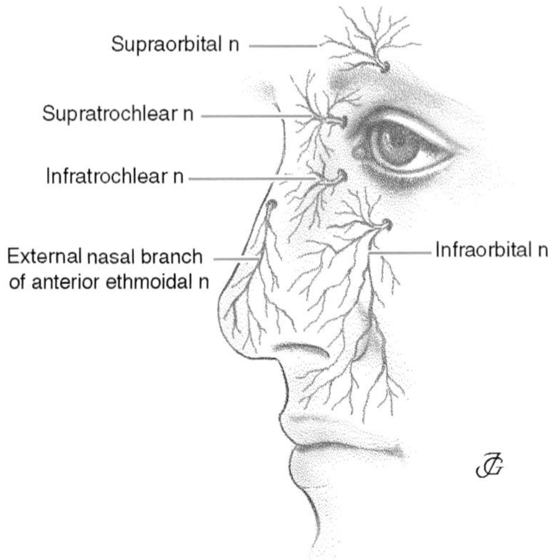

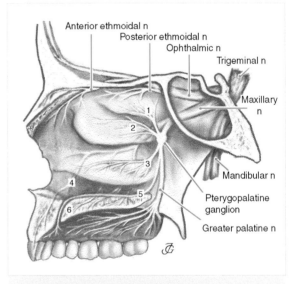

Fig. 1.56 Nerve supply of the external nose by four branches of the ophthalmic nerve.

Sensory Innervation

The sensory innervation of both the external pyramid and the nasal cavity is derived from the trigeminal nerve (▶ Fig. 1.55). See also ▶ Fig. 10.57 for more details.

Sensory Innervation of the External Pyramid

The external pyramid receives its nerve supply through five different nerves. Four of them originate in the ophthalmic nerve (V1) and one in the maxillary nerve (V2), as shown in ▶ Fig. 1.56:

- Supraorbital nerve: nasal root, upper eyelid, conjunctiva, forehead, frontal sinus
- Supratrochlear nerve: bony pyramid, upper eyelid, conjunctiva, frontal sinus
- Infratrochlear nerve: bony and cartilaginous pyramid, eyelids, conjunctiva, and lacrimal sac
- External nasal branch of the anterior ethmoidal nerve: medial part of cartilaginous pyramid and the lobule
- Infraorbital nerve: lateral part of cartilaginous pyramid and lobule, cheek, upper lip, and lower eyelid

As always in the nasal domain, there is a wide overlap between the distributional areas of these five nerves. Local anesthesia of the external nose is therefore carried out by blocking the exits of the supraorbital, infraorbital, and anterior ethmoidal nerve (see ▶ Fig. 10.56).

Fig. 1.57 Nerve supply of the nasal cavity.
1, 2 = posterior superior lateral nasal branches; 3 = posterior inferior lateral nasal branches; 4 = anterior superior alveolar nerve; 5 = nasopalatine nerve; 6 = incisive nerve

Sensory Innervation of the Nasal Cavity

A large number of nerves contribute to the nerve supply of the nasal cavity. They are derived from all three main branches of the trigeminal nerve (▶ Fig. 1.57).

- *Superior–anterior*: anterior ethmoidal nerve
- *Superior–posterior*: posterior ethmoidal nerve and nasal nerves (posterior superior lateral nasal branches and posterior superior medial nasal branches to the lateral wall and septum, respectively)
- *Inferior–anterior*: anterior superior alveolar nerve, nasopalatine nerve (to septum)
- *Inferior–posterior*: nasal nerves (posterior inferior nasal branches of the greater palatine nerve)

The ethmoidal nerves are derived from the ophthalmic nerve (V1). All other branches are derived from the maxillary nerve (V2). Fibers of many maxillary nerve branches (posterior superior lateral and medial nasal branches) traverse the pterygopalatine ganglion without synapsing before entering the nasal cavity through the sphenopalatine foramen. Hence these branches are often described as branches of the pterygopalatine ganglion. The nasopalatine nerve is the largest of the posterior superior medial nasal branches and continues as the incisive nerve through the incisive canal to the anterior portion of the hard palate.

There is again an extensive overlap (and also a certain variation, e.g., as a result of previous surgery) between the areas supplied by these different nerves.

The fibers of the parasympathetic system (see following text) run together with the sensory fibers. Most fibers of the sympathetic system follow the blood supply, but some are also distributed via sensory nerves.

The Incisive Nerve and the Maxilla–Premaxilla Approach

In making an anterior–inferior septal tunnel, the mucoperiosteum of the septal base and nasal floor is elevated from the bone. In this procedure, the incisive nerve may be severed. This may produce anesthesia of the palatal mucosa just posterior to the incisor teeth. The incisive nerve is the terminal branch of the nasopalatine nerve (▶ Fig. 1.57). This nerve courses through the deep layers of the periosteum in a groove on the vomer, and in the perichondrium of the septal cartilage. Its final branch enters the incisive canal under the premaxillary wing about 12 mm dorsal to the piriform aperture (▶ Fig. 1.58). It leaves this canal just behind the first incisor tooth and innervates a small triangular medioventral area of palatal mucosa (▶ Fig. 1.59). The greater palatine artery runs upward in the incisive canal to contribute to the vascular supply of the septum. Normally there are two incisive canals, a left one and a right one. For further details, see ▶ Fig. 1.76 and ▶ Fig. 1.77; page 33.

Damage to the incisive nerve is sometimes unavoidable in extensive septal surgery if the premaxilla and anterior nasal spine have to be completely dissected. Fortunately, only a minority of patients notice and complain of a temporary loss of sensitivity in the medial anterior part of the palate. In cases with limited pathology of the premaxillary area, laceration of the nerve can be avoided by making the inferior tunnel from above (see page 165).

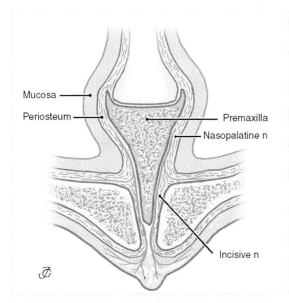

Fig. 1.58 Nasopalatine nerves and incisive nerve in relation to the premaxilla and incisive canal.

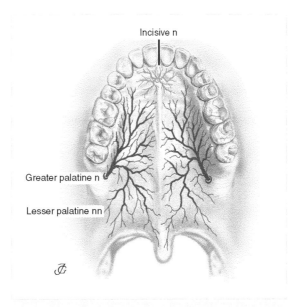

Fig. 1.59 Innervation of the palate.

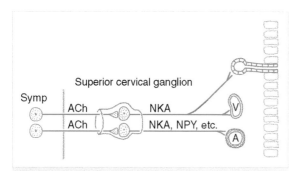

Fig. 1.60 Sympathetic innervation of the nasal mucosa with its neurotransmitters. (Modified from Lundblad.)
ACh = acetylcholine; NKA = neurokinin A; NPY = neuropeptide Y; V = vein; A = artery.

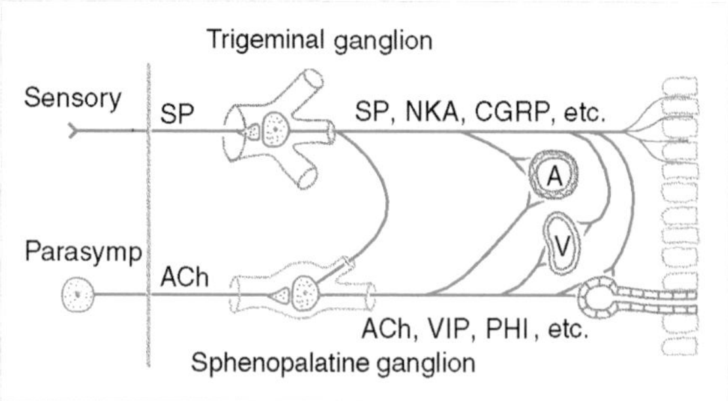

Fig. 1.61 Sensory and parasympathetic innervation of the nasal mucosa with its neurotransmitters. (Modified from Lundblad.) A = artery; CGRP = calcitonin gene-related peptide; ggl = ganglion; PHI = peptide histidine isoleucine amide; SP = substance P; V = vein.

Motor Nerve System

The nerve supply of the nasal musculature is derived from the facial nerve, in particular its buccal and zygomatic branches. Innervation of the dilating muscles is part of a reflex arc consisting of mechanoreceptors of the lung, viscerosensory nerve fibers, the inspiratory breathing center in the medulla oblongata, and the facial nerve fibers to the nasal musculature.

Sympathetic Innervation

The sympathetic innervation of the mucosal lining of the nasal cavity, including the turbinates, originates in a center in the thoracic part of the spinal cord. The preganglionic fibers reach the sympathetic trunk and synapse in the superior cervical ganglion, acetylcholine (ACh) being the neurotransmitter (▶ Fig. 1.60). Postganglionic fibers are distributed to the nose via blood vessels as perivascular plexuses, and via the internal carotid nerves along the ICA. From these nerves, the deep petrosal nerve branches out in the foramen lacerum and joins the greater petrosal nerve. The combined nerve travels as the nerve of the pterygoid canal (vidian nerve) through the pterygoid canal to the pterygopalatine fossa. The sympathetic fibers pass through the pterygopalatine ganglion without synapsing and are distributed to the nasal mucosa along the sensory nerves (i.e., the posterior superior lateral and medial nasal branches of the maxillary nerve). The majority of the fibers terminate in the walls of the arterioles, venules, and venous sinoids, and have a vasoconstrictive effect. A minority terminate at the nasal glands and modify secretion.

Parasympathetic Innervation

The parasympathetic fibers for the nasal cavity originate in the superior salivatory nucleus and leave the brainstem via the sensory root of the facial nerve, the intermediate nerve. These fibers leave the facial nerve in the greater petrosal nerve, which joins the deep petrosal nerve to form the nerve of the pterygoid canal (vidian nerve, see previous text). In the pterygopalatine fossa, the fibers synapse in the pterygopalatine ganglion (neurotransmitter: ACh, vasoactive intestinal peptide [VIP], peptide histidine isoleucine amide [PHI], etc.) and are distributed to the nasal mucosa along the sensory nasal nerves just like the sympathetic nerve fibers (▶ Fig. 1.61). In the mucosa, they dilate small vessels and stimulate secretion by the nasal glands. Pterygopalatine ganglion is the official term according to the *Terminologia Anatomica*; however, in literature the ganglion is often called the sphenopalatine ganglion.

Olfactory Organ

The olfactory organ is located in the superior nasal passage on the upper middle part of the middle turbinate and the adjoining area of the septum. In humans, the olfactory region is a very irregular area with a somewhat yellow-brownish color with a total surface of some 100 to 500 mm². Its size and shape show very large individual variation (▶ Fig. 1.62). In general, the olfactory region decreases with age. Due to its irregularity, it is almost impossible to distinguish it from the respiratory region of the nasal mucosa. On average, however, the olfactory region does not extend further than 2.0 to 2.5 cm below the lamina cribrosa.

The olfactory region consists of two to three layers of columnar cells with small (Bowman's) glands in between. In contrast to the main mucosa of the nasal cavity, there is no basement membrane. Similar to other sensory organs, the cells are of two different types: sensory and supporting. The sensory cells are long and slender. On top they are provided with 8 to 18 hairs that protrude into a thin layer of mucus. Their base extends into a nerve fiber with several neurotubules, which transport the signal to the central olfactory system. Unlike other sensory organs, there is no synapse between the sensory cell and the nerve fiber. Groups of nerve fibers covered by basal cells at the base of the epithelium combine to form so-called

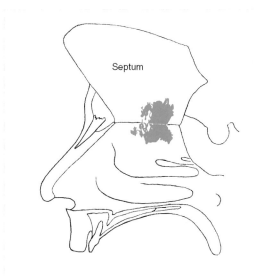

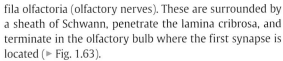

Fig. 1.62 Olfactory region on the most cranial area of the lateral nasal wall and septum. (After Brunn.)

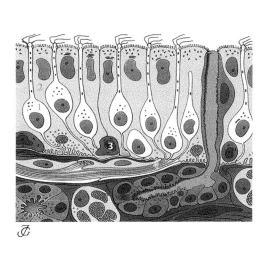

Fig. 1.63 Olfactory epithelium showing (1) ciliated receptor cells, (2) supporting cells bearing microvilli, (3) basal epithelial cells, (4) axons, and (5) Bowman glands.

fila olfactoria (olfactory nerves). These are surrounded by a sheath of Schwann, penetrate the lamina cribrosa, and terminate in the olfactory bulb where the first synapse is located (▶ Fig. 1.63).

For the nasal surgeon, it is of utmost importance to recognize that olfactory cells and nerve endings are present at the upper part of the middle turbinate. Resection of the middle turbinate may therefore deprive the patient of a part of his olfactory sense. Resection of the middle turbinate as a routine procedure in surgery for nasal polyps and sinusitis must, therefore, be condemned.

1.2 Histological Features of the Main Nasal Structures and Their Implications for Nasal Surgery

This chapter is devoted to the functional anatomy and histology of the most important nasal structures. Special attention is paid to the consequences of the anatomical and histological features for the practice of nasal and sinus surgery.

The data presented here are from the research carried out in the Department of Anatomy of Utrecht University Medical Centre (Heads: Prof. Dr. B. Hillen, Prof. Dr. RLAW Bleys) by fellows of the Department of Otorhinolaryngology (Zhai et al 1995 and 1996; Hafkamp et al 1999; Popko et al 2007; and Bleys et al 2007).

All histological sections are from adult Caucasian noses. Some of them were dissected to study different macroscopic anatomical issues. The other specimens were fixated in 10% neutral buffered formalin, washed in buffered

phosphate 0.1 M at pH 7.4 for 1 day, decalcified with 5% HNO_3 for 7 days, dehydrated in increasing concentrations of alcohol for 5 days, and put in xylene for 3 days. They were then embedded in paraffin or in carboxymethylcellulose and frozen to -20 °C. An adhesive tape was then fixed to the surface of the paraffin block. Subsequently, the specimens were sectioned with a microtome (PMV 200) into serial sections of 25 μm thickness at 150 or 250 μm intervals in different planes (coronal, transverse, or parallel to the nasal dorsum).

The sections were then stained with a modified Mallory–Cason trichrome technique (MC), hematoxylin and eosin (H&E), or a combination of the MC method and resorcin-fuchsin (MC-RF). Finally, together with the tape they were mounted on glass slides for microscopic study.

MC staining was used in the majority of the sections, as this method allows a fine differentiation between the various histological tissues. MC-RF staining was used to distinguish between fibrous structures.

In the studies of the perichondral envelope of the septal and the lobular cartilages, the tissues were stained according to the MC, Azan, Herovici, Verhoeff–van Gieson, and Lawson methods, as well as by immunohistochemistry to demonstrate the presence of collagen type I and II.

1.2.1 Septum

Septal Cartilage: Chondrocytes and Extracellular Matrix

In the periphery we find the young chondrocytes. They are numerous, small, flat, and oriented parallel to the surface. In the intermediate zone they are less numerous and more ovaloid, and their axis runs more perpendicular to

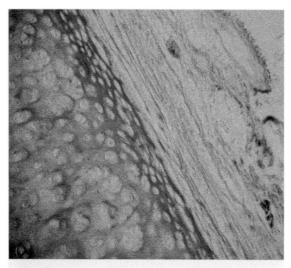

Fig. 1.64 Septal cartilage (MC staining). In the periphery of the septal cartilage, we find numerous young, small, and flat chondrocytes, which are oriented parallel to the cartilaginous surface. In the intermediate zone, they are less numerous and more ovaloid, and their axis runs more perpendicular to the surface.

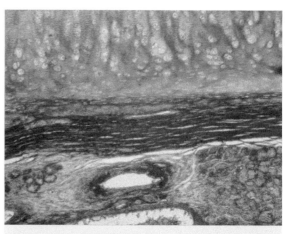

Fig. 1.65 Septal cartilage (MC staining). The extracellular matrix of the septal cartilage shows a distinct difference in composition between the peripheral and central zones. The cells in the periphery are surrounded by homogeneous material with a high bluish-stained collagen type II.

the surface. The lowest density of chondrocytes is found in the central zone. Here, they are spheroidal and more or less aligned in columns perpendicular to the cartilaginous surface (▶ Fig. 1.64 and ▶ Fig. 1.65).

The extracellular matrix of the septal cartilage shows a distinct difference in composition between the peripheral and central zones. The cells in the periphery are surrounded by homogeneous material with a high collagen type II content and higher density of young collagen fibers as compared to the more central zones. There are no elastic fibers in the cartilage (▶ Fig. 1.65).

Septal Cartilage: Perichondrium

The perichondrium of the septal cartilage consists of a homogeneous layer of collagen type I fibers and elastic fibers. The elastic fibers have a network-like arrangement. Clearly distinguishable zones in the septal perichondrium have been previously suggested (by ourselves) but could not be observed. The suggested existence of a dense inner and a loose outer layer was probably due to a processing artifact (▶ Fig. 1.66).

Chondrospinal Junction

The base of the cartilaginous septum widens slightly at the level of the anterior nasal spine. Various paraseptal cartilages, each in its own perichondrial envelope, lie adjacent to this pear-shaped broadening. In this specimen (▶ Fig. 1.67 and ▶ Fig. 1.68), the medial paraseptal cartilages are positioned horizontally, the lateral ones more vertically. Their perichon-

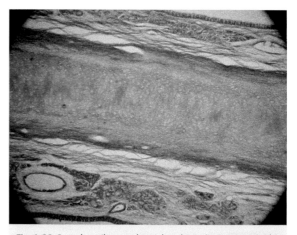

Fig. 1.66 Septal cartilage and perichondrium (MC staining). The existence of a dense inner and a loose outer perichondral layer is suggested but is probably due to a processing artifact.

drium holds them together. The form and position of the paraseptal cartilages provide the cartilaginous septum with a broader base that rests on the surface of the anterior nasal spine. The cranial part of the anterior nasal spine widens like the bow of a ship, providing a pedestal for the septum. The septum and the spine are separated by a relatively wide gap of about 0.5 mm, which is filled with loose connective tissue. This allows a certain degree of mobility. At the chondrospinal area, stability is thus combined with a certain amount of mobility.

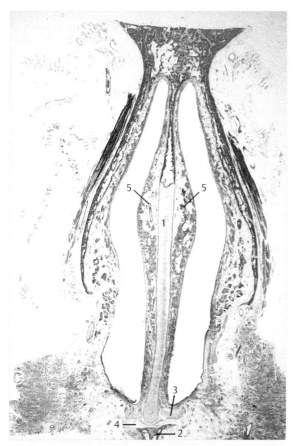

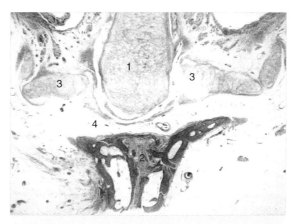

Fig. 1.68 Chondrospinal junction (high magnification of detail of ▶ Fig. 1.67). Base of the cartilaginous septum (1); anterior nasal spine (2); two large, horizontally positioned and two small, vertically positioned paraseptal cartilages (3); wide junctional gap with loose connective tissue fibers (4).

Fig. 1.67 Chondrospinal junction (coronal section, MC staining). Cartilaginous septum (1); anterior nasal spine (2); paraseptal cartilages (3); junctional gap with loose connective tissue (4); septal turbinates (5).

Chondropremaxillary Complex

At the chondropremaxillary complex, the cartilaginous septum is thinner in the middle than at its cranial and caudal end. Its base shows a considerable bilateral broadening, the processus lateralis ventralis. The left and right premaxillary bones are unified in the midline. The unified premaxilla has two wings that serve as a pedestal for the septal cartilage. Two almost vertically positioned paraseptal cartilages cover the lateral side of the junction. They are kept in place by tight perichondrium that surrounds each of them individually. The narrow gap between the cartilage and the bone is filled with dense connective tissue. Three types of fiber can be recognized: lateral fibers, which run from the perichondrium of the septal cartilage to the periosteum of the lateral wall of the premaxilla; medial fibers, which run from the perichondrium of the septal cartilage into the "joint area"; and "crossing" fibers, which traverse the junction and terminate in the premaxilla bone or its periosteum. The function of all these structures seems to be to provide maximal stability and rigidity (▶ Fig. 1.69, ▶ Fig. 1.70, ▶ Fig. 1.71, and ▶ Fig. 1.72).

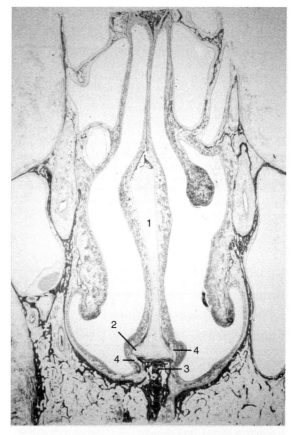

Fig. 1.69 The chondropremaxillary complex (coronal section, MC staining). Cartilaginous septum (1) with its processus lateralis ventralis (2), premaxilla (3), and paraseptal cartilages (4).

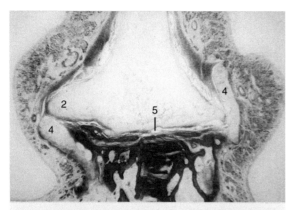

Fig. 1.70 Chondropremaxillary complex (high magnification of detail of ▶ Fig. 1.69). Processus lateralis ventralis (2); paraseptal cartilages in different positions (4); narrow gap between the septum and the premaxilla filled with dense connective tissue fibers (5).

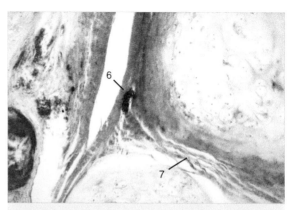

Fig. 1.71 Chondropremaxillary complex (high magnification of detail of ▶ Fig. 1.69). Lateral fibers (6); medial fibers (7).

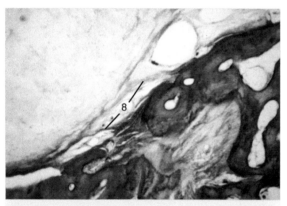

Fig. 1.72 Chondropremaxillary complex (high magnification of detail of ▶ Fig. 1.69). Crossing fibers between the base of the septal cartilage and the premaxilla (8).

Chondroperpendicular and Chondrovomeral Junction

Chondroperpendicular Junction

The posterior margin of the cartilaginous septum is fixed into a shallow groove of the anterior margin of the perpendicular plate. The type of junction between the septal cartilage and the perpendicular plate is unique in the human body. It is the only "articulation" where cartilage-covered and noncartilage-covered bone join. The septal perichondrium is continuous with the periosteum of the perpendicular plate. This stands to reason, as the perpendicular plate is the ossified posterior part of the primitive cartilaginous septum (▶ Fig. 1.73). Consequently, a posterior (subperiosteal) tunnel can be easily elevated from an anterior–superior (subperichondrial) tunnel.

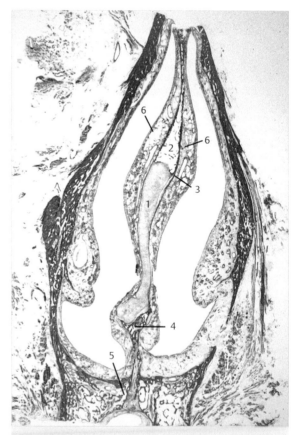

Fig. 1.73 Chondroperpendicular junction (coronal section at the level of the premaxilla and the incisival canal, MC staining). Cartilaginous septum (1); perpendicular plate (2); continuity between perichondrium and periosteum (3); premaxilla (4); Incisive canal (5); septal turbinates (6). Note the bone marrow in the perpendicular plate.

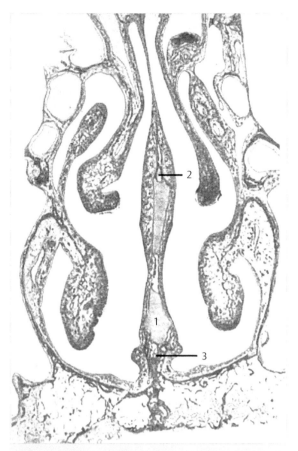

Fig. 1.74 Chondrovomeral junction (coronal section at the level of the ethmoid bone, MC staining). Cartilaginous septum (1); perpendicular plate (2); vomer (3).

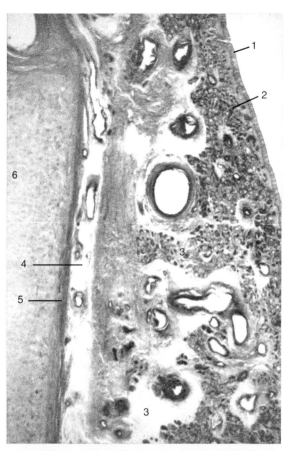

Fig. 1.75 Septal mucoperichondrium (coronal section, MC staining). Pseudostratified columnar ciliated epithelium (1); lamina propria with mucous cells and serous glands (2); parenchyma (3); outer perichondrial layer with loose fibers (4); inner perichondrial layer with dense fibers (5); septal cartilage with relatively few chondrocytes and connective tissue fibers in the center and a higher density of cells and elastic fibers in the periphery (6).

Chondrovomeral Junction

The pear-shaped posterocaudal margin of the cartilaginous septum is fixed into a groove of the vomer. The junction is characterized by a very narrow gap with connective tissue fibers that are organized in a similar way to the chondropremaxillary junction. There are relatively more crossing fibers, however, which may explain why, during surgery, a mucosal tear may occur more easily at the chondrovomeral junction. The chondrovomeral junction allows some rotation when pressure is applied on the nasal dorsum, thus decreasing the risk of a fracture (▶ Fig. 1.74).

Mucoperichondrium

The mucoperichondrium consists of several different layers: (1) pseudostratified columnar ciliated epithelium with goblet cells and openings of the seromucous glands; (2) the lamina propria, or parenchymal layer, of varying thickness with seromucous glands, arterioles, venules, and nerve fibers; and (3) the perichondrium, consisting of connective tissue fibers running parallel to the cartilage. In the perichondrium, two layers may be distinguished: an outer layer of loosely arranged fibers with small arterioles, venules, and nerves; and an inner layer of densely packed fibers adjacent to the cartilage (▶ Fig. 1.75).

If, during surgery, the mucoperichondrium is elevated in the proper plane—that is, under the inner perichondrial layer—then no damage will occur to vessels (no bleeding), nerves (branches of the nasopalatine nerve, incisive nerve), special structures (vomeronasal organ), or submucosal organelles.

Incisive Nerve

The incisive nerve is a final branch of the nasopalatine nerve. It runs in a posterior–anterior direction in a narrow groove along the vomer parallel to its anterior

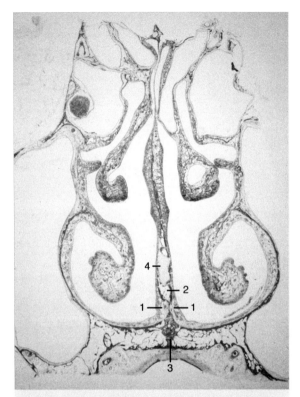

Fig. 1.76 Incisive nerve (coronal section at the middle of the nasal cavity, MC staining). Incisive nerve (1); vomer (2); bony palate (3); sphenoidal process of the cartilaginous septum (4).

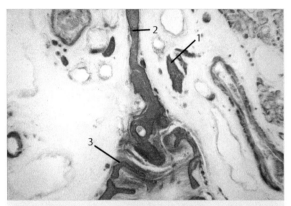

Fig. 1.77 Incisive canals. Incisive nerves (1); vomer (2); bony palate (3).

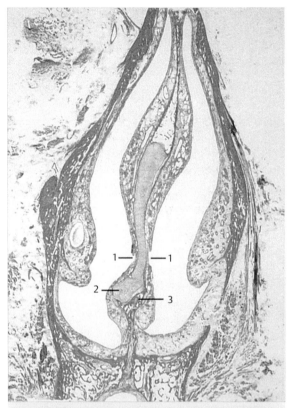

Fig. 1.78 Vomeronasal organ (coronal section just posterior to the premaxilla, MC staining). Bilateral mucosal pit or opening (1); cartilaginous septum (considerably dislocated in this case) (2); premaxilla (3). Note the septal turbinates and turbinate-like tissue inside the bony pyramid and at the nasal floor.

border. It then passes under the wing of the premaxilla, curving down into the incisive canal of the premaxilla together with the artery and vein, and innervating a small triangular area behind the front teeth. In the septum, it is situated within the superficial layers of the periosteum (▶ Fig. 1.76 and ▶ Fig. 1.77). If, during septal surgery, a superior subperiosteal tunnel is elevated at the proper level (i.e., under the deepest periosteal fibers), no damage to the incisive nerve will occur. However, if an inferior subperiosteal tunnel is made (e.g., in the maxillary–premaxillary approach), the nerve may be severed. As a result, some patients may notice a temporary sensory impairment in a small area behind the front teeth. This can be avoided only if the undertunneling is strictly limited to the lateral wall of the premaxilla and not continued laterally on the nasal floor.

Vomeronasal Organ

The vomeronasal organ (organ of Jacobson) is a rudimentary chemosensory organ found in most mammals and the majority of humans. It is located at the base of the anterior cartilaginous septum in the lamina propria of the mucosa adjacent to the perichondrium. The organ is able to perceive chemical signals with a sexual or territorial significance, called pheromones. It starts as a mucosal

depression at the ventral part of the septal base (▶ Fig. 1.78). Its posterior part deepens, and the lips of the pit fold over to form a tunnel that runs within the perichondrium in a dorsal direction (▶ Fig. 1.79). It then forms a small duct of variable length (2 to 10 mm), which terminates in a small pouch (▶ Fig. 1.80). Both duct and

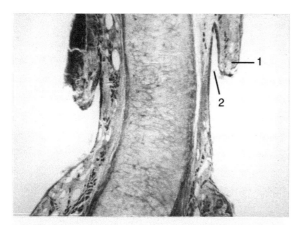

Fig. 1.79 High magnification detail of ▶ Fig. 1.78. Opening with posterior lip (1); beginning of the duct (2).

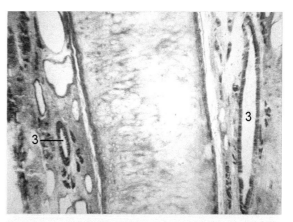

Fig. 1.80 High magnification detail of ▶ Fig. 1.78. Vomeronasal organ (coronal section, MC staining). Vomeronasal organ lined with a high columnar epithelium lying within the perichondrium of the septal cartilage (3).

pouch are lined with a high columnar cell epithelium. In contrast to most mammals, the vomeronasal organ in man is situated in the lamina propria adjacent to the perichondrium, not in the cartilage or bone.

Septal Pathology

Septal Deviation and Basal Crest

A high deviation of the perpendicular plate and cartilaginous septum to one side, and a basal crest to the other side, is a common type of pathology. A classic example is shown in ▶ Fig. 1.81 and ▶ Fig. 1.82. The perpendicular plate and the cranial part of the cartilaginous septum are deviated to the right, whereas the septal base is dislocated to the left. The anterior nasal spine is somewhat asymmetric, the left wing being larger than the right. There is extensive scarring at the chondrospinal junction. Several pieces of cartilage are present. It is unclear whether they represent (dislocated) paraseptal cartilages, or new posttraumatic cartilaginous growth.

Vomeral Crest

Vomeral crests generally occur at the more posterior parts of the anterior septum. They usually consist of a bony (vomeral) and a cartilaginous part. The latter derives from the base of the cartilaginous septum and/or a dislocated sphenoidal process, as shown in ▶ Fig. 1.83 and ▶ Fig. 1.84. They often end in a spur.

Vomeral Spur

Vomeral spurs or spines may occur at the junction of the cranial margin of the vomer, the caudal margin of the perpendicular plate, and the posterior border of the cartilaginous septum. They are found at the posterior septum at the level of the middle of the inferior turbinate, where they often impact the conchal parenchyma. They usually consist of a bony (vomeral) part and a dislocated outgrowth of the sphenoidal process of the cartilaginous septum (▶ Fig. 1.85 and ▶ Fig. 1.86).

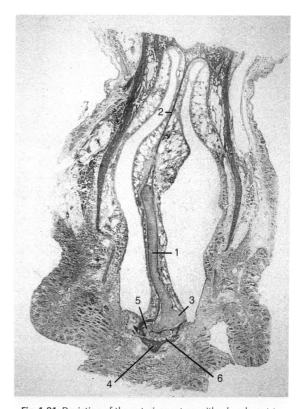

Fig. 1.81 Deviation of the anterior septum with a basal crest to the opposite side (coronal section at the level of the anterior nasal spine, MC staining). Cartilaginous septum (1); perpendicular plate (2); dislocated septal base (3); anterior nasal spine (4); chondrospinal junction with scar tissue and multiple pieces of cartilage (5). Note the septal turbinates and the turbinate-like tissue on the inside of the nasal bones.

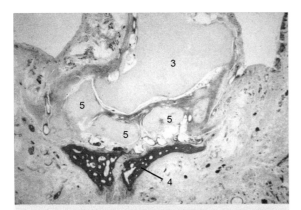

Fig. 1.82 High magnification of detail of ▶ Fig. 1.81. Dislocated septal base (3); premaxilla (4); chondrospinal junction with scar tissue and several (dislocated) pieces of cartilage (5).

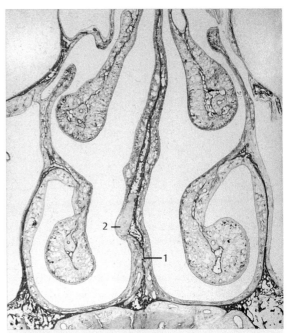

Fig. 1.83 Vomeral crest (coronal section at the level of the sphenoidal process of the cartilaginous septum, MC staining). Vomer (1); superimposed dislocated sphenoidal process (2).

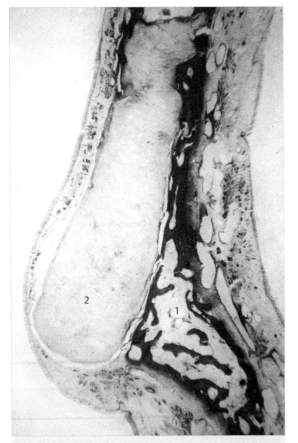

Fig. 1.84 High magnification of detail of ▶ Fig. 1.83. Vomer (1); sphenoidal process with its perichondrial envelope (2).

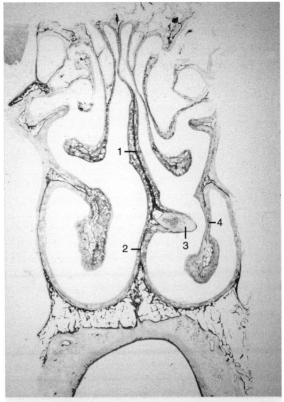

Fig. 1.85 Vomeral spur (coronal section at the posterior part, MC staining). Perpendicular plate (1); vomer (2); dislocated sphenoidal process of cartilaginous septum (3); impression in the inferior turbinate (4).

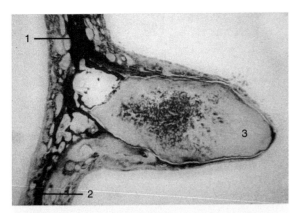

Fig. 1.86 High magnification of detail of ▶ Fig. 1.85. Perpendicular plate (1); vomer (2); dislocated sphenoidal process of cartilaginous septum (3).

1.2.2 Turbinates

Humans have three or four protruding turbinates with a bony skeleton on each lateral nasal wall (▶ Fig. 1.87). These are combined with mounds (intumescentias) with a turbinate-like parenchyma. These are mainly located on the septum (septal turbinate) and on the lateral nasal wall in front of the middle turbinate (▶ Fig. 1.78, ▶ Fig. 1.81, and ▶ Fig. 1.87). Of the protruding lateral turbinates, the inferior, middle, and superior turbinate are invariably present in all human beings. A small, rudimentary fourth lateral turbinate, the supreme turbinate, is found in only about 30% of the population (▶ Fig. 1.87). The inferior turbinate is a "maxilloturbinate" because it is part of the maxillary bone. The middle, superior, and supreme turbinates, on the other hand, are part of the ethmoidal complex. Accordingly, they may be called "ethmoidal turbinates."

As a result of these protruding turbinates and the various thickenings, the anterior part of the nasal cavity (area 3 and 4) has the form of a slit. This geometry increases the turbulence of inhaled air and enhances the contact of the inspired air with the mucosa and the olfactory organ.

Inferior Turbinate

The inferior turbinate is part of the maxilla. It is comparable to the maxilloturbinates in mammals. Its bony skeleton consists of a curved lamella of solid, more or less spongiotic bone. A bulla within the inferior turbinate is extremely rare. The inferior turbinate has a large amount of parenchyma and an extensive vascular bed with many venous sinoids or capacitance vessels. As a consequence, the inferior turbinate may congest to more than twice its normal size in its resting state (▶ Fig. 1.88). The angle between the lateral nasal wall and the turbinate bone varies greatly from about 20° ("laterally positioned") to 90° ("medially positioned"), as illustrated in ▶ Fig. 1.89. Compare also ▶ Fig. 1.45.

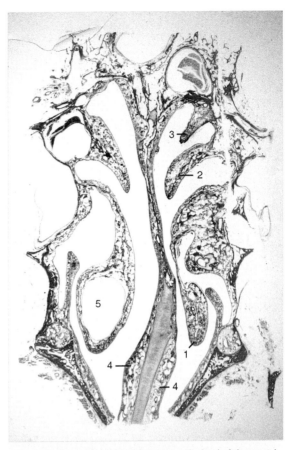

Fig. 1.87 The turbinates (axial section at the level of the cranial part of the middle nasal passage, MC staining). Middle turbinate (1); superior turbinate (2); supreme turbinate (3) on the left; septal turbinates (4); bullous middle turbinate on the right (5). Note the obstruction of the left middle meatus with impression and atrophy of the middle turbinate due to a septal deviation.

Middle Turbinate (Concha Bullosa)

The middle turbinate is the first ethmoidoturbinate. Its skeleton is part of the ethmoid bone. The presence of a cell or small sinus in its anterior part with an ostium at its medial side is seen in about 25% of the population (▶ Fig. 1.90 and ▶ Fig. 1.91).

Septal Turbinate

The septal turbinate is a localized thickening of the mucosa of the septum in area 4, opposite the anterior and middle part of the middle turbinate (▶ Fig. 1.92). It has previously also been called "intumescentia" or "tuberculum" septi. Like the other turbinates, the septal turbinate may hypertrophy according to physiological demands and as a result of pathology. Compare ▶ Fig. 1.47, ▶ Fig. 1.78, ▶ Fig. 1.81, and ▶ Fig. 1.87.

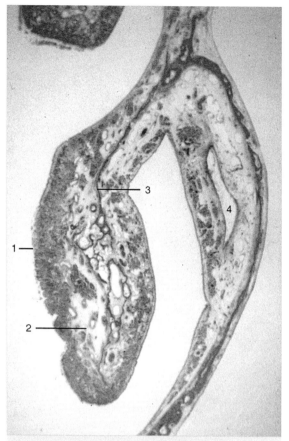

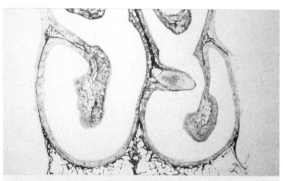

Fig. 1.89 Inferior turbinates (coronal section at the posterior part of the nasal cavity; detail of ▶ Fig. 1.85, MC staining) demonstrating a huge difference between the angle of attachment of bony lamella of the inferior turbinates, almost 90° on the right, 40° on the left.

Fig. 1.88 Inferior turbinate (coronal section through its anterior part, MC staining). Ciliated mucosa (1); extensively vascularized parenchyma (2); turbinate bone, partially spongiotic (3); lacrimal duct (4).

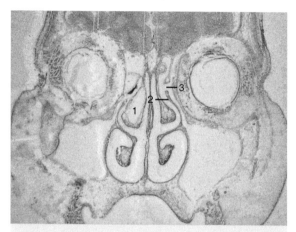

Fig. 1.90 Concha bullosa (coronal section at the level of the ostia of the maxillary sinuses; MC staining). Bullous middle turbinate or concha bullosa (1); uncinate process (2); ostium of the maxillary sinus (3).

1.2.3 Bony Pyramid

Junction between the Triangular Cartilage and Nasal Bones

The upper border of the triangular cartilage is rigidly attached to the lower margin of the inner wall of the bony pyramid. The bone overlaps the cartilage for about 1 to 3 mm, as can be seen in ▶ Fig. 1.93. The cartilage is tightly fixed to the inside of the bone (▶ Fig. 1.94). A traumatic dislocation of the cartilage from the bone is therefore difficult to correct. Each nasal bone has its own periosteal envelope. Both periostea fuse at the internasal suture. As a consequence, it is impossible to create a subperiosteal tunnel on the bony dorsum, contrary to what has often been claimed. As soon as the periosteum is elevated, it will tear.

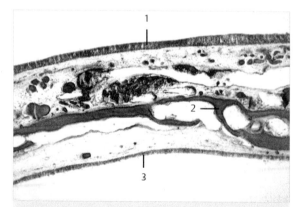

Fig. 1.91 Wall of a concha medial bullosa (MC staining). Outer mucosa with columnar ciliated epithelium (1); bony wall (2); inner ciliated mucosa (3).

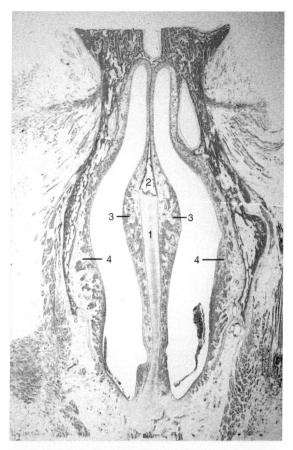

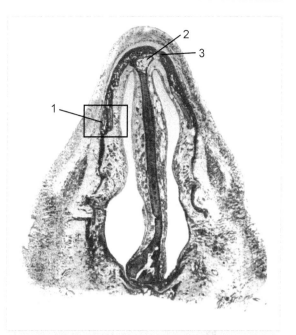

Fig. 1.93 Junction between the cartilaginous and bony vault (coronal section at the level of the anterior nasal spine, MC staining). The bony pyramid overlaps the cranial end of the triangular cartilage (1). Note the broadening and partial ossification of the cranial end of the septum at the K area (2); internasal suture (3).

Fig. 1.92 Septal turbinate (coronal section of the anterior part of the nasal cavity, MC staining). Cartilaginous septum (1); perpendicular plate (2); septal turbinates (3); turbinate-like tissue on the lateral nasal wall (4). Note the opening of the vomeronasal organs at the septal base.

1.2.4 Cartilaginous Pyramid

Septolateral Cartilage: Cartilaginous Septum and Triangular Cartilages

The cartilaginous septum and the two triangular cartilages comprise a single anatomical structure, the dorsolateral cartilage (▸ Fig. 1.95). The two triangular cartilages constitute a vault that is supported by the septum. The dorsum of the cartilaginous vault is more or less flat or slightly grooved. The lower part of the triangular cartilage forms the mobile lateral wall of the valve area. The lower margin of the triangular cartilage is overlapped by the medial part of the lateral crus of the lobular cartilage. The intercartilaginous area consists of loose connective tissue with some sesamoid cartilages, allowing the lateral nasal wall to move during respiration (▸ Fig. 1.95). Above the perichondrium of the cartilaginous vault is a thin sheet of loose connective tissue.

Undermining of the dorsal skin in surgery should be performed in this plane because the nasal muscles, vasculature, and nerve supply lie immediately above. The inside of the cartilaginous pyramid is covered with mucosa, whereas the vestibule and its cul de sac are lined with skin (see also ▸ Fig. 1.96 and ▸ Fig. 1.97).

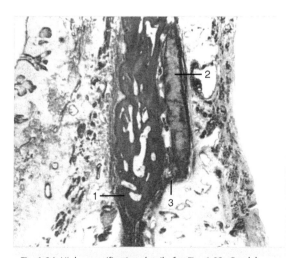

Fig. 1.94 High magnification detail of ▸ Fig. 1.93. Caudal margin of bony vault (1); cranial margin of triangular cartilage (2); tight junction between cartilage and bone (3).

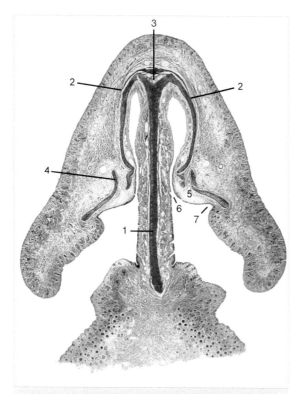

Fig. 1.95 Cartilaginous vault and lobule (coronal section, HE staining). The cartilaginous septum (1) and the two triangular cartilages (2) forming one structure; dorsal groove of cartilaginous vault (3); lateral crus of lobular cartilage overlapping the lower margin of the triangular cartilage (4); intercartilaginous area with loose connective tissue and sesamoid cartilages (5); valve (6); cul de sac (7).

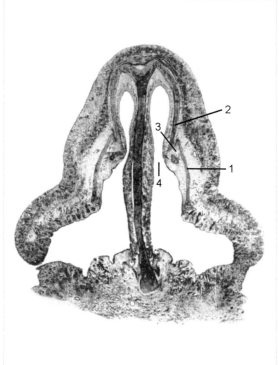

Fig. 1.96 Intercartilaginous joint area (coronal section, MC staining). Lateral crus of lobular cartilage (1) overlapping the lower margin of the triangular cartilage (2); intercartilaginous area with loose connective tissue and sesamoid cartilages (3); valve (4).

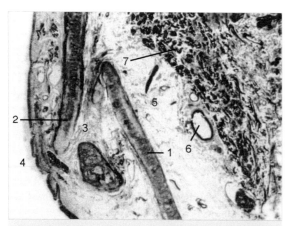

Fig. 1.97 High magnification of detail of ▶ Fig. 1.96. Lateral crus of lobular cartilage (1) overlapping the lower margin of the triangular cartilage (2); intercartilaginous loose connective tissue with sesamoid cartilage (3); valve (4); plane of undermining of the skin (5), vasculature (6), and musculature (7).

Valve Area

The lower margin of the triangular cartilage (limen nasi) constitutes the nasal valve, the mobile part of the lateral wall of the valve area (area 2). The valve area is the narrowest region of the internal nose. In the Caucasian leptorrhine nasal pyramid, the angle between the caudal margin of the triangular cartilage and the septum measures only about 15°. In mesorrhine and platyrrhine noses, it is considerably larger. The valve area is the major region of nasal resistance and acts as an accelerator of inspired air. As a consequence, the airstream becomes more turbulent, which improves contact between the air and the mucosa (see page 54). Since the caudal end of the triangular cartilage moves in and out with respiration, it has been compared with a valve. Actually, it is not a valve in the strict sense of the word; rather it is a variable isthmus which acts as a resistor and a diffusor or turbulizer.

The lateral nasal wall (valve) should be mobile, moving in and out with respiration. On the other hand, it must be rigid enough to withstand the negative intranasal pressure during inspiration, and prevent inspiratory collapse. The special relationship between the triangular and lobular cartilage and

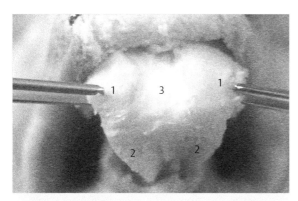

Fig. 1.98 Macrodissection of a fresh specimen of the interdomal and intercrural region using the external approach. Dome (1); medial crus (2); interdomal area (3).

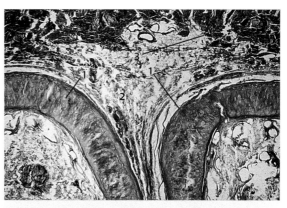

Fig. 1.99 Interdomal area (transverse section through the lobular tip, RF staining). Domes (1); interdomal area; no transverse interdomal fibers resembling a ligament; most fibers run parallel to the cartilage (2); musculature (3).

the anatomy of the lateral lobular wall makes this structure mobile yet rigid. In most cases, the cranial margin of the lateral crus of the lobular cartilage slightly overlaps the medial part of the triangular cartilage. This adds to the rigidity. At the same time, the intercartilaginous area consists of loose connective tissue with a few small sesamoid cartilages. This allows inward and outward movement of the lateral wall. The intercartilaginous area thus acts more or less as a joint, while the lateral soft-tissue area serves as a hinge (see page 13). The cul de sac also plays a role in this system, as inspiratory air hitting the cul de sac will narrow the valve slightly (▶ Fig. 1.96 and ▶ Fig. 1.97).

1.2.5 Lobule

Interdomal Area

The area between the domes of the lobular cartilages is filled with relatively dense connective tissue. On macroscopic dissection, a sling of connective tissue extending in a cranial direction and covering the triangular paraseptal soft-tissue area (paraseptal cleft) can be seen (▶ Fig. 1.98). However, microscopic study reveals that there are no transverse interdomal fibers. Most fibers run parallel to the cartilage following their curvature (▶ Fig. 1.99 and ▶ Fig. 1.100). Whereas several authors have postulated an interdomal "tip-supporting" ligament (or "Pitanguy ligament"), no such structure appears to exist. Nevertheless, loosening up the interdomal area too much should be avoided, as this may lead to postoperative broadening and drooping of the tip.

Intercrural Area

The area between the two medial crura is filled with relatively loose connective tissue. All fibers run parallel to the cartilage. There are no transverse fibers interconnecting the crura, as has been suggested by certain authors. There

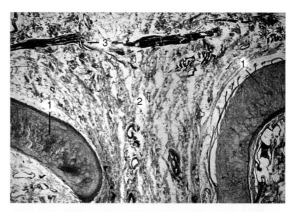

Fig. 1.100 High magnification of same area as ▶ Fig. 1.99 (RF staining). Domes of the lobular cartilages (1); connective tissue fibers running parallel to the cartilage (2); fibers of the transverse part of nasalis muscle (3). Note the small interdomal vessels.

is no such thing as an intercrural ligament (▶ Fig. 1.101 and ▶ Fig. 1.102).

Septocrural Area

The septocrural area consists of relatively loose connective tissue. Contrary to assumptions in the literature, there are no fibers directly connecting the caudal end of the septum to the medial crura. There is no such thing as a septocrural membrane (▶ Fig. 1.103 and ▶ Fig. 1.104).

Alae

The alae consist of a thick outside skin with numerous sebaceous glands, a thick subcutaneous layer, a muscular layer, the lateral crus of the lobular cartilage, and the relatively thin skin with glands and hairs covering the vestibule (▶ Fig. 1.104 and ▶ Fig. 1.105).

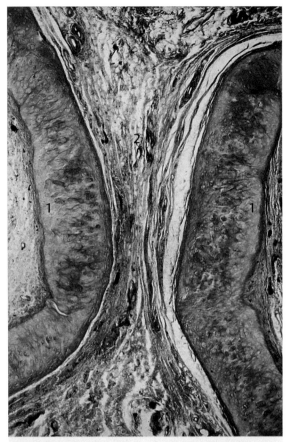

Fig. 1.101 Intercrural area (transverse section at the level of the columella, RF staining). Medial crura (1); connective tissue fibers following the course of the cartilage. No transverse intercrural fibers (2).

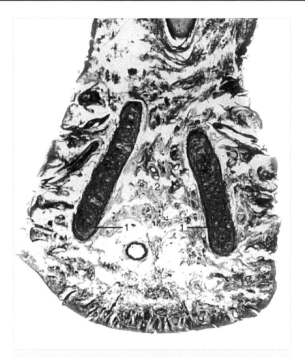

Fig. 1.102 Intercrural area (coronal section through the lower part of the columella, RF staining). Medial crus (1); intercrural loose connective tissue, no intercrural fibers (2). Note the columellar artery.

1.2.6 Lobular Cartilages

Cartilage

In the lobular cartilages, the difference between the small, flat chondrocytes lying parallel to the surface in the peripheral zone and the larger cells arranged palisade-like perpendicular to the surface in the central zones is more distinct than in the septal cartilage (▸ Fig. 1.106).

Perichondrium

The perichondrium of the lobular cartilages consists of a homogeneous layer of collagen fibers and elastic fibers. In the lateral crus, the outer perichondrium is distinctly thicker than the inner perichondrium. Thickness measurements have shown a statistically significant difference (Bleys et al 2007). This may be related to the difference between the forces that are applied to the outer and the inner side of the lateral crus of the lobular cartilage. Muscle fibers of the dilator nasi attach to the outside only (▸ Fig. 1.107).

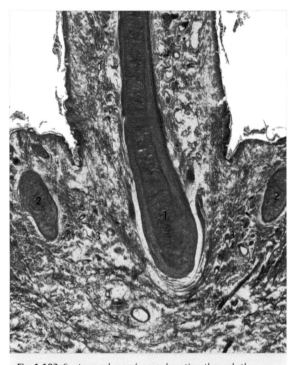

Fig. 1.103 Septocrural area (coronal section through the anterior part of the lobule, RF staining). Caudal end of the septum with its perichondrium (1); medial crura (2); septocrural connective tissue (3).

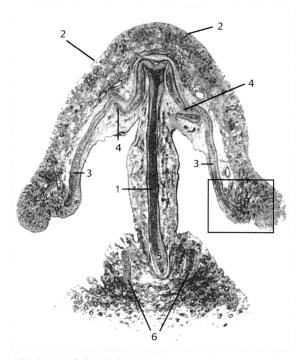

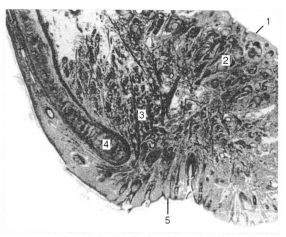

Fig. 1.105 High magnification of detail of ▶ Fig. 1.104. Thick outside skin with numerous sebaceous glands (1); subcutaneous tissue (2); intermingling fibers of the dilator naris (3); lateral crus of the lobular cartilage (4); vestibular skin with glands and hairs (5).

Fig. 1.104 Lobule and alae (coronal section through the anterior part of the lobule, MC staining). Septum (1); triangular cartilage (2); lateral crus of lobular cartilage (3); intercartilaginous area with sesamoid cartilage (4); caudal end of septum (5); medial crura (6).

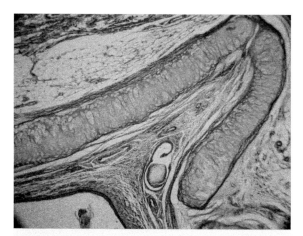

Fig. 1.106 Lateral crus of lobular cartilage (MC staining). In the lobular cartilages, the difference between the peripheral small and flat chondrocytes that are lying parallel to the surface and the larger chondrocytes in the central zones that are positioned palisade-like and perpendicular to the surface is even more distinct than in the septal cartilage. See also ▶ Fig. 1.64.

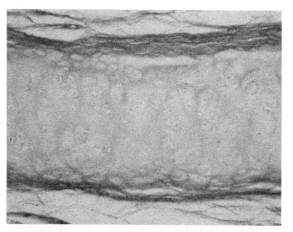

Fig. 1.107 Lateral crus of lobular cartilage (MC staining). The perichondrium of the lobular cartilages consists of a homogeneous layer of collagen fibers and elastic fibers. The outer perichondrium is distinctly thicker than the inner one. This is very likely related to the difference between the forces that are applied to the outer and the inner side of the lateral crus.

1.3 Nasal Development and Growth

1.3.1 The Phases

Two phases should be distinguished in nasal ontogenesis: the developmental phase, and the growth phase.

Developmental or Morphogenetic Phase

The developmental phase is the period of embryonic life during which the nose and related structures are formed. This phase lasts roughly from the third week to the third month after conception. At the third week, the maxillary and mandibular processes begin to develop, and the nasal olfactory placode becomes visible. At about the third month, formation of the nose, maxilla, and mandible is completed.

Growth Phase

In the subsequent growth phase, the dimensions of the nose and related structures increase. Simultaneously, changes in the anatomical relationships of the various nasal structures occur, while several cartilaginous structures become partially or completely ossified. The nose grows rapidly in the first few years of life but growth gradually slows down. A second period of growth occurs during puberty. The growth phase may be divided into the following more or less arbitrary periods: prenatal, neonatal, childhood, and pubertal.

1.3.2 Developmental Phase

The nose and midface are formed by the two maxillary and mandibular processes and the frontonasal prominence between the fourth and eighth week of postovulatory age.

Age 4 Weeks (Length 3–5 mm)

The olfactory placode (or nasal placode) becomes visible as a convex thickening of the surface ectoderm. It transforms into the fovea nasalis and then forms the nasal sac. From then on, a frontonasal prominence starts to develop in a caudal direction. Simultaneously, the two maxillary and mandibular processes grow from lateral to medial (see ▶ Fig. 1.108).

Age 5 to 6 Weeks (Length 5–6 mm)

The frontonasal prominence divides into a medial and a lateral nasal process. The maxillary processes first fuse with the lateral nasal folds and then extend and fuse with the medial folds. The two mandibular processes also fuse at this stage. The openings between the maxillary and mandibular processes form the primitive mouth

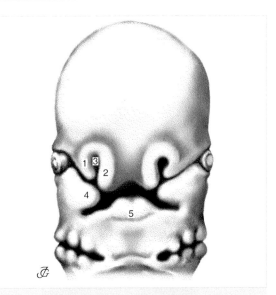

Fig. 1.108 The human face at 5 to 6 weeks of embryonic life (length 5 to 6 mm). 1 = lateral nasal process; 2 = medial nasal process; 3 = primary nasal cavity; 4 = maxillary process; 5 = mandibular process. (After Diewert 1983.)

(▶ Fig. 1.108). If the fusion between the maxillary process and the nasal processes is incomplete, a cleft will remain. The result will be a cleft lip and/or palate.

Age 6 to 7 Weeks (Length 12–18 mm)

The anterior nares are formed and the grooves between the various processes gradually disappear. The primitive nasal cavity is formed as well as a transverse furrow between the frontonasal prominence and forehead. The nasal pyramid becomes recognizable.

Age 7 to 8 Weeks (Length 22 mm)

The nasal capsule is formed, consisting of a median septal part and two lateral parts. The septum starts to develop in a caudal direction. Three transverse prominences appear on the lateral wall of the nasal cavity to become the three main turbinates (▶ Fig. 1.109).

Age 2 to 2.5 Months (Length 3–4 cm)

Ossification of the maxillary and palatine processes starts.

Age 3 to 3.5 Months (Length 10–12 cm)

The nasal capsule and turbinates are still cartilaginous (▶ Fig. 1.110).

Age 4 to 4.5 Months (Length 15–18 cm)

Ossification of the nasal capsule and of the lateral part of the inferior turbinate begins (▶ Fig. 1.111).

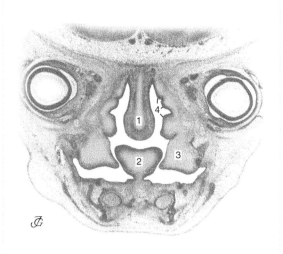

Fig. 1.109 Coronal section at 7 weeks (length 22 mm). 1 = septum; 2 = tongue; 3 = palatine process; 4 = buds of superior, middle and inferior turbinates. (After Arredondo de Arreola et al 1996.)

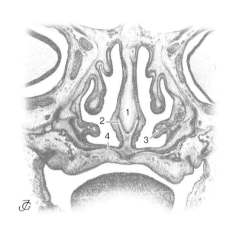

Fig. 1.110 Coronal section at 3.5 months (length 18 cm). 1 = septum; 2 = vomeral alae; 3 = beginning of ossification of turbinates; 4 = ossification of maxilla. (After Arredondo de Arreola et al 1996.)

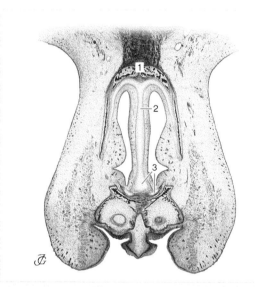

Fig. 1.111 Coronal section at about 4 months (length 18 cm). 1 = nasal bones with underlap of upper margin of triangular cartilages; 2 = septolateral cartilage; 3 = septal cartilage with processus lateralis ventralis and paraseptal or vomeronasal cartilage. (After Lang 1988.)

1.3.3 Growth Phase

Face and Nose

At birth, the facial part of the skull is smaller than its cranial part. By adulthood they are about the same size. The neurocranium reaches 90% of its adult dimensions by the age of 6 years. The viscerocranium, on the other hand, continues to grow until 18 to 20 years of age. The external nasal pyramid becomes more prominent, higher, and longer. The maxilla and the mandible grow in a ventral direction.

Nasal growth rate is high in embryonic life and during the first months after birth. It then gradually decreases until the onset of sexual maturation, when it strongly accelerates. This pubertal growth spurt continues until age 16 to 17 years in girls and 16 to 18 years in boys, then rapidly declines. Nasal growth rate generally follows the same pattern as the growth velocity of the skeleton as a whole as measured by body length (▶ Fig. 1.112). During adult life, the nose continues to grow slowly, in contrast to body length.

Septum

The septum develops from the medial wall of the nasal capsule between the seventh to eighth week and the second to third month of embryonic life. In the beginning, it is completely cartilaginous; later, some parts start to ossify. At birth, the vomer, maxillary crest, and palatine crest are bony. After birth, the posterior part of the septum gradually ossifies from cranial to caudal and from caudal to cranial directions. The septum, in particular its anterior part, demonstrates rapid growth in neonatal life and in early childhood. Its growth then gradually slows down.

The septum plays a decisive role in the ventral growth of the nasal pyramid, the nasal cavity, and the midface. This has been shown clearly by the work of Scott (1950)

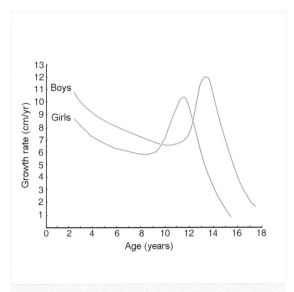

Fig. 1.112 Growth rate of body length in relation to age in boys and girls. (After data from Tanner and Davies 1985.)

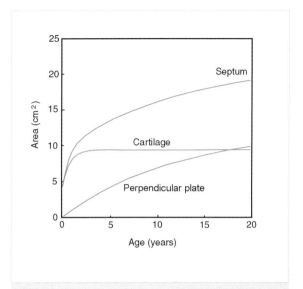

Fig. 1.113 Growth of cartilaginous septum, perpendicular plate, and septum as a whole between 0 and 20 years. In contrast to body length, there is no growth spurt of the septum in puberty. (After van Loosen et al 1996.)

and Sarnat and Wechsler (1967), and by the elaborate experiments on rabbits by Verwoerd and collaborators in the 1980s and 1990s. While the growth of the more caudal part of the septal cartilage influences the outgrowth of the midface, the growth of its anterior and ventral part determines the prominence and length of the nasal pyramid. This has also been demonstrated in patients who have suffered a septal injury in early childhood (Huizing 1966; Pirsig 1977, 1992; Grymer 1997).

Cartilaginous Septum

The cartilaginous septum grows rapidly in the first 2 years of life. Its growth then slows down and almost stops after the age of 3 years (▶ Fig. 1.113 and ▶ Fig. 1.114). At that point, the cranial and posterior part of the cartilaginous septum starts to ossify by enchondral ossification in an anterior and caudal direction, thereby forming the perpendicular plate. This process continues in adult life, though at a slower pace. The basal margin of the septal cartilage is fitted into a groove formed by the two fusing premaxillae and the anterior part of the vomeral lamellae (see ▶ Fig. 1.41).

Perpendicular Plate

The perpendicular plate is formed by intracartilaginous ossification of the cranial and posterior part of the cartilaginous septum (▶ Fig. 1.115 and ▶ Fig. 1.116). This process starts in the sixth month in the region of the crista galli, and slowly proceeds in a caudal and anterior direction. Growth of the perpendicular plate continues at a fast pace until the age of 10 years. It then slows down

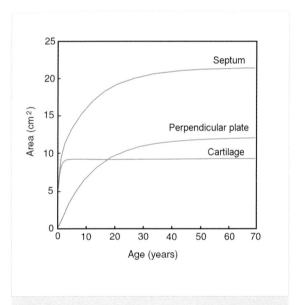

Fig. 1.114 Growth of cartilaginous septum, perpendicular plate, and septum as a whole between 0 and 70 years. (After van Loosen et al 1996.)

but continues until approximately the age of 40 years (▶ Fig. 1.113 and ▶ Fig. 1.114). At puberty, the process of ossification has reached the vomer. A small strip of cartilage from the cartilaginous septum remains between the perpendicular plate and the vomer, the so-called sphenoidal process of the cartilaginous septum (▶ Fig. 1.117).

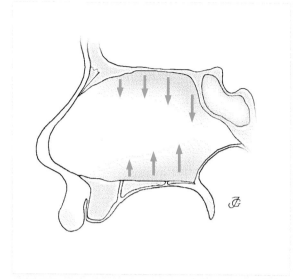

Fig. 1.115 Ossification of the perpendicular plate and vomer at about 1 to 3 years.

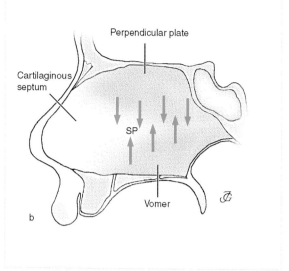

Fig. 1.116 Ossification of the perpendicular plate and vomer at about 10 to 17 years.

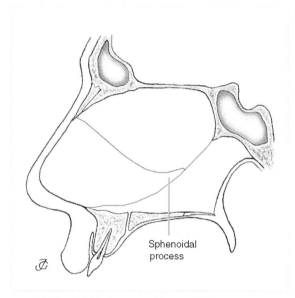

Fig. 1.117 Sphenoidal process of the cartilaginous septum.

Vomer

The vomer ossifies by intramembranous ossification between the 12th postovulatory week and birth. The ossification process takes place from caudal to cranial. Two lamellae are formed. The cranial–anterior parts of these lamellae are V-shaped and hold the posterior part of the cartilaginous septum. The posterior parts or alae enclose the rostrum sphenoidale. At 6 to 8 years of age, the perpendicular plate and vomer fuse. Around puberty, the vomer meets the premaxilla.

Premaxilla

The premaxilla, previously called the intermaxillary bone (see blue box), is formed by two ossification centers that emerge at about 8 to 9 weeks of age. They fuse about 1 week later. Then, from the posterior part of the cranial half, a wing starts to develop on both sides. These premaxillary alae continue to grow throughout childhood and particularly during puberty. The premaxilla fuses with the maxillary bones in the first year of life. Later in puberty, it fuses with the anterior end of the vomer. Since this is where the upper incisor teeth develop, early trauma to this area may lead to irregularities in the position or eruption of the upper teeth.

The intermaxillary bone was a topic of fierce debate in the second half of the 18th century. The leading anatomists of the time, in particular Petrus Camper of Groningen, were of the opinion that the intermaxillary bone is missing in humans. In this respect, humans were believed to differ from the great apes and all higher developed mammals. The "missing intermaxillary bone" was generally accepted as proof that humans were created by God and had not descended from the apes. It was Goethe who, in 1783, discovered that the intermaxillary bone is present in humans too but fuses with the maxillary bones. (Hellmich and Hellmich, 1982)

Cartilaginous Vault

The triangular cartilages originally extend under the nasal bones up to the roof of the ethmoid bone (▶ Fig. 1.111). Their cranial margins lose their connection with the anterior skull base and gradually retreat in a caudal direction. By adulthood, they still underlap the bony vault by 2 to 5 mm (see ▶ Fig. 1.20).

Bony Vault

The medial part of the bony pyramid originates from intracartilaginous ossification of the upper part of the cartilaginous nasal capsule. Its lateral part is the result of ossification of the nasal process of the maxillary bones. In adult life, the nasal bones partially fuse in the midline.

1.3.4 Disturbance of Development and Growth—Consequences for Nasal Pathology and Surgery

Disturbance of Nasal Development

Genetic and exogenic factors may interfere with nasal morphogenesis in many ways. The most well known malformations are discussed next.

Cleft Lip and Palate

Incomplete fusion of the maxillary process and the lateral nasal process results in a unilateral or bilateral cleft lip and/or palate. It is associated with characteristic deformities of the nasal pyramid, lobule, septum, turbinates, and nasal cavity (as described in Chapter 2 and illustrated in ▶ Fig. 2.26, ▶ Fig. 2.27, ▶ Fig. 2.28, ▶ Fig. 2.29, ▶ Fig. 2.30, and ▶ Fig. 2.31). The disturbance of growth that leads to this malformation occurs in the second month of embryonic life (see ▶ Fig. 1.108). The earlier the embryologic development becomes distorted, the more severe the anomaly.

Nasal Bifidity

Incomplete fusion of the two medial nasal processes causes bifidity of the nose. This malformation may vary from a minor vertical groove in the columella or between the two domes to severe bifidity of the lobule and the cartilaginous and bony vault (see ▶ Fig. 2.27).

Medial Nasal Fistula, Cyst, and Glioma

Incomplete fusion of the two medial nasal processes may allow squamous epithelium and brain tissue to become entrapped in the midline. This may result in a medial nasal cyst and a fistula extending endocranially. Another well-known consequence of this developmental disturbance is a nasal glioma.

Nasal Proboscis

The whole nose or one half of it consists of a russel-like structure, usually involving the eye and its adnexa. This serious malformation results from a lesion of the olfactory plate and/or the forebrain at or before the fifth postovulatory week.

Nasal Agenesis

Nasal agenesis is a very rare anomaly in which the external nose does not develop and the nasal cavity is totally or partially obliterated.

Choanal Atresia

The choanae are obliterated by a membrane, a bony lamella, or a combination of the two. The obliterating bony lamella is part of the palatine bone and usually runs upward at a slightly oblique angle.

Nasal and Midface Hypoplasia

For reasons that usually remain obscure, the nasal pyramid and midface do not develop normally. The external nose is small in all its dimensions and the midface is retruded. The condition is described in Chapter 2 (▶ Fig. 2.32, ▶ Fig. 2.33, ▶ Fig. 2.34; page 77).

Disturbance of Nasal Growth

Several events may interfere with the growth of the nose in a more or less serious way. The most well known factors are discussed next.

Intrauterine Growth Disturbance

Although relatively rare, nasal growth may be disturbed during intrauterine life. The congenitally deviated nose is the most, well-documented example (see ▶ Fig. 9.1).

Birth Trauma

Vaginal birth causes some kind of deformation of the external nose and septum in a fairly large proportion of neonates. In most cases, the deformity is corrected spontaneously as a result of the elasticity of the tissues. In some children, however, it leads to a deviated septal-pyramid syndrome or a low-wide pyramid syndrome in later life (see Chapter 2, page 70).

Childhood Trauma

The primary cause of a large percentage of nasal deformities seen in adults is (repeated) trauma of the septum and/or external pyramid in early childhood. The most common late consequences are a deviated nose and an underdeveloped pyramid and midface. These effects have been clearly documented in studies on identical twins by

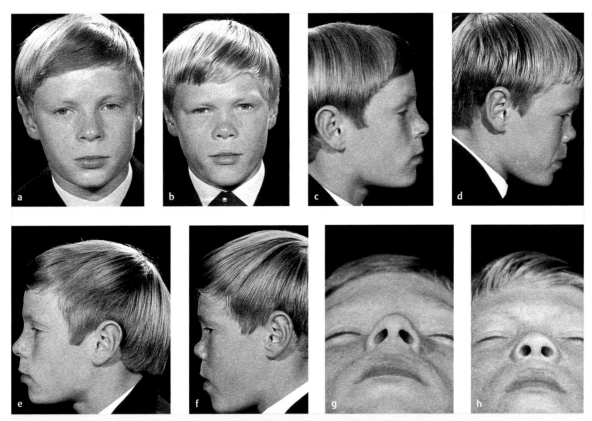

Fig. 1.118 Characteristic impairment and retardation of nasal growth in identical twins at the age of 14 years.
The boy on the right **(b)** suffered from nasal trauma with subsequent septal infection (small abscess) at the age of 8 years. The abscess was drained but the defect was not repaired. When we compare him with his twin brother on the left **(a)** 6 years later, we notice a typical retardation of nasal growth.
a, b In the boy on the right **(b)** the height of the nasal pyramid is much less than in his twin brother.
c, d In the boy on the right **(d)** the length and prominence of the external nose are limited; the bony and cartilaginous pyramid is broader and saddling; the lobule is low and wide; the tip is underprojected; the columella is short and somewhat retracted; the nasolabial angle is increased.
e, f In the boy on the right **(f)** the length and prominence of the external nose are limited; the bony and cartilaginous pyramid is broader and saddling; the lobule is low and wide; the tip is underprojected; the columella is short and somewhat retracted; the nasolabial angle is increased.
g, h In the boy on the right **(h)** the lobule is severely underprojected and wide; the columella is short and somewhat retracted.
From Huizing 1966.

Huizing (1966), Pirsig (1992), and Grymer (1997). The earlier (and the more destructive) the trauma, the more severe the growth disturbance and the ultimate nasal pathology.

Childhood Septal Abscess

A septal abscess in childhood poses the greatest threat to normal nasal growth. Unless treated by septal reconstruction as soon as possible, it will lead to severe disturbance of the outgrowth of the septum, pyramid, and midface. A characteristic example of the growth disturbance caused by trauma and septal abscess in childhood is presented in ▶ Fig. 1.118.

1.4 Surgical Physiology

Six different nasal functions may be recognized, in their phylogenetic order:
1. Olfaction
2. Respiration
3. Climatization (heating and humidification of inspired air)
4. Defense of the respiratory tract
5. Speech production
6. Facial expression and beauty

When, during the process of evolution, air became the medium of life instead of water, the nose developed. This required the development of a special tract with new provisions: the respiratory tract. At its entrance, a chemical sense developed—the olfactory organ—that differs from that within the mouth of sea animals. Moreover, an elaborate system to prepare the inhaled air in an optimal way for the lower respiratory tract developed, its functions including heating, humidification, and partial cleansing of particles. For that particular purpose, the nose consists of two parts: a right and a left. They work together but independently.

The human nose consists of an external and an internal nose. Only human beings and some types of ape have an external nose. From a physiological point of view, the external nose or nasal pyramid should first be considered as a regulator of airway resistance and airflow, as well as an organ of defense (function as an air filter). The reason that the external nose evolved in a plane in front of the face is not fully clear. It was probably an adaptation to changes in the conditions of life. The differences in the shape of the external nose between various human races suggest that adaptation to climatic conditions played a major role. Anthropological studies have revealed a close relationship between morphological features of the human nasal skeleton and the geographical climate, resulting in variations in nasal morphology. This connection emphasizes the fact that, in the context of evolution, adequate respiratory function of the nose is essential for ideal pulmonary gas exchange.

The internal nose is the actual and original nasal organ. The basic tasks of olfaction, climatization of inspired air, and defense take place within the three different functional segments of the internal nose (▶ Fig. 1.119). The anterior segment is the inflow of the nose. It includes the vestibulum, isthmus, and the anterior part of the nasal cavity. Physically, it functions as a flow manifold, nozzle, and diffuser, providing maximum contact between air and mucosa. The anterior segment, including the nasal valve area, is responsible for alteration of the nasal airflow. The airflow pattern is disrupted, spreading the air over the mucosa of the adjoining turbinates to allow optimal respiratory function within the middle functional segment.

1.4.1 Olfaction

Olfaction serves a variety of purposes. It helps locate food as well as water, and find a partner of the other sex. It also warns against the approach of enemies and the danger of environmental gases. The sense of smell is fully mature at birth, indicating its utmost importance in the mother–child relation.

"In surgery, function should prevail over form."

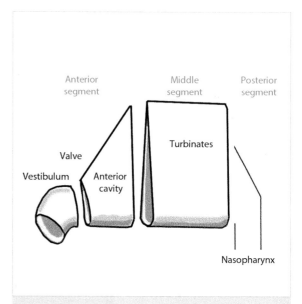

Fig. 1.119 Schematic representation of the functional anatomy of the human nasal organ.

The nose is an organ with a number of highly important functions. When operating on this organ, the nasal surgeon may be pursuing various goals: curing nasal disease, reconstituting normal nasal function and form, or enhancing facial expression and beauty. In surgery, curing disease and improving nasal function must always prevail over enhancement of beauty, no matter how important and legitimate this objective might be in a given case. In nasal surgery, function should never be sacrificed for beauty.

The organ of smell is located in a narrow cleft of 1 to 2 mm in the anterior part of the superior nasal passage above the level of the middle turbinate, both on its lateral (ethmoidal) and medial (septal) wall (▶ Fig. 1.120). The surface area of the olfactory epithelium varies between individuals. In adults it usually covers about 200 to 400 mm². Even at birth it may be up to 500 mm². The olfactory epithelium contains about 20 million receptor cells. These cells are connected to unmyelinated fibers that, in small bundles, traverse minor openings in the anterior skull base (i.e., the lamina cribrosa of the ethmoid bone). In addition, tubular serous glands (Bowman's glands) are present.

The human olfactory epithelium is renewed every 60 days by apoptosis, dead cells being replaced by basal cells. The axons grow in a site-specific manner, meaning that the new axons grow to the places vacated by the old ones.

Odors must be either fat soluble or water soluble to be perceived. The total number of different odors that man is able to distinguish has been estimated at several million. The human species is nevertheless a very poor smeller compared to most mammals. For instance, the olfactory area in dogs is thirty times larger than in humans.

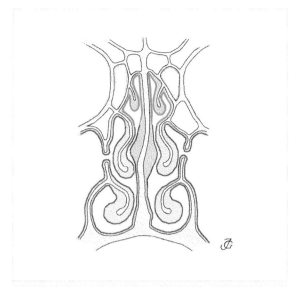

Fig. 1.120 Olfactory epithelium in the anterior part of the upper nasal passage or olfactory cleft, on the septum and the medial wall of the ethmoid bone.

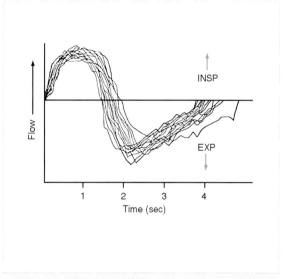

Fig. 1.121 Normal breathing cycle at rest. 1 = inspiratory phase; 2 = midcycle rest; 3 = expiratory phase; 4 = intercycle rest; INSP = inspiration; EXP = expiration. (From Cole 1982; data from Proctor and Hardy 1949.)

As only small amounts of air usually reach the olfactory region, in sensory analysis, the airflow is intensified by sniffing (the air is sucked in short bursts through the nose).

Loss of smell is a common complaint in ENT patients. Damage to the olfactory organ or nerve fibers (e.g., due to [viral] infections or anterior skull base fracture) may result in perceptive anosmia or hyposmia. Conductive anosmia or hyposmia may occur in cases when the inspired air fails to reach the otherwise intact sensory segment. Since the olfactory organ is located high within the nasal cavity and its access is narrow, conductive anosmia or hyposmia are common findings in rhinological practice.

Both types of disturbed olfaction may be differentiated by olfactory testing before and after decongestion of the mucosa caudal to the olfactory cleft.

1.4.2 Respiration

The major nasal function is breathing. The nose constitutes the first part of the respiratory tract and fulfills three major tasks within this system:
1. It provides the major part of respiratory resistance.
2. It facilitates close contact between air and mucosa due to changes in airflow patterns (increased turbulence and decreased velocity), allowing sufficient climatization.
3. It acts as the first line of defense for the protection of the lower respiratory tract.

Parameters of Breathing

The frequency of breathing in adults at rest is about 16 breaths per minute. According to ventilatory demands, it increases during exercise and decreases during sleep.

The volume of air inhaled in a single breath averages 500 mL. The total volume of air inhaled per day thus equals some 12,000 L. It is interesting that in humans, daily intake of air is approximately 12,000 L (= 12 m^3), whereas daily intake of water is about 2 kg, and that of food, 1 kg. All this air will be heated up to the body temperature of 37°C and humidified up to 100% relative humidity. The majority of air conditioning takes place within the nasal airways.

The velocity of the airstream depends on the force of respiration and the cross-sectional area and geometric shape of the nose at a given area. During normal inspiration, airflow velocity is 2 to 3 m/s within the nostril and 12 to 18 m/s within the nasal valve area (see also ► Fig. 1.127).

Respiratory Cycle

The normal breathing pattern consists of four main phases: inspiration, midcycle rest, expiration, intercycle rest (► Fig. 1.121). During breathing, graphical recording of the pressure changes at the level of the nostril, by means of a nozzle or by body plethysmography, may disclose abnormalities of the respiratory cycle. Pressure at the external nasal ostium equals 8 to 15 mm water at inspiration, and 2 to 4 mm less at expiration. It has been suggested (Cottle 1968, Heinberg and Kern 1974) that certain anomalies of the breathing pattern (e.g., a midcycle rest) might indicate imminent cardiopulmonary disease. However, a correlation between abnormalities of the respiratory cycle and cardiac disease has not been established yet.

Nasal Resistance and Its Effects

In nasal breathing, 50 to 60% of the total resistance of the respiratory tract is caused by the nose, in particular by the nasal valve area and the turbinates. During mouth breathing, the resistance of the upper airways decreases to less than 20% of total airway resistance. The nose creates a difference between the environmental air pressure and pressure within the lower respiratory tract. The major site of high nasal resistance is the nasal valve area, including the heads of the inferior and middle turbinates. The contribution to total nasal resistance by the nasal valve area, on the one hand, and the turbinates on the other, critically depends on individual nasal anatomy (e.g., ethnic factors, age, gender), the physiological state of the mucosa during the nasal cycle, and pathological abnormalities.

It is interesting to speculate for what purpose within phylogenetic development of the respiratory tract the nose has been added as a resistor of such magnitude. Two effects may be distinguished: pulmonary as well as cardiac effects, and local effects in the nose itself.

> "There is no real difference between structure and function: they are two sides of the same coin. If structure does not tell us anything about function it means we have not looked at it correctly."
> Szent-Gyorgyi

Pulmonary and Cardiac Effects of the Nasal Resistor

The most important pulmonary and cardiac effects of the nasal resistor are: a wider opening of the peripheral bronchioli and alveolar ventilation, allowing a more profitable gas exchange; and higher negative thoracic pressure resulting in better venous cardiac and pulmonary backflow. The nose also represents a source of nitric oxide, reaching the lower airways by inhalation and considered to be responsible for homeostasis of the bronchial tone and vasculature.

Local Effects in the Nose

Local effects result from the fact that the major nasal resistor, the nasal valve area, is located at the entrance of the nasal cavity. The nasal valve is a three-dimensional region, thus the term nasal valve area should be preferred. The nasal valve area is a triangular narrowing comprising the more or less rigid anterior septum and the soft tissue overlying the piriform aperture and nasal floor, the mobile caudal end of the triangular cartilage (valve), and the more or less swollen head of the inferior turbinate (▶ Fig. 1.122 and ▶ Fig. 1.123). It is remarkable that this area is the narrowest segment of the entire nasal cavity.

This anatomical–physiological narrowing at the entrance of the functional nasal segment causes a considerable increase in velocity of the inspired air (Bernoulli's law) from 2 to 3 m/s at the nostril to 12 to 18 m/s at the valve area. As a result, the outer layers of the laminar

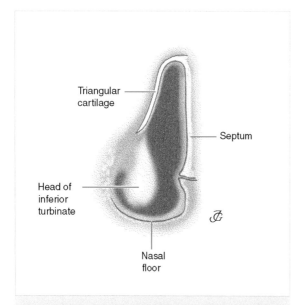

Fig. 1.122 The nasal valve area is the main nasal resistor. It consists of the mobile caudal margin of the triangular cartilage (the valve proper), the more or less swollen head of the inferior turbinate, and the semirigid septum and floor of the piriform aperture.

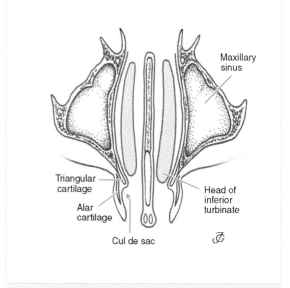

Fig. 1.123 The contribution of the inferior turbinate to the resistance of the valve area is variable. It depends on the degree of swelling of its head.

airstream become turbulent as Reynolds number is exceeded (see page 391). The valve area thus functions as an accelerator and consequently as a "diffuser" or "turbulizer" of the inspired air.

The anterior nasal segment, including the nasal valve area and the turbinates, plays a crucial role in air conditioning. The nasal valve area is responsible for alterations in nasal airflow: the airflow pattern is disrupted, spreading the air over the entire mucosa of the turbinates to allow heating and humidification of the inspired air. It acts as a diffuser, where turbulence increases and velocity decreases. When inhaled air passes the nasal valve area, the laminar airflow changes into a turbulent one, intensifying the contact between air and mucosa. Variations in the airflow pattern (velocity, flow, vortices, path lines) vary the degree of contact of the inhaled air with the surrounding mucosa. The kinetic energy of turbulent airflow allows maximal contact between the inhaled air and the mucosa. In laminar airflow, the direction of flow is parallel to the mucosal surface, with only the air film closest to the surface touching the nasal mucosa. In turbulent airflow, however, all of the air comes in contact with the mucosa due to mostly three-dimensional, random, and unsteady movements of the particles. There is a very close relationship between intranasal air conditioning and airflow patterns. Lower parts of the respiratory tract play a minor role in air conditioning (Lindemann 2006).

It is noteworthy that the increase in air temperature and humidity is higher within the short distance (about 1 cm) of the anterior segment than along the entire length of the middle turbinate (about 4 cm) (Keck 2000).

Resistors and Geometry of the Nose

When studying the dynamic behavior of the airstreams passing through the human nose, the physical laws postulated by Bernoulli (1738), Venturi (1788), Hagen-Poiseuille (ca. 1830), and Reynolds (1889) can be observed to hold. In connection with this topic, we refer to the section in the Appendix on physical laws governing airstreams. However, these laws of fluid physics apply to flow through a circular tube. The nasal cavity presents a completely different geometrical structure. As previously discussed, it consists of three anatomically and physiologically different segments. The anterior segment consists of three elements: an almost horizontal ovaloid opening (nostril), a funnel-shaped widening with various protrusions and pouches (vestibule), and a more or less triangular narrowing (valve area). The specific characteristics of the anterior segment are summarized in ▶ Table 1.2, ▶ Table 1.3, and ▶ Table 1.4.

The middle segment of the nasal cavity is a more or less trapezoid-shaped slit with very irregular lateral walls (▶ Table 1.5). The posterior segment or downstream area consists of the posterior end of the turbinates, the anterior wall of the sphenoidal sinuses, and the choanal opening (▶ Table 1.6).

Table 1.2 Geometrical data and resistors of the nostril (first element of the anterior nasal segment)

Nostril	
Position:	Horizontal
Shape:	Ovaloid
Cross-sectional area:	90 mm^2
Resistors:	Protruding ends of medial crura

Table 1.3 Geometrical data and resistors of the vestibule (second element of the anterior nasal segment)

Vestibule	
Position:	Oblique
Shape:	Funnel
Cross-sectional area from caudal to cranial:	90 → 120 → 60 mm^2
Resistors:	Protruding end of lateral crus Cul de sac

Table 1.4 Geometrical data and resistors of the valve area (third element of the anterior nasal segment and the transition between the anterior and middle nasal segment)

Valve area	
Position:	Oblique
Shape:	Triangular
Cross-sectional area:	50–70 mm^2
Resistors:	Valve (lower margin of triangular cartilage) Head of inferior turbinate Septum, floor of valve area

Table 1.5 Geometrical data and resistors of the middle nasal segment of the nasal cavity

Nasal cavity	
Shape:	Trapezoid-like slit
Cross-sectional area:	40/130/80 mm^2
Resistors:	Laterally: inferior, middle, and superior turbinates Medially: septal turbinates, septal folds

Table 1.6 Geometrical data and resistors of the posterior nasal segment

Choana	
Shape:	Ovaloid
Cross-sectional area:	80 mm^2
Resistors:	Tails of inferior and middle turbinates Anterior wall of sphenoidal sinus

All these segments, with their cross-sectional areas, specific geometry, and walls act as resistors and directors of airflow. They determine the course of the inspiratory and expiratory airstream and its velocity and turbulence behavior.

Pathway and Velocity of Inspiratory and Expiratory Airflow

The route taken by inspired and expired air has been the subject of numerous studies for more than a century and a variety of experimental and numerical models has been used for the analysis of airflow. The first investigators at the end of the 19th century thought that the pathway of both the inspiratory and expiratory airstream was through the inferior nasal passage. Later, experiments on cadaver specimens and other models demonstrated that the inspiratory airstream takes a higher, curved course, while the expiratory airstream follows the lower nasal passage (Paulsen 1882, Franken 1894, Goodale 1896, Courtade 1903, Mink 1920, Proetz 1951). Van Dishoeck (1936) demonstrated in model experiments that the course of the inspiratory airstream was influenced by the position of the nostril: the smaller the nasolabial angle, the higher the course. More recently, the inspiratory airstream has been further analyzed by others (Swift and Proctor 1977, Mlynski et al 2001 and others) applying noselike models in fluid dynamics experiments.

Nowadays, numerical models for airflow simulation play an increasingly important role. Numerical simulation is a method displaying a real environment (e.g., the human nose) within a computational model. Computational fluid dynamics (CFD) is a numerical simulation application to study various flow dynamics. The appropriate fluid flow physics are applied to the virtual nose model, resulting in a prediction of the fluid dynamics. It allows airflow patterns within the entire human nose to be displayed and analyzed and, if desired, simulations of

the intranasal climate as well (Lindemann et al 2006, Keck and Lindemann 2010).

Inspiratory Airflow

The inspiratory airstream mainly follows the middle nasal passage (▶ Fig. 1.124 and ▶ Fig. 1.125). When passing through the external ostium, vestibule, and valve area, the air follows an upstream course that runs almost parallel to the nasal dorsum. After traversing the valve area, the airflow takes a more horizontal course. It hits the heads of the middle and inferior turbinates, enters the middle and, to a lesser extent, inferior nasal passages, and finally curves downward towards the choana and nasopharynx.

This relatively cranial course of inspiratory airflow is caused by the special anatomy of the external nose: the horizontal position of the nostril, the funnel shape of the vestibule, the position and configuration of the valve area, and the slope of the nasal dorsum. After passing the narrow valve area, the airflow becomes more turbulent for reasons already discussed (▶ Fig. 1.126). The relatively cranial course of the inspiratory airflow and the turbulence of the outer sheets of air promote longer and better contact between air and mucosa, as well as better contact with the olfactory area.

In laminar airflow, the direction of flow is parallel to the mucosal surface, with only the air film closest to the surface touching the nasal mucosa. The increased kinetic energy of the turbulent airflow allows an intensified contact between inhaled air and mucosa. The highest volume flows and flow velocities can be obtained in the center of the nasal cavity, followed by the inferior and middle meatus. The highest air pressure is detected at the heads of the inferior and middle turbinates. The areas surrounding the turbinates show vortices of low velocity with turbulence. Therefore, the turbinates seem to be responsible for the close contact between air and nasal wall (Lindemann et al. 2005).

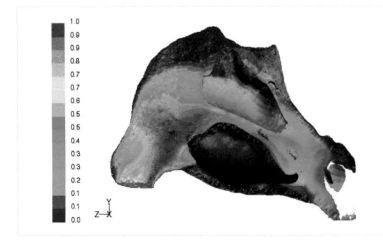

Fig. 1.124 Inspiratory contours of velocity magnitude (m/s) in a 3D nose model (lateral view).

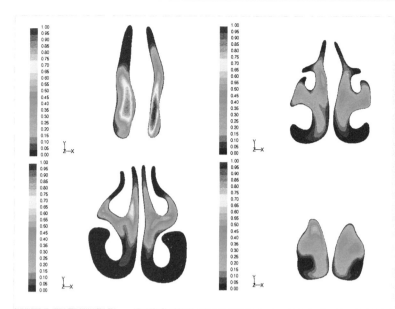

Fig. 1.125 Inspiratory contours of velocity magnitude (m/s) displayed on coronary cutting planes from anterior to posterior.

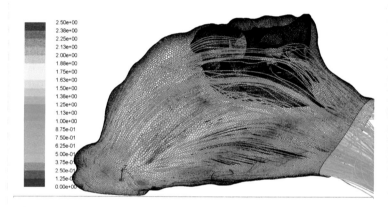

Fig. 1.126 Inspiratory airflow as path lines colored by velocity magnitude (m/s) (lateral view).

In addition to anatomical factors, the force of inspiratory breathing also plays an important role. The higher the inspiratory force, the higher the velocity of the airstream passing the narrow valve area. Consequently, the degree of turbulence of the air is increased, and the route taken by the air through the nasal cavity is more cranial. This is the case when we take a short, forced breath (sniff) to smell better.

Within the olfactory region, a slow, turbulent airflow with static vortices is prevalent, allowing intense contact between the inhaled air and the epithelium of the olfactory region (Lindemann et al. 2006).

The velocity of air during inspiration measures about 2 to 3 m/s at the nostril. It increases slightly in the vestibule, and then suddenly increases to 12 to 18 m/s at the valve area (▶ Fig. 1.127). Beyond the valve area, air velocity again decreases. In the nasal cavity it measures about 2 to 4 m/s.

Expiratory Airstream

The expiratory airstream takes a more caudal course through the nasal cavity, and mainly follows the inferior nasal passage. This is caused by the almost vertical position and relatively large diameter of the choana. The expiratory airflow is of the laminar type. The pressure differences from posterior to anterior are relatively small. Consequently, airflow velocity is low so Reynolds number is not attained. During expiration, the existing inspiratory turbulent airflow predominates in the posterior and middle nasal segment, and is bundled and transformed into a laminar one.

Physiology of the Valve Area

The nasal valve area constitutes the transition between the external and internal nose. It is a relatively narrow area measuring 50 to 70 mm^2. It is the major contributor

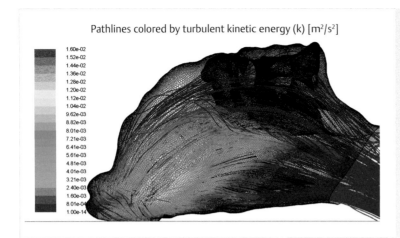

Pathlines colored by turbulent kinetic energy (k) [m²/s²]

Fig. 1.127 Inspiratory airflow as path lines colored by turbulent kinetic energy (k) [m²/s²] (lateral view).

to nasal resistance, and consequently, a major regulator of nasal airflow. For the detailed anatomy of this area the reader is referred to ► Fig. 1.34 and ► Fig. 1.35.

Mink (1902, 1903, 1920) was the first to use the term *nasal valve*, in contrast to the 19th century anatomists (Zuckerkandl 1892), who spoke of the *ostium internum*, or *isthmus nasi*. Mink wrote that "the nose is provided with a valvular device... " and that "the valve rules the inflow of ambient air." Later authors, such as Van Dishoeck (1936, 1965) and Williams (1972), supported this concept. Bridger (1970) and Bridger and Proctor (1970) introduced the term *flow-limiting segment*, and compared the area with a Starling resistor (a semirigid tube with a collapsible segment). Haight and Cole (1983) located the resistive site "confined to a segment of a few millimeters at the junction of the compliant cartilaginous vestibule with the rigid bony cavity." They found nasal resistance increased from about 1.0 to 6.0 cm $H_2O/L/s$ at a distance between 2.0 and 2.5 cm from the posterior margin of the nostril. They also found that the head of the inferior turbinate is an important contributor to this resistive area (► Fig. 1.128). The latter was confirmed by Jones et al (1988) in patients before and after "radical trimming" or "anterior trimming" of the inferior turbinates, and later again by Shaida and Kenyon (2000). Today, we prefer the term *valve area* to *valve* because it has become evident both in experiments and in clinical practice that the resistive area is a three-dimensional region and comprises several elements (Kaspenbauer and Kern 1987). Of these, the mobile caudal margin of the triangular cartilage and the more or less swollen head of the inferior turbinate are the most important. Other factors are the cartilaginous septum and the soft tissue covering of the floor of the piriform aperture. The valve proper is influenced by a number of anatomical and physiological factors, as we will discuss in the following text.

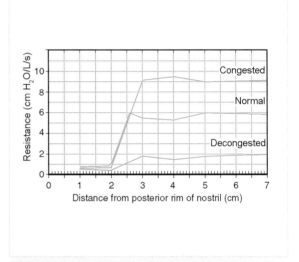

Fig. 1.128 Nasal resistance at different distances from the posterior rim of the nostril. In the normal nose, a strong increase in resistance occurs at 2.0 to 6.0 cm (i.e., the valve area). In the congested nose, this increase in resistance is considerably greater due to swelling of the head of the inferior turbinate. In the decongested nose, there is only a limited increase in nasal resistance. (Data from Haight and Cole 1983.)

Forces Acting on the Valve Area

The medial wall (septum) and the floor of the valve area are semirigid structures. The lateral wall, however, is somewhat flaccid and mobile. It moves inward during inspiration and outward during expiration. The magnitude of inward movement during inspiration depends on two factors (► Fig. 1.129):

1. The transvalvular pressure difference (difference between the pressure in the intranasal valve area and environmental air pressure), and
2. The compliance/rigidity of the lateral wall.

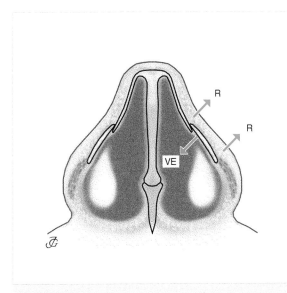

Fig. 1.129 Forces acting on the valve area during inspiration. VE = Venturi effect: the negative intravalvular pressure caused by increased air velocity; R = rigidity of the various anatomical components of the lateral nasal wall.

The magnitude of the transvalvular pressure difference, on the one hand, is determined by the force of inspiration and the cross-sectional area of the valve area. The narrower the valve area, the higher the velocity of inspired air and the greater the transnasal pressure difference (relative negative intravalvular pressure due to the so-called Venturi effect; see ▶ Fig. 10.54). The compliance of the lateral wall of the valve area, on the other hand, depends on four different factors. First factor is the dimension and thickness of the triangular cartilage and the presence or absence of returning of its lower margin. Second factor is the relationship between the lower margin of the triangular cartilage and the lobular cartilage (a greater degree of overlap will increase the rigidity of the lateral nasal wall). The third factor is the rigidity of the overlying connective tissue layers, skin, and the lateral soft-tissue area (hinge area) with its sesamoid cartilages. Finally, contraction of the nasal musculature (in particular the dilator, nasalis, and apicis nasi muscles) contributes to compliance of the lateral wall of the valve area (▶ Table 1.7).

Effect of Pathology at the Valve Area

The valve area is the most critical functional area of the nose. A limited stenosis at this area has great consequences for inspiratory breathing. Any narrowing will cause an increase in the transnasal pressure gradient, causing a greater degree of inward suctioning of the lateral wall and valvular collapse if its rigidity is not sufficient to counteract the negative pressure. It is well known that a minor septal deviation or convexity, or abnormal congestion of the head of the inferior turbinate, may be enough to induce this sequence of events. The same applies to pathological weakening of the lateral nasal wall after surgery or trauma.

Nasal Cycle

The human nose exhibits spontaneous changes in unilateral nasal resistance. When these changes are periodical and reciprocal we speak of a "nasal cycle" (Eccles 1997). The nasal cycle is caused by dilatation and constriction of the capacitance vessels in the nasal mucosa, in particular the inferior turbinates, in a rhythm of 3 to 5 hours. When the right nasal cavity is in a congested state, the left side is decongested, and vice versa. As a result, total nasal resistance and airflow will remain unchanged. This phenomenon is called the nasal cycle (▶ Fig. 1.130). Eccles pointed out that we are not dealing with a real cycle but a reciprocal (3:1) relationship of the resistance of both nasal cavities.

The nasal cycle was accidentally discovered by Kayser (1895) and has been an object of study ever since. The most important contributions have been from Lillie (1923), Heetderks (1927), Stocksted (1952, 1953), Keuning (1968), Masing (1969), Hasegawa and Kern (1978), and Eccles et al (1996, 1997, 2000).

The nasal cycle is controlled by the adrenergic system. It is regulated by a central modulating system located in the brainstem but is also influenced by local factors. The use of vasoconstrictive nose drops temporarily abolishes the mechanism. During nasal infection, the amplitude of the nasal cycle is increased.

In earlier studies, a nasal cycle was reported to be present in about 80% of adults with a normally functioning nose, as well as in children above the age of 3 to 5 years. Eccles et al (1997), applying more strict criteria, found a

Table 1.7 Activity of the nasal muscles during quiet breathing, after exercise, and during sniffing; the activity of the depressor septi muscle was not determined in this study (data from Bruintjes et al. 1996)

Muscle	Quiet breathing	After exercise	Sniffing
Procerus	—	±	±
Levator labii superioris	±	+	±
Pars transversa musculi nasalis	±	+ +	+
Pars alaris musculi nasalis	±	+ +	+ +
Dilator naris	±	+ + + +	+ +
Apicis nasi	±	+ + + +	+ +

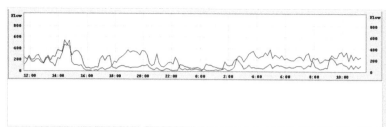

Fig. 1.130 Exemplary long-term rhinoflowmetry over 24 hours with normal nasal breathing, representing the nasal cycle. Red curve = right side; blue curve = left side; X-axis = time in hours; Y-axis = nasal respiratory volume at the maximum speed of inspiration in mL/s. (After data by Prof. G. Mlynski.)

real cycle to exist in only 20 to 40% of the adult population. It was also demonstrated in mammals.

The nasal cycle is present in all positions of the head and body. It has no effect on ciliary beat, but mucociliary transport may be influenced. The purpose of the nasal cycle is not well understood. A relation with homolateral pulmonary function has often been suggested but never proven. Eccles et al (1996) postulated that it serves as a defense. They hypothesize that in the congestion phase, the muscles around the venous sinusoids contract and squeeze out exudates. This would help cleanse the nose and enhance defense by releasing immunoglobulins and mediators.

Individuals with normal nasal function usually do not notice the alternating process of congestion and decongestion of the nasal mucosa. In pathological conditions, however, the nasal cycle may influence symptoms. Some patients complain of an alternating (left–right) breathing obstruction in the late (vasodilatory) phase of an infectious rhinitis, such as a common cold. Others notice a unilateral rhythmic obstruction on the side of a septal deviation.

A long-term assessment of nasal function and of the nasal cycle is still difficult to acquire. Therefore, the recently developed "long-term rhinoflowmetry" might present a new means to further investigate the nasal cycle.

Nasal Muscle Function

Electromyographical studies have shown that all nasal muscles are active at inspiration, in particular the nasalis, dilator naris, and apicis nasi muscles (e.g., van Dishoeck 1937, Bruintjes et al 1996). Contraction of these muscles widens the nostrils and increases rigidity of the lateral nasal wall, thus counteracting the risk of valvular collapse. Some muscle fibers insert at the cartilaginous structures of the lateral nasal wall; others end in the subcutaneous tissues.

All muscles attaching at the lateral nasal wall are "openers," not "compressors." Sea animals like the sea lion open their nares when surfacing by contracting the nasal muscles. When submerging, the muscles relax and the nostrils are closed.

In nasal surgery we try to preserve the nasal musculature as far as we can. Undermining of the dorsal skin should be as deep as possible—that is, immediately above the perichondrium and periosteum. In lobular surgery,

the attachments of the muscle fibers to the cartilages (in particular those of the dilator muscle to the lateral crus) should not be cut.

1.4.3 Air Conditioning (Heating and Humidification)

The Mucosa as the Essential Organ of the Nose

Laymen think of the external nasal pyramid as the nose. Rhinosurgeons look at it as a three-dimensional complex structure that is made up of various anatomical–physiological components. They recognize the nasal mucosa as one component without always realizing that this mucosal lining of both nasal cavities performs most nasal functions. Intranasal air conditioning of the inhaled air and defense of the respiratory tract are the specific tasks of the mucosa, submucosa, and the parenchymal tissue of the turbinates. Therefore, the lateral wall of the nasal cavity is provided with a number of irregular protrusions—the turbinates—enlarging the functional nasal mucosa to a total surface area of about $150\,cm^2$.

Thus, the precious and irreplaceable nasal mucosa must be respected as much as possible in nasal surgery. Damage to the mucosa should strictly be avoided when performing septal and pyramid surgery, and even more importantly, when operating on the turbinates. Whenever possible, incisions in the mucosa should be avoided. Any approach is made through skin incisions. When a mucosal incision is unavoidable (e.g., draining a posterior hematoma), a horizontal incision is preferred over a vertical one, as a vertical mucosal scar may interrupt mucociliary transport.

One of the major functions of the nose, or rather the nasal mucosa, is to heat inspired air to almost body temperature (37°C) and humidify it to maximum saturation with water before arriving at the lower respiratory tract. For this purpose, the nasal organ is equipped with a large surface of mucosa with an extensive submucosal vascular network, a high density of secretory glands, and a rich nerve supply. The turbinate system was also developed to serve this task. The same applies, to some extent, to the nasal valve area, as it enhances the exchange of heat and water by changing nasal airflow from a laminar pattern to a more turbulent one within its narrow passage. This emphasizes the very close relationship between intranasal air conditioning and airflow patterns (e.g., velocity, flow, vortices, path lines): the intranasal climate is mainly determined by airflow behavior within the nasal cavity. This is comparable with weather formation in nature.

The anterior nasal segment in particular, including the valve area and the turbinates, plays a crucial role in air conditioning. The space between the valve area and the head of the middle turbinate is the most effective part of the nasal cavity at heating and humidifying inhaled air.

When considering air conditioning, the expiration phase should not be neglected. Conditioning depends on *both* heating the air during inspiration *and* heat recovery during expiration. The crucial factor for water transfer from expired air to mucosa seems to be the temperature difference between the mucosal surface and the respiratory air.

The nasal surgeon should be aware of these physiological mechanisms and try to restore them when they are compromised by pathology or previous surgery.

Heating and Humidification

Several in vivo investigations revealed that an air temperature of about 31 to 34°C and a relative humidity of about 90 to 95% after inspiration could be observed within the nasopharynx (Keck and Lindemann 2010). However, nasal heating and humidification are not complete at this level. Further warming and humidification up to 37°C and 100% relative humidity occurs to a minor extent within the lower airways.

Due to the fact that most of the conditioning takes place within the anterior nasal segment, short-term exposure to cold, dry air or warm, humid air does not impair nasal air conditioning (Keck et al 2001). The nose has a large reserve for heating and humidification. The temperature difference between the mucosal surface and the respiratory air is a crucial prerequisite for heat exchange between the two. The temperature of the nasal mucosa depends on the phase of the respiratory cycle and the exact intranasal detection site. The mean mucosal temperature during respiration ranges from 30°C at the end of inspiration to 34°C at the end of expiration (Lindemann et al 2002). This temperature gradient between the mucosal surface and inspired as well as expired air is essential for effective heat and water transfer.

During inspiration, the warmer nasal wall heats the cooler air; during expiration, the cooler wall cools down the warmer air. In addition, water is regained from saturated and warmed expired air in the cooler mucosa. Thereby, water is preserved for humidification of air during the following inspiration. Thus, the loss of heat and water is reduced (Keck and Lindemann 2010).

There is also a close relationship between nasal airflow patterns and nasal mucosal temperature (Lindemann et al 2006). In regions of turbulent airflow, temperature changes are more pronounced than in regions of laminar airflow. This fact again confirms the close relation between airflow and intranasal air conditioning.

Nasal surgeons should not forget that any surgical intervention at the head of the inferior turbinate alters the valve area, and may lead to considerably disturbed air conditioning.

Mucosal Temperature and Perception of Nasal Patency

Difficulty in nasal breathing is a common complaint. At present, we mainly rely on a good clinical examination to identify the underlying problem causing nasal obstruction (Scadding et al 2011). For medicolegal or insurance purposes and for clinical trials, more objective means of measuring nasal patency and/or flow are often warranted, but data often correlate poorly with the subjective feeling of nasal obstruction. The feeling of nasal obstruction may have an underlying anatomical, mucosal, or physical etiology. Anatomical and mucosal causes of nasal obstruction are well known, but physical factors related to nasal obstruction are less studied. The existence of cold receptors in the nasal cavity has been verified. The subjective perception of nasal flow actually seems to be related to the activation of these receptors. For example, L-menthol causes a subjective improvement of nasal patency due to vapor action on the sensory nerve endings of the nasal mucosa, without objectively increasing measured nasal patency values (Eccles, Lindemann et al 2008). Additionally, there is a negative correlation between mucosal temperature and rhinometrical airflow volumes: high nasal flow is associated with low mucosal temperature (Lindemann et al. 2009).

The physiological perception of nasal airflow could be based on the cooling of the nasal mucosal surface by the air jet. This supports the hypothesis that the presence of nasal thermoreceptors plays an important role in the perception of nasal patency. These findings emphasize the fact that adequate heat and water exchange seems to be necessary for the perception of airflow and the feeling of a free nose.

1.4.4 Defense

The nose is provided with a number of different mechanisms to protect the airways: mechanical, humoral, and cellular defense.

Mechanical defense. The first line of mechanical defense consists of the vibrissae at the nostril and the vestibule. They protect the airways against incoming larger objects such as insects, although only to a limited extent. The second line of mechanical defense is the mucous blanket covering the mucosal membranes, in which smaller particles are entrapped and subsequently transported to the nasopharynx by the coordinated movements of the MCT. The third barrier is the epithelial lining, being a physical barrier between the lumen and the nasal tissue.

Humoral defense is provided by the production of immunoglobulins (IgA and IgG) and various enzymes at the level of the nasal mucosa. The role of humoral defense mechanisms in airway homeostasis becomes apparent in patients with dysfunction of Ig production, resulting in recurrent respiratory tract infections.

Cellular defense is mediated by a large variety of cells that may be recruited to help counteract the effects of allergens, viruses, bacteria, molds, etc. Eosinophils are the hallmark of allergic rhinitis, but are also attracted to the nasal mucosa in some forms of nonallergic rhinitis and rhinosinusitis with or without nasal polyps.

Filtering of the Air

Nasal cleansing of particles involves several processes. *Filtration* is removal of particles from respiratory air. *Deposition* is removal of particles by sedimentation on the nasal mucosa. *Retention* is the capture of mainly gaseous particles of the air. *Clearance* means removal of deposited particles on the mucosa by ciliary activity.

Nasal deposition depends on the attributes of the inspired particles (hygroscopic or hydrophobic, size, aerodynamic diameter, surface, density, and other chemical variables). Particles with a diameter between 0.4 and 3.0 µm mostly pass the nasal airways and are mainly deposited in the bronchial airways. Particles with a diameter smaller than 0.4 µm and bigger than 10 µm are mainly filtered in the nose (e.g. Keck et al 2002).

As a result of gravity and turbulence of the inspired air, some of the particles that are present in inhaled air will be deposited on the mucous layer covering the mucosal membranes. Larger and heavier particles will be deposited sooner and thus more anteriorly. They are entrapped in the upper layer of the mucous blanket. When insoluble, they are transported with a relatively high speed (0.5 to 2.0 cm/min) towards the pharynx by ciliary movement, and swallowed. To this end, the mucous layer consists of two sheets: an upper, more viscous and sticky gel in which the foreign particles are entrapped; and a lower liquid layer that allows ciliary movement. Soluble particles may dissolve in the deeper periciliary mucous layer and affect the mucosa.

Similar to climatization, particle filtration depends on respiratory parameters such as breathing frequency and tidal volume.

Cilia

Movements of the cilia covering the columnar cells of the mucosa are the driving force behind transportation of mucus towards the nasopharynx (MCT). A normal ciliary beat consists of an effective and a recovery stroke. During the effective stroke, the cilium is stretched and reaches the gel layer with its tip. This leads to propulsion of the upper viscous layer of mucus. In the recovery stroke, the cilium curves and bends backward to its rest position in a

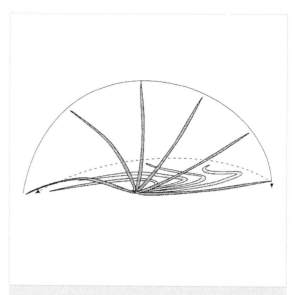

Fig. 1.131 Effective and recovery strokes of the ciliary beat and their different planes. (From Schuil 1994.)

plane parallel to the epithelial surface. It then enters a short rest phase (► Fig. 1.131). The effective stroke of various neighboring cilia and cells is coordinated in a synergistic way. The mechanism behind this ciliary coordination or metachron is not yet elucidated.

Under normal circumstances, ciliary beat frequency (CBF) is 8 to 11 Hz at the normal nasal mucosa temperature of 33 to 34°C. An increase in CBF leads, within a certain range, to an enhancement of MCT (Boek et al 1999). CBF is sensitive to a large number of influences, however. Desiccation of the mucosa leads to immediate abolishment of ciliary activity and loss of cilia. Temperature increase produces, within a certain range, an increase in CBF. Changes in pH (between 6.5 and 7.5) and osmolarity (between 300 and 400 mol) have no effect (Ingels et al 1991).

Various mediators and neuropeptides that play a role in nasal (patho)physiology have been found to inhibit or enhance ciliary activity (Schuil et al 1994). Our present knowledge is summarized in ► Table 1.8. Several pharmaceutical products applied to the nose for diagnosis and treatment have also been shown to affect ciliary beat (► Table 1.9). In particular, reference is made to the preservative benzalkonium chloride, a frequent ingredient in nasal sprays.

Mucociliary Transport (MCT)

The superficial viscous mucous layer covering the nasal mucosa is propelled at a speed of 0.5 to 2.0 cm/min in a dorsal direction by the to-and-fro movements of the cilia. These cilia symbolically move as ears of corn in the wind. MCT velocity may vary considerably. It may be influenced by various factors such as the quality of the mucous

Table 1.8 Effect of the most important mediators and neuropeptides on CBF

	No effect	Inhibition	Enhancement
Histamine	+ (in vitro)		+ (in vivo)
Leukotriene C4	+ (in vitro)		
Prostaglandin D2	+ (in vitro)		
Prostaglandin E2		+ (in vitro)	
Substance P	+ (in vitro)		+ (in vivo)
CGRP			+ (in vitro)
Nitric oxide			+ (in vitro)
Interleukin 13		+ (in vitro)	

Abbreviations: CBF, ciliary beat frequency; CGRP, calcitonin gene–related peptide.

layers, CBF and ciliary coordination, and turbulence of the inspired air.

For an ideal functioning of the MCT, a temperature of 37°C and a relative humidity of 100% is required. If there is insufficient heat and humidity, the ciliary cells stop functioning after a short time. The bacterial colonization is facilitated under these conditions and infections may result. Therefore, MCT and intranasal air conditioning are also closely related.

It is scientifically presumed that cilia have a sensory function in addition to their purely mechanical function. If applied, for example, bitter substances such as nicotine or quinine have contact with ciliary cells, consecutively the calcium concentration within the cells increases. The cells are activated and the CBF is increased in order to remove pollutants from the nasal mucosa.

The methods used to examine cilia and to measure CBF and MCT in clinical practice are discussed on page 121.

The nasal surgeon should keep in mind the importance of this defense mechanism. He must try to restore it as far as possible, a normal breathing pattern should be restored and the nasal mucosa preserved.

Humoral Defense

The nasal mucosa is provided with extensive and complicated mechanisms of humoral defense that have not yet been elucidated.

Immunoglobulins. IgA and, to a lesser extent, IgG are considered to play a major role in nasal defense. Secretory IgA concentration in nasal mucus is very high at 0.5 to 2.2 g/L—higher than in saliva or intestinal secretions.

Table 1.9 Effect on CBF of some pharmaceuticals topically used in the nose (after data by Ingels, Boek, and Schuil)

Pharmaceutical agent	No effect	Inhibition	Enhancement
Topical anesthetics			
Cocaine 3%		+ +	
Cocaine 7%		+ + + (stasis)	
Lidocaine 1%		+ +	
Lidocaine 4%		+ + + (stasis)	
Vasoconstrictors			
Xylometazoline 0.1%		+	
Oxymetazoline 0.05%		+	
Preservatives			
Benzalkonium chloride		+	
Saline 0.9%		+	
Saline 7.0%		+ + + (stasis)	
Antifungals			
Amphotericin B		+ + +	
Itraconazole		+ + +	
Other			
Corticosteroids		+	
Carbachol			+
Salbutamol			+

Abbreviations: CBF, ciliary beat frequency.

Its concentration is not related to serum IgA level. IgG seems to play a smaller role. Its concentration only amounts to 0.2 g/L. IgM concentration in nasal secretions is very low. Immunoglobulins are produced in the nasal mucosa by plasma cells and B lymphocytes.

Histamine is the most potent compound, which is released by mast cells and basophils during the immediate phase of the (IgE-mediated) allergic reaction. It is responsible for the most important symptoms in allergic rhinitis: nasal congestion, secretion, and sneezing.

Leukotrienes (LTB4, LTC4) play a similar role to histamine during immediate allergic reactions. They are also involved in the continuing "inflammatory" response.

Prostaglandins (PGD2, PGE2) are another group of mediators produced by mast cells during the allergic response. Their role is not yet elucidated.

Interleukins are a group of cytokines produced by cells in the nasal mucosa and are part of the inflammatory spectrum seen in rhinitis and rhinosinusitis. Interleukins are released upon activation of lymphocytes, mast cells, neutrophils, eosinophils, epithelial cells, and fibroblasts present in nasal tissue. Several major interleukins have been identified, and the most important ones at present seem to be IL-4, Il-5, IL-8, IL-12, IL-13, and IL 17. The wide variety of functions of this growing family of cytokines are still under exploration, but several have redundant and heterogeneous effects on epithelial cells, fibroblasts, mast cells, endothelial cells, and sensory nerves residing in the nasal mucosa.

Activation of endothelial and epithelial cells leads to upregulation of the expression of *adhesion molecules*, which are responsible for the influx of inflammatory cells at the site of immune stimulation by microbial or environmental triggers. So far, three main groups of adhesion molecules have been described: selectins, integrins, and the immunoglobulin superfamily.

Cytokines may have proinflammatory potential, but some, such as IL-10 and transforming growth factor-beta (TGF-B), have anti-inflammatory actions. These so-called anti-inflammatory cytokines are considered to protect the upper airways against inflammatory damage.

Cellular Defense

The nasal mucosa, submucosa, and secretions contain numerous types of cells that play a role in the different types of respiratory mucosal defense.

Dendritic cells reside in the nasal mucosa. They capture pathogens and allergens, migrate to the draining lymph nodes, and present parts of the pathogens and allergens to T and B lymphocytes. In this way, an adequate immune response is initiated, on both a cellular and a humoral level.

Eosinophils are the most well known. Their number in the mucosa, submucosa, and in nasal secretions is specifically increased in allergic rhinitis (IgE-mediated allergy). Their number is related to the severity of symptoms.

Their granules contain various proteins, toxins, and enzymes.

Mast cells were found long ago to play a role. They are present in the submucosa and, in allergic reactions, migrate to the mucosal surface, where they degranulate and release a great number of substances, such as histamine, platelet activating factor (PAF), different enzymes, and cytokines. Some of these enzymes induce the release of prostaglandins (PGD2, PGE2) and leukotrienes (LTB4, LTC4).

Basophils are also present in the submucosa, but they increase in number and migrate to the mucosal surface in allergic challenge. They release histamine and LTC4, among others.

Plasma cells are recruited in various conditions. They play a dominant role in the production of immunoglobulins.

T lymphocytes are scattered in high numbers in allergic conditions. CD4 (helper cells) strongly prevail over CD8 (suppressor) cells. When activated, they produce various cytokines.

B lymphocytes are among the producers of IgE.

Nasal Reflexes

The basic functional role of the nose in human physiology is also illustrated by the large number of nasal reflexes. Some of them are pure defensive reflexes; others are signs of the complex relationship between the nose and other physiological systems.

Naso–Nasal Reflex (Sneezing)

The sneezing reflex is the most important sensory (trigeminal) defensive reflex. It may occur as a reaction to a wide range of physical and chemical nasal stimuli. Even bright light can cause sneezing (photic sneezing), which can be observed in 17 to 35% of people. Its causes are not yet clarified. However, an autosomal dominant inheritance, the so-called ACHOO syndrome (Autosomal Dominant Compelling Helio-Ophthalmic Outburst of Sneezing [Collie et al 1978]) is assumed. The most common theory is an abnormally close course of the optic nerve to the trigeminal nerve. In cases of sudden brightness, action potentials are conducted along the optic nerve, stimulating the trigeminal nerve as well. This is perceived cerebrally as an irritation of the nasal mucosa, finding its expression as a sneeze.

Sneezing occurs in three phases. In the first phase, air is deeply inhaled. The breath is held briefly (second phase), and then the expiratory muscles suddenly contract (the third phase). The air is strongly exhaled against a closed glottis. The larynx and pharynx are then opened and a short explosive expiration follows through the nose (and mouth). Simultaneously, via local and central parasympathetic efferent pathways, nasal vasodilatation and secretion are induced. The airflow velocity reaches over 45 m/s. This sneezing "reflex" is not a real reflex as it is neurally too complex and can be deliberately influenced. It is eliminated by local and general anesthesia.

Naso(Laryngo)bronchial Reflex (Nasopulmonary Reflex)

A second reflex with a defensive nature is the nasopulmonary reflex. This reflex has been studied for a long time and its significance is still a matter of dispute. It is an ipsilateral reflex, with the sensory trigeminal nerve endings of the nasal mucosa as its afferent, and vagal fibers as its efferent, pathway. Nasal stimulation, for example cold air, may induce a reduction in breathing—even apnea—and laryngeal and bronchial constriction. This naso(laryngo)bronchial reflex may play an important role in breathing distress, especially in the elderly. Several studies have demonstrated that nasal obstruction or nasopharyngeal packing may cause a decrease in arterial oxygen saturation and an increase in blood carbon dioxide. The nasal surgeon and the ENT doctor applying a tamponade (particularly a Bellocq type) for epistaxis should be aware of this phenomenon.

In allergic rhinitis and in sinus disease, (sino)nasal inflammation and bronchial pathology interact in various ways. Neural pathways are clearly involved, with mediators like substance P being upregulated in bronchi after nasal stimulation. In addition, the systemic circulation plays a role in this nasobronchial interaction by transporting cytokines, such as IL-5 released in the upper airways to the blood, resulting in enhanced bone marrow synthesis of inflammatory cells and upregulation of adhesion molecules on bronchial endothelial cells. In addition, allergens that are deposited in the nasal mucosa enter the submucosal area and blood vessels, leading to activation of systemic basophils. Clinically, these immunologic phenomena translate into a close interaction between (sino) nasal inflammation and bronchial pathology, both in allergy as well as in rhinosinusitis. Conversely, bronchial asthma or chronic obstructive pulmonary disease (COPD) have a negative impact on (sino)nasal disease, with more severe inflammation and symptoms and a worse outcome after functional endoscopic sinus surgery (FESS) (Hellings et al 2010).

Corporonasal Reflex (Diving Reflex)

The diving reflex is a protective mechanism in all lung-breathing creatures when immersed in water. The brain receives information that the airways are under water. Stimulation of the parasympathetic nervous system due to immersion of, for example, the face, chest, feet, and back in cold water leads to reduced breathing (even apnea), bradycardia, and centralization of the blood-stream ("blood shift"). Hereby, the oxygen consumption of vital organs is reduced.

Apart from the above-described reflexes, several other nasal reflexes have been described and studied. These reflexes are clinically less important. Therefore, they are only listed in brief.

Nasocardiac Reflex (Cranial Nerve V–Cranial Nerve X)

Strong stimulation of the nasal mucosa produces bradycardia and a reduction of cardiac output with lowering of the blood pressure.

Nasovascular Reflex

Nasal stimulation causes peripheral vasoconstriction.

Genitonasal Reflex

Sexual arousal and orgasm cause swelling of the nasal mucosa, particularly of the turbinates.

Gastronasal Reflex (Cranial Nerve X–Parasympathicus)

Strong gastric stimulation by irritation (e.g., alcohol, coffee) or gastritis may cause nasal secretion and vasodilatation on the homolateral (left) side of the nose.

1.4.5 Speech

The nose and the paranasal cavities are an essential part of the speech-production apparatus. The nasal cavity is one of the resonators that play a role in production of some vowels and several consonants. Typical examples are "m" and "n," the so-called nasal consonants.

The amount of nasal resonance is called "nasalance." Previously, it was common to speak of "rhinolalia clausa" when nasal resonance was decreased, and of "rhinolalia aperta" when nasal resonance was present in consonants requiring closure of the nasopharynx by the soft palate.

Many rhinological patients suffer from decreased nasalance because of nasal obstruction due to mucosal swelling, polyposis, or septal deformity. Surgery may have a considerable effect on their speech and singing. Professional (and amateur) singers may benefit considerably from functional reconstructive nasal surgery.

1.4.6 Facial Beauty and Facial Expression

The nose plays a dominant role in concepts of facial beauty and expression. In almost all cultures, we find indications of the dominant role that the shape of the nose plays in life. A nose perceived as beautiful enhances facial beauty and helps make a person attractive. A deformed or damaged nose may be perceived as ugly.

Beauty

Different cultures have developed different concepts of nasal beauty. We find evidence of this in the special "rules" that were conceived for describing ideal body proportions, and from works of art.

When discussing beauty, it is of utmost importance to take into consideration the many ethnic differences in the shape of the face and nose. The faces and noses of blacks and Asians are very different from those of the Caucasians. The rhinoplasty surgeon should be aware of this and should attempt to preserve some ethnic character when performing an operation.

Aversion to One's Own Nose

Many patients visit the nasal surgeon because they dislike their nose. In many cases their problem is understandable: a deviated pyramid, a large hump, a severe saddle, etc. Mostly, their complaints are not only cosmetic; function is impaired too. Where there is no real "deformity" but a minor "abnormality" or nothing more than a "variation," the surgeon should be warned. A careful analysis of the "problem," sometimes including a psychological analysis, is then required. Nothing is more disappointing, both for the patient and the doctor, than a patient who is dissatisfied with a "good" result. According to recent studies, a significant number of patients with aesthetic nasal complaints have symptoms of a body dysmorphic disorder (BDD).

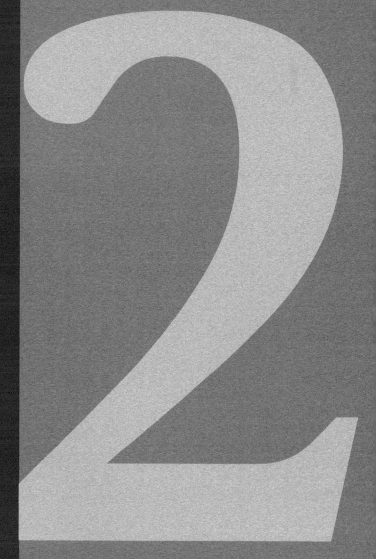

Chapter 2
Pathology and Diagnosis

2 Pathology and Diagnosis

2.1 Nasal Syndromes

In health and disease, signs and symptoms frequently occur in more or less fixed combinations. We then speak of a syndrome (in Greek, "syndrome" = "come together"). In the domain of functional corrective nasal surgery, we suggest distinguishing the following syndromes:

2.1.1 Deviated Pyramid Syndromes

The "deviated nose" is characterized by a deviation of the external nasal pyramid in combination with a deformity of the nasal septum. In the great majority of patients, the underlying cause is mechanical trauma with a lateral, frontolateral, or laterobasal impact. A genetically deviated nose has been observed in some families. In rare cases, a deviated nose is of intrauterine origin. Patients with a deviated external nose generally have both functional and aesthetic complaints.

Depending upon which part of the pyramid is deviated, we distinguish four types:
- *Deviated pyramid*
  - The bony and cartilaginous pyramid and lobule deviate to the same side.
- *C-shaped pyramid*
  - The bony pyramid deviates to the right, the cartilaginous pyramid to the left.
- *Reversed C-shaped pyramid*
  - The bony pyramid deviates to the left, the cartilaginous pyramid to the right.

- *Deviated cartilaginous pyramid*
  - The cartilaginous pyramid is deviated, whereas the bony pyramid is in the midline.

Deviated Pyramid

Both the bony and the cartilaginous pyramid, and usually the lobule as well, deviate to one side (▶ Fig. 2.1 and ▶ Fig. 2.2). When the nasion–stomion line is drawn, deviation of all parts of the nasal pyramid becomes obvious.

The bony pyramid leans to one side. It is asymmetric, with a short, steep slope on the side of the deviation (due to an infraction of the nasal bone) and a long, shallow slope on the opposite side.

The cartilaginous pyramid is deformed in a similar way. The triangular cartilages are asymmetric, especially when the trauma occurred in childhood. Some sagging of the cartilaginous dorsum may be present.

The lobule often leans to the same side. The tip deviates to the side of the deviation. The columella is oblique, with its upper (ventral) part leaning to the side of the deviation. It may also be broadened, due to dislocation of the caudal end of the septum. The alae differ in length and the nostrils are asymmetric. These lobular asymmetries are usually automatically corrected by repositioning of the septum and the cartilaginous pyramid. Only in patients with a long-standing severe deviation might additional lobular surgery be needed.

The septum may show a variety of deformations. The anterior septum is usually dislocated to the side of the deviation, whereas its posterior part is either in the

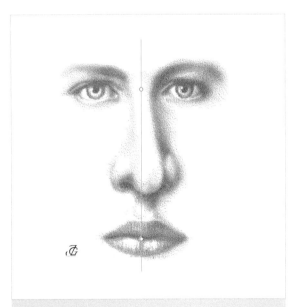

Fig. 2.1 Deviated pyramid.

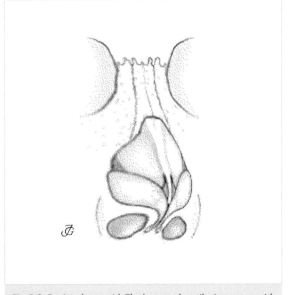

Fig. 2.2 Deviated pyramid. The bony and cartilaginous pyramid, including the lobule, deviate to one side.

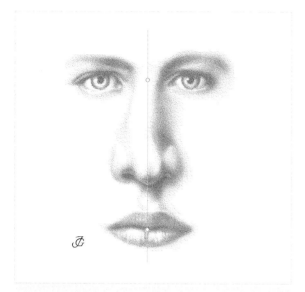

Fig. 2.3 C-shaped deviation of the pyramid.

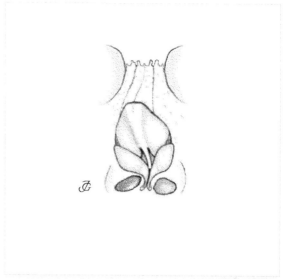

Fig. 2.4 C-shaped deviation of the pyramid. The bony pyramid deviates to the right, the cartilaginous pyramid and lobule lean to the left.

midline or deviated to the contralateral side. The caudal septal end often protrudes into the vestibule, and the valve area may be narrowed by a septal convexity or fracture. A basal bony–cartilaginous crest and/or a vomeral spur deformity are common.

Breathing is generally impaired on both sides, the most severe symptoms occurring on the side of the valvular obstruction.

C-Shaped Pyramid

The bony pyramid deviates to the right, whereas the cartilaginous pyramid leans to the left. The lobule usually leans to the same side as the cartilaginous pyramid (▶ Fig. 2.3 and ▶ Fig. 2.4). This type of deformity is also called a "twisted" nose.

The deformities of the various parts of the pyramid and the septum are similar to the ones described earlier. They may occur in different combinations, however.

Reversed C-Shaped Pyramid

The bony pyramid deviates to the left, whereas the cartilaginous pyramid leans to the right. The lobule usually deviates to the same side as the cartilaginous pyramid (▶ Fig. 2.5 and ▶ Fig. 2.6).

Deviated Cartilaginous Pyramid

The bony pyramid is straight and symmetrical, whereas the cartilaginous pyramid and lobule are deviated and asymmetrical (▶ Fig. 2.7 and ▶ Fig. 2.8). The cartilaginous septum deviates to the same side, and its caudal end is usually dislocated to the side of the deviation and protrudes into the vestibule and nostril. The valve area is mostly obstructed by a fracture or a convexity of the

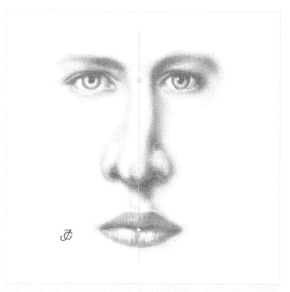

Fig. 2.5 Reversed C-shaped deviation of the pyramid.

septal cartilage. The posterior septum is normal or deviated. Inspiratory breathing is usually impaired, especially on the side of the narrowed valve area.

2.1.2 Hump Nose (Dorsal Nasal Deformity)

The nasal dorsum is convex. This may concern the bony pyramid, the cartilaginous pyramid, or both the bony and the cartilaginous pyramid. The nasal tip is often relatively low or depressed. A hump may occur as a single

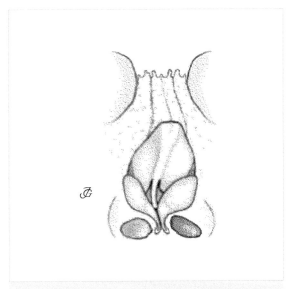

Fig. 2.6 Reversed C-shaped deviation of the pyramid. The bony pyramid deviates to the left, the cartilaginous pyramid and lobule lean to the right.

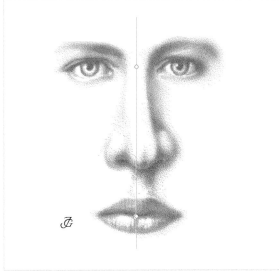

Fig. 2.7 Deviated cartilaginous pyramid.

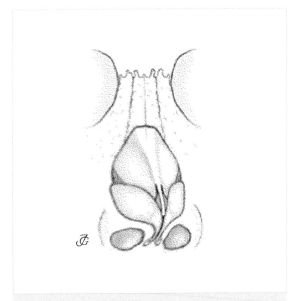

Fig. 2.8 Deviated cartilaginous pyramid. The bony pyramid is normal, the cartilaginous pyramid and lobule are deviated.

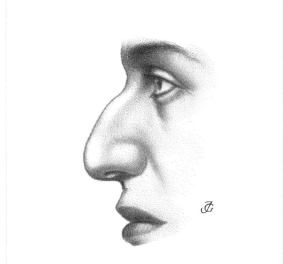

Fig. 2.9 Bony and cartilaginous hump. Both the bony and cartilaginous pyramid are convex and projecting.

deformity or variation. It may also occur in combination with various types of septal and pyramidal pathology. A hump itself usually only causes aesthetic complaints. We distinguish the following types:

- *Bony and cartilaginous hump*
  - Both the bony and the cartilaginous dorsa are convex (humped). The maximum convexity is usually located at the K area (▶ Fig. 2.9).
- *Bony hump*
  - The convexity is confined to the bony pyramid (see ▶ Fig. 2.48).
- *Cartilaginous hump*
  - The convexity is limited to the cartilaginous dorsum (see ▶ Fig. 2.49).
- *Relative hump (pseudohump)*
  - The bony dorsum is projecting due to saddling of the cartilaginous pyramid (see ▶ Fig. 2.50).

These different types of humps are discussed and illustrated in more detail in the section on Humps page 82.

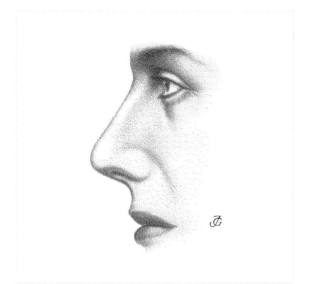

Fig. 2.10 Prominent-narrow pyramid syndrome. The entire external nasal pyramid is prominent, narrow, and long; the dorsum may be straight, slightly convex, or show a bony and cartilaginous hump; the lobule is narrow and projecting; the nasolabial angle is large.

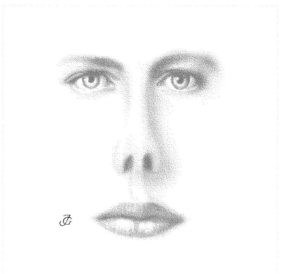

Fig. 2.11 Prominent-narrow pyramid syndrome. The external pyramid is narrow and prominent; the lobule is narrow and projecting.

2.1.3 Prominent-Narrow Pyramid Syndrome (Tension Nose)

The prominent-narrow pyramid syndrome is characterized by a (abnormally) prominent and narrow external nasal pyramid. It is of genetic ethnic origin, and rather common in Caucasians. It is seen more frequently in females than in males. The prominent-narrow pyramid syndrome is essentially a pronounced form of leptorrhine (▶ Fig. 2.10, ▶ Fig. 2.11, and ▶ Fig. 2.12).

The entire external pyramid is narrow and prominent. Its length and height are greater than normal. The bony dorsum is straight or slightly humped, and the overlying skin is usually thin. The cartilaginous pyramid is narrow and prominent, and its dorsum is often slightly convex. The frontonasal angle is relatively small, and the nasolabial angle is larger than normal. The piriform aperture is high and narrow. The clinical nasal index is less than 70. The skull is dolichocephalic. Retrognathism of the mandible is a frequent feature. The valve area is narrow and high and easily collapsible. The lobule is narrow and projecting. The tip is narrow and may be pulled down slightly by the tension of the stretched alae and columella. There is a positive "OO phenomenon" (see ▶ Fig. 2.142). By puckering the lips, as when pronouncing the vowel sound "OO," the tip is drawn down and backward due to the tension (overstretch) of the columella and the upper lip.

The columella is relatively long and slender; the alae are thin and (over)stretched. The nares are more or less

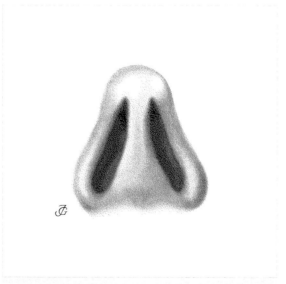

Fig. 2.12 Prominent-narrow pyramid syndrome. The nostrils are slitlike and their axis almost vertical; the columella is long and narrow; the alae are thin and stretched.

slitlike and their axis is almost vertical instead of oblique. As a consequence, the alae may collapse on inspiration. The septum is usually normal, although small deformations may be present. The upper lip is usually short, and retrognathism of the mandible is common.

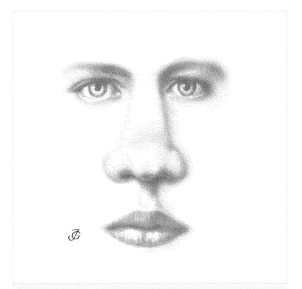

Fig. 2.13 Low-wide pyramid syndrome. The external nasal pyramid is low and wide; the bony and cartilaginous pyramids are depressed and low; the nasal bones are thick; the lobule is low and wide.

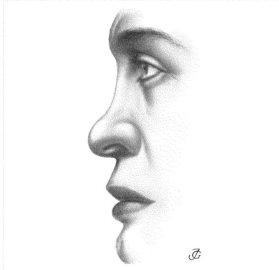

Fig. 2.14 Low-wide pyramid syndrome. The bony and cartilaginous pyramids are low; the nasal bones are thick; the lobule is low, wide, and underprojected.

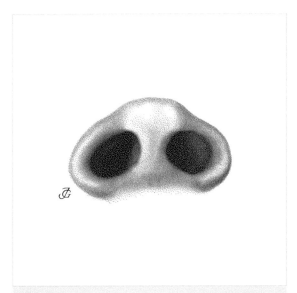

Fig. 2.15 Low-wide pyramid syndrome. The lobule is underprojected and broad. The tip is flat and depressed; the columella is short and retracted; the nostrils are wide and rounded; the alae are ballooning.

Patients with prominent-narrow pyramid syndrome may ask for surgery for aesthetic reasons. However, there may also be functional reasons; for example, breathing impairment due to inspiratory collapse of the alae and/or obstruction of the valve area.

Cottle has named the prominent external pyramid the "tension nose." He pointed out that the soft tissues are under tension as a result of the strong ventral growth of the septum and bony pyramid in comparison to the soft tissues.

2.1.4 Low-Wide Pyramid Syndrome (Saddle Nose)

The low-wide pyramid syndrome or saddle nose is a very common nasal syndrome that may be either congenital (congenital nasal hypoplasia) or the result of severe septal pathology (trauma, septal abscess, inadequate septal surgery). The bony pyramid is broad and lacks prominence (▶ Fig. 2.13 and ▶ Fig. 2.14). The dorsum is flat. The nasal bones are usually thick. The bony pyramid is more or less round or trapezoid rather than pyramidal. The cartilaginous pyramid is low and wide. The clinical nasal index is more than 85.

The cartilaginous dorsum sags, lacking support and projection (▶ Fig. 2.13 and ▶ Fig. 2.14). This is due to a defective anterior septum and scarring of the soft tissues. The triangular cartilages are often atrophic. The fibrous connections between the cartilaginous and the bony pyramid may have been lost, making the lower margins of the nasal bones visible.

The lobule is underprojected, lacking support. Its shape resembles that of the lobule in childhood (▶ Fig. 2.15). This is partially due to causative trauma or infection, and partially the result of disturbed nasal growth. Because of the absence of (septal) support, the tip can easily be pressed downward—the so-called rubber nose

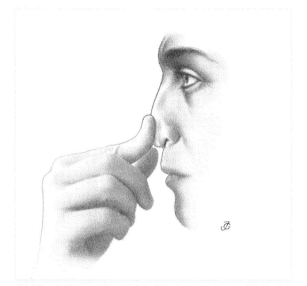

Fig. 2.16 Low-wide pyramid syndrome. The lobule and tip lack projection and support. The lobule is easily compressed by pressing with the finger on the tip (the so-called rubber nose).

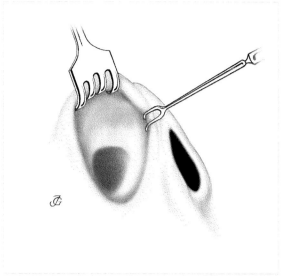

Fig. 2.17 Low-wide pyramid syndrome. The valve is low and very wide due to loss of the cartilaginous septum and retraction of the soft tissues of the septum.

phenomenon (▶ Fig. 2.16). The tip is broad and flat. The columella is short and retracted, especially at its base. The alae are more convex and thicker than normal. The nostrils are round and ballooning.

The vestibule and the valve area are broad and low (▶ Fig. 2.17). The valve angle is depressed and considerably increased, sometimes even up to 90°.

Patients with low-wide pyramid syndrome usually have both functional and aesthetic complaints. Their breathing is often disturbed, although their nasal passages are wide enough. Because of deformity of the vestibule and the valve area, the inspiratory airstream will be less turbulent than normal. This may compromise the air-conditioning and cleansing functions of the nose. The mucosa is usually of poor quality. The cilia may be partially missing, and mucociliary clearance is impaired, leading to local infection, crusting, and bleeding. All these factors will, to some degree, negatively influence nasal function.

Apart from being part of a syndrome, saddling and sagging may also occur in isolation as a symptom. We distinguish the following five types of saddle nose:
- *Bony saddle*
  - The bony pyramid is concave whereas the cartilaginous dorsum is normal (see ▶ Fig. 2.52).
- *Cartilaginous saddling or sagging*
  - The cartilaginous dorsum is concave and depressed, while the bony dorsum is normal (see ▶ Fig. 2.53 and ▶ Fig. 2.54).
- *Linea nasalis dorsalis*
  - A linea nasalis dorsalis is a pathological horizontal crease over the cartilaginous dorsum just above the lobule (see ▶ Fig. 2.58).

- *Dorsal step*
  - The cartilaginous pyramid is detached from the bony pyramid. The junction between the triangular cartilages and the nasal bones is disrupted (see ▶ Fig. 2.55 and ▶ Fig. 2.56).
- *Sagging of the supratip area*
  - The area just cranial to the tip is depressed (see ▶ Fig. 2.57).

2.1.5 Ski-Slope Nose

The so-called ski-slope nose is a common "postsurgical look" and one of the most well-known complications of rhinoplasty. The nasal dorsum is more or less sloping due to excessive lowering of the bony and cartilaginous dorsum, especially in the region of the K area (▶ Fig. 2.18; see also ▶ Fig. 6.71, ▶ Fig. 6.72, ▶ Fig. 6.73, and ▶ Fig. 6.74). The surgeon did not take into account that the dorsal skin over this region is thinner than over the cartilaginous dorsum (see ▶ Fig. 1.31). Sagging of the cartilaginous dorsum due to inadequate fixation of the cartilaginous septum may also play a role. A ski-slope deformity can be prevented by: (1) limiting the amount of reduction of the lower part of the bony dorsum; (2) fixing the cartilaginous septum to the premaxilla (or the anterior nasal spine) and the columella to prevent sagging of cartilaginous dorsum; and (3) transplanting some crushed septal cartilage under the skin in the K area.

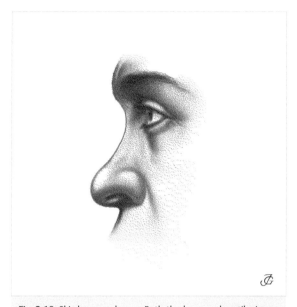

Fig. 2.18 Ski-slope syndrome. Both the bony and cartilaginous pyramids are concave. This syndrome is seen after excessive reduction of a bony and cartilaginous hump. The dorsum is usually more or less irregular on palpation and may have an "open roof" (see ▶ Fig. 2.19 and ▶ Fig. 2.20).

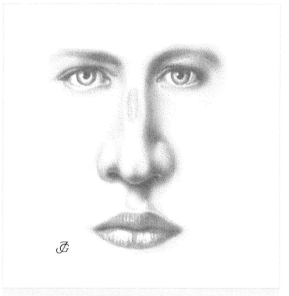

Fig. 2.19 Open roof syndrome. Defect of dorsum (open roof) visible and palpable through the skin.

2.1.6 Open Roof Syndrome

Open roof syndrome is characterized by neuralgic symptoms that are caused by a traumatic defect in the bony (and cartilaginous) dorsum. The most common cause is resection of a bony and/or cartilaginous hump with subsequent closure of the dorsum. Cottle was the first to describe this syndrome as an entity.

Its main symptoms are tenderness of the bony dorsum, pain when wearing eyeglasses, and pain on inspiring cold air. On examination, an irregular defect in the bony dorsum and K area can be seen and palpated through thin and adherent skin with telangiectasias (▶ Fig. 2.19 and ▶ Fig. 2.20).

The symptoms are caused by a defect in the bony roof and damage to the external nasal branches of the anterior ethmoidal nerve (see ▶ Fig. 1.56). As a result of the defect, the outside skin and the inside nasal mucosa are in direct contact, which may induce neuralgia. Evidence supporting this pathogenetic explanation is the fact that symptoms disappear after secondary closure of the dorsum through osteotomies and interposition of a layer of connective tissue or soft cartilage between the skin and the bony defect.

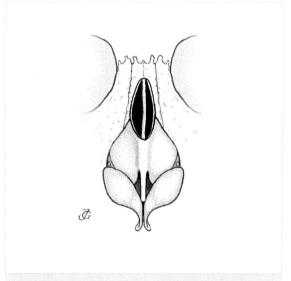

Fig. 2.20 Open roof syndrome. Defect of bony and cartilaginous dorsum due to resection of a bony and cartilaginous hump.

2.1.7 Lobular Inspiratory Insufficiency Syndrome ("Alar Collapse")

Lobular inspiratory insufficiency syndrome is characterized by collapse of the lateral wall of the lobule during the inspiratory phase of breathing. As a result of negative pressure on inspiration, the lateral nasal wall is sucked inward and collapses. This condition was already recognized as a pathological entity in the second half of the 19th century and was called "alar collapse" (▶ Fig. 2.21). Alar collapse is a misleading term, however, and has induced many surgical mistakes. The collapse of the mobile lateral nasal wall is, in many cases, not due to alar weakness. The most common causes are as follows:

- Slitlike nostrils, as in the prominent-narrow pyramid syndrome (see ▶ Fig. 2.12)
- Narrowing of the nostrils and/or vestibules due to an abnormally broad columella (see ▶ Fig. 2.87), protrusion of the medial crura (see ▶ Fig. 2.88), a protruding, dislocated caudal end of the septum (see ▶ Fig. 2.100), or alar pathology (see ▶ Fig. 2.78, ▶ Fig. 2.79, ▶ Fig. 2.80, ▶ Fig. 2.81, ▶ Fig. 2.82, ▶ Fig. 2.83, and ▶ Fig. 2.84)
- Narrowing of the valve area due to pathology of the septum, triangular cartilage, or inferior turbinate (see ▶ Fig. 2.102 and ▶ Fig. 2.104)

All these kinds of pathology, sometimes in combination, may lead to collapse of (parts of) the lateral wall of the lobule. For this reason, we prefer to speak of the "lobular

Table 2.1 Main causes of lobular inspiratory insufficiency

Nostril	Slitlike nostrils (prominent-narrow pyramid syndrome)
Nostril vestibule	Broad columella Protruding medial crura Dislocated and protruding caudal septal end
Vestibule	Protruding lateral crus
Valve area	Stenosis due to: • septal pathology • synechiae • triangular cartilage pathology • hyperplasia of inferior turbinate head

inspiratory insufficiency syndrome." ▶ Table 2.1 gives an overview of the most frequent causes.

2.1.8 Middle Meatus Obstructive Syndrome

Middle meatus obstructive syndrome is characterized by a set of symptoms that may occur when the middle meatal passage is obstructed. The main symptoms of this syndrome are:

- Headaches, varying from vague pressure feelings to pain, usually localized at the level of the bony pyramid and radiating in a frontal and orbital direction (anterior or posterior ethmoidal neuralgic syndrome)
- Sinusitis as a result of obstruction of the ostia of the maxillary and frontal sinus and anterior ethmoidal cells
- Impaired breathing
- Hyposmia

Obstruction of middle meatal areas has diverse causes, both anatomical and pathological. Analysis of the factors contributing to the syndrome is of utmost importance in selecting the mode of treatment. The following anatomical features may be involved: the septum, middle turbinate, uncinate process, ethmoidal bulla, infundibulum ethmoidale, and the mucosa overlying these structures. ▶ Table 2.2 gives an overview of the most common causes.

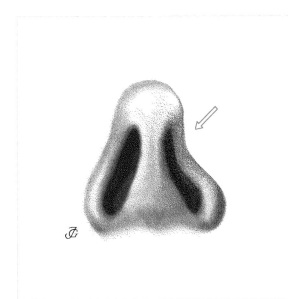

Fig. 2.21 Lobular inspiratory insufficiency syndrome. The lateral wall of the lobule(s) collapses on inspiration. This syndrome may be caused by slitlike nostrils, narrowing of the naris and/or vestibule, the caudal part of the septum, or pathology of the valve area.

Table 2.2 Main conditions that may contribute to middle meatus obstructive syndrome

Septum	Deviation or thickening opposite the middle turbinate
Middle turbinate	Concha bullosa or spongiosa lateral curling
Uncinate process	Long and/or medially curled
Ethmoidal bulla	Large Ventral location
Infundibulum	Narrow
Mucosa	Swelling Polypoid degeneration

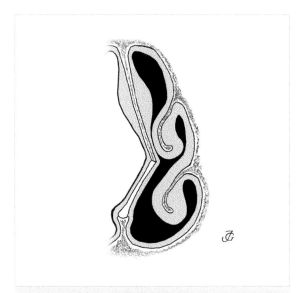

Fig. 2.22 Middle meatus obstructive syndrome. Obstruction of the middle meatus by a septal deviation.

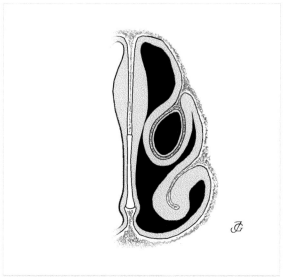

Fig. 2.23 Middle meatus obstructive syndrome. Obstruction of the middle meatus by a bullous middle turbinate.

Septum: A deviation or a thickening of the septum in area 4 at the level of the head of the middle turbinate can easily lead to temporary or permanent contact between the septal and turbinate mucosa. Septal surgery may be helpful in these cases (▶ Fig. 2.22).

Middle turbinate: A concha bullosa is a normal anatomical variation found in about 25% of the population. The turbinate skeleton may be very thick and spongiotic. In combination with other conditions, these variations can play a major role in the development of an obstructive syndrome (▶ Fig. 2.23). Middle turbinate surgery might then be indicated.

Uncinate process: The uncinate process may follow a medial instead of a lateral course. Its end may also be curved medially downward, suggesting the presence of a second, more laterally localized, medial turbinate. These variations can easily contribute to obstruction of the middle meatus.

Ethmoidal bulla: The size and location of the ethmoidal bulla shows considerable interindividual variation. When large and relatively more ventral than average, it may be in more or less permanent contact with the middle turbinate or the lateral wall of the infundibulum. In this case, it will obstruct the entrance to the infundibulum.

Infundibulum ethmoidale: The depth and width of the infundibulum may be another cause of middle meatus obstruction syndrome.

Nasal mucosa: Allergy, hyperreactivity, and infection will induce mucosal swelling. This may lead to contact between the septum and the middle turbinate as well as to obstruction of the infundibulum and ostiomeatal complex. In chronic conditions, hyperplasia and polypous degeneration may result.

In mild cases, conservative treatment (antibiotics, corticosteroid sprays) is prescribed. Polyps resistant to conservative treatment have to be resected, and infundibulotomy and/or anterior ethmoidectomy may be indicated. A septal deformity and concha bullosa may be addressed during the same surgical procedure.

2.1.9 Wide Nasal Cavity Syndrome ("Empty Nose" Syndrome)

Wide nasal cavity syndrome or "empty nose syndrome," as Stenquist and Kern 1996 have named it, is characterized by an abnormally wide nasal cavity with crusting and a variety of complaints. It is usually secondary to extensive surgery of the inferior and/or middle turbinate (▶ Fig. 2.24 and ▶ Fig. 2.25).

Patients with wide nasal cavity syndrome suffer from a variety of complaints: a feeling of nasal obstruction in spite of normal breathing; nasal irritation and itching; headaches and pressure feelings; radiating pain on inspiring cold air; crusting; and minor blood loss. The severity of these complaints varies considerably from person to person. Some patients have only minor symptoms, whereas others are real "nasal cripples."

On examination, the nasal cavity is abnormally spacious, lacking (part of) one or both turbinates. Mucosal pathology varies greatly. In some patients, the mucosa is dry and pale because of metaplasia; in others, it is red because of chronic infection. Crusting may range from absent to severe. The symptoms are caused by abnormal air currents due to disturbed anatomy and loss of the mucosa and its serous and mucus glands. In many cases,

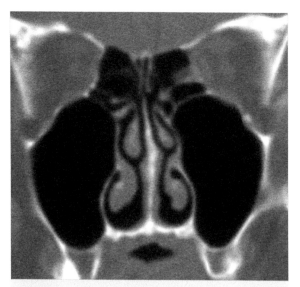

Fig. 2.24 Wide nasal cavity syndrome, or empty nose syndrome. Coronal CT scans before bilateral infundibulotomy and resection of the inferior turbinates.

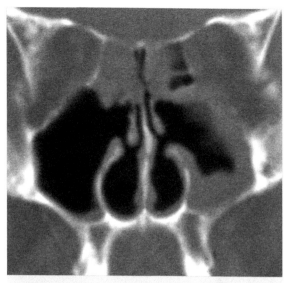

Fig. 2.25 Wide nasal cavity syndrome, or empty nose syndrome. Coronal CT scans after bilateral infundibulotomy and resection of the inferior turbinates. Note the reactive swelling of the mucosal lining of the ethmoids and left maxillary sinus to compensate for the abnormally wide space.

however, the discrepancy between the degree of the anatomical disturbance and the severity of the symptoms is difficult to understand.

2.1.10 Dry Nose Syndrome

Dry nose syndrome is found in primary and secondary atrophic rhinitis. Primary atrophic rhinitis may occur as part of a systemic syndrome or may be of unknown origin. Secondary atrophic rhinitis is much more common. It is mostly iatrogenic, resulting from a loss of normally functioning mucosa following electrocoagulation, chemocautery, or laser treatment of the inferior turbinates. Septal surgery without proper septal reconstruction may be an additional factor. Symptoms include nasal irritation, itching, and a feeling of dryness. Some crusting and epistaxis may also occur.

2.1.11 Cleft Lip– and Cleft Palate–Nose

A cleft lip and/or cleft palate is one of the most common congenital anomalies. Its treatment is one of the most difficult challenges to the maxillofacial and nasal surgeon. The deformity consists of a unilateral or bilateral defect of the upper lip, alveolar process of the maxilla, and/or palate. Unilateral clefts are much more common than bilateral clefts.

The incidence of cleft lip and palate varies considerably by region and ethnic group. According to recent literature, the incidence lies between 0.3 per million (Native Americans, Japanese) and 2.5 per thousand (black Nigerians and South Africans).

A positive family history can be found in about a quarter of cases. External factors are assumed to play a causative role in other cases. When they occur before the sixth week of gestation, they may lead to a complete syndrome. When occurring later, but before the 10th to 12th week, an isolated palatal defect will occur (see Chapter 1, page 44).

In patients with a cleft lip, all nasal elements and adjacent structures are more or less affected.

The bony and cartilaginous pyramid are asymmetrical and lean slightly to the noncleft side (NCS; ► Fig. 2.26 and ► Fig. 2.27).

The piriform aperture is asymmetrical, the aperture on the cleft side (CS) being lower and narrower. The anterior nasal spine deviates to the CS or may be missing. The premaxilla is severely deviated to the CS with its median axis up to 40° (► Fig. 2.28).

The lobule is deviated to the CS and strongly asymmetrical. The tip is bifid and flat and deviates to the CS. The dome and lateral crus on the CS are severely depressed, less convex, and more caudally located; the ala is elongated, flat, and displaced in a lateral and caudal direction; the vestibule is narrow and has a more horizontal axis.

The columella is short, broad, and oblique. Its upper end leans to the CS; its base is retracted. The medial crus on the CS is somewhat displaced in a caudal direction and looks shorter than the opposite medial crus (► Fig. 2.29).

The septum is severely deformed. Its caudal end is dislocated to the NCS and may thereby narrow the vestibule on this side. More posteriorly, the cartilaginous septum, vomer, and perpendicular plate are strongly deviated to the CS, obstructing the valve area and the nasal cavity. At

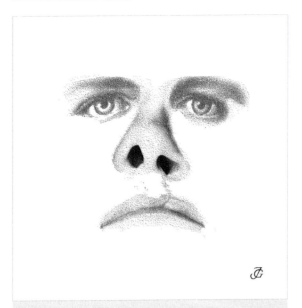

Fig. 2.26 Cleft lip- and cleft palate-nose on the left side. The bony and cartilaginous pyramid lean slightly to the NCS. The lobule is severely deformed: the dome and ala on the CS are depressed, the alar base is lower, the nostril is more horizontal.

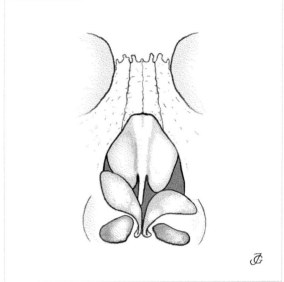

Fig. 2.27 Cleft lip- and cleft palate-nose on the left side. The bony pyramid leans to the NCS, whereas the cartilaginous pyramid and lobule deviate to the CS. The lobule is severely asymmetrical. The ala on the CS is flattened and displaced, and the lateral crus of the lobular cartilage is lower, less convex, and located more caudally.

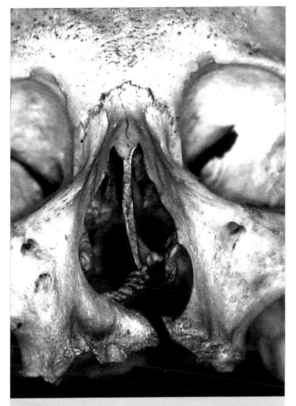

Fig. 2.28 Cleft lip- and cleft palate-nose on the left side. Skull. The piriform aperture on the CS is lower and narrower. The anterior nasal spine and the premaxilla are strongly deviating to the CS. A pronounced crest and spur are present on the CS. The bone of the inferior turbinate on the CS is lower and more lateral than on the NCS. Photo courtesy Prof. Pirsig.

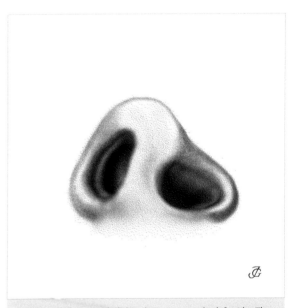

Fig. 2.29 Cleft lip- and cleft palate-nose on the left side. The lobule is severely asymmetrical: the dome and lateral crus on the CS are depressed and rotated in an anterior direction. The nostril is ovaloid and has an almost transverse axis. The vestibule is narrow. The columella is short and deviating to the CS. The caudal septum is deviating to the NCS

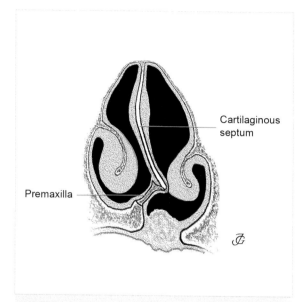

Fig. 2.30 Cleft lip- and cleft palate-nose on the left side. Septal deformity at the level of the premaxilla. The premaxilla deviates to the CS at a 45° angle. The cartilaginous septum and vomer are deviating to the left. A huge crest is present at the chondropremaxillary and chondrovomeral junction. The inferior turbinate is located lower and is somewhat compressed.

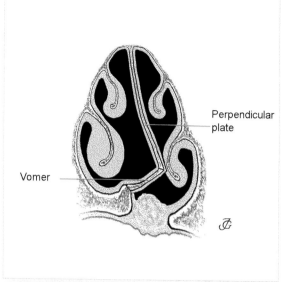

Fig. 2.31 Cleft lip- and cleft palate-nose on the left side. Deformity of the septum and turbinates at the level of the vomer. The perpendicular plate and vomer deviate to the CS. A pronounced crest and spur are usually present at the chondrovomeral and the perpendicular–vomeral junction. The inferior turbinate on the CS is compressed and positioned lower. The inferior turbinate on the NCS usually demonstrates compensatory hypertrophy.

the chondropremaxillary– and perpendicular–vomeral junction, a pronounced cartilaginous and bony crest and spur are present. Due to these skeletal distortions, the inferior part of the vomer is part of the nasal floor on the NCS (▶ Fig. 2.30 and ▶ Fig. 2.31).

The depressed ala usually contributes to stenosis of the valve area. The inferior turbinate on the CS is lower and compressed in a lateral direction. Its bony lamella is lower than normal. On the NCS, the inferior turbinate is usually compensatory hypertrophied. The middle turbinate on the CS is generally somewhat more slender than on the NCS.

2.1.12 Congenital Nasal Hypoplasia (Nasomaxillary Dysplasia, Binder Syndrome)

This syndrome is characterized by congenital underdevelopment of all nasal structures in combination with maxillary hypoplasia or retrusion. It is relatively rare and sporadic. In most cases, the cause is unclear. The bony and cartilaginous pyramids are low, wide, and underprojected. The lobule is flat and wide. The nostrils vary greatly in shape from round to square, and have a transverse axis. The tip is broad and sometimes bifid, the columella is short and broad, and the alae are abnormally convex (▶ Fig. 2.32 and ▶ Fig. 2.33). The septum is underdeveloped in an anterior and caudal direction and may be

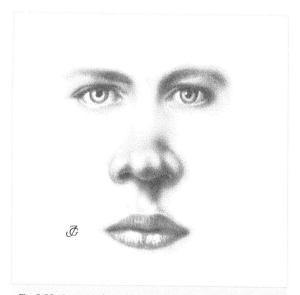

Fig. 2.32 Congenital nasal hypoplasia. The bony pyramid, cartilaginous pyramid, and lobule are low, wide, and short.

partially missing. The maxillary bones are hypoplastic and the midface is retruded (▶ Fig. 2.34). The anterior nasal spine is usually missing. This syndrome is sometimes called Binder syndrome (Binder 1962).

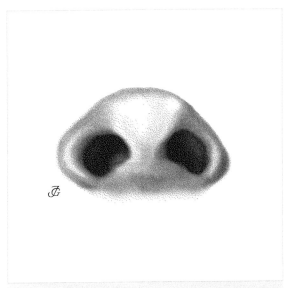

Fig. 2.33 Congenital nasal hypoplasia. The nostrils are square; the tip is broad and sometimes bifid; the columella is short and broad; the alae are round and abnormally convex.

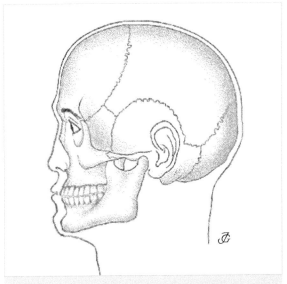

Fig. 2.34 Congenital nasal hypoplasia. The midface is underdeveloped and retruded.

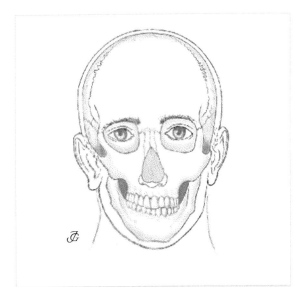

Fig. 2.35 Facial asymmetry. Asymmetry of the middle and lower thirds of the face, suggesting a severely deviating external nasal pyramid. In reality, there is only a limited septal and pyramidal deviation.

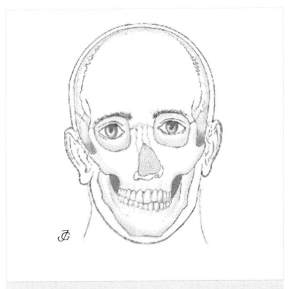

Fig. 2.36 Facial asymmetry. A similar case to ▶ Fig. 2.35, showing a combination of a deviation of the nose to the left and a concavity of the face to the right.

2.1.13 Facial Syndromes

Facial Asymmetries

The following facial asymmetries may be distinguished: the long-face syndrome, the short-face syndrome, maxillary protrusion, maxillary retrusion (midface hypoplasia), mandibular prognathism, and mandibular retrognathism. In this section, we restrict ourselves to a discussion of the syndromes that significantly affect the analysis and surgical correction of nasal deformities.

Left–Right Facial Asymmetry

Various elements of the skull and face are asymmetrical between the right and the left. Two examples are presented in ▶ Fig. 2.35 and ▶ Fig. 2.36, where the middle and lower part of the face is concave on the right. The external ear canal and auricle on the right are located

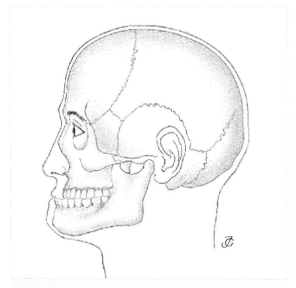

Fig. 2.37 Retroposition of the maxilla.

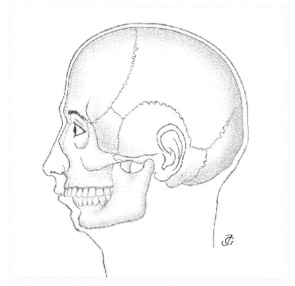

Fig. 2.38 Retroposition of the mandible.

lower than on the left side. The maxillary bones are asymmetrical, with a relative retroposition on the right. The mouth is displaced to the right, the left corner being somewhat lower than the right. The mandible is asymmetrical. The chin is displaced to the right. Because of the severe facial asymmetry, it is difficult to determine whether the nose is in the midline or deviated. For instance, when the trichion–nasion–stomion–gnathion line is drawn, the nose seems to be deviating to the left. When the trichion–nasion–tip line is drawn, the external pyramid appears straight. Both cases stress the importance of careful facial analysis. It is crucial to determine the position of the external pyramid in relation to the other facial structures.

Maxillary and Mandibular Retrusion

Maxillary Retrusion (Retroposition)

The maxilla is bilaterally or unilaterally retropositioned with respect to the frontal bones and the nasal pyramid. Bilateral retroposition of the maxilla and cheek accentuates the degree of prominence (projection) of the nose in relation to the face. Unilateral retropositioning may give (or accentuate) the impression that the external nose is leaning to that side. Retroposition of the maxilla may be examined clinically by studying the face from above with a flat object on both cheeks (▸ Fig. 2.37). Exact measurements may be made by X-ray cephalometry.

Mandibular Retrusion (Retroposition or Retrognathia)

Retrusion of the mandible, or retrognathia, is a common feature of the dolichocephalic skull. It is frequently seen in Caucasians (▸ Fig. 2.38). Retroposition of the mandible visually accentuates the prominence of the nasal pyramid. In these patients, "let-down" of the pyramid is therefore often combined with mentoplasty.

2.1.14 Nasal Neuralgias

Nasal or sinus disease is the most common cause of facial pain and headache. Branches of the palatine nerve become irritated, producing pain and pressure sensations that may be felt in a wide area of the head. It is customary for laymen and doctors alike to suspect some kind of "sinusitis." In many cases, however, the cause is found in the septum and the turbinates. Two syndromes may be distinguished as follows:
1. Pterygopalatine neuralgia or Sluder syndrome
2. Anterior and/or posterior ethmoidal neuralgia

Pterygopalatine Neuralgia (Vidian Neuralgia or Sluder Syndrome)

Branches of the pterygopalatine nerve (posterior–superior and posterior–inferior lateral nasal branches or posterior septal branches) become irritated by pressure or infection. The most common symptoms are *homolateral*-deep pain or pressure feelings localized paranasally and around the orbit, sometimes radiating towards the forehead and the back of the skull. It is often combined with increased homolateral secretion and nasal blockage. This type of cephalic neuralgia was first described as a specific entity by Greenfield Sluder (1908, 1913, 1927) and is therefore often referred to as Sluder syndrome. It is also called Vidian neuralgia.

Its most common cause is impaction of a septal deformity (usually a spur) into the posterior part of the inferior turbinate. Other causes may be a new growth, a foreign body, or an infection of the posterior–inferior half of the nasal cavity.

Diagnosis of pterygopalatine neuralgia is confirmed by the immediate relief of symptoms when the pterygopalatine ganglion is anesthetized (preferably with crystalline cocaine on the tip of a cotton wool applicator; see page 133 and ▶ Fig. 3.5). The more precisely localized the anesthesia, the better this type of neuralgia can be distinguished from other types, such as ethmoidal neuralgia. If a septal impaction is suspected as the likely cause of the Sluder-type of neuralgia, a test with local decongestion may be tried before applying anesthesia. If the pain stops when the turbinate is simply detached from the septum, the pain can be attributed to the septoturbinate contact. Septal surgery is often an effective treatment.

Anterior (Posterior) Ethmoidal Neuralgia

A similar syndrome may occur when branches of the anterior or posterior ethmoidal nerve are involved. Pain and pressure feelings are then perceived in and around the bony pyramid and nasal root, paranasally, medially, and posteriorly in the homolateral orbit and the forehead. Ophthalmic symptoms frequently occur, especially tearing. The syndrome may then be called Charlin syndrome or nasociliary neuralgia (Charlin 1930). Its most common cause is obstruction of the middle nasal passage or the infundibulum, as discussed and illustrated in the section on middle meatus obstructive syndrome (see page 73). Another variant of anterior ethmoidal neuralgia is open roof syndrome.

2.2 Nasal Symptoms—The Most Common Deformities, Abnormalities, and Anatomical Variations

The human nose is subject to a wide array of deformities, abnormalities, and anatomical variations.

Deformity: Whether we are dealing with a deformity is rarely a matter of discussion. Congenital malformations of the nose like those in cleft-lip patients, nasal hypoplasia, or bifidity are clearly deformities. The same applies to acquired anomalies of the nose as may occur after trauma, infection, or new growth. Deviated nose, saddle nose, open roof, retracted columella, and septal deviation, to name a few, are considered deformities.

Abnormality: An abnormality may be defined as a "pathological anatomical change." Frequently, an abnormality implies functional disturbance. This is not always the case, however. Generally, a slight posttraumatic sagging of the cartilaginous dorsum, flaccid alae, or an over-projected tip are abnormalities.

Anatomical variation: Deciding when an anatomical condition should be considered an anatomical variation may be more difficult, as this is often a matter of personal opinion. Many variations are, to a certain extent, dependent on race, gender, or age, and have therefore to be considered within the normal range.

2.2.1 Pathology and Variations of Nasal Dimensions

The human external nose may vary considerably in all its dimensions. Interindividual differences are determined by ethnic factors, gender, age, and pathological influences due to injury and infection. We define these differences in terms of: size (small–large), length (long–short), height, prominence (prominent–low), and width (wide–narrow) (▶ Fig. 2.39).

Long Nose (▶ Fig. 2.40)

The distance nasion–tip is abnormally large, often in combination with excessive height. The pyramid may be prominent and narrow, and the tip is often drooping. The nasolabial angle is more acute than average. A long nose may be caused by genetic as well as endocrine factors. The external nasal pyramid tends to lengthen with increasing age. A long nose may also result from surgery when a dorsal hump has been resected without shortening nasal length.

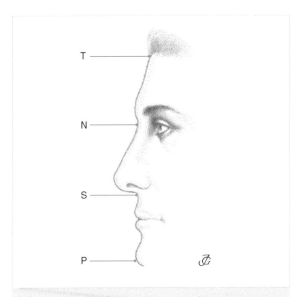

Fig. 2.39 Normal facial dimensions. T = trichion; N = nasion; S = subnasale; P = pogonion. The distance T–N equals N–S equals S–P.

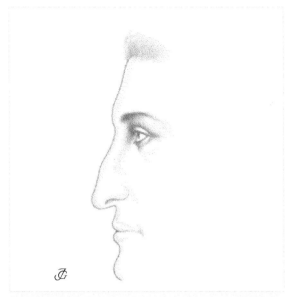

Fig. 2.40 Long nose. The nasion–tip distance is abnormally large compared to the trichion–nasion distance and subnasale–pogonion distance.

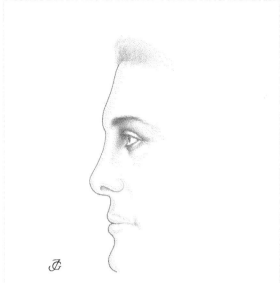

Fig. 2.41 Short nose. The nasion–tip distance is abnormally small compared to the trichion–nasion distance and subnasale–pogonion distance.

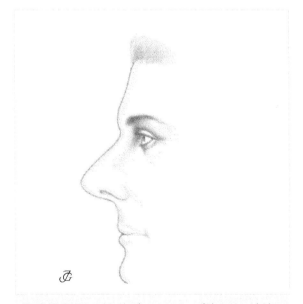

Fig. 2.42 Prominent nose. The projection of the pyramid (the dorsum–nasal base line distance) is larger than normal.

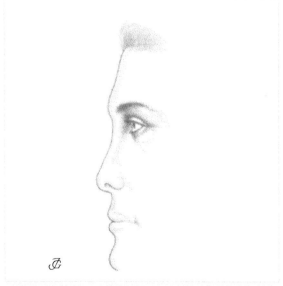

Fig. 2.43 Low nose. The projection of the pyramid (the dorsum–nasal base line distance) is smaller than normal.

Short Nose (▶ Fig. 2.41)

The distance nasion–tip is shorter than normal. This is always combined with diminished height. The pyramid is generally wide and less prominent than normal. The nasolabial angle is relatively large. A short nose is seen in patients with congenital nasal hypoplasia or impaired nasal growth. It may also occur after surgery where the nasal tip has been upwardly rotated too much.

Prominent Nose (▶ Fig. 2.42)

The projection (prominence, salience) of the external nasal pyramid is greater than normal. Usually, the nose is long and narrow.

Low Nose (▶ Fig. 2.43)

The projection of the nasal pyramid is less than normal. In most cases, the nose is also short and wide. A low nose

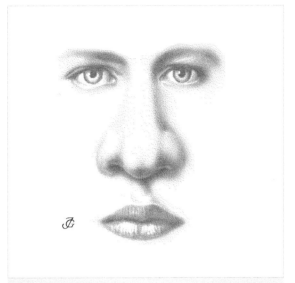

Fig. 2.44 Wide nose. The width of the pyramid (the distance between the left and right baselines) is larger than normal.

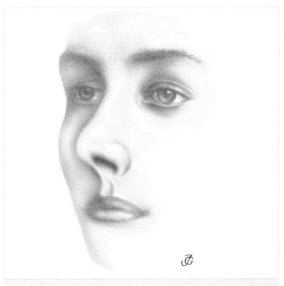

Fig. 2.45 Narrow nose. The width of the pyramid (the distance between the left and right baselines) is smaller than normal.

is often combined with a concave nasal dorsum. We then speak of a saddle nose, a sagging dorsum, or low-wide pyramid syndrome (see also ▶ Fig. 2.13, ▶ Fig. 2.14, ▶ Fig. 2.15, ▶ Fig. 2.16, and ▶ Fig. 2.17).

Wide Nose (▶ Fig. 2.44)

The width (horizontal dimension) of the nasal pyramid is abnormally large. In most cases, the bony pyramid, the cartilaginous pyramid, and the lobule are unusually wide. Usually, the nose is both shorter and less prominent than normal.

Narrow Nose (▶ Fig. 2.45)

The width of the nasal pyramid is small. This condition is generally combined with a greater length and prominence. We then speak of prominent-narrow pyramid syndrome (see also ▶ Fig. 2.10, ▶ Fig. 2.11, and ▶ Fig. 2.12).

"Greek Nose" (▶ Fig. 2.46)

The forehead and nasal dorsum are almost in line. The frontonasal angle is almost 180°. This profile was adopted in ancient Greece as the ideal and was used in sculptures of gods and heroes.

2.2.2 Humps

A hump is a convexity of the nasal dorsum. When both the bony and the cartilaginous pyramid are involved, we speak of a hump nose. To a certain extent, a hump nose may be considered a syndrome (see page 67), though a hump may also occur in isolation as a deformity or

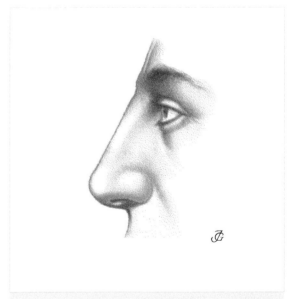

Fig. 2.46 "Greek" nose. The nasofrontal angle is almost 180°.

variation. Sometimes it is seen along with pathology of the septum and pyramid. We distinguish the bony hump, the cartilaginous hump, a combination of these two, and the relative hump or pseudohump.

Bony and Cartilaginous Hump (▶ Fig. 2.47)

Both the bony and the cartilaginous dorsum are convex (humped). The maximum convexity is usually located at the K area. This type of hump may be of genetic or

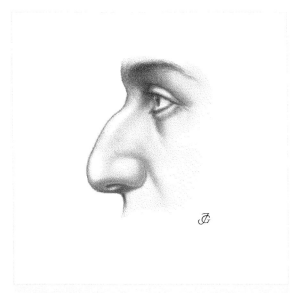

Fig. 2.47 Bony and cartilaginous hump. Both the bony and cartilaginous dorsum are abnormally convex.

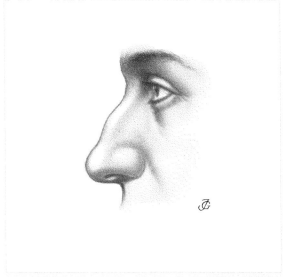

Fig. 2.48 Bony hump. The bony dorsum is abnormally convex and projecting.

traumatic origin. In some ethnic groups, a convex nasal dorsum is normal.

Bony Hump (▶ Fig. 2.48)

The convexity is confined to the bony pyramid. A bony hump is usually due to previous trauma or to inadequate surgery.

Cartilaginous Hump (▶ Fig. 2.49)

The convexity is limited to the cartilaginous dorsum. A cartilaginous hump is usually of traumatic origin. It may also be of genetic origin, or occur as a side effect of inadequate lobular surgery, resulting in loss of tip projection.

Relative Bony Hump (▶ Fig. 2.50)

The bony dorsum seems overprojected due to saddling of the cartilaginous pyramid. The convexity of the bony dorsum is relative, which means we are dealing with a pseudohump. The condition is often misdiagnosed by both patient and doctor. The underlying cause is usually a defective anterior septum. Treatment must therefore consist of septal reconstruction with an additional transplant, rather than resection of the pseudohump.

2.2.3 Saddling and Sagging

Saddling (a saddle) and sagging denote concavity of the nasal dorsum. This is often due to extensive pathology, such as the low-wide pyramid syndrome (see page 70). It may be an isolated deformity, or it may occur in combination with other types of pathology. We distinguish the

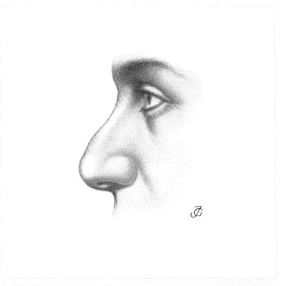

Fig. 2.49 Cartilaginous hump. The cartilaginous dorsum is abnormally convex and projecting.

bony saddle, the cartilaginous saddle or sagging, the linea nasalis dorsalis, the dorsal step, and sagging of the supratip area.

Bony and Cartilaginous Saddle Nose (▶ Fig. 2.51)

Both the bony and cartilaginous dorsum are concave. The pyramid is broad and low. A bony and cartilaginous saddle nose is one of the most common nasal deformities. It may produce both functional and aesthetic complaints. The most

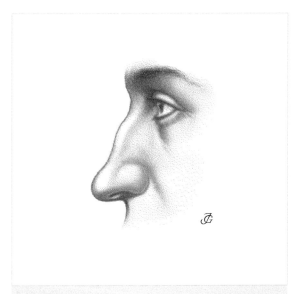

Fig. 2.50 Relative bony hump. The bony dorsum seems overprojected due to sagging of the cartilaginous dorsum.

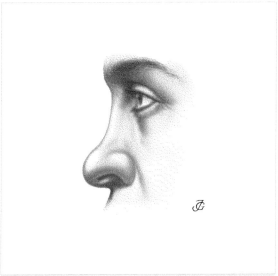

Fig. 2.51 Bony and cartilaginous saddle nose. Both the bony and cartilaginous dorsum are abnormally concave and low.

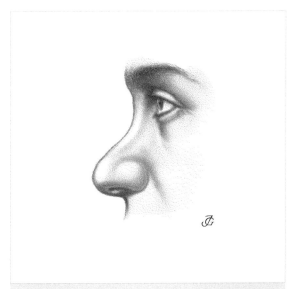

Fig. 2.52 Bony saddle. The bony dorsum is abnormally concave and low.

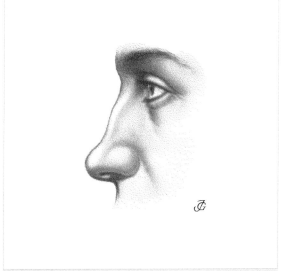

Fig. 2.53 Cartilaginous saddle. The cartilaginous dorsum is abnormally concave and low.

common causes are destruction of the anterior septum by infection and/or severe trauma in childhood, and severe frontal trauma with impression of the external pyramid.

Bony Saddle (▶ Fig. 2.52)

The bony pyramid is concave, while the cartilaginous dorsum is normal. This is a relatively rare type of pathology. It may result from a traumatic frontal impression of the bony pyramid, or arise after over-resection of a bony hump.

Cartilaginous Saddle (▶ Fig. 2.53)

The cartilaginous dorsum is concave, while the bony pyramid is normal. This is the most common type of saddling. It is invariably related to septal pathology. A defective anterior septum due to trauma, infection, or inadequate surgery is the most common underlying cause.

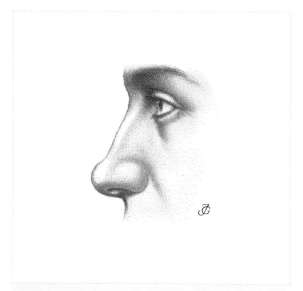

Fig. 2.54 Cartilaginous sagging. The cartilaginous dorsum is slightly depressed due to loss of support.

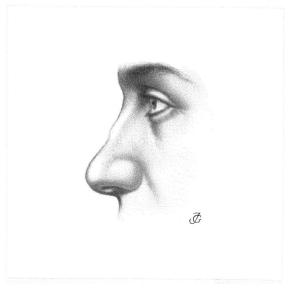

Fig. 2.55 Dorsal step. The continuity between the bony and cartilaginous pyramid is disrupted, leading to a local depression.

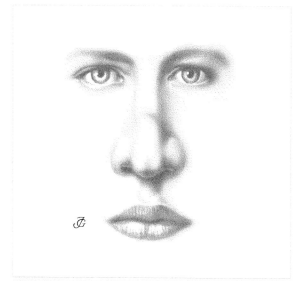

Fig. 2.56 Dorsal step. The continuity between the bony and cartilaginous pyramid is disrupted, leading to a local impression.

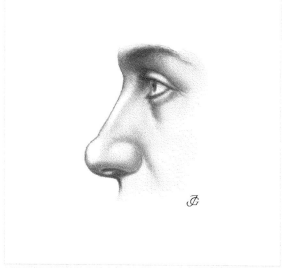

Fig. 2.57 Sagging of the supratip area.

Cartilaginous Sagging (▶ Fig. 2.54)

Sagging of the cartilaginous dorsum is a minor variant of saddling and has the same origin.

Dorsal Step (▶ Fig. 2.55 and ▶ Fig. 2.56)

The bony and the cartilaginous pyramid are detached at the K area. The continuity between the bony and the cartilaginous part of the nose is disrupted. A "step" is present at the junction between the nasal bones and the triangular cartilages, usually caused by frontal trauma with impression of the cartilaginous pyramid and septum. A dorsal step may cause considerable cosmetic complaints.

Sagging of the Supratip Area (▶ Fig. 2.57)

The area just cranial to the tip is depressed. This may be the result of localized trauma or may occur after septal and lobular surgery.

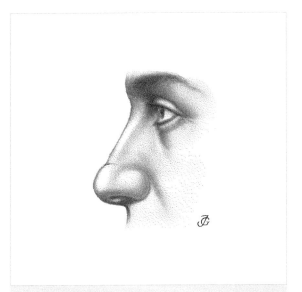

Fig. 2.58 Linea nasalis dorsalis. A horizontal crease in the skin just cranial to the lobule.

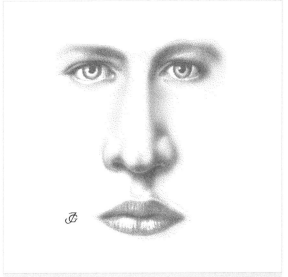

Fig. 2.59 Asymmetry of the bony pyramid. The bony pyramid has unequal lateral walls in terms of size and/or position.

Linea Nasalis Dorsalis (▶ Fig. 2.58)

The linea nasalis dorsalis is a horizontal crease in the skin of the cartilaginous dorsum just cranial to the lobule. It is seen in patients with chronic secretory rhinitis as a result of permanent sniffing and wiping of the nose. It may also occur as a minor variant of sagging of the cartilaginous dorsum.

2.2.4 Bony and Cartilaginous Pyramid

Other important conditions affecting the bony and/or cartilaginous pyramid that occur as isolated symptoms or in combination with other pathology are: asymmetry of the pyramid, irregularity of the bony pyramid, a lateral "step," a defect of the bony pyramid, an open roof, asymmetry of the cartilaginous pyramid, disruption of the triangular–bony junction, and atrophy of the cartilaginous pyramid.

Asymmetry of the Bony Pyramid (▶ Fig. 2.59)

The two sides of the bony pyramid are unequal in terms of position and length. This is often seen in patients with a deviated pyramid with impression of one of the bony walls. This asymmetry is caused by trauma or inadequate repositioning of the bony pyramid after osteotomies.

Irregularity of the Bony Pyramid (▶ Fig. 2.60)

The bony dorsum or the lateral bony wall is irregular. Irregularities do not always cause symptoms and might

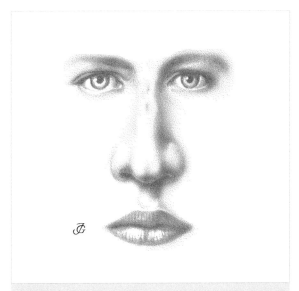

Fig. 2.60 Irregularity of the bony pyramid.

only be noticed on palpation. In some cases, they are clearly visible, and tender on palpation. Irregularities can be made more evident by stretching the overlying skin. They are usually caused by traumatic fractures, but may also be due to incomplete or asymmetrical hump removal with insufficient smoothing of the dorsum. Furthermore, they may result from inadequate repositioning of the bony walls after osteotomies.

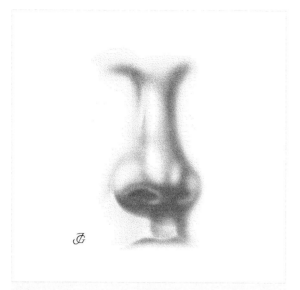

Fig. 2.61 Lateral step. On the lateral wall of the bony pyramid, a ridge is visible and palpable.

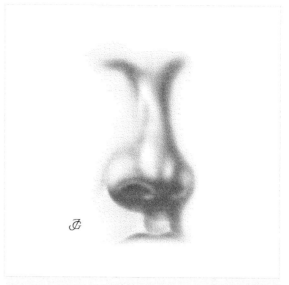

Fig. 2.62 Defect of the bony pyramid. A defect of the lateral wall or dorsum of the bony pyramid is visible and/or palpable.

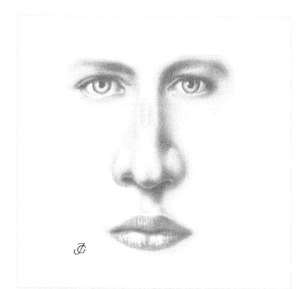

Fig. 2.63 Open roof. A defect of the bony dorsum. This abnormality is usually caused by a hump resection without proper reconstruction of the dorsum.

Lateral Step (▶ Fig. 2.61)

On the lateral bony wall, a ridge or groove is visible and/or palpable. This deformity is mostly caused by a high lateral osteotomy and (too much) infraction of the bone.

Defect of the Bony Pyramid (▶ Fig. 2.62)

A defect of the bony pyramid may occur after severe trauma with multiple fractures and dislocation or necrosis of bony fragments.

Open Roof (▶ Fig. 2.63)

The bony dorsum is defective. This is most commonly due to a hump resection without adequate closure of the resulting defect of the bony pyramid. An open roof is usually diagnosed by palpation. Large defects are sometimes visible too. Various neuralgic symptoms may occur. We then speak of an "open roof syndrome" (see page 72).

Asymmetry of the Cartilaginous Pyramid (▶ Fig. 2.64)

The lateral walls (i.e., triangular cartilages) are unequal in position and length. The cartilaginous septum is usually deformed, too; it is either dislocated or defective. Both function and nasal aesthetics are impaired. This asymmetry results mostly from trauma or impaired nasal growth.

Dorsal Step (see ▶ Fig. 2.55 and ▶ Fig. 2.56)

A dorsal step is due to disruption of the junction between the triangular cartilages and the nasal bones. The attachment of the cranial margin of the triangular cartilage to the undersurface of the caudal border of the nasal bone is disrupted. A depression at the upper part of the triangular cartilage is visible and palpable.

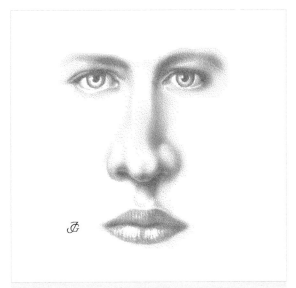

Fig. 2.64 Asymmetry of cartilaginous pyramid.

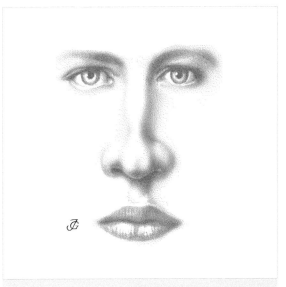

Fig. 2.65 Atrophy of the cartilaginous pyramid.

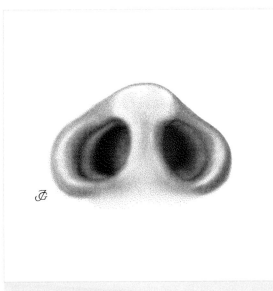

Fig. 2.66 Low and wide lobule.

Atrophy of the Cartilaginous Pyramid (▶ Fig. 2.65)

The triangular cartilages are atrophied and partially missing, having been replaced by scar tissue. The lateral soft or hinge area may be scarred, atrophied, and retracted. The lateral wall of the valve is weakened and collapsible, which may cause impairment of inspiratory breathing. This pathology is usually the result of (repeated) trauma, a dorsal hematoma, and/or infection.

2.2.5 Lobule

Low, Wide Lobule (▶ Fig. 2.66)

The lobule is low and wide at all levels (tip, nares, and base). The tip is broad and underprojected or depressed. The alae are convex, the columella short, the nostrils more or less round. The vestibules are wide and low. The tip index is large. A low and wide lobule is normal among black people and, to a lesser degree, Asians. In Caucasians, it is only seen in newborns and infants. The condition may also be caused by retardation of nasal growth after trauma or a septal abscess at a young age (see also page 49 and ▶ Fig. 1.118a-h).

High, Narrow Lobule (▶ Fig. 2.67)

The lobule is prominent and narrow, the tip narrow and pointed, the alae long and stretched, and the columella long. The nostrils are narrow and the vestibules high and narrow. The tip index is small. A high, narrow lobule is common in Caucasians, especially in combination with dolichocephaly (see also ▶ Fig. 2.11 and ▶ Fig. 2.12).

Tip

Broad Tip (▶ Fig. 2.68)

The tip is broad and usually round (ballooning). The domes are wide, convex, and sometimes far apart. The skin is generally thick. This variation has no functional consequences.

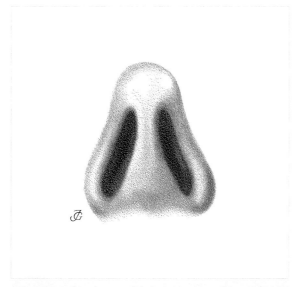

Fig. 2.67 High and narrow lobule.

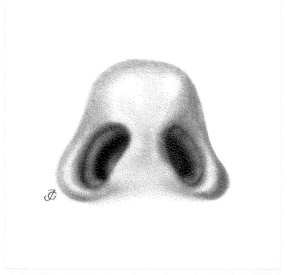

Fig. 2.68 Broad tip.

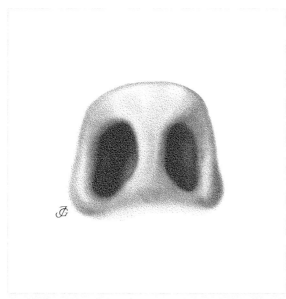

Fig. 2.69 Square tip.

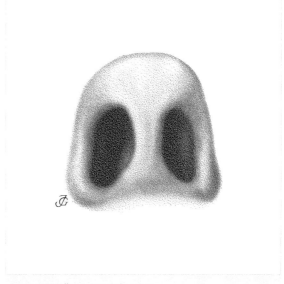

Fig. 2.70 Bulbous (amorphous) tip.

Square Tip (▶ Fig. 2.69)

The tip is broad and square. The domes are wide and more or less double angulated. The skin is usually thick. Nasal function is not impaired.

Bulbous (Amorphous) Tip (▶ Fig. 2.70)

The tip is massive and undefined because of a thick skin and an abnormally large amount of subcutaneous connective, fatty, and glandular tissue. The lobular cartilages are usually large and thick. Nasal function is usually not compromised.

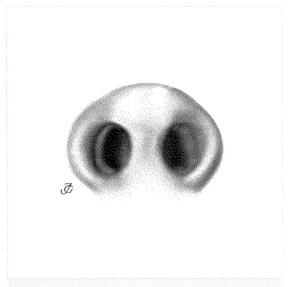

Fig. 2.71 Ball tip.

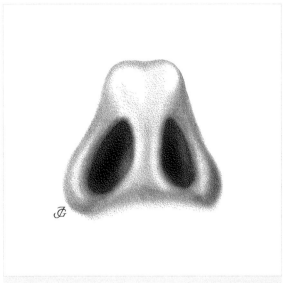

Fig. 2.72 Bifid tip, double tip, distended tip.

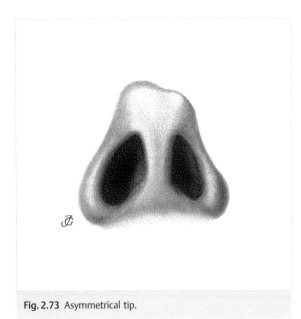

Fig. 2.73 Asymmetrical tip.

Ball Tip (▶ Fig. 2.71)

The tip is round both in its horizontal and vertical dimension due to round and wide domes.

Bifid Tip, Double Tip, Distended Tip (▶ Fig. 2.72)

The tip is double, and the distance between the two domes is abnormally large. Between the two domes is a vertical groove or depression of the skin that may continue in a vertical columellar groove. Bifidity of the nasal tip is a congenital anomaly caused by incomplete fusion of the two nasal processes in embryonic life. Complaints due to a bifid tip are only aesthetic in nature.

Asymmetrical Tip (▶ Fig. 2.73)

The tip is asymmetrical due to differences in the size and position of the two domes. Asymmetry of the tip may be congenital but may also result from inadequate tip or lobular surgery. Cleft lip is another well-known cause.

Overprojected Tip (▶ Fig. 2.74)

The tip is abnormally prominent (projected) in relation to the level of the cartilaginous and bony pyramid. An overprojected tip may occur as an isolated congenital abnormality. It may also be associated with a prominent narrow lobule with a long columella and slitlike nostrils.

Underprojected Tip (▶ Fig. 2.75)

The tip is abnormally low (depressed) in relation to the cartilaginous and bony pyramid. An underprojected tip may occur as an isolated congenital abnormality. It may also be due to retraction of the columella and the membranous septum as a result of a defective anterior septum.

Upwardly Rotated Tip (▶ Fig. 2.76)

The nasolabial angle is abnormally large. This may occur as a congenital anomaly in individuals with a very short nose. It is also seen after rhinoplasty cases in which the nose was shortened too much.

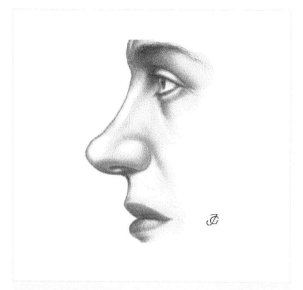

Fig. 2.74 Overprojected tip.

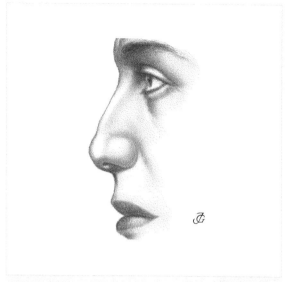

Fig. 2.75 Underprojected tip.

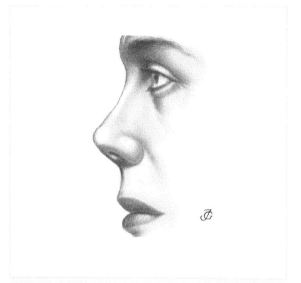

Fig. 2.76 Upwardly rotated tip.

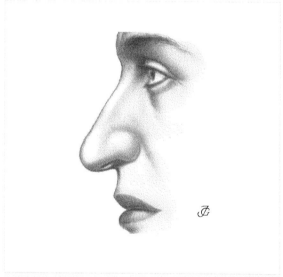

Fig. 2.77 Hanging (pendant, drooping) tip.

Hanging (Pendant, Drooping) Tip (▶ Fig. 2.77)

The tip is low and hanging, and the nasolabial angle is abnormally small. This is seen in the elderly, particularly in males, and is caused by increasing laxity of the soft tissues. It is also seen as a complication following rhinoplasty. It may occur for various reasons; for example, after an external approach by retraction of the columella and membranous septum, or due to loss of support of the domes following the luxation technique.

Alae

Thin Alae (▶ Fig. 2.78)

The alae are thin, usually long, and less convex than average. They are more or less "stretched" and often flaccid as a result of pronounced growth of the septum. Thin and flaccid alae, especially when combined with slitlike nostrils, easily collapse on inspiration. Thin alae are generally part of a prominent, narrow lobule.

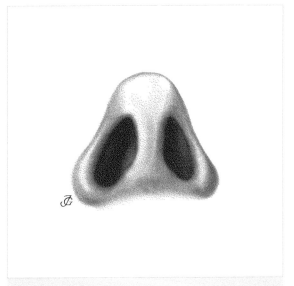

Fig. 2.78 Thin alae.

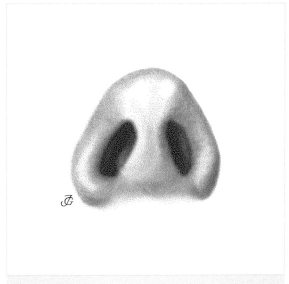

Fig. 2.79 Thick alae.

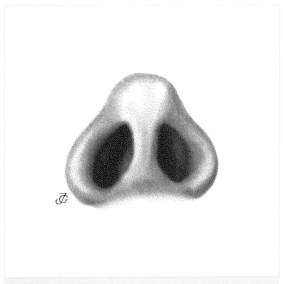

Fig. 2.80 Convex (ballooning) alae.

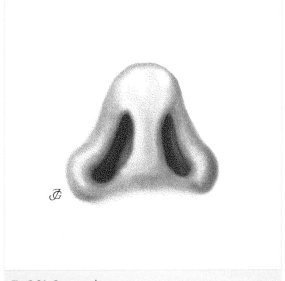

Fig. 2.81 Concave alae.

Thick Alae (▶ Fig. 2.79)

The alae are thick and usually short. This is mainly due to the thickness of the skin and the subcutaneous tissue. The condition may be part of a low, wide lobule, though it also occurs in isolation.

Convex (Ballooning) Alae (▶ Fig. 2.80)

The alae are strongly curved or ballooning, and the lateral crus is abnormally convex.

Concave Alae (▶ Fig. 2.81)

The alae are concave and may show a deep furrow. In pronounced cases, inspiratory collapse may occur.

Asymmetrical Alae (▶ Fig. 2.82)

The alae are asymmetrical, either as part of a congenital malformation, or as a result of trauma or surgery. A unilateral cleft lip is the most common cause. In this entity, the ala is shorter and abnormally convex while the alar base is located in a more cranial position.

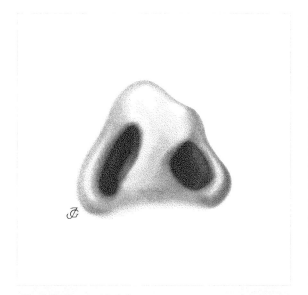

Fig. 2.82 Asymmetrical alae.

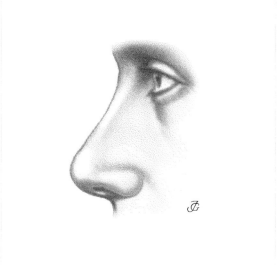

Fig. 2.83 Pronounced horizontal alar groove.

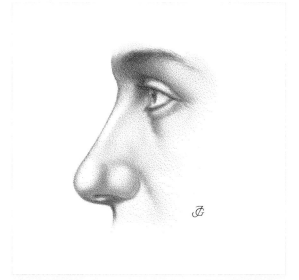

Fig. 2.84 Pronounced vertical alar groove.

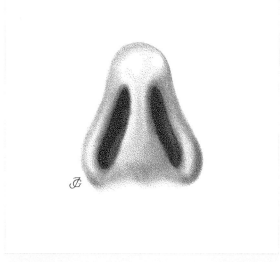

Fig. 2.85 Long columella.

Pronounced Horizontal Alar Groove (▶ Fig. 2.83)

The ala shows a horizontal groove. This may be due to a congenital concavity of the lateral crus, or the result of over-resection of cartilage from its cranial margin.

Pronounced Vertical Alar Groove (▶ Fig. 2.84)

The ala shows a vertical groove at the transition between the dome and the lateral crus. This is usually congenital but may also result from cutting through the dome in lobular surgery.

Columella

Long Columella (▶ Fig. 2.85)

The columella is long and generally narrow. This abnormality is seen in the prominent-narrow pyramid syndrome (see page 69).

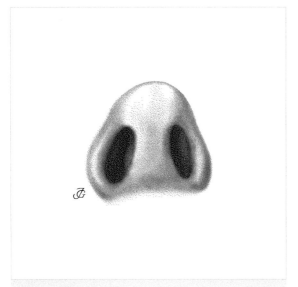

Fig. 2.86 Short columella.

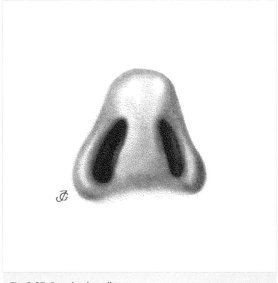

Fig. 2.87 Broad columella.

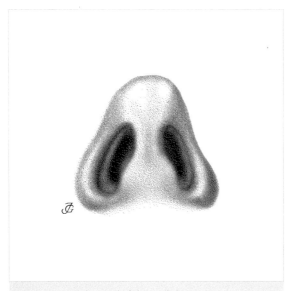

Fig. 2.88 Protruding end of the medial crura.

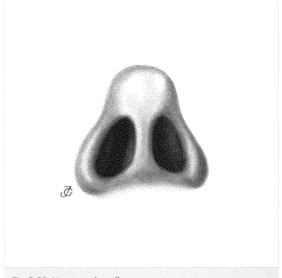

Fig. 2.89 Narrow columella.

Short Columella (▶ Fig. 2.86)

The columella is short and usually broad. This is seen in the congenitally wide, low lobule, and as part of the low-wide pyramid syndrome (see page 70).

Broad Columella (▶ Fig. 2.87)

The columella is abnormally broad and usually short. This variation is almost always congenital. The two medial crura are far apart, separated by an abnormal amount of connective tissue. A broad columella may show a vertical columellar groove (see ▶ Fig. 2.94).

Protruding End of Medial Crura (▶ Fig. 2.88)

The end of one or both medial crura is abnormally curled and protrudes into the vestibule. Inspiratory breathing may be impaired, especially when this abnormality is combined with a narrow nostril, a dislocated caudal end of the septum, or a thin, flaccid ala.

Narrow Columella (▶ Fig. 2.89)

The columella is narrow and usually long. This variation is seen in Caucasians in the prominent-narrow pyramid syndrome.

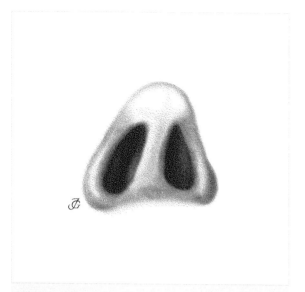

Fig. 2.90 Oblique columella.

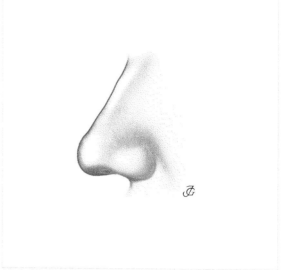

Fig. 2.91 Retracted (hidden) columella.

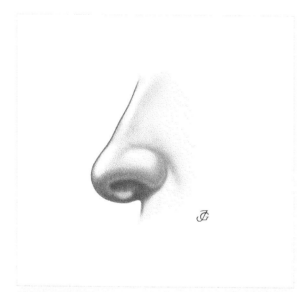

Fig. 2.92 Hanging ("showing") columella.

Oblique Columella (▶ Fig. 2.90)

The most common cause of an oblique columella is dislocation of the caudal end of the septum. It is also seen in congenital asymmetries of the lobule such as in cleft-lip patients, or following surgery.

Retracted (Hidden) Columella (▶ Fig. 2.91)

The columella, in particular its base, is retracted in a cranial direction. Its lower margin is above the level of the alar rim. When the nose is examined from the side, the columellar base is "hidden" by the ala. The nasolabial angle is smaller than normal. Retraction of the columella may be caused by a defective caudal septal end, scarring of the membranous septum, or by a fractured or resected anterior nasal spine. A midcolumellar retraction may be caused by undesired scarring of a horizontal columellar incision, as in the external approach.

Hanging ("Showing") Columella (▶ Fig. 2.92)

The columella is abnormally low in relation to the alae. Its lower part is usually curved to some extent, or "hanging." When the nose is inspected from the side, too much of the columella is visible. This may cause cosmetic complaints. Nasal function is not impaired. A hanging columella may be of congenital origin or the result of lobular surgery.

Asymmetrical Columella (▶ Fig. 2.93)

The left and right halves of the columella are unequal in level or width. This may be caused by asymmetry of the medial crura or by dislocation of the caudal end of the septum. An unequal lower margin of the columella is usually a complication of surgery, for example asymmetrical suturing of the infracartilaginous incision or asymmetrical septocolumellar sutures.

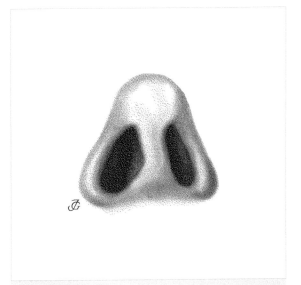

Fig. 2.93 Asymmetrical columella.

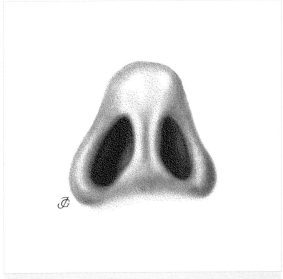

Fig. 2.94 Bifid columella.

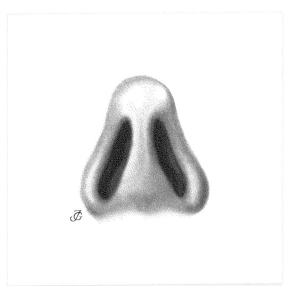

Fig. 2.95 Narrow (slitlike) nostril.

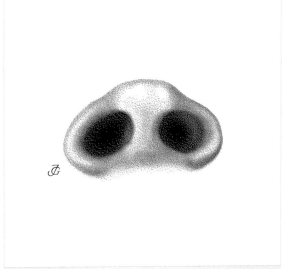

Fig. 2.96 Wide nostril.

Bifid Columella (▶ Fig. 2.94)

The columella shows a more or less pronounced vertical groove between the medial crura. This is a sign of incomplete fusion of the left and right nasal primordium during development. The condition is similar to the bifid tip. These developmental abnormalities are often seen together.

Nostrils (Nares)

Narrow (Slitlike) Nostril (▶ Fig. 2.95)

The nostrils are narrow and elongated, resembling a slit to a certain degree. This is seen in Caucasians as part of a prominent, narrow lobule.

Wide Nostril (▶ Fig. 2.96)

The nares are wide and often circular or, to some extent, square. This is seen among black people and Asians, and in the pathologically low, wide lobule.

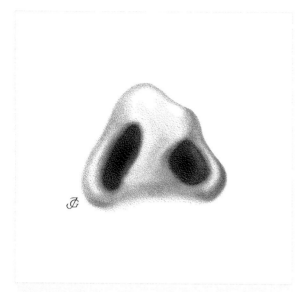

Fig. 2.97 Asymmetrical nostrils.

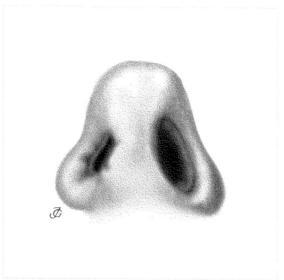

Fig. 2.98 Stenosis of the nostril.

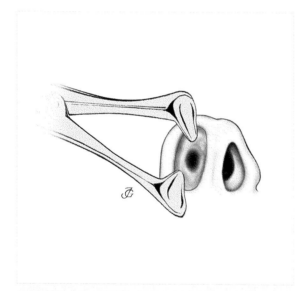

Fig. 2.99 Stenosis of the vestibule (scarring).

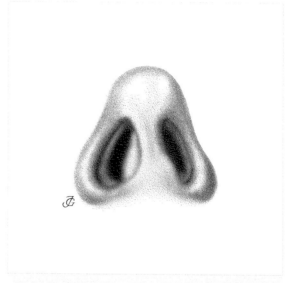

Fig. 2.100 Stenosis of the vestibule (subluxation).

Asymmetrical Nostrils (▶ Fig. 2.97)

The nares are asymmetrical in size, shape, and/or position. The columella is asymmetrical and oblique. This is seen in congenital anomalies, particularly in cleft-lip patients, and in cases with traumatic deformities of the anterior septum and cartilaginous pyramid.

Stenosis of the Nostril (▶ Fig. 2.98)

Stenosis of the nostril is seen in congenital malformations, such as cleft-lip. Another common cause is soft-tissue trauma (e.g., traumatic avulsion of the ala, dog bites, accidental caustic damage from treating epistaxis). It may also occur following surgery when too many incisions have been made in the vestibule, particularly when they have been inadequately sutured.

Vestibule

Stenosis of the Vestibule (▶ Fig. 2.99 and ▶ Fig. 2.100)

The most common cause of vestibular stenosis is dislocation of the caudal part of the cartilaginous septum. Other causes are congenital malformations, such as cleft lip, and

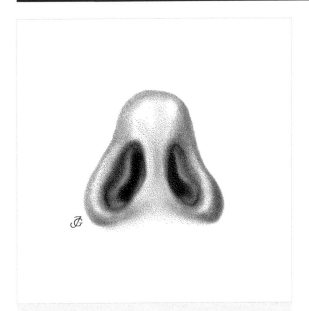

Fig. 2.101 Protrusion of the lateral crura.

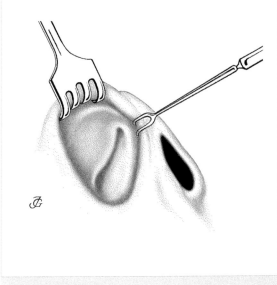

Fig. 2.102 Narrow valve area.

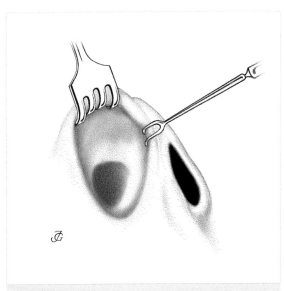

Fig. 2.103 Wide valve area.

scarring following soft-tissue trauma. Vestibular deformities are often combined with deformities of the nostril, columella, and valve area. Breathing, especially inspiration, is usually severely disturbed.

Stenosis of the vestibule may be caused by dislocation and protrusion of the septal caudal end (subluxation).

Protrusion of the Lateral Crura (▶ Fig. 2.101)

The lower margin of the lateral crus protrudes into the vestibule. This may cause inspiratory collapse of the vestibule. It may occur after lobular modifying surgery, or

when the connection between the lobular cartilage and the triangular cartilage is disrupted.

2.2.6 Valve Area

Narrow Valve Area (▶ Fig. 2.102)

The valve area is narrow and high, and the valve angle is abnormally small (less than 20°). This is seen in Caucasians in prominent-narrow pyramid syndrome. Other common causes are septal deviations and convexities, abnormalities of the triangular cartilage, and too much infraction of the lateral bony wall after osteotomy.

Wide Valve Area (▶ Fig. 2.103)

The valve area is wide and low, and the valve angle is abnormally large. A wide valve area is normal in black people and Asians. In Caucasians, a wide valve area is a common feature of low-narrow pyramid syndrome or saddle nose. In these cases, the valve area is usually more circular than triangular. The valve angle is large and may even measure 80 to 90°. This is seen in patients with a missing anterior septum with retraction of the soft tissues that have replaced the septal cartilage. Nasal breathing may be subjectively disturbed because of an abnormal inspiratory airstream.

Obstructed Valve Area (▶ Fig. 2.104)

The nasal valve area may be obstructed for a number of reasons. Narrowing of the valve area may be related to the septum, triangular cartilage, nasal mucosa, or head of the inferior turbinate, or to synechiae, scarring of the

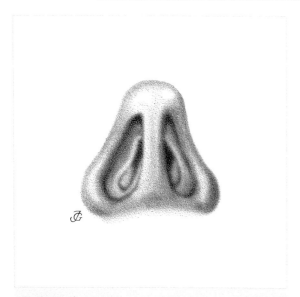

Fig. 2.104 Obstructed (narrow) valve area.

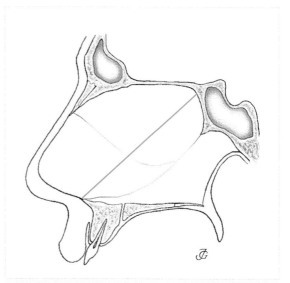

Fig. 2.105 Gray's line. Septal fractures anterior to this line tend to be vertically oriented, whereas those posterior to this line are usually horizontally oriented.

vestibule, nasal form (high, narrow pyramid), or a combination of these pathologies. (For a clear overview, see Kern 1978.) Inspiratory breathing is impaired even in minor pathology.

2.2.7 Septum

Pathology of the septum ranks high among the deformities of the human body. It has been stated that a normal septum is rare. Fortunately, many septal deformities do not cause functional complaints. The degree and location of the deformity determine the likelihood and severity of symptoms.

Classification of Septal Pathology

Classification of septal deformities may be based on their morphology, localization, etiology, and complaints (functional effects).

Morphology

From the very beginning of rhinology as a clinical science in the last quarter of the 19th century, it has been common practice to describe septal deformities on the basis of their morphological character. Terms such as septal deviations, crests, spurs (spines), and convexities are generally accepted. These descriptive terms are understood by every rhinologist and should therefore not be replaced by complicated systems. Some authors have tried to integrate the various deformities in a simple system, for example Mladina (1987), who has proposed a division into seven classes.

Localization

Septal deformities may be distinguished on the basis of their location. We may thus speak of a basal crest, a posterior spine, or an anterior deviation. In this respect, one may add the Cottle area where the deformity is localized (see page 15). An alternative is to use specific anatomical terms to indicate the location of the deformity, such as nostril, vestibule, valve area, middle (inferior) meatus, infundibulum, and choana.

Etiology

Septal pathology may also be classified in terms of its cause: genetic, developmental, traumatic, or infectious. Traumatic deformities may be classified into frontal, lateral, basal, frontolateral, or basolateral, according to the (likely) impact of the injury. Vernon Gray has drawn attention to the fact that fractures ventral to an imaginary line drawn from the anterior wall of the sphenoid bone to the anterior nasal spine (Gray's line) are mostly vertically oriented, and those dorsal to this line are mostly horizontally oriented (▶ Fig. 2.105).

Function

Finally, septal deformities may be subdivided on the basis of the leading symptom. Although instructive, this is not common practice.

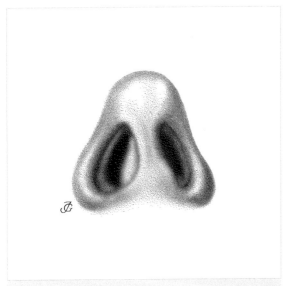

Fig. 2.106 Dislocated caudal septal end.

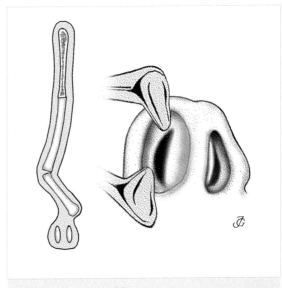

Fig. 2.107 Single vertical fracture.

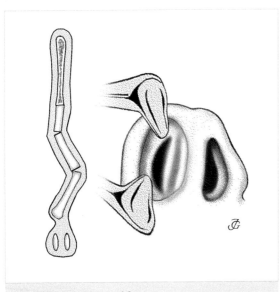

Fig. 2.108 Multiple vertical fractures.

Specific Septal Pathology

Dislocated Caudal Septal End (▶ Fig. 2.106)

The caudal end of the cartilaginous septum is dislocated to one side, so that it protrudes into the vestibule and the nostril. This is a common type of pathology. It may lead to breathing obstruction, vestibulitis with crusting, and to cosmetic complaints. A caudal septal dislocation is often combined with a vertical septal fracture at the level of the valve area on the opposite side. It is generally caused by trauma with a (baso)lateral impact. If the causative injury occurred in childhood, the septum may show excessive growth in the caudal direction, causing an ugly protrusion into the nostril.

Single Vertical Fracture (▶ Fig. 2.107)

The cartilaginous septum is fractured in a craniocaudal direction due to an injury with a lateral or laterobasal impact on the cartilaginous part of the external pyramid. The vertical fracture line is usually located at the level of the piriform aperture (i.e., the valve area) on the side of the impact. A vertical fracture is usually associated with dislocation of the caudal end of the septum to the other side. The external pyramid shows deviation of the cartilaginous pyramid to the opposite side. Severe inspiratory breathing obstruction, or even total blockage of the airway, is a common symptom. Local irritation, infection, crusting, or bleeding as a result of abnormal air currents is regularly seen.

Multiple Vertical Fractures (▶ Fig. 2.108)

The septum shows two or three nearly vertical fractures posterior to each other. This type of septal deformity is usually caused by frontal trauma with its impact on the lower half of the external pyramid. The cartilaginous dorsum is impressed (sagging) and twisted ("crooked nose"). In patients with a double vertical septal fracture, the first fracture line is usually located at the valve area, the second at the septoperpendicular junction. In cases with three fractures, the second is found 1 to 2 cm posterior to the first, while the third is located at the chondroperpendicular junction.

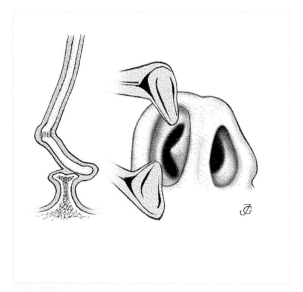

Fig. 2.109 Horizontal fracture.

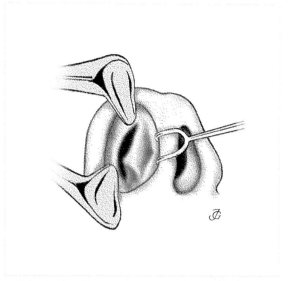

Fig. 2.110 Mixed fracture.

Horizontal Fracture (▶ Fig. 2.109)

The cartilaginous septum is fractured in dorsoventral direction as a result of lateral nasal trauma to the bony part of the external pyramid. The fracture line is located at the septal base at the level of the chondropremaxillary and the chondrovomeral junctions. A horizontal fracture is usually associated with a basal crest and a spur on the same side, and a high deviation of the cartilaginous and bony septum in area 3 and 4 to the other side. The external pyramid generally shows deviation of the bony and cartilaginous pyramid to the opposite side. Breathing obstruction is common if the deformity is severe. Neuralgic symptoms may occur in cases where the septum impacts into the inferior or middle turbinate (Charlin syndrome, see page 80).

Mixed Fracture (▶ Fig. 2.110)

The septum is fractured both vertically and horizontally. Various different types of mixed fracture may occur, depending upon the severity of the trauma.

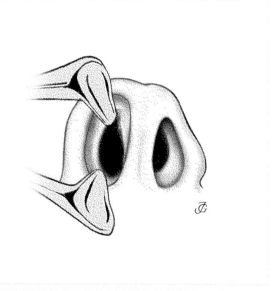

Fig. 2.111 High cartilaginous deviation.

High Cartilaginous Deviation (▶ Fig. 2.111)

The superior part of the cartilaginous septum is deviated. This type of pathology often goes together with a basal crest. The cartilaginous pyramid is often deformed. Deviations of this type in areas 2 and 4 mostly cause functional complaints. Those in area 3 usually cause few symptoms.

Convexity–Concavity of the Cartilaginous Septum (▶ Fig. 2.112)

The cartilaginous septum is bent. When a convexity occurs at the valve area (area 2), it usually causes severe breathing obstruction.

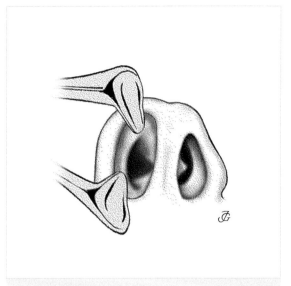

Fig. 2.112 Convexity–concavity of the cartilaginous septum.

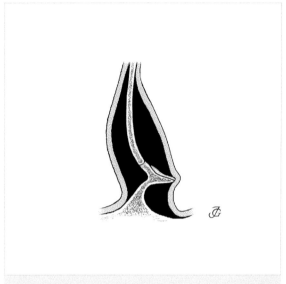

Fig. 2.113 Vomeral spur or spine.

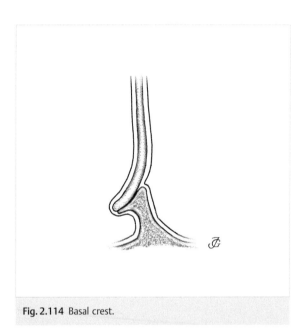

Fig. 2.114 Basal crest.

Vomeral Spur or Spine (▶ Fig. 2.113)

A spur or spine is a sharp and localized pyramid-like protrusion usually located on the vomer (vomeral spur). A spur is generally the prolongation of a basal crest on the same side. It is often combined with a high bony deviation to the other side. A vomeral spur mainly consists of bone. On its cranial side, some cartilage derived from the sphenoidal process of the septal cartilage is frequently present. A spur rarely interferes with breathing. However, it frequently causes a nasal hyperreactivity syndrome with pain or pressure feelings (Sluder syndrome, see page 79) when it impinges in the inferior turbinate.

Basal Crest (▶ Fig. 2.114)

A crest is a sharp ridge. Septal crests are most frequently located on the septal base (basal crest), particularly at the chondropremaxillary and the chondrovomeral junction. They usually continue posteriorly into a vomeral spur. A basal crest is often combined with a high deviation of the septum to the other side. It usually consists of an inferior bony part (premaxilla, maxillary crest, and vomer) and a superior cartilaginous part. Crests rarely interfere with breathing. When they are in permanent contact with the inferior turbinate, they may cause symptoms of hyperreactivity (mucosal swelling with hypersecretion, obstruction, and sneezing) and homolateral pain or pressure feelings.

High Bony Deviation (▶ Fig. 2.115)

The cranial part of the perpendicular plate is deviated. This is usually combined with deformity of the septal cartilage, a basal crest, and deviation of the bony and cartilaginous pyramid.

Septal Perforation (▶ Fig. 2.116)

For a discussion of the pathology and the symptoms of septal perforation, we refer to page 200.

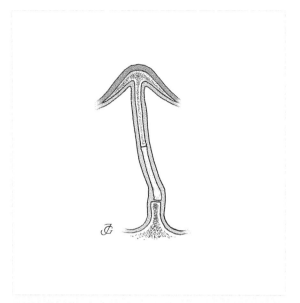

Fig. 2.115 High bony deviation.

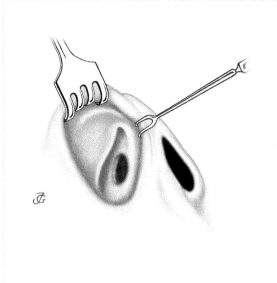

Fig. 2.116 Septal perforation.

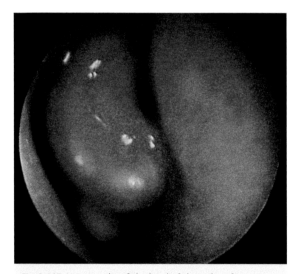

Fig. 2.117 Hypertrophy of the head of the right inferior turbinate.

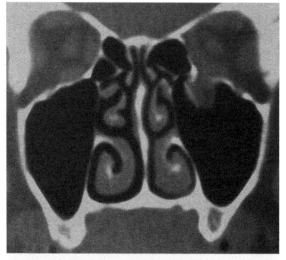

Fig. 2.118 Protrusion of the right inferior turbinate due to the horizontal position of the turbinate bone.

2.2.8 Turbinates

Compensatory Hyperplasia

Compensatory hyperplasia is a well-known turbinate symptom. It is a physiological reaction that serves to diminish the size and normalize the configuration of the breathing space in the pathologically wide nasal cavity (▶ Fig. 2.117). In patients with a septal deviation, it is a characteristic observation. It occurs both in the inferior and middle turbinate.

Protrusion of the Turbinate

Protrusion or abnormal medial position of the turbinate is a rather frequent normal anatomical variant. It is sometimes not easily diagnosed on rhinoscopy. Generally, a coronal CT scan clearly reveals this type of variation.

In the *inferior turbinate*, the position of the turbinate is more horizontal than average. The angle between the turbinate bone and the lateral nasal wall is larger than normal, even up to 90° (▶ Fig. 2.118).

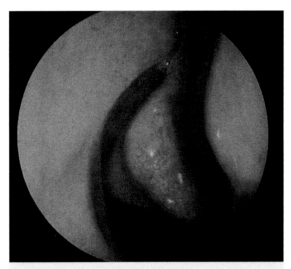

Fig. 2.119 Paradoxically curved right middle turbinate.

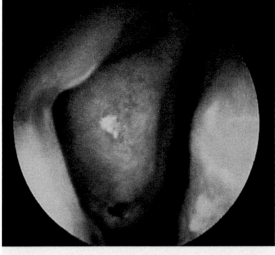

Fig. 2.120 Bullous middle turbinate on the right. Note the ostium at the lower end.

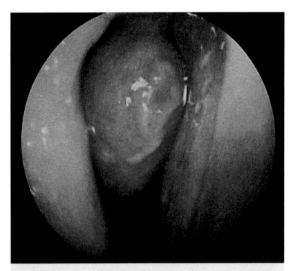

Fig. 2.121 Hypertrophy of the entire inferior turbinate on the right.

In the *middle turbinate*, a number of variations may occur, such as medial ("paradoxical") curving of the caudal or ventral end, and duplication (▶ Fig. 2.119).

Concha Bullosa

The turbinate bone contains a cell that is filled with air and lined with mucosa. It may have an ostium.

In the *middle turbinate*, one or more cells are present in about a quarter of the population. In fact, we are dealing with ethmoidal cells. Such cells may be very large, hence the name bulla. Usually, a bulla is filled with air

(▶ Fig. 2.120). However, as a result of infection, its ostium may become closed so that it fills with mucus or pus. A bullous middle turbinate may cause obstruction of the middle meatus and cause symptoms as mentioned earlier (see also page 73).

A cell in the *inferior turbinate* is very rare. Only a few cases have been described.

Hyperplasia of the Turbinate Head

Hyperplasia of the turbinate head is a very common type of pathology observed in most patients suffering from allergic rhinitis, nasal hyperreactivity, or chronic infection.

In the *inferior turbinate*, the hypertrophic head protrudes in a medial and anterior direction and may obstruct the valve area.

In the *middle turbinate*, hypertrophy is often combined with polypous degeneration of the mucosa. The middle meatus is obstructed, and drainage and ventilation of the paranasal sinuses may be compromised. Facial neuralgia may result.

Hyperplasia of the Whole Turbinate

Hyperplasia of the whole turbinate is an even more common symptom of allergic rhinitis, nasal hyperreactivity, or chronic infection.

In the *inferior turbinate*, this is a very common type of pathology that causes permanent nasal obstruction to differing degrees, and requires treatment (▶ Fig. 2.121).

The same applies to the *middle turbinate*. In this case, the hypertrophy is usually a symptom of a more extensive pathological syndrome.

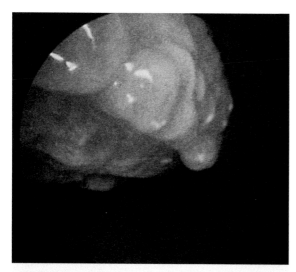

Fig. 2.122 Degenerated mucosa of the tail of the right inferior turbinate.

Hyperplasia of the Turbinate Tail

This is frequently seen in patients with chronic sinusitis and postnasal discharge. Due to continuous irritation and infection, the mucosa degenerates with the formation of polypoid, papillomatous, or fibrous new growth (▶ Fig. 2.122).

2.3 Diagnosis and Documentation

2.3.1 Making the Diagnosis

There are four basic steps to diagnosis in reconstructive nasal surgery:
1. Recording the patient's complaints and taking the medical history
2. Examining the nose and related structures
3. Arranging photography and imaging and taking measurements when required
4. Performing function tests

Completion of these diagnostic steps generally requires two or three office visits. The findings are reviewed prior to surgery on the day the patient is admitted to hospital. The final diagnosis is made at surgery after topical anesthesia and mucosal decongestion have taken effect.

The *first visit* is devoted to listening to the patient's complaints, taking a general medical and rhinological history, and conducting an initial examination of the nose and related structures. Arrangements for photography, imaging (CT and/or MRI), and function tests (e.g., rhinomanometry, acoustic rhinometry, and olfactometry) are made (see page 114). The preliminary diagnosis and a

preliminary plan of treatment are discussed. Generally, however, we limit the information that is given at this stage. We explain to the patient that we will discuss the findings and the treatment at length at the next visit, when the results of all examinations are available. A standard leaflet about nasal surgery procedures may be handed out, provided that the patient is informed about the operation that is most likely indicated.

The *second visit* is focused on the results of the photography, imaging, and function tests. The complaints are reviewed and the examination of the nose and analysis of the face are repeated. Endoscopy is carried out (after decongestion). The findings are then summarized and a treatment proposal is made and explained. The advantages and disadvantages of general versus local anesthesia are discussed. At this time, the benefits and risks of surgery should be discussed (see following text). The patient is also informed about the practical aspects of surgical intervention (e.g., hospital admission or day surgery, length of stay, postoperative care and follow up, rules to be adhered to when back home, period of not working, etc.). It is advisable to write down in the patient's medical record the most important considerations and decisions in order to avoid later misunderstandings. In some cases, we like to read them aloud to the patient while writing.

Treatment Plan

A treatment plan is drawn up and discussed with the patient. The surgical procedure is explained, including the risks and benefits of the operation, as extensively dealt with in the section on Preoperative Care on page 128. An information leaflet and consent form are handed to the patient. It is advisable to have a relative of the patient present during this second visit to help avoid any misunderstandings.

Visual Analogue Scoring of Complaints and Rating Scales of Quality of Life

Visual Analogue Scoring Scale

Over the past two decades, it has become more and more common to express the degree of a patient's complaints in numbers instead of using adjectives such as "light," "moderate," "severe," "very severe," and so on. Staging the severity of a complaint on a numeric scale, a so-called visual analogue scale (VAS), allows a more scientific evaluation of the effect of a certain treatment. Numbers allow a statistical analysis, so that the effect of a therapy can be expressed quantitatively. Scales ranging from 1 to 5 or from 1 to 10 are both generally accepted. Using this method, the effect of a surgical procedure can be quantified and the effectiveness of a new drug can be compared with that of placebo, for example. Also, the use of a VAS

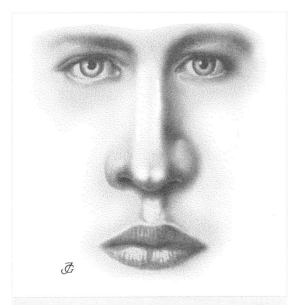

Fig. 2.123 Inspection of the external nose using reflection of light. Note the bilateral and symmetrical dorsal reflex lines and dome reflexes.

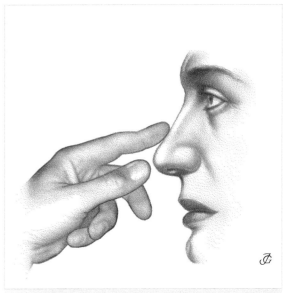

Fig. 2.124 The bony and cartilaginous pyramid is examined by gently stroking with the index finger.

may be helpful in treating an individual patient. We use this method to investigate the effect of a conservative treatment, for example the effect of a corticosteroid spray on breathing obstruction caused by turbinate hyperplasia. When the effect appears to be insufficient, this will help both the surgeon and the patient to decide on a surgical reduction of the turbinate.

Quality of Life Scale

Similarly, it has become customary to test the results of treatment using a "quality of life scale." Patients are asked to rate various aspects of health and well-being numerically before and after therapy.

> "The patient must be interviewed... By means of questions it is possible to learn a great deal concerning the illness, which enables better treatment."
> (Rufus, leading physician at Ephesus Medical School, 1st century AD)

2.3.2 Examination

Inspection and Palpation

In medical examination, *inspection* precedes palpation. However, when examining the nose, inspection and palpation are usually carried out simultaneously. Inspection requires a light, which is not too bright, so that shadow effects and light reflexes remain visible. It is important to illuminate the nose from different angles by moving the patient's head. This is the best way to visualize scars, irregularities, asymmetries, dimples, and grooves. Special attention is drawn to reflection lines and shadow areas (▶ Fig. 2.123).

There are two ways to *palpate* the nose: by gently stroking, and gently pressing. Stroking gently with the index finger will reveal irregularities and defects of the skin, bone, and cartilage. The quality of the feeling gives information about the thickness and condition of the skin and the subcutaneous tissues. Both index fingers, or one index finger and the thumb, are used to palpate for symmetry. Gentle pressure is applied to investigate the stiffness, mobility, and support of the various nasal structures. The bony dorsum is examined with the index finger (▶ Fig. 2.124), the bony pyramid with two or three fingers (▶ Fig. 2.125 and ▶ Fig. 2.126). The cartilaginous dorsum and the nasal tip (domes) are examined for projection and support by applying gentle (rhythmic) downward pressure with the index finger (▶ Fig. 2.127). The columella and the position of the caudal end of the septum are examined by lifting the tip with the thumb (▶ Fig. 2.128). The ala is examined by gentle palpation between the index finger and the thumb (▶ Fig. 2.129). All elements of the external pyramid should be examined in the front view, both side views, and the base view (see box Specific Aspects of the Nasal Pyramid to be Examined).

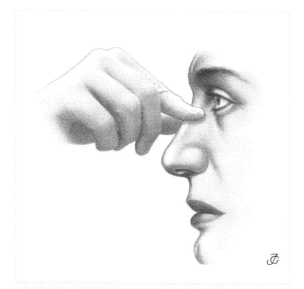

Fig. 2.125 The pyramid is examined with the index finger and thumb, or with both index fingers.

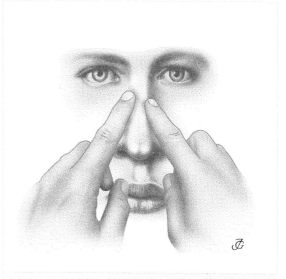

Fig. 2.126 The skin over the bony pyramid is moved to and fro with both index fingers to investigate whether the skin is freely mobile over the bony skeleton.

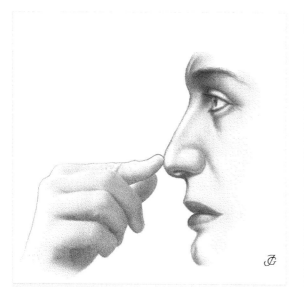

Fig. 2.127 The projection and support of the cartilaginous dorsum and tip are tested by gentle pressure with the index finger.

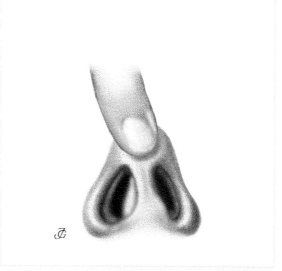

Fig. 2.128 The position of the caudal end of the septum and the columella is examined by lifting the tip with the thumb.

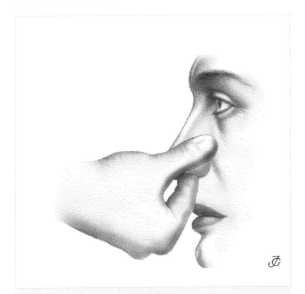

Fig. 2.129 The lateral crus and dome are examined for size, shape, thickness, and rigidity with the index finger and thumb.

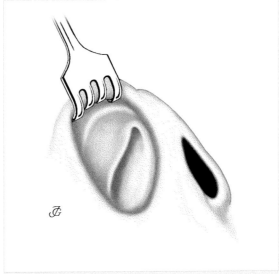

Fig. 2.130 The vestibule and valve area are inspected using a blunt, four-pronged hook.

Specific Aspects of the Nasal Pyramid to be Examined

Front view
• Length and width in relation to face

Side view
• Length in relation to forehead and chin
• Prominence (projection) of bony pyramid, cartilaginous pyramid, and tip
• Angles: frontonasal and nasolabial
• Profile: humps, saddling, sagging, irregularities
• Columellar position and columellar base in relation to alar rim
• Grooves and dimples

Base view
• Projection of lobule and tip
• Width, configuration, and symmetry of nares, columella, alae, vestibulum, and valve

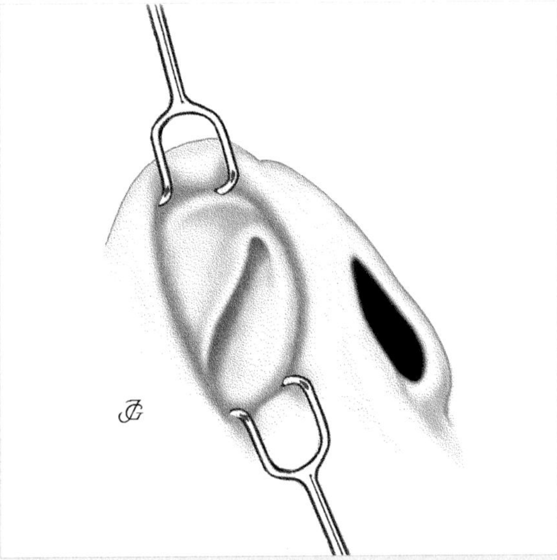

Fig. 2.131 The vestibule is inspected using two blunt, two-pronged dull retractors.

2.3.3 Examination of the Internal Nose

Inspection and Palpation

Inspection and palpation of the internal nose starts with inspection (and, if indicated, palpation with a cotton wool applicator) of the nostrils, vestibules, and valve areas. This is done as follows:

• Without instruments during normal breathing, and at forced inspiration (see breathing tests);
• With an alar retractor (▶ Fig. 2.130); or
• By using two blunt hooks or retractors to simultaneously inspect the lateral and the medial wall of the vestibule (▶ Fig. 2.131).

Note

A nasal speculum is not the proper instrument to inspect the vestibulum and valve area as it distorts their anatomy.

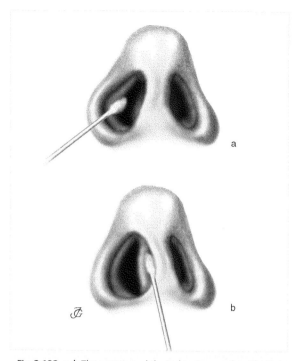

Fig. 2.132 **a, b** The septum and the turbinates may be palpated with a cotton wool applicator.

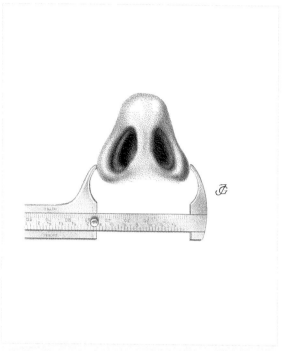

Fig. 2.133 A caliper is used to measure nasal dimensions and indices.

Anterior Septum

The position of the caudal end of the cartilaginous septum is examined by pushing the nasal tip and columella upward with the thumb. In this way, dislocation and a protrusion of the caudal end of the septum may be visualized (▶ Fig. 2.128). The position of the base, cartilaginous septum, and their relation to the nasal spine and premaxilla may be studied by retraction of the columella to the other side with a blunt hook, and by palpation with a slender cotton wool applicator (▶ Fig. 2.132**a, b**).

Valve Area

The valve area is examined first without instruments and then using an alar retractor or one or two blunt, two-pronged retractors. The ala should not be lifted too high to avoid alteration of the valvular configuration (▶ Fig. 2.130 and ▶ Fig. 2.131).

Posterior Septum and Turbinates

The posterior septum, turbinates, ethmoidal infundibulum, frontal recess, and sinus ostia are examined as follows. First, the various areas are inspected using a nasal speculum. The mucosal membranes are then decongested (and anesthetized) with small gauzes soaked in xylometazoline 0.1% (and lidocaine 4%). Nasendoscopy with a 0° and/or 30° endoscope is then carried out. Finally, certain

structures may be palpated with a cotton wool applicator or a probe. This is helpful in several respects: to better diagnose defects of the cartilaginous and bony septum; to examine the quality of the margins of a septal perforation; to determine whether we are dealing with mucosal hyperplasia or polyposis; and to confirm the presence of turbinate hyperplasia and concha bullosa.

2.3.4 Analysis of Nose, Face, and Dentition

In nasal surgery, we are operating upon a part of the face. The characteristics of the external nasal pyramid strongly affect our judgment of the face, just as the dimensions of the face highly influence our judgment of the nose. Asymmetries and abnormal dimensions of the face play a major role in our perception. Thus, when examining nasal deformities, abnormalities, and variations, we have to analyze the nose in relation to the face. A normal, straight nasal pyramid will only give the impression of being normal and nondeviating when the face is symmetrical. The projection of the nasal pyramid depends upon the prominence of the forehead, maxilla, and especially the chin. We use a caliper to take measurements of certain nasal and facial dimensions as part of the examination procedure (▶ Fig. 2.133). The most informative parameters of the nose are height, length, width, and prominence. The most important angles are the frontonasal and the nasolabial angles. The most useful indices are the clinical nasal index and the tip index.

Proportions

The facial proportions may be visualized (and measured) by drawing four horizontal and six vertical lines on the front view photograph of the patient (see Chapter 1, ▸ Fig. 1.2, and ▸ Fig. 1.3).

Angles

The frontonasal and nasolabial angle may be drawn and measured on the profile photograph (see ▸ Fig. 1.11**a, b**).

Dentition

Examining the patient's dentition is an essential part of a rhinological investigation. Special attention is paid to the number and position of the incisor and canine teeth. When elements in the upper jaw are missing, this may be combined with a deformity of the premaxilla and the anterior septum. Sometimes, a dislocated (canine) tooth is present in the base of the septum. Trauma to the premaxillary area in early childhood is a common cause of malpositioning of the anterior upper teeth.

Dental occlusion is another aspect to be examined. Usually, malocclusion disorders are due to a disturbance of the maxillary–mandibular relationship. Indirectly, this has an impact on the visual position of the external nasal pyramid in the face (see also the section on facial syndromes (see page 78). In patients with an evident dental abnormality, referral to a maxillofacial surgeon is indicated. Nasal surgery might then have to be preceded by orthognathic surgery.

2.3.5 Imaging

The position of the maxilla and the mandible (chin) in relation to the other structures, in particular the external nasal pyramid, may be analyzed on lateral and fronto-occipital standard radiographs, or on standard photographs. The procedure is described next.

Steps

- A vertical line is dropped through the subnasale at a right angle to the Frankfort horizontal line (line from infraorbital margin to the upper margin of the bony external ear canal). In the "ideal" face, this line will touch the pogonion. If this is not the case, this indicates retrusion or protrusion of the maxilla and/or mandible.
- A second line is drawn at a tangent to the nasal dorsum. The angle between this line and the vertical line (nasofacial angle) is normally 30 to 40°. In a prominent nose it is larger, in a low nose smaller.

- A third line is drawn from the nasal tip to the pogonion. The angle between this line and the nasal dorsal line (nasomental angle) is normally 120 to 130°. In a patient with mandibular retrusion or a prominent nasal pyramid, this angle is smaller. Normally, the upper lip is 1 to 2 mm posterior to this line, and the lower lip 2 to 4 mm.
- A fourth line is drawn at a tangent to the gnathion, passing through the innermost curve at the junction of the neck and submental area. Normally, this line forms an angle (mentocervical angle) of 80 to 95° with the vertical line and an angle of 110 to 120° with the nasomental line.

For more general aspects of facial and nasal proportions, as well as definitions of the various points, lines, and angles used in nasal analysis, the reader is referred to Chapter 1, page 2.

Radiographs

Standard radiographs have been the gold standard for some eight decades in screening for facial trauma (orbital floor, orbital rim, zygoma), nasal fractures, and diseases of the paranasal sinuses. Nowadays, coronal CT scanning has superseded standard radiography, as pathology and anatomical variations can be imaged in greater detail according to requirements. The recently introduced cone beam CT scanning has proven an equally effective technique with a smaller radiation load.

CT Scans

CT scanning has greatly improved rhinological diagnosis and follow-up of treatment. This applies, first of all, to sinus disease. However, in several nasal disorders, CT scans may be of great help too. The following are well-known examples:
- Deformities of the bony and cartilaginous pyramid (coronal and axial planes)
- Septal pathology (coronal plane)
- Turbinate anatomy (concha bullosa) and turbinate pathology (coronal plane)
- Complications of dorsal transplants and implants (coronal and oblique planes)
- Designing a custom-made prosthesis in patients with a large septal perforation (sagittal plane)

▸ Fig. 2.134 presents an example of the value of a pre-operative CT scan in a patient with breathing obstruction. The coronal scan shows severe septal pathology with deviation of the cranial part of the perpendicular plate to the right that is easily missed in rhinoscopy, and compensatory hyperplasia of the left inferior turbinate.

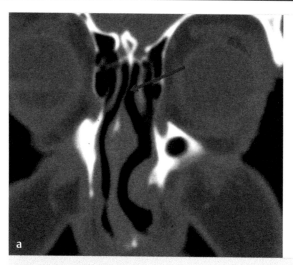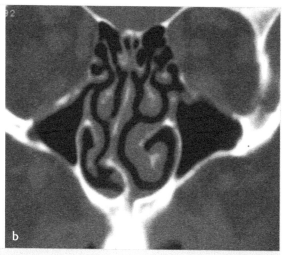

Fig. 2.134 a, b CT scans may be very helpful in making a correct diagnosis. Note the high deviation (arrow) of the perpendicular plate to the right, an abnormality that is usually difficult to see on endoscopy. Also note the compensatory hypertrophy of the left inferior turbinate. (Courtesy Prof. Clement.)

MRI

Magnetic resonance imaging is of limited value in reconstructive nasal surgery except for demonstrating and diagnosing soft-tissue swelling and tumors.

2.3.6 Photographic Diagnosis and Documentation

Taking color photographs in four or five standardized positions is an essential step in analyzing the external nose, face, and head. These photographs are obligatory for all patients in whom the appearance of the external pyramid is (or may become) changed by surgery. In the first place, they may be of great help in explaining the pathology and the planned surgical treatment to the patient before the final decision to go ahead is taken (see previous text). Secondly, these photos are of utmost importance in evaluating the result. Photographs are also important for the follow-up of deformities and abnormalities. Photographic follow-up of a traumatic septal pyramid deformity during childhood and pubertal growth may be of great help in decision-making. If the deformity increases with time, we may decide to operate at an earlier age. Similarly, photographic documentation is crucial for the follow-up of scars, retractions, irregularities, or

postoperative sagging of the dorsum. Finally, if a dissatisfied patient brings a lawsuit against the doctor, the preoperative and postoperative photographs may be crucial for the defense (see boxes: Indications for Preoperative and [Usually 6 month-] Postoperative Photographs in Patients Undergoing Surgery and Main Indications for Follow-up Photography).

> **Indications for Preoperative and (Usually-6-Months-) Postoperative Photographs in Patients Undergoing Surgery**
>
> **Before and after surgery**
>
> Adults:
> • pyramid and lobular surgery
> • surgery of adjacent structures
>
> Children:
> • septal surgery
> • pyramid and lobular surgery
> • surgery of adjacent structures

Follow-up of deformities, abnormalities, and variations

Congenital:
- nasal hypoplasia
- cleft-lip syndrome
- bifidity, etc.

Posttraumatic:
- deviations
- sagging and saddling
- humps
- irregularities, etc.

Postinfectious:
- scars
- saddling and sagging
- retractions, etc.

Postsurgical:
- infection
- scars
- sagging and saddling
- retractions
- irregularities, etc.

Technique of Standard Nasal Photography

Medical photography must be performed according to certain standards. Otherwise, the required information may be distorted by technical variations, while postoperative and preoperative photos are not comparable. The following rules should be adopted.

Computerized Photography

Use of computer-stored images has become increasingly popular recently. This way of storing data certainly offers many practical advantages. However, digitized photographs might be modified, and may therefore not be accepted as proof in medicolegal cases. In some countries, courts have, in fact, rejected computer images presented as proof by the defending surgeon. Some surgeons use computer images to analyze and discuss nasal deformities or variations with the patient in the same way as standard photographs. However, some also use the possibilities afforded by a computer to demonstrate to the patient the modifications that might be achieved by surgery. We would warn against this, as it may give the patient the false impression that what can be done on a computer screen can be duplicated by surgery. One of the greatest mistakes a surgeon can make is to present a patient with a printout of a computer-modified image.

Patient Positioning and Preparation

- The patient sits up straight on a small, revolving stool.
- Eyeglasses are removed. The front view photographs are taken both with and without spectacles.
- The forehead should be free of overhanging hair.
- Earrings are removed.

Lighting and Background

The patient's face is lit by indirect light to avoid shadow effects. The background must be even and preferably colored, either light blue or a light or medium shade of green.

Requirements

All photographs have to be taken according to a number of internationally accepted rules. Otherwise they may give a false impression and cannot be compared.

Standard Positions

Generally, four standard positions are used:
1. Front view
2. Left side view
3. Right side view
4. Base view

Many surgeons also like to have a left and right oblique view. These exposures provide extra information about the lateral nasal wall. In patients with a deviated pyramid, a view from above may also provide extra information.

All photographs should fill the frame more or less completely.

Front View (▶ Fig. 2.135)

- The patient has to look straight into the camera.
- The whole face, including the hair, ears, and chin, must be depicted.
- Both auricles should be equally visible.
- The line through the inferior margin of both orbits must be horizontal.

If these requirements are not met, the position of the nasal pyramid in the face will be incorrectly documented.

Base View (▶ Fig. 2.136)

- The head is deflected backward so that the nasal tip is projected just between the eyebrows. This is of extreme importance. If this requirement is not met, the preoperative and postoperative projection of the lobule cannot be compared.
- The upper lip is depicted completely, whereas the chin and ears are not. For this reason, the base view is usually printed twice as large as the other photographs.

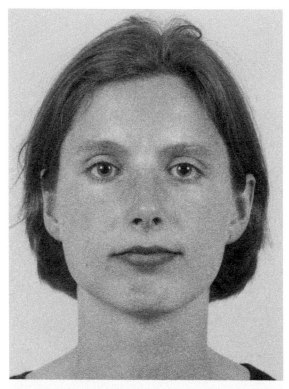

Fig. 2.135 Front view depicting hair, ears, and chin. The auricles are equally visible. A line runs through the inferior margin of both orbits horizontally.

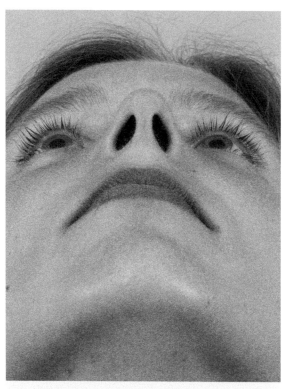

Fig. 2.136 Base view showing the nasal tip at the level of the eyebrows. Only the nasal base and upper lip are depicted.

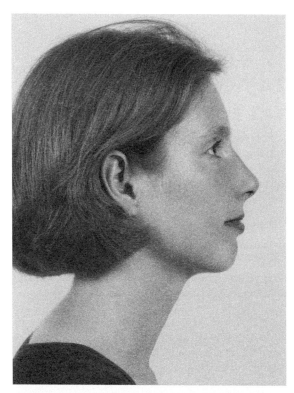

Fig. 2.137 Right side view depicting hair and chin. The line from the lower orbital rim to the tragus is horizontal. Only the nearest eyebrow is visible.

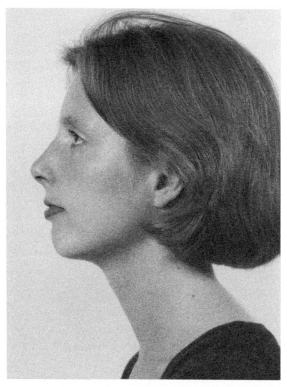

Fig. 2.138 Left side view.

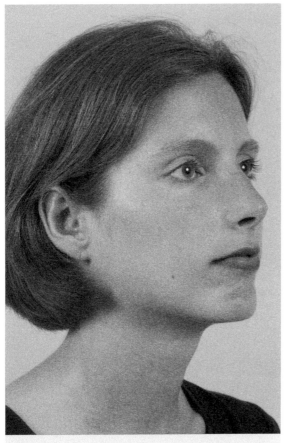

Fig. 2.139 Right oblique view.

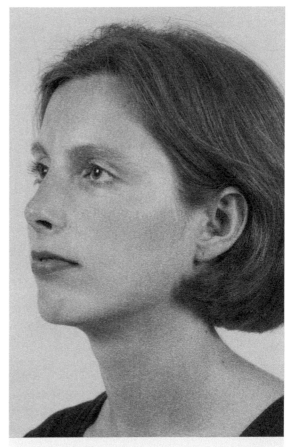

Fig. 2.140 Left oblique view.

Side View, Left and Right (▶ Fig. 2.137 and ▶ Fig. 2.138)

- The subject is positioned at 90° to the camera by turning the stool. The head is upright. The hair and chin have to be depicted.
- The line drawn from the lower orbital rim to the tragus must be horizontal.
- The nearest eyebrow should be completely visible, whereas the contralateral eyebrow must be invisible.
- The nasal tip is depicted free from the frame at about one-third of the horizontal dimension. The posterior half of the head is thus not shown.

Oblique Side View, Right and Left (▶ Fig. 2.139 and ▶ Fig. 2.140)

- The body and head are in the same position as for the side view, except that the head is turned 135° instead of 90°.

2.4 Function Tests

2.4.1 Breathing Tests

Nasal breathing can be investigated by simple observational tests that can be carried out in the office as part of a rhinologic examination, and by more sophisticated quantitative tests such as rhinomanometry, acoustic rhinometry (not a real breathing test), measurement of inspiratory peak flow, and anemometry, which require special instruments.

Observational Tests

Observational tests are carried out as part of our standard rhinological examination since they are not time-consuming and do not require special instruments. They are not quantitative, however, and their outcome cannot be recorded. Some of them were suggested over a century ago, such as the observation of alar movement and of breathings sounds.

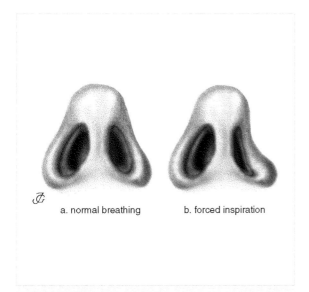

Fig. 2.141 a, b The nostrils and alae are observed during normal and forced inspiration for inspiratory insufficiency of the lateral nasal wall ("alar collapse").

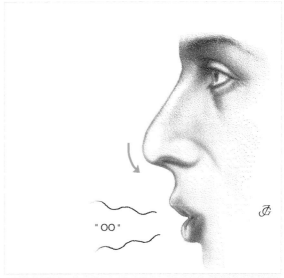

Fig. 2.142 Positive "OO phenomenon." When the lips are puckered, as by pronouncing the vowel sound "OO," the tip is drawn down and backward.

Breathing Sounds

- *Normal respiration:* The patient is asked to breathe quietly through the nose while the examiner listens to the inspiratory and expiratory breathing sounds. At the same time, the examiner observes the movements of the lateral nasal wall. This is first performed with both nostrils open, then with the right and left nostril closed alternately. This may be done by gently sealing the nostril with the inside of the thumb in such a way that the lobule is not distorted.
- *Forced inspiration:* The sequence is repeated during forced inspiration. The examiner carefully watches the movements of the alae and looks for any retraction of the lateral nasal wall (▶ Fig. 2.141**a, b**).
- This simple test must be performed in all patients who complain of inspiratory breathing obstruction. It is the only way to determine the level of functional stenosis of the anterior nasal segment (area 1, nostril and vestibule, and area 2, valve area).

OO Phenomenon

In a tension nose (see page 69), the tip is narrow and may be pulled down slightly by the tension of the stretched alae and columella (positive "OO phenomenon"). By puckering the lips, as when pronouncing the vowel sound "OO," the tip is drawn down and backward due to the tension (overstretch) of the columella and the upper lip (▶ Fig. 2.142).

Columella Narrowing Test (Nostril Test)

The lower half of the columella is narrowed by means of a forceps to examine the effect of widening the nostril and vestibule on inspiration. The patient is asked whether this influences breathing, while the observer studies how narrowing the columella affects alar movement (▶ Fig. 2.143).

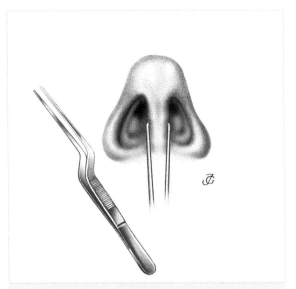

Fig. 2.143 Columella narrowing test. The lower half of the columella is narrowed with a forceps to test alar insufficiency.

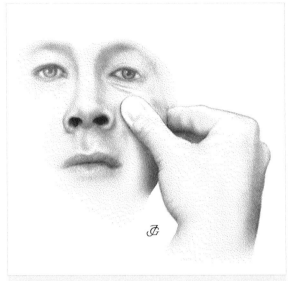

Fig. 2.144 Cottle test. The lateral lobular wall is pulled laterally and slightly upward to examine inspiratory valvular insufficiency.

Valve Opening Test (Cottle Test)

The skin over the upper margin of the piriform aperture is pulled laterally and slightly upward in order to widen the valve area (▸ Fig. 2.144). The patient is asked if this affects inspiratory breathing, while the examiner observes the effect on the valve area. This simple test may corroborate the existence of a valve problem. Most patients suffering from valvular stenosis have already discovered the positive effect of this maneuver. They sometimes apply it to help in falling asleep, using tape or a finger. It is important to use the thumb or one finger. Otherwise, the whole nasal entrance will be opened, whereby the test loses its specificity.

Cotton Ball Test/Breathe-Right Nasal Strip

The effect of artificially widening the valve area can also be determined by the "cotton ball test" or by applying a Breathe-Right nasal strip.

A small ball of cotton wool is positioned with a bayonet forceps at the valve angle to study the effect of widening the valve area (▸ Fig. 2.145). Alternatively, a Breathe-Right nasal strip may be used. A positive outcome of this test suggests that widening the valve by septal pyramid surgery, valve surgery, or a spreader graft will very likely improve nasal breathing.

Quantitative Tests

History

The importance of nasal breathing was not fully recognized until the 1870s. The first measurements of nasal breathing

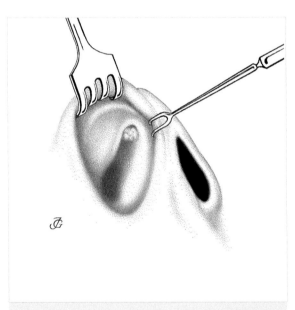

Fig. 2.145 Cotton ball test. A cotton ball is positioned at the valve angle to examine the effect of widening the valve area.

date from the last decades of the 19th century. In 1889, Zwaardemaker introduced the first clinical breathing test using a calibrated cold mirror to measure and compare the amount of air exhaled through the right and left nostrils.

In the first half of the 20th century, various manometric techniques were developed. The development of the pneumotachograph made dynamic recording of respiration possible, which led to the development of modern rhinomanometry in the 1960s. Thanks to the work of several pioneers in different countries (e.g., Cottle, Spoor, Masing, Bachmann, Broms, Kern, and Cole), rhinomanometry gradually became a standardized technique. This method allows the recording of nasal pressure in relation to inspiratory and expiratory flow in an XY diagram. Following various improvements, the technique was finally standardized by the "International Standardization Committee on Objective Assessment of the Nasal Airway" (ISCOANA) in 1984 and 2005 (Clement et al 1984, Clement and Gordts 2005). Acoustic rhinometry was devised as a method to measure the cross-sectional area and volume of the nasal cavity by Hilberg, Jackson, and Pedersen in 1989. It is thus not a breathing test per se, but informs us about the geometry of the nasal cavity. It was further developed by Lenders and Pirsig in 1990 and Tomkinson and Eccles in 1998. A report on its use and standardization can be found in the 2005 ISCOANA report.

In more recent years, measurement of nasal peak inspiratory flow (NPIF) has been added as a simple, although less reliable, method that may be used for clinical screening purposes.

Finally, anemometry is a method that measures air velocity over time, but is not directly proportional to resistance or flow.

Objective Breathing Tests

Rhinomanometry

Rhinomanometry has become a standardized technique and the most commonly used quantitative breathing test.

It measures the relationship between flow and pressure for each nasal cavity separately. Different methods have been suggested: anterior versus posterior rhinomanometry and active versus passive rhinometry. Active anterior rhinomanometry has become the method of choice.

Active Anterior Rhinometry (AAR)

In active anterior rhinomanometry, the pressure difference (Δp) between the nostril and the nasopharynx is measured as a function of airflow (.V) for each nasal cavity separately. An airtight transparent mask is placed over the nose of the test subject. The mask is connected to a pneumotachograph, which measures airflow through the tested side. The pressure difference between the nostril and the nasopharynx is measured through a tube that is fitted airtight to the nostril of the other side (▶ Fig. 2.146). The subject is examined in a sitting position and is asked to breathe quietly. The pressure–flow relationship of four to five breathing cycles is averaged by a computer with a sample frequency of at least 50 Hz and registered by an XY recorder. Graphic representation uses the mirror-imaging technique. Airflow (in cm^3/s) is recorded on the ordinate, the pressure gradient (in Pascal [Pa]) on the abscissa. Inspiration is shown on the right of the rhinomanogram, expiration on the left (▶ Fig. 2.147). It is important to follow the recording online during the testing to check for any leakage and irregular breathing.

According to the international standard, resistance is given at the fixed pressure difference of 150 Pa. In a normal nose, the median value for unilateral inspiratory

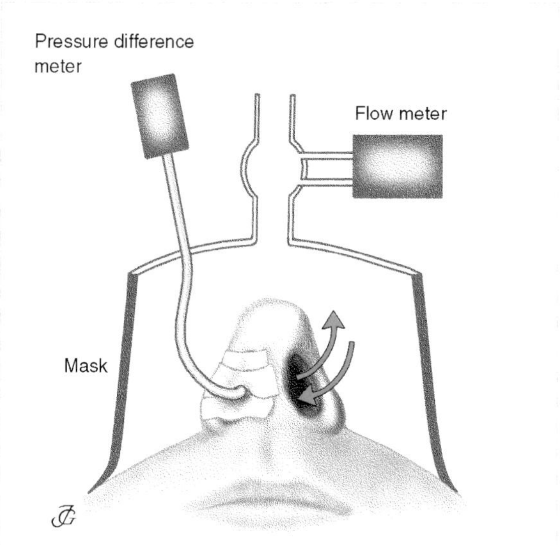

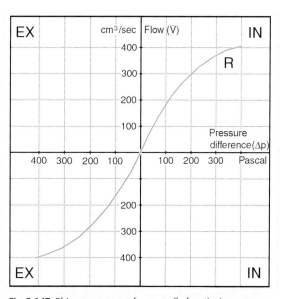

Fig. 2.146 Active anterior rhinomanometry. The subject is tested in a sitting position. The pressure–flow relationship during quiet breathing is measured independently for both nasal cavities. An airtight mask is fitted over the nose to measure flow through the side to be tested. A tube is sealed to the nostril of the opposite side to measure the pressure gradient between the nostril and the nasopharynx of the test side.

Fig. 2.147 Rhinomanogram of a normally functioning nose according to the internationally accepted standard. XY recording of airflow (cm^3/s) and pressure difference (Pa) of five breathing cycles for the right nasal cavity, as found in a normal nose. Inspiration on the right, expiration on the left.

nasal resistance is 0.36 Pa/cm^{-3}/s (range: 0.34–0.40) in the nondecongested nose and 0.26 Pa/cm^{-3}/s (range: 0.25–0.30) in the decongested nose. If necessary, resistance can also be given at 75 Pa or 100 Pa, but this should be clearly stated. Total nasal resistance may be calculated from the pressure values obtained for the left and right nasal cavity according to the formula:

$$R_{tot} \frac{R_1 \times R_r}{R + R_1} \qquad (2.1)$$

Active anterior rhinomanometry using a mask has a number of advantages over other methods: it is well tolerated and it allows measurement of both nasal cavities independently; it is a dynamic way of testing nasal breathing; and it measures nasal flow at different pressures during active respiration.

To obtain reliable and reproducible results, the following requirements should be met:

- The mask must be wide enough to not deform the nasal lobule. At the same time, it has to be narrow enough to be airtight.
- The tube by which the pressure gradient is measured must be attached airtight to the nostril by adhesive tape without distorting the lobule.

Diagnostic Value of Rhinomanometry

Rhinomanometry is an important diagnostic tool. It provides objective information about nasal resistance by determining flow versus pressure gradient. When performed lege artis, it follows the laws of fluid dynamics and is by definition correct (▶ Fig. 2.148).

This objective information, however, does not always correlate well with the subjective findings of the patient. In a small percentage of cases, patients may report breathing difficulties or doctors may find pathology while rhinometric values are normal. Conversely, rhinomanometry may produce an abnormal outcome even though the patient has no complaints (▶ Fig. 2.149).

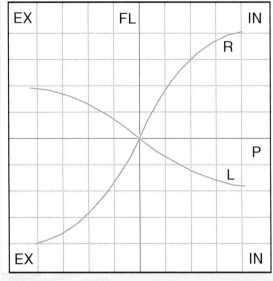

Fig. 2.148 Pressure–flow curve in a patient with a septal deviation on the left; subnormal pressure–flow curve on the right.
Inspir. Rl = 1.5 Pa/cm^{-3}/s at 150 Pa
Inspir. Rr = 0.6 Pa/cm^{-3}/s at 150 Pa

Rhinomanometry only provides general information about nasal resistance in relation to the dynamics of breathing. As it only records flow and pressure gradient, it does not give information about the localization of the obstruction.

The only exceptions are cases of alar collapse. Here, rhinomanometry not only informs us about the location of the collapse, but also about the pressure at which it occurs (▶ Fig. 2.150).

Rhinomanometry is not applicable in:

- Very young children
- Complete unilateral obstruction, and
- Patients with a septal perforation

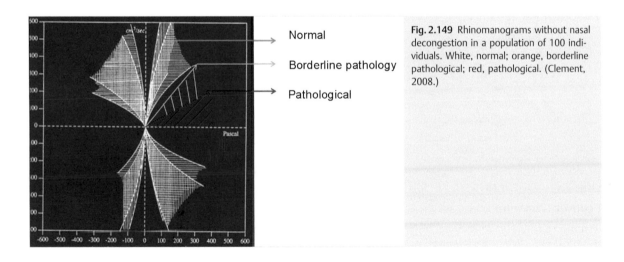

Fig. 2.149 Rhinomanograms without nasal decongestion in a population of 100 individuals. White, normal; orange, borderline pathological; red, pathological. (Clement, 2008.)

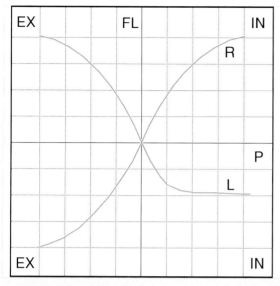

Fig. 2.150 Inspiratory collapse of the anterior nasal segment on the left; subnormal pressure–flow curve on the right.
Inspir. Rl = 0.8 Pa/cm^{-3}/s at 150 Pa and 1.6 Pa/cm^3/s at 300 Pa
Inspir. Rr = 0.6 Pa/cm^{-3}/s at 150 Pa and 0.7 Pa/cm^{-3}/s at 300 Pa

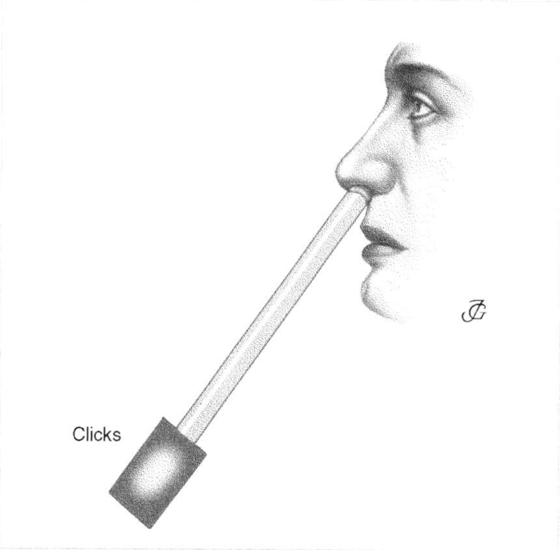

Fig. 2.151 Acoustic rhinometry. The geometry of the nasal cavity is determined by analyzing the reflection of acoustic clicks presented to the nasal cavity through a nosepiece.

Other Rhinomanometric Techniques

In *active posterior rhinomanometry*, pressure measurements are made with a tube posterior to the base of the tongue while the subject breathes through the nose with the mouth closed. Since many patients do not tolerate a tube in the back of the mouth, this is not advised as a standard method.

In *passive rhinomanometry*, a fixed amount of air (250 cm^3) is blown through a nasal cavity via a nozzle by external means, while the subject is holding his or her breath. The amount of pressure needed is measured. This method does not represent normal breathing, and differences between inspiration and expiration are not established.

Anemometry

Anemometry measures temperature changes of inhaled and exhaled air at the level of the nostril over time, giving a rough estimate of nasal patency changes over time. It is a semiquantitative, indirect method that is used mainly in sleep apnea studies to measure the nasal cycle.

There may be many therapies; there is only one diagnosis.

Objective Nonbreathing Tests

Acoustic Rhinometry

Acoustic rhinometry allows measurement of the cross-sectional area and the volume of the nasal cavity. It provides us with a curve that represents an estimate of the cross-sectional area of the nasal cavity as a function of distance from the nostril. A click is presented to the nasal cavity through a nose piece that is positioned parallel to the sagittal plane and at 45° to the coronal plane (▶ Fig. 2.151). The reflected signal is recorded within the range of 0.1 to 10 kHz. The test is performed while the patient is seated and holding his or her breath.

Two types of nose pieces exist:
1. The conical nose piece is introduced into the vestibule. As it distorts the vestibule to a certain extent, it is not recommended when measuring the nasal valve area. In measuring the effect of nasal challenge; however, this disadvantage does not cause a problem.
2. The anatomical plateau-shaped nose piece allows a rather airtight seal with minimal or no distortion of the ostium externum, especially when applied with some Vaseline. Its disadvantage is that several models are needed to fit different sizes and shapes of nostrils (adults, children etc.).

The normal acoustic rhinometric curve has a characteristic W-configuration showing two minimal cross-sectional areas (MCA). The first one, MCA 1, is at about 1.5 cm and represents the end of the nose piece and its junction with the nose (Tomkinson and Eccles 1998). The second one, MCA 2, corresponds with the valve area (i.e., the nasal valve and the head of the inferior turbinate), the flow-limiting segment (▶ Fig. 2.152 and ▶ Fig. 2.153). According to the ISCOANA (International Standardization Committee for the Objective Assessment of the Upper Airways), only MCA 2 is clinically relevant because MCA 1 is considered an artifact due to the nose piece.

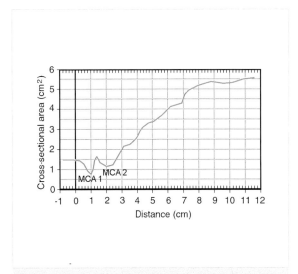

Fig. 2.152 Acoustic rhinogram. The normal curve shows the cross-sectional area of the internal nose in relation to the distance from the sound source. MCA 1 was formerly considered to represent a part of the nasal valve. Nowadays it is assumed to be an artifact due to the nose piece. MCA 2 corresponds to the head of the inferior turbinate is now called MCA (ISCOANA).

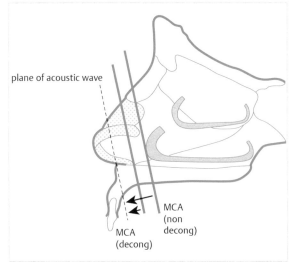

Fig. 2.153 Position of MCA in a nondecongested and a decongested nose. MCA moves forward after decongestion because it induces a shortening of the acoustic wave (arrows).

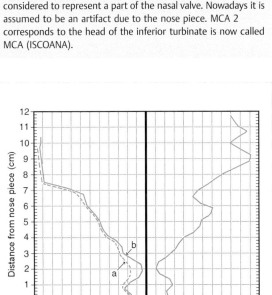

Fig. 2.154 Acoustic rhinogram before (b) and after (a) decongestion on the right side in a patient with hyperplasia of the head of the inferior turbinate. After decongestion the distance to MCA is reduced.

The last part of the curve is ascending, and shows the squared diameter of the nasal cavity versus distance. The method actually reduces the real cross-sectional area of the nose, which is slitlike and very irregular, to a circular cross-section with the area πr^2 in which r is the hydraulic radius.

To distinguish between a mucosal and a septal narrowing, acoustic rhinometry is carried out before and after mucosal decongestion (▶ Fig. 2.154 and ▶ Fig. 2.155).

The great advantage of acoustic rhinometry is its simplicity. It is fast and noninvasive, and can therefore also be used in young children (Djupesland 1999). A short tube and a special nozzle is then required.

Diagnostic Value of Acoustic Rhinometry

Rhinomanometry and acoustic rhinometry are complementary tools. The first is a dynamic method that records nasal pressure in relation to inspiratory and expiratory flow; the second is a static method that measures the cross-sectional area and volume of the nasal cavity. Acoustic rhinometry has the following limitations:

- It cannot be used when the nasal cavity is blocked.
- Only obstructions at the level of the valve area and in the anterior part of the nasal cavity can be measured reliably.
- The method loses its sensitivity with distance: pathology beyond 4 cm cannot be determined.
- Pathology posterior to an obstruction cannot be measured because the acoustic energy of the clicks is not high enough to measure reliably behind a stenosis.
- It cannot record alar and valvular collapse, as these are dynamic phenomena that occur on inspiration when the negative pressure in the vestibule or valve area, respectively, exceed a certain limit.
- It cannot be applied in patients with a septal perforation.

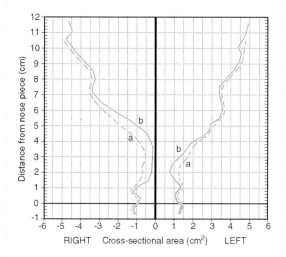

Fig. 2.155 Acoustic rhinogram in a patient with a septal deviation on the right before (b) and after (a) decongestion. The first part of the right nasal cavity is almost completely blocked. After decongestion, the stenosis has decreased, but there is still a considerable difference between the right and left side, indicating an anatomical deformity.

Measuring Nasal Inspiratory Peak Flow

An inspiratory flow meter is used to measure nasal inspiratory peak flow (NIPF). A disadvantage of this method is that the mucosa may be sucked inward on forced inspiration. Nonetheless, several authors have claimed a good correlation with the outcome of rhinomanometry. Although the latter is to be preferred, peak flow measurements might be used to measure the effect of surgery or long-term medication. An advantage of measuring NIPF is that the apparatus is rather inexpensive and easy to handle. The patient can take it home and document his or her own breathing obstruction.

2.4.2 Olfactometry

Unlike audiometry in otology, olfactometry has not (yet) become a routine examination in rhinological patients. In some clinics, every patient's smell is tested prior to rhinoplastic surgery. One reason for this is to avoid a medicolegal conflict if a patient claims a decreased sense of smell postoperatively. In patients with polyposis, hyposmia or anosmia is usually a major complaint. Olfaction tests may then be useful to show the effects of surgery. At present, the UPSIT test (University of Pennsylvania Smell Identification Test) and the "Sniffin' Sticks" test are the best tests available.

Screening Tests

Screening tests are helpful to distinguish between normal and impaired olfactory function. The most commonly used method is the "Sniffin' Sticks" test. It is available as a short test with 3 or 5 odor probes, or a more elaborate test with 12 odors (Kobal et al 1996, Hummel et al 1997, Mueller et al 2006). The odor is presented by removing the cap of a pen containing an odorant, which is held under both nostrils for about 3 seconds. The patient has to identify the odor from four choices.

Threshold and Identification Tests

Threshold and identification tests are used to assess olfactory functions in more detail.

The *threshold test* is carried out by a forced choice procedure with the patient blindfolded. Usually, a dilution series of 16 steps is used. At each step, three sticks are offered, one of them bearing the odorant (usually n-butanol or phenylethyl alcohol, which have negligible effects on trigeminal nerve endings) and the other two bearing only solvent. The concentration of the odorant is increased in a stepwise manner until it is correctly identified twice in a row. The concentration is then lowered until the test person is unable to correctly identify the offered odorant. In this way, the olfactory threshold is determined.

The *discrimination test* is performed in a similar way. The test person is offered three sticks, two of which release the same odor whereas the third has a different odor.

2.4.3 Measuring Air-Conditioning Capacity
Humidifying Capacity

The humidifying capacity of the nose can be determined by measuring the relative humidity of the inspired and expired air. This may be done at different levels of ambient humidity. At present, humidity measurements have not been introduced in clinical practice as the implications of such measurements are not clear.

Warming-Up Capacity

The same applies to measuring the warming-up capacity of the nose. Tests to determine the humidifying and the warming-up capacity of the nose will be introduced in the future.

2.4.4 Measuring Nasal Defense

Since the nose is the main defense organ of the respiratory tract, we need tests to study its protective functions. The tests should measure the following known aspects of nasal defense:

- Ciliary beat frequency (CBF) and ciliary ultrastructure
- Mucus composition and rheologic properties
- Mucociliary transport (MCT)
- Cellular defense
- Humoral defense

Cilia and Ciliary Activity

Ciliary function may be examined directly by measuring CBF, and studying ciliary structure by transmission electron microscopy (TEM). Indirectly, it may be tested by measuring MCT.

Ciliary Beat Observation and Measurement of Ciliary Beat Frequency

Ciliary function can be examined by phase-contrast microscopy or by studying ciliary beat using a photo-electric method. This is always done when primary (or secondary) ciliary dyskinesia is suspected. A brush or a small biopsy is taken from the medial surface of the inferior turbinate without the use of any local anesthetic or decongestants, as these drugs are known to affect ciliary activity. The brush or biopsy is best stored and examined in Locke-Ringer solution (sodium chloride, potassium chloride, calcium chloride, magnesium chloride, sodium bicarbonate, and dextrose in water), not in isotonic (0.9%) saline (Boek et al 1999). If no ciliary movement is seen, the cilia are studied morphologically by means of TEM.

Transmission Electron Microscopy

A more precise diagnosis of primary ciliary dyskinesia (PCD) can be made by TEM of the cilia. When structural anomalies like missing dynein arms are observed, the diagnosis of ciliary akinesia is very likely. The ultimate diagnosis of PCD is established by ciliogenesis in vitro, a technique that is only available in a limited number of institutions worldwide. Nasal nitric oxide (NO) measurement may, however, represent a good alternative and an elegant screening test for PCD. Low levels of nasal NO make a diagnosis of PCD very likely.

Mucociliary Transport Testing

Nasal clearance is tested by measuring MCT time. A small amount of an inert compound is deposited just posterior to the head of the inferior turbinate (or on the septum at the level of the valve area). The time that elapses until the test substance arrives in the nasopharynx is measured. In a normally functioning nose, MCT time varies from 8 to 12 minutes. This large variation diminishes the value of the test.

The substances most commonly used to measure MCT are dyes (such as charcoal, methylene blue, or edicol orange), a sweet-tasting substance like saccharine, or radioactive technetium. The test substance must not interact with mucus or the mucosal membrane, and it must be easily detectable in the nasopharynx. The arrival of a dye in the nasopharynx is established by posterior rhinoscopy using a rigid endoscope. When saccharine is used, the test subject is asked to inform the examiner as soon as he or she notices a sweet taste. The transport of technetium is determined by measuring radioactivity with a gamma camera. The combination of charcoal and saccharine is most commonly used in a clinical setting. Radioactive technetium is advocated for research purposes, as it is the most sensitive method.

Charcoal–Saccharine Test

A small amount of charcoal and saccharine is deposited just posterior to the head of the inferior turbinate. The method records the time elapsing until the charcoal becomes visible in the choana (as observed by posterior rhinoscopy with a rigid 70° endoscope) and/or until the saccharine is tasted. The method is simple but not very precise.

Technetium Test

This technique is a more precise method and is therefore preferred for clinical research. In daily practice, however, this method is less suitable. It is more cumbersome and requires the assistance of a department of nuclear medicine.

2.4.5 Allergy and Hyperreactivity Testing

The diagnosis of allergic rhinitis is based on the presence of two or more nasal symptoms and the demonstration of sensitization, preferably by skin prick testing. The patient is asked about any of the following reactions:
- Nasal symptoms like nasal congestion, rhinorrhea, secretions, and itchy nose
- Ocular symptoms like itchy eyes, tearing and/or conjunctival vascular dilation
- Bronchial symptoms like cough, shortness of breath, and wheezing
- Cutaneous problems like atopic eczema, itchy and red skin
- General problems like impaired sleep, disturbed concentration and/or reduced physical activity

The patient is also interviewed about abnormal nasal responses to specific stimuli such as temperature changes, air pollution (smoke, dust), food, drink, and light.

Allergy testing is an integral part of the routine diagnosis of patients with nasal mucosal disease. Skin prick testing (SPT) remains the diagnostic procedure. When there is discrepancy between history and SPT outcomes, or when SPT is not feasible or available, allergen-specific IgE should be determined. Allergen provocation is only advocated in patients where the association between allergen exposure and induction of symptoms needs to be clarified, such as occupational disease, or prior to starting immunotherapy.

Hyperreactivity may be tested by provocation of the nasal mucosa with histamine (histamine diphosphate 330 μg/nostril), methacholine, or cold dry air. These tests have not yet come into clinical practice due to their time-consuming nature.

Techniques Used in Nasal Provocation

The solutions to be used are prepared and administered according to the guidelines of the IRS as published in 2000.[1]

Nasal response is assessed by determining symptom scores (using a VAS scale) in combination with objective measurement of nasal patency, the amount of secretion, and the number of sneezes.

Several methods can be used to quantify the effects of provocation on nasal patency and airflow: anterior or posterior rhinomanometry, acoustic rhinometry or PNIF. Each method has its intrinsic advantages and disadvantages that should be taken into account.

---

[1] It is advised to follow the recommendations of the Standardization Committee on Objective Assessment of the Nasal Airway. See Clement PA. Committee report on standardization of rhinometry. Rhinology 1984;22:151–55 and Consensus report on acoustic rhinometry and rhinomanometry. Rhinology 2005;43:169-79.

Chapter 3

Surgery—General

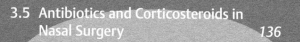

3 Surgery—General

3.1 Concepts of Functional Reconstructive Nasal Surgery

3.1.1 Surgery for Function and Form

The primary objective of nasal surgery should be to restore nasal function. The nose evolved to facilitate smelling and breathing, to detect odors, to control the inspiratory and expiratory airstream, to humidify and warm inspired air, and to serve as the first line of defense of the respiratory tract. These functions are taken care of by the interaction between the inspired air and the mucous membranes. This interaction is made possible by the complex airflow through the nose, determined by the geometry of the internal nose and by its external form. Therefore, all nasal surgery deals with function and aesthetics at the same time.

Nowadays, a large proportion of all nasal surgery is done in pursuit of the elusive goals of beauty and happiness. It is telling that most books on nasal surgery that have appeared over the past decades are devoted to cosmetic rhinoplasty. No matter how legitimate the pursuit of beauty may be, the nasal surgeon should be aware of the limits of surgery. If a person's nose is considered "normal" with respect to their ethnic origin, gender, and age, changing its features may run counter to medical ethics. Even in today's civilization, the primary objective of nasal surgery must be to restore function. The goal of functional improvement must always be given priority over that of enhancing beauty (▶ Fig. 3.1).

> "There could be something insincere about changing a nose." Arthur Miller "After the Fall" (1964)

3.1.2 Concepts

Nasal surgery or rhinoplasty should be functional and reconstructive. In the words of Kern, we must try to "recreate normality." We attempt to restore function by reconstructing normal anatomy.

> "In functional reconstructive nasal surgery we try to recreate normality." Eugene B Kern

Septal deformities are corrected and septal defects are reconstituted; a deviated bony and cartilaginous pyramid is straightened; a distorted nasal valve is corrected; irreversible hypertrophy of a turbinate is reduced. All tissues are handled conservatively and preserved whenever possible. Resections should be limited. Tissue is only removed where necessary for repositioning and reconstruction. A special effort is made to preserve mucosal membrane, the functional organ of the nose. If the turbinates are to be reduced, the required reduction in volume is achieved by a method that ensures preservation of their function.

3.1.3 Basic Principles

To achieve our goals of reconstituting function and form, we apply the following three basic principles:

1. *The septum and pyramid are corrected in one procedure.* Apart from exceptional cases, septal and pyramid pathology are addressed in one procedure. A deviated pyramid is nearly always combined with some type of septal pathology. The bony pyramid can therefore only be successfully repositioned after mobilization and repositioning of the septum. Similarly, deformities of the cartilaginous pyramid can only be adjusted after mobilization of the septum. A saddle nose is another example. First, the septum has to be rebuilt to provide support for the dorsum, tip, and columella. Second, the pyramid is mobilized and repositioned. Finally, the lobule is modified as required, and adjusted to the new septum and pyramid. If a transplant is to be inserted to augment the nasal dorsum, this is performed as the final step.

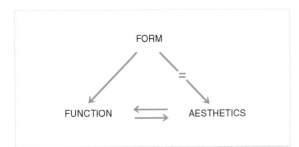

Fig. 3.1 Interrelationship between form, function, and aesthetics in nasal surgery. Aesthetics and form are identical, while function is dependent on form. Function and aesthetics usually complement each other; however, they may be in opposition. In this case, surgery for function should prevail over surgery for aesthetics.

2. *The lobule is preferably modified in the same procedure as the septum and the external pyramid.* In most cases, it is advisable to correct the lobule together with the septum and pyramid in the same surgical procedure. Limited and moderate modifications such as narrowing the tip, increasing or decreasing tip projection, and upwardly rotating the tip can be performed very well in the same operation. In patients with a more severe lobular deformity, it is better to postpone lobular surgery for a second operation. In special cases, additional dorsal augmentation (saddle nose) or additional lobular refinement may be indicated at a later stage. This type of refinement surgery should not be carried out before healing is completed (i.e., not earlier than 9 to 12 months after the previous operation).

3. *In patients with extensive pathology, surgery may be performed in two stages.* In cases with extensive pathology (e.g., cleft-lip nose, congenital hypoplasia, or severe saddle nose), surgery is planned from the beginning in two or even three stages. This may also be advisable in difficult revision cases. The septum and pyramid are then addressed in the first operation and the lobule in the second.

3.2 Endonasal versus External Approach

3.2.1 Historical Development

Surgery of deformities of the external nasal pyramid commenced in the second half of the 19th century using external incisions (Dieffenbach, Berlin 1845). The introduction of the endonasal approach to correct a dorsal hump and a bulbous prominent tip by John Orlando Roe of Rochester, New York (1887) was a great step forward. This method was further developed by others, in particular Jacques Joseph in Berlin in the first decade of the 20th century.

In the 1920s, Réthi of Budapest and Gillies of London introduced an approach to the nasal dorsum through an incision at the lobular base. Although this method did not have many followers, it was never completely forgotten (e.g., Šerçer 1957, 1962; see page 396).

In the 1970s, when almost all nasal surgeons were satisfied with the endonasal approach to various nasal deformities, the external approach was reintroduced. Within a few years, the "open approach" became very popular because it allows "open structure surgery." The external approach through a midcolumellar incision proved to be a great step forward, particularly in correcting lobular pathology.

3.2.2 Advantages and Disadvantages of the Two Different Approaches

Both the endonasal and the external approach have their advantages and disadvantages. Which method to use in an individual case depends on various factors: first, the type of pathology and the surgical goals; and second, the surgeon's personal preference and surgical experience.

> There is no such thing as a "typical" or "standard" rhinoplasty.

In general, surgery should be performed with as little trauma as possible provided that access to the surgical field is sufficiently wide to work safely. Since the endonasal approach is less traumatic to the columella, nasal tip, and dorsum, we could say: *"What can be done endonasally should be done endonasally."*

Although avoiding external incisions is an additional argument in favor of the endonasal approach, stab incisions for osteotomies and broken columellar incisions for the open approach have proven free from significant problems. The external approach is therefore preferred when a wide overview of the pathology of the lobule, dorsum, and anterior septum is required, and when wide access to the septum is necessary, for instance to suture the mucosa in closing a septal perforation.

3.2.3 Which Approach to Use When?

Septum

The best approach to the septum is the endonasal route using the caudal septal incision (CSI). This method combines the advantages of an endonasal incision with optimum access to all parts of the septum, including posteriorly.

However, the external approach can also be applied very well to deformities of the anterior septum. This particularly applies to reconstruction of the anterior septum, as shown by Rettinger (1993).

Bony and Cartilaginous Pyramid

A deviated pyramid is generally best corrected by the endonasal approach. Combining a CSI with a bilateral intercartilaginous incision (IC) provides excellent access to most types of septal pyramid pathology, such as the deviated nose, the hump nose, the saddle nose, and the prominent-narrow pyramid syndrome. Nowadays, many surgeons feel more secure using the open approach when dealing with dorsal problems. The excellent overview that it provides makes subtle and accurate corrections easier.

Lobule

In modifying the lobule, particularly in patients with more pronounced lobular pathology, the external approach offers several advantages. The direct view allows a more atraumatic dissection and better adjustment and modification of the cartilages. The external approach is the method of choice in patients with pronounced lobular abnormalities and in most revision cases.

3.2.4 Sequence of the Surgical Steps

In corrective nasal surgery, the sequence of the surgical steps is of great importance. There are no fixed rules, however. In our opinion, there is no such thing as a "standard" or "typical" rhinoplasty as we find described in some older textbooks. The way we deal with the problem depends on the pathology, the patient's history, and the surgical goals. The sequence of steps depends first of all on the surgical approach: the endonasal or the external (or open) approach.

Endonasal Approach

The usual sequence of steps when using the endonasal approach is as follows:
1. Mobilization and repositioning of the septum
2. Correction of the bony and cartilaginous pyramid: hump resection (if indicated), osteotomies, and repositioning
3. Additional septal surgery: septal reconstruction and fixation to adapt the septum to the new pyramid
4. Lobular surgery: modification of the lobular structures and adjustment of the lobule to the new pyramid

External Approach

The usual sequence of steps when using the external approach is as follows:
1. Exposure of the lobular structures and cartilaginous dorsum
2. Mobilization and repositioning of the septum
3. Correction of the bony and cartilaginous pyramid
4. Reconstruction of the septum
5. Modification of the lobule

It is a matter of personal preference whether the lobular surgery is carried out before or after performing osteotomies and repositioning the bony pyramid. If a bloodless field has been achieved, the pyramid is usually corrected first. Then, the lobule is adjusted to the new situation.

3.3 Preoperative and Postoperative Care

3.3.1 Preoperative Care

Discussing the Benefits and Risks of Surgery

Both the patient and the doctor want the results of surgery to be excellent. However, operations are not always as successful as both parties would like them to be. This certainly applies to functional reconstructive and aesthetic nasal surgery. Some patients may be disappointed. In certain cases, this might lead to a conflict, or even a complaint or lawsuit. Rhinological surgeons who are experienced in writing expertise reports in such cases have noted that the majority of patient–doctor conflicts are due to insufficient preoperative consultation, misunderstanding, and unrealistic expectations of the patient, rather than due to surgical failures. It is therefore of utmost importance to spend enough time ensuring that the patient understands the benefits and risks of surgery in his or her case. Modifying the patient's nose on a computer screen and suggesting or promising that the postoperative result will be the same may induce false expectations.

Informing the Patient

An *information leaflet* may help the patient understand the various modalities of nasal surgery and the way that surgery and preoperative and postoperative care are organized. In many countries, the surgeon is obliged to present such a leaflet to the patient. The patient should also understand that nasal surgery involves modifying living tissues, which means that the desired results can never be promised. The leaflet should also provide information about the potential complications.

Obtaining Informed Consent

Over the past decades, it has become more and more customary to have the patient sign an informed consent form. On this form, the patient declares that he or she has been informed about the type of surgery, the chances of success, and possible complications. Whether an informed consent form is used depends on the national legal situation and personal preference. It safeguards both parties and may prevent later uneasy discussions. In some countries, proposals to introduce an informed consent form have been turned down, as it was thought to cause too much anxiety in patients.

Risks to be Discussed

The risks to be discussed or mentioned in an information leaflet or informed consent form have always been a matter of discussion. In many countries, it is generally accepted that complications occurring in more than 1% of cases must be mentioned. In our opinion, very serious complications with a lower incidence than 1% (e.g., meningitis or blindness) should also be discussed.

Planning the Surgery

The surgical plan is discussed with the patient. The approach (endonasal or external) and the steps that are to be taken to achieve the goals are mentioned and explained.

If autogeneic cartilage might be needed for reconstruction or augmentation, the surgeon explains the choice of the donor site and discusses the consequences of the additional surgery. The patient is explicitly asked to give his or her consent for this part of the procedure as well. The need for internal dressings, as well as postoperative taping and splinting, is also discussed. The likelihood of developing certain postoperative complaints and inconveniences is mentioned. These include temporary mouth breathing, swelling of the eyelids and upper lip, possible ecchymoses, pressure headache, and some bleeding immediately after the operation.

In cases with extensive pathology, such as a bony and cartilaginous saddle nose, surgery in two phases may be indicated. In a two-phase operation, the septum and pyramid are addressed in the first operation, while the lobular work and additional augmentation is performed at the second stage 9 to 12 months later.

In patients with crusting, septal perforation, or ozena, it is advisable for the patient to start applying antibiotic–corticosteroid ointment (e.g., Terracortril) in the nasal cavities a week before surgery.

Antibiotics

Depending on the case, antibiotic treatment is started the day before surgery (see page 137).

Premedication

The premedication is ordered (see page 132).

Cutting the Vibrissae and Preparing the Surgical Field

At the start of the surgery the nasal cavity is cleaned using suction or cotton wool applicators. The vibrissae are cut and in special cases (e.g., transplants, revision cases), the vestibule is disinfected.

3.3.2 Postoperative Care

Immediate Postoperative Care

Medication

Postoperative medication is directed at alleviating pain and headache, preventing infection, and reducing swelling. When an antibiotic course has been started preoperatively, it is continued for 3 to 7 days, depending on the pathology and the type of surgery performed. A sleeping tablet may be administered in the first days as sleep is usually disturbed because of nasal blockage.

Pain/Headache

Pain or headache is treated by paracetamol or a similar drug upon request (usually 500 mg, 1 to 4 times daily). Normally, however, rhinoplasty does not produce pain. Most patients only suffer from headaches and pressure feelings that subside on the second and third postoperative day. If they have distinct pain, infection should be considered, particularly when a septal or dorsal transplant (or implant) has been used. Stent and tapes must then be removed carefully before the nose is inspected and palpated. Depending on the case, the internal dressing may be removed partially or completely. For treatment of the most common infectious complications (septal abscess, dorsal abscess, paranasal abscess, sinusitis), the reader is referred to Chapter 9, page 357.

Swelling

Swelling may be counteracted by administering systemic corticosteroids, but this is rarely indicated. Antihistamines may be used in patients who have an allergy. In other cases, they are not effective.

Fever

Some elevation of temperature (38.0 to 38.5°C) in the first 2 days is normal. Infection should be suspected when the temperature exceeds 38.5°C, is higher on the second day than on the first day, or takes a zigzag course. Another alarming sign is pain. The surgical field should then be inspected. Appropriate measures have to be taken, as previously discussed.

Later Postoperative Care

Internal Dressings

The length of time that internal dressing should stay in the nose has always been a matter of discussion. It depends on the type of surgery (and thus the purpose of the dressing) and the type of dressing applied. The various types of dressing materials are discussed in

129

Chapter 10 (page 372). Internal dressings with an important support function (supporting repositioned nasal bones or a reconstructed cartilaginous pyramid and septum) are usually kept in place for 3 to 5 days. Dressings to prevent bleeding and swelling may be removed earlier (after 1 to 2 days). It has often been claimed that patients suffer greatly from internal dressings and their removal. This is not the case in our experience. The disadvantages can be greatly reduced by using soft or coated materials, applying ointment on gauzes, and lubricating dressings with isotonic saline before removing. Internal dressings are preferably removed with the patient in a recumbent position. After removal, the nasal cavities and vestibules are gently cleansed of secretions and crusts using suction and cotton wool applicators with some ointment. Once the nose has been cleansed, instructions are given on the use of saline nasal washings, decongestive nose drops (gradually decreasing dosage), and ointment is applied to the vestibules over the next days.

Tapes

The use of external tapes and the timing of their removal will depend on the type of surgery and the surgical goals. The purpose of applying tapes is to reduce swelling, prevent hematomas, and hold the various structures in their new position. Thus, the more extensive the surgery and the structural modifications, the more taping is used and the longer the tapes have to stay in place. When eyelid tapes have been applied, they are removed on the first day (upper eyelid) and the second day (lower eyelid). Tapes

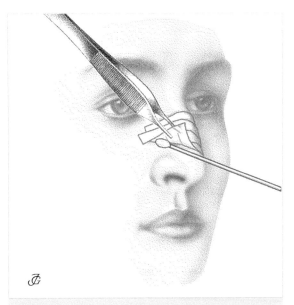

Fig. 3.2 External taping is removed in a lateral-to-medial rolling movement to avoid detaching the skin from the underlying tissue, using cotton wool applicators soaked in benzine.

fixing the skin to the underlying tissues usually stay in place for 3 to 5 days. They are then removed and usually replaced by fresh tapes. The same applies to the tapes that are used to help keep the bone and/or cartilaginous pyramid in its new position, as well as to the tapes that are applied to maintain modifications made by lobular surgery.

The doctor should allow ample time to remove the tapes very carefully. The patient is treated in a recumbent position, and every effort is made to ensure ample illumination of the surgical field. The tapes are rolled off the skin to avoid detaching the skin from the underlying tissues. This is done from a lateral to a medial direction using cotton wool applicators soaked in benzine to dissolve the glue (▶ Fig. 3.2).

Stent

A stent is used for the same reasons as tapes. In addition, a stent protects against trauma in the healing phase. Generally, therefore, a stent is removed on the third to fifth day, but it is adjusted or replaced by a fresh one if it does not fit properly. If osteotomies have been carried out, it may be wise for the patient to wear the stent for some weeks.

Sutures

Nonabsorbable sutures are generally removed after 5 to 7 days. Sutures used to close incisions may be removed earlier than those used to fix tissues in their new position. Resorbable sutures are generally left in place. However, if they are superficial, it may take rather a long time for them to dissolve. If they cause crusting, they are removed.

Endonasal Splints

Splints are removed after 1 to 2 weeks following mucosal local anesthesia and decongestion. If they cause complaints such as bleeding, crusting, or pain, they may be removed earlier. They may also be left in place longer, although there is rarely any reason to do so.

Patient Advice

The patient must not wear heavy glasses for 4 to 6 weeks after mobilization of the bony pyramid. Patients who are dependent on vision aids should wear their glasses on a small stent (▶ Fig. 3.3).

Sports should be avoided for several weeks. Sports with body contact (such as soccer or rugby) must be avoided for at least 6 to 8 weeks, unless a special protective device is worn (▶ Fig. 3.4).

Work can usually be resumed after 2 to 3 weeks. This time frame is, of course, highly dependent on the type of work. For example, someone in the public eye, such as a TV newscaster, will need more time before resuming professional activities than an office worker.

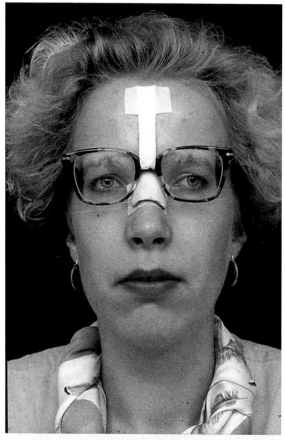

Fig. 3.3 A small stent is placed over the bony dorsum to protect the repositioned bony pyramid from dislocation by glasses.

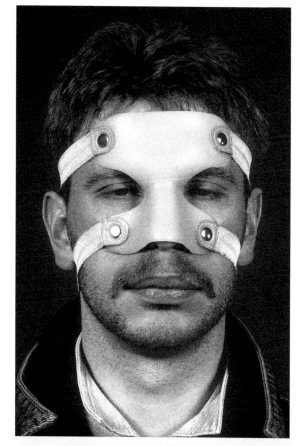

Fig. 3.4 Protective device worn during sports in the first 2 months after surgery.

Follow-Up

Healing Phase

A combination of surgical and social factors will determine how long a patient has to stay in hospital. Most aftercare, such as removal and replacement of tapes and stent, removal of sutures and splints, and nasal cleansing can easily be carried out on an outpatient basis. "Self-treatment" (e.g., removal of tapes) in the first 2 weeks should be avoided, in our experience.

The healing process is monitored at regular intervals. It is checked every 5 to 7 days during the first 2 to 3 weeks after discharging the patient. Progress is then checked after 1 month, 3 months, and finally 6 months to assess the functional and aesthetic results. After 6 months, standard postoperative photographs are taken and function tests are conducted to assess the final result.

Long-Term Follow-Up

The importance of long-term follow-up after nasal and sinus surgery cannot be emphasized enough. Unfortunately, many good early results of nasal surgery tend to deteriorate with time. The 3-month or 6-month postoperative photographs presented at meetings and in books do not tell the whole truth. Reality is different. Accepting reality is the first step toward improving one's personal results and the outcome of techniques in general.

Discussing Risks

When discussing risks, it is important to relate them to one's own figures. For example, the physician could tell the patient that ophthalmological complications such as impairment of vision have been described in the literature, but that such complications have never occurred in his or her own practice.

> **Patient–Doctor Conflicts**
>
> The majority of patient–doctor conflicts appear to be due to insufficient preoperative consultation, misunderstanding, and unrealistic expectations by the patient, rather than to surgical failures.

3.4 Anesthesia and the Bloodless Surgical Field

3.4.1 Local or General Anesthesia?

Nasal surgery can be performed under local or general anesthesia. Nowadays, most patients and surgeons prefer general anesthesia. However, certain procedures such as septal, turbinate, and lobular surgery can be carried out just as well under local anesthesia. Even osteotomies can be performed under local anesthesia.

Local anesthesia may be chosen on the following conditions:

- The psychological state of the patient must be normal.
- Sufficient premedication has to be administered.
- Local anesthesia must be complete.
- Surgery under local anesthesia should not last more than about 1.5 hours.
- Verbal communication with the patient should be possible during the operation.

If all of these requirements are met, local anesthesia may be preferable, as it usually involves less bleeding and postoperative morbidity is usually lower.

3.4.2 Local Anesthesia

Premedication

A combination of drugs is administered. There are many combinations that have proven their effectiveness. The objective of premedication is to avoid anxiety and facilitate surgery. Nowadays, anesthetists have various drugs at their disposal to control the state of the patient during surgery. Therefore, premedication can be best given in cooperation with an anesthetist. An additional reason for this policy is that local anesthesia can then be easily converted to general anesthesia if required.

Monitoring

As premedication may cause adverse general side effects, the most important physical parameters (pulse rate, blood pressure, blood oxygen saturation) are monitored. Moreover, an intravenous infusion with physiological saline is applied to allow additional administration of drugs if necessary.

Music

It is advisable to offer patients the option to wear headphones so that they can listen to music. They may be asked to bring their own CDs of easy-listening music. The sound should not be switched on before local anesthesia is complete. While anesthetizing, we remain in verbal contact with the patient.

There are several advantages to playing music: It dampens pain sensations, and the patient does not hear the noise of the operating theater and the conversation between the surgeon and the assistants. The latter may be especially desirable in a training clinic.

Principles and Technique of Local Anesthesia and Vasoconstriction

Block anesthesia is preferred over surface and infiltration anesthesia since it requires a lower dosage of drugs and does not interfere with nasal form, as infiltration anesthesia may. The following nerves are to be blocked:

- *Endonasally*: The anterior and posterior ethmoidal nerves, the pterygopalatine nerves, and the ascending palatine nerves
- *Extranasally*: The infraorbital nerves and the supraorbital nerves

Vasoconstriction is achieved by subcutaneous or submucosal infiltration at all areas where incisions are to be made, as well as paranasally, at the lobular base, and at the nasal root.

Notes

1. Pain sensations are limited by using already anesthetized areas as the access for further injection.
2. Subcutaneous infiltration of the external nose, especially the lobule, is avoided so as not to interfere with form. Subcutaneous infiltration is only given paranasally, at the lobular base, and at the nasion.

On the Use of Cocaine

Cocaine is a very potent but toxic anesthetic. It is more effective than the anesthetics developed later such as procaine, tetracaine, and lidocaine. At the same time, cocaine produces vasoconstriction, unlike modern anesthetics, such as lidocaine, which cause vasodilation. Cocaine was introduced as a local anesthetic, in ophthalmology by Koller, and in the pharynx and larynx (and consequently also in the nose) by Jellinek in Vienna in 1884. Despite its toxic side effects, many nasal and sinus surgeons still prefer cocaine to more modern anesthetics. For intranasal application, 200 to 300 mg is considered the maximum dose. Cocaine should be applied slowly and combined with a vasoconstrictive agent to decrease the rate of resorption. Most surgeons, like ourselves, use adrenaline for that purpose, although the combination of cocaine and adrenaline increases the risk of hypertensive and cardiac reactions. The systemic toxic effects of cocaine that may occur are cardiac arrhythmias (ventricular tachycardia and fibrillation). Euphoric excitement and restlessness followed by tremors and convulsion may occur. Central nervous system reactions can be counteracted by an intravenous injection of 10 to 30 mg diazepam.

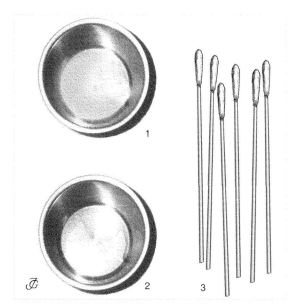

Fig. 3.5 Side-table with: (1) cup with 200 mg crystalline cocaine; (2) cup with 15 drops of adrenaline (epinephrine) 0.1%; (3) cotton wool applicators. A separate table is used to avoid mixing up drugs for surface application with those for injection.

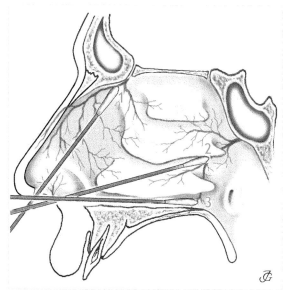

Fig. 3.6 Anesthesia and vasoconstriction of the septum, turbinates, and lateral nasal wall is performed with cotton wool applicators soaked in adrenaline (epinephrine) 0.1% and crystalline cocaine, which is applied at the entrance of the anterior ethmoidal nerve (1), pterygopalatine nerve (2), and ascending palatine nerve (3).

Endonasal Block Anesthesia

Endonasal block anesthesia and vasoconstriction is achieved by applying cotton wool applicators with crystalline cocaine and adrenaline (epinephrine) 0.1% to where the anterior ethmoidal nerve, pterygopalatine nerve, and ascending palatine nerve enter the nose.

Steps

- A small side table (▶ Fig. 3.5) is laid with:
  ○ A small cup containing 200 mg crystalline cocaine
  ○ A small cup containing 15 drops of adrenaline 0.1%
  ○ Cotton wool applicators
- The cotton tip is dipped first in the adrenaline solution and then in the crystalline cocaine.
- The first applicator is gently inserted parallel to the nasal dorsum in the direction of the anterior ethmoidal nerve (▶ Fig. 3.6). The second is gently applied in the middle nasal meatus, lateral to the middle turbinate. As the mucosa is still sensitive, the applicators are not forced into their final position at this stage.
- After preliminary decongestion and anesthesia, the tip of the first applicator is positioned at the spot where the anterior ethmoidal nerve enters. The second applicator is positioned against the lateral nasal wall, lateral to the tail of the middle turbinate. This is done to anesthetize the fibers coming from the pterygopalatine ganglion.
- A third applicator may be applied on the nasal floor at the posterior end of the hard palate, where branches of

the ascending palatine nerve enter the nose. Blocking of these nerve endings is advised for turbinate surgery, resection of a posterior septal spur, and in narrowing the nasal cavity by submucosal implantation.

Local Infiltration

Lidocaine HCl 1% with adrenaline 1:100,000 is injected with a 3-mL syringe using a 16-mm/0.5-mm (orange) needle in the vestibular area and using a 40-mm/0.8-mm (green) needle for paranasal injection.

Steps

- Infiltration (0.5 mL) of the membranous septum and the caudal end of the septum, using the short, fine needle (▶ Fig. 3.7)
- Infiltration at the site of the vestibular, intercartilaginous, and infracartilaginous incisions, using the short, fine needle; generally, two to three blebs per incision will suffice (▶ Fig. 3.8, ▶ Fig. 3.9, and ▶ Fig. 3.10)
- Bilateral infiltration (1.0 mL) of the nasal base using the already anesthetized area to insert the long needle (▶ Fig. 3.11)
- Bilateral infiltration (about 1.0 mL) paranasally, using the already anesthetized areas to insert the long needle; from this point, the infraorbital nerve can be blocked as well, if desired (▶ Fig. 3.12)
- Infiltration (0.5 to 1.0 mL) of the nasion to block the descending branches of the supraorbital nerve with the short, fine needle (▶ Fig. 3.12)

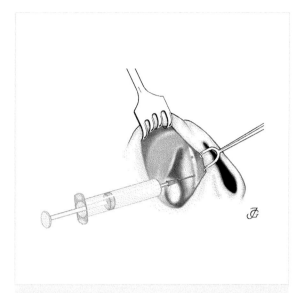

Fig. 3.7 The caudal septal end is subcutaneously infiltrated before making a CSI.

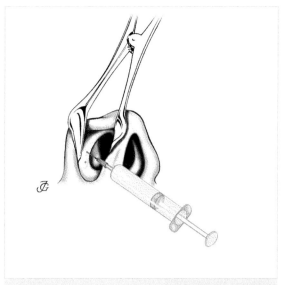

Fig. 3.8 Subcutaneous infiltration of the vestibular skin anterior to the ascending branch of the piriform aperture for the vestibular incision.

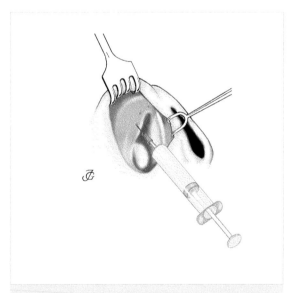

Fig. 3.9 Subcutaneous infiltration of the skin at the caudal margin of the triangular cartilage for the IC incision.

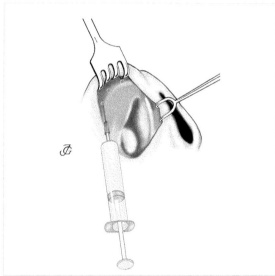

Fig. 3.10 Subcutaneous infiltration at the caudal margin of the lobular cartilage for the infracartilaginous incision.

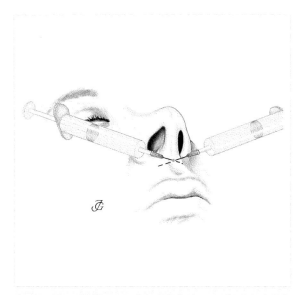

Fig. 3.11 Local infiltration of the lobular base is shown.

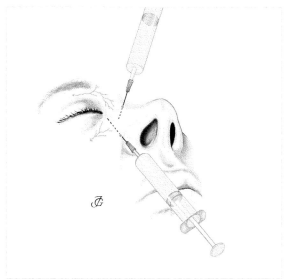

Fig. 3.12 Subcutaneous infiltration of the paranasal area and the nasal root blocks the branches of the infraorbital and supraorbital nerves.

3.4.3 General Anesthesia

Principles

A stable general anesthesia is essential for a bloodless surgical field. General anesthesia should be stabilized before additional local anesthesia and vasoconstriction can be applied. The level of the general anesthesia should remain the same until the very end of the operation.

Systolic blood pressure is stabilized around 100 mm Hg. The patient is positioned with the head about 40 cm above the level of the feet (anti-Trendelenburg position).

Additional local vasoconstriction and anesthesia are applied according to the rules that have been agreed upon with the anesthetist. In some cases (e.g., patients with hypertension or a history of cardiac disease), the use of vasoconstrictors may be contraindicated. This will have to be discussed prior to surgery. The cocaine–adrenaline mixture may then be substituted by a local application of xylometazoline 0.1%.

Additional Vasoconstriction and Local Anesthesia

Endonasal Topical Anesthesia and Vasoconstriction

Small gauzes soaked in a solution of cocaine 3% with epinephrine 1:20,000 are carefully applied endonasally in areas 5, 4, and 3. The gauzes are prepared on a separate table to avoid confusion with the topical anesthetic.

Local Infiltration of the Vestibule and Nasal Base, and Paranasally

Lidocaine HCl 1% with epinephrine 1:100,000 is injected at the caudal end of the septum into the nasal base, paranasally, and in those places where incisions will be made as described previously. Blocking the infraorbital and supraorbital nerves is not necessary in general anesthesia. Altogether, 5 to 7 mL will usually be sufficient.

In cases where time-consuming septal and lobular surgery has to be carried out, it is advisable to reinforce the paranasal infiltration before osteotomies are performed.

3.4.4 The Bloodless Surgical Field

A bloodless field is of paramount importance in nasal surgery. Less bleeding ensures a better view and less trauma. It is therefore mandatory to take all possible measures to reduce bleeding. In our surgery we place emphasis on:
1. The position of the patient (head up)
2. Lowering of blood pressure
3. Local vasoconstriction and anesthesia
4. Surgical dissection in anatomical planes
5. Compression of soft tissues during the operation

Patient Position

The patient is positioned with the level of the head about 40 cm above the feet. The head is also slightly rotated backward and positioned on a stabilizing cushion. Care is taken not to rotate the neck too much so as to avoid obstruction of venous backflow in the neck.

Lowering of Blood Pressure

The need for hypotension is discussed with the anesthetist. In general, a systolic blood pressure of 100 to 110 mm Hg is usually sufficient to control bleeding when it is combined with the other measures discussed here.

Local Vasoconstriction and Anesthesia

Local vasoconstriction and additional anesthesia are administered to the nasal mucosa, areas where incisions are made, paranasally, and at the lobular base (see previous text on techniques). Local application of a cocaine–adrenaline mixture to the nasal mucosa will prevent mucosal bleeding for about 1.5 hours. Local infiltration of areas where incisions are planned with a lidocaine–adrenaline mixture greatly enhances a bloodless approach, while paranasal and infralobular infiltration is of great help in hump resection, osteotomies, and lobular surgery.

Surgery in Anatomical Planes

Dissection should be performed in anatomical planes as much as possible. Sometimes, cutting through tissues cannot be avoided, for example when making incisions, in hump removal, and when dissecting scar tissue. These areas need local infiltration to reduce bleeding. To avoid unnecessary tissue damage and bleeding, the septum is approached subperichondrially and subperiosteally, and the nasal dorsum is undermined at the level of the loose connective tissue layer just above the perichondrium and the periosteum. Lateral osteotomies are preferably performed subperiosteally, while medial osteotomies are made intraseptally. In this way, bleeding will be prevented as much as possible.

Compression of Tissues

Compression of the tissues during surgery, especially in its final stages, is of great help in diminishing bleeding and preventing postoperative hematomas and edema. Temporary dressing of the nasal cavity after the first phase of septal surgery while working on the pyramid and lobule may also be of great help.

3.5 Antibiotics and Corticosteroids in Nasal Surgery

Whether patients undergoing nasal surgery require preoperative and/or postoperative administration of antibiotics and corticosteroids is still a matter of dispute. Our decision making in this respect is usually opinion based. The literature is not unanimous. Weimert and Yoder 1980 concluded from their prospective randomized study that the incidence of infectious complications is not sufficient

Table 3.1 Use of antibiotics and corticosteroids in functional reconstructive nasal surgery

	Antibiotics	Corticosteroids
Septal surgery		
primary	-	-
revision	(1)	-
severe scarring	1	-
transplant	2	-
Septum-pyramid surgery		
osteotomies	1	(+)
hump resection	(1)	-
transplant	2	-
Lobular surgery		
as an isolated procedure	-	-
Narrowing of the nasal cavity		
using transplant material	2 or 3	-
Concomitant sinus disease	2	–/+

to warrant the use of prophylactic antibiotics. Schäfer and Pirsig 1988, on the contrary, saw a distinctly higher rate of infectious complications in their study in septorhinoplasty patients in those who did not receive prophylactic antibiotics compared with those who did (5 versus 1 serious infection and 9 versus 3 moderate infections). Lilja et al 2011 administered 1500 mg Cefuroxim IV prior to septoplasty and found an infection rate of 2.2% compared to 8.3% in unprotected patients. An overview of the literature until 2008 was published by Georgiou et al.

▶ Table 3.1 and box Antibiotic and Corticosteroid Schemes summarize our protocol for the use of antibiotics and corticosteroids in nasal surgery.

Antibiotic and Corticosteroid Schemes

Antibiotic regimens
1. Amoxicillin + clavulanic acid 500/125
   3 dd 625 mg i.v. → oral 3–5 days
2. Amoxicillin + clavulanic acid 500/125
   3 dd 625 mg
   In combination with Flucloxacillin
   4 dd 500 mg i.v. → oral 5–6 days
   In patients allergic to amoxicillin:
   erythromycin 4 dd 500 mg

Corticosteroid schemes
1. Prednisolone (oral)
   20–20–20–15–15–10–10–5–5–5 mg
2. Prednisolone
   60–60–60 mg

3.5.1 Antibiotics

Systemic Antibiotics

On the basis of a number of studies, we may draw the following conclusions:

- In primary surgery of the septum and/or the lobule, there is no need for systemic antibiotic prophylaxis.
- When osteotomies are performed, antibiotics may be used to prevent infections.
- When transplants (especially allogeneic or heterotopic) are used in reconstruction, the use of a broad spectrum antibiotic is indicated.

3.5.2 Corticosteroids

Studies on the use of systemic and topical corticosteroids (Hoffman et al 1991, Kittel and Masing 1976) have shown that corticosteroids decrease the degree of postoperative swelling. This is not sufficient reason, however, to administer corticosteroids following nasal surgery except in special circumstances, such as patients with allergy or nasal polyposis.

Chapter 4

Incisions and Approaches

4

4 Incisions and Approaches

4.1 General

4.1.1 Terminology

Incisions, Approaches, and Techniques

There is often confusion about the terms *incision*, *approach*, and *technique*.

- An *incision* is an opening made in the skin or mucosa that allows us to gain access to a certain area or anatomical structure. For instance, the caudal septal incision gives access to the septum, or the intercartilaginous incision serves as an entrance to the nasal dorsum.
- An *approach* is a surgical method used to arrive at a certain structure so that it may be modified. For instance, an anterosuperior septal tunnel is used as an approach to the cartilaginous septum, or undermining of the skin of the nasal dorsum is a means to approach a bony hump.
- A *technique* is a surgical procedure or method by which an anatomical structure is mobilized, repositioned, or modified. For instance, the let-down technique is used to lower a prominent pyramid, or the inversion technique is used to narrow the nasal tip. Generally speaking, a technique is a method by which tissues are repositioned, modified, or resected.

Misnomers

From an anatomical or a semantic point of view, the names of the following incisions are incorrect.

Hemitransfixion: anatomically incorrect. This incision is not a half transfixion but an incision of the skin overlying the caudal end of the cartilaginous septum. We use "caudal septal incision."

Transfixion incision: linguistic misnomer. The word *transfixion* already implies that the tissues are cut through (Latin: transfigo, -fixi, -fixum = to stab).

Hemitransfixion incision: anatomically as well as linguistically incorrect (see previous text).

Marginal incision: causes confusion when used to denote the incision that follows the caudal border of the lobular cartilage (see ▶ Fig. 4.8). We use "infracartilaginous incision." The term *rim incision* is reserved for an incision at the rim of the nostril (see ▶ Fig. 4.18).

Glabellar incision: anatomically incorrect. This incision is not made at the glabella. It is made in a horizontal wrinkle at the depth of the frontonasal angle.

4.1.2 External versus Internal Incisions

Internal incisions are preferable to external incisions. External incisions are often said to become "almost invisible" when the tissues are handled delicately and sutured precisely. This may be true, but a completely invisible internal scar is always preferable to an almost invisible external one.

Therefore, external incisions are avoided unless they are inevitable. For instance, the columellar inverted V incision is inevitable in the external approach.

4.1.3 Basic Principles

When making an incision, we apply the following basic principles:

- *A rigid underlayer is preferable.*

  Incisions are preferably made at places where a cartilaginous or bony underlayer is present. The cartilage or bone will prevent undesired retraction of connective tissue during the healing process. Therefore, very little soft-tissue retraction is seen at a caudal septal incision, whereas unwanted scarring may result from a columellar incision, transfixion, vestibular incision, or intercartilaginous incision.

- *Incisions are made at right angles to the skin.*

  Incisions are generally made at right angles to the skin or mucosa for optimal healing. It is advisable to slightly stretch soft tissues while making an incision.

- *Incisions must be made with a sharp knife.*

  The belly of the blade is used, not its (pointed) tip. If a disposable blade has been used on rigid tissues, a fresh one should be used if further incisions are needed.

- *Incisions should be of sufficient length.*

  Incisions should be as short as possible, but long enough to provide sufficient access to the structures and allow the required maneuvers. If an incision is too conservative, the instruments will have to be forced in. This usually tears the edges, causing the wound to heal irregularly. This applies especially to incisions used for osteotomies, rasping, and inserting transplants. Incisions are only rarely continuous. All risk of postoperative stenosis must be avoided. There may be some exceptions, however. In surgery of the valve and the cartilaginous dorsum, the intercartilaginous incision may be connected with the caudal septal incision to obtain a sufficiently wide overview. Care must then be taken to restore normal anatomy when suturing.

- *Incisions are closed apart from endonasal stab incisions.*
  Suturing helps to adjust and fixate the tissues in their new position, avoid postoperative bleeding, and prevent scarring and stenoses (see Chapter 9, page 358, page 359, ▸ Fig. 9.71, ▸ Fig. 9.72, and ▸ Fig. 9.73). Stab incisions are usually closed by one suture or a small tape (e.g., Steristrip). The number of stitches applied depends not only on the length of the incision, but also on whether the incision was made solely to gain access or also to modify certain structures and their relationships. Changing the relationship between structures may require more sutures.
- *Suture materials—a matter of consideration.*
  The choice of suture material may be a matter of dispute. A thin monofilament artificial fiber, atraumatically mounted on a round needle, is probably the best. These stitches have to be removed after 3 to 5 days, however. When used in the vestibule, painless removal is usually difficult. We therefore use resorbable material for endonasal sutures.

4.2 Main Incisions

4.2.1 Caudal Septal Incision (Hemitransfixion)

The caudal septal incision (CSI), also known as the hemitransfixion, is made about 2 mm above and parallel to the caudal margin of the cartilaginous septum. It provides access to the septum, premaxilla and anterior nasal spine, nasal dorsum, columella, and floor of the nasal cavity.

A right-handed surgeon makes the CSI on the right side, even if the caudal septal end is dislocated to the left. Since the surgeon is standing on the right side of the patient, a right-sided approach means that the instruments can be introduced and maneuvered from the right.

Steps

- The columella clamp is opened and introduced with the right hand. It is gently closed over the septum and then slowly withdrawn until it slips from the septum. To avoid ischemia, the clamp is then fixed by turning the screw. The columella should not be clamped too securely for too long.
- In experienced hands, a nasal speculum may be used instead of a columella clamp.
- With the left hand, the columella clamp is moved to the left. It is then moved in a cranial direction to expose the caudal septal end and stretch the overlying soft tissues (▸ Fig. 4.1).
- The alar protector is introduced into the right nostril by the assistant.

- The caudal septal end is identified by palpation with the back of the handle of the knife.
- An incision is made in the skin parallel to the caudal septal margin at a distance of about 2 mm using a No. 15 blade. The incision should follow the full length of the caudal margin of the septal cartilage. Some surgeons like to incise from below, as shown in ▸ Fig. 4.1. Others prefer to cut from above or to combine a cut from below and from above. Care is taken to not cut into the nostril. The assistant is continually protecting the nostril rim opposite the blade.
- Skin, subcutaneous fibers, and perichondrium are gently cut through by multiple delicate strikes of the knife until the cartilage is reached.
- The last perichondrial fibers are scraped away in all directions with the No.15 blade, a Cottle knife, and/or pointed, slightly curved scissors (▸ Fig. 4.2).
- Care is taken to not cut into the cartilage, as this may cause bending of the caudal end.
- The columella clamp is removed.
- The caudal septal end is dissected from its ventrocaudal corner down to the anterior nasal spine with pointed, slightly curved scissors (see ▸ Fig. 5.4, ▸ Fig. 5.5, ▸ Fig. 5.6).

Suturing

The CSI is closed by two or three 5–0 or 4–0 atraumatic sutures, or by two or three 2–0 or 3–0 septocolumellar (SC) sutures.

Access

The caudal septal incision provides access to the following areas: (1) septum; (2) premaxilla and anterior nasal spine; (3) nasal dorsum; (4) columella; and (5) floor of the nasal cavity.

Septum: Depending on the pathology, the septum is approached by elevating the mucoperichondrium and the mucoperiosteum as discussed in Chapter 5 (page 159).

Premaxilla and anterior nasal spine: The premaxilla and the anterior nasal spine may be exposed by the maxilla-premaxilla–approach as illustrated in ▸ Fig. 5.17 and ▸ Fig. 5.18.

Nasal dorsum: The dorsum may be approached by undermining the skin as illustrated in ▸ Fig. 4.5.

Columella: Access to the columella, in particular the intercrural space, may be obtained by creating a columellar pocket as discussed in Chapter 7 (see ▸ Fig. 7.68).

Floor of nasal cavity: The floor of the nasal cavity may be approached by elevating its mucoperiosteum using the MP approach (see ▸ Fig. 5.17, ▸ Fig. 5.18).

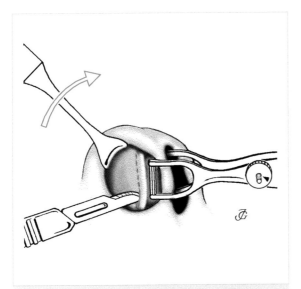

Fig. 4.1 The caudal septal incision (CSI) or "Hemitransfixion" is the universal approach to the septum, dorsum, columella, and nasal floor.

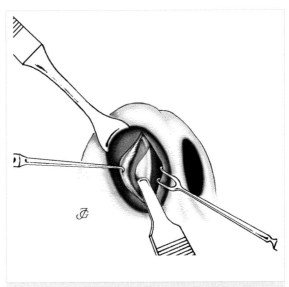

Fig. 4.2 The caudal end of the septum is exposed by scraping aside the last perichondrial fibers with a Cottle knife or pointed, slightly curved scissors.

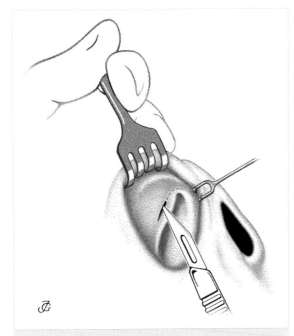

Fig. 4.3 The intercartilaginous (IC) incision used as an approach to the nasal dorsum and the lobule. It may be made using a No. 15 or a No. 11 blade.

4.2.2 Intercartilaginous Incision

The intercartilaginous (IC) incision is a cut made in the vestibular skin just cranial to the caudal margin of the triangular cartilage. The IC incision gives access to the cartilaginous and bony dorsum and allows retrograde undermining of the lobule.

Steps

- The ala is retracted in a lateral and cranial direction with the left hand using an uneven four-pronged hook. The middle finger is used to provide counterpressure, stabilization, and exposure of the valve area (▶ Fig. 4.3).
- The caudal margin of the triangular cartilage is identified with the back of the knife handle. The medial part of the caudal margin is examined for the presence of returning.
- An incision is made from lateral to medial just above the caudal border of the triangular cartilage using a No. 15 or No. 11 blade. The incision starts halfway along the lower end of the cartilage and continues just past the valve angle.
- A No. 15 blade is used to incise the skin only.
- When a No. 11 blade is used, the loose intercartilaginous connective tissue is cut at the same time. The blade is moved like a saw, cutting parallel to the triangular cartilage. The incision does not join with the CSI. A small tongue of tissue is kept intact between the ends of the two incisions (▶ Fig. 4.4). The IC and the CS incisions are only joined when wide access to the dorsum is required, for example in surgery of the cartilaginous vault and the nasal valve, for removal of a hump, and when inserting a large dorsal transplant.
- The ala is lifted by the four-pronged hook to open the incision. Blunt, slightly curved scissors are introduced with the points downward. The skin of the dorsum may now be undermined using gentle spreading movements in the plane between the subcutis and the perichondrium (▶ Fig. 4.5).

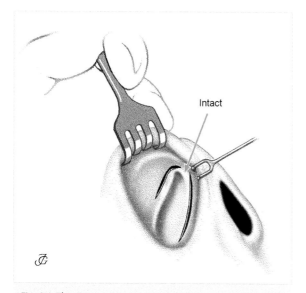

Fig. 4.4 The IC incision is not joined with the CS incision except for special purposes. A small tongue of skin is kept intact between the two incisions.

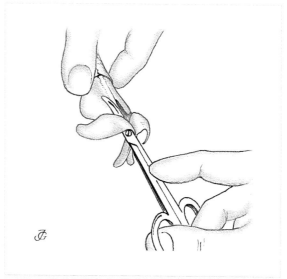

Fig. 4.5 Access to the dorsum is gained by supraperichondrial undermining in a cranial direction.

Note

The length of the IC incision depends on the kind of surgery to be performed. A (bilateral) incision of about 10 mm is long enough to undermine the dorsal skin for repositioning the bony pyramid. A 10-mm incision also suffices for inserting crushed cartilage or a small cartilaginous transplant. If the transplant is large, the approach has to be made wider, while the skin has to be undermined over a broader area. For transplants in the supratip and tip area, a very small cut just above the valve angle may be sufficient.

Suturing

The IC incision is generally closed by two or three 5–0 or 4–0 atraumatic resorbable sutures. After valve surgery, more stitches may be required. If upward rotation of the tip is desired, suturing may be done in an oblique fashion by "advancing sutures" This means pulling the tissues above the incision in a medial and cranial direction.

Access

The intercartilaginous incision provides access to: (1) the nasal dorsum and the cartilaginous and bony vault; (2) the valve; and (3) the lobule.

Nasal dorsum and cartilaginous and bony vault: The dorsum (cartilaginous and bony vault) may be approached by undermining the dorsal skin according to the technique shown in Chapter 6 (► Fig. 6.3 and ► Fig. 6.62; page 214 and page 235).

Valve: The valve may be exposed as shown in Chapter 6 (► Fig. 6.90 and ► Fig. 6.91; page 249).

Lobule: Access to the lobular structures may be gained by retrograde undermining of the lobular skin as illustrated in ► Fig. 7.4.

4.2.3 Vestibular Incision

The vestibular incision is a slightly curved cut made in the vestibular skin just lateral to the margin of the piriform aperture. It is used as an approach to the paranasal area, the piriform aperture, and the lateral wall of the nasal cavity.

Steps

- The skin of the vestibule is stretched using a short speculum (left hand), holding its blades in a vertical position (► Fig. 4.6).
- A slightly curved incision 7 to 8 mm in length is made with the No. 15 blade just lateral to the transition between the vestibular skin and the nasal mucosa. The belly of the knife is used. Only the skin is incised, as cutting through the subcutaneous tissues may cause abundant bleeding from the angular artery.
- The subcutaneous tissue is loosened up by gentle spreading movements in a craniocaudal direction using blunt, slightly curved scissors (► Fig. 4.7). In this way, the angular artery is pushed aside and remains undamaged. The dissection is continued up to the maxilla and the piriform aperture. The incision should be wide enough to accommodate the chisels that are to be used for osteotomies.
- If narrow osteotomes (2 mm wide "micro-osteotomes") are used, a vestibular incision will not be needed.

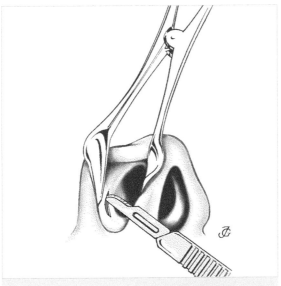

Fig. 4.6 The vestibular incision to approach the paranasal area, the piriform crest, and the lateral wall of the nasal cavity.

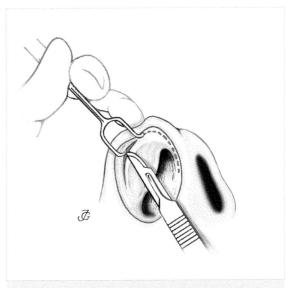

Fig. 4.8 The infracartilaginous incision to deliver the lobular cartilage in the external approach and the luxation technique.

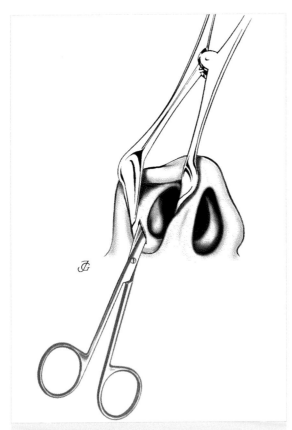

Fig. 4.7 The loose connective tissue fibers are dissected up to the maxilla and the piriform aperture.

Access

The vestibular incision provides access to: (1) the paranasal area; (2) the piriform aperture; and (3) the lateral wall of the nasal cavity.

Paranasal area: The paranasal area may be approached (for instance to perform lateral and transverse osteotomies) as described in Chapter 6 (page 229 and illustrated in ▶ Fig. 6.46, ▶ Fig. 6.47, ▶ Fig. 6.48, and ▶ Fig. 6.49).

Piriform aperture: The lateral and cranial margin of the piriform aperture may be exposed as shown in Chapter 6 (page 229; ▶ Fig. 6.46, ▶ Fig. 6.47, ▶ Fig. 6.48, and ▶ Fig. 6.49).

Lateral wall of the nasal cavity: Access to the lateral wall of the nasal cavity and the inferior turbinate may be gained according to the techniques described in Chapter 8 (see page 311).

4.2.4 Infracartilaginous Incision

The infracartilaginous incision is an incision at the caudal margin of the lateral crus, dome, and medial crus of the lobular cartilage (▶ Fig. 4.8). It is also called the "marginal incision," though this name may give rise to some misunderstanding, as previously discussed. In our opinion, the term *marginal incision* should be reserved for an incision at the rim of the nostril (see ▶ Fig. 4.18). The infracartilaginous incision does not follow the margin of the nostril but the inferior margin of the lobular cartilage. It gives access to the lobular cartilages and the cartilaginous vault. It is used in the external approach as well as in the luxation technique to deliver the lobular cartilages. It may also be used as the sole incision for access to the domes and lateral crura of the lobular cartilage.

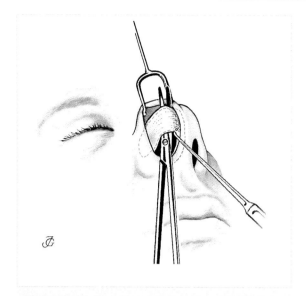

Fig. 4.9 The lobular cartilage is dissected free using small curved scissors, and delivered with a round hook that is poked through the caudal margin of its dome.

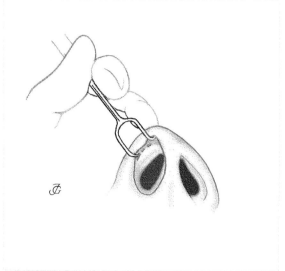

Fig. 4.10 The lateral infracartilaginous incision as an approach to the lateral wall of the lobule and cartilaginous pyramid.

The Infracartilaginous Incision As Used in the External Approach

Steps

- The infracartilaginous incision is usually made from medial to lateral.
- The transcolumellar inverted V incision is continued upward over the medial crura, then laterally at the caudal margin of the domes and lateral crura (see ▶ Fig. 4.12). Care is taken not to damage the rim of the cartilage.
- The cartilage is exposed by supraperichondrial dissection with pointed, slightly curved scissors or small angulated scissors (see ▶ Fig. 4.13). See also Chapter 7 (page 264).

The Infracartilaginous Incision As Used in the Luxation Technique

Steps

- The incision is made from lateral to medial.
- The lower half of the (right) ala is everted with a sharp–dull two-pronged hook (dull–sharp hook for the left ala), while the middle finger of the left hand exerts the necessary counterpressure. The caudal margin of the lateral crus is identified.
- The skin is incised from lateral to medial by gentle strokes with a No. 15 blade. Care is taken to avoid cutting into the caudal rim of the cartilage. The back of the blade is therefore kept in contact with the cartilage.

- As soon as the first millimeters of the incision have been made, the hook is repositioned. The sharp prong is placed into the upper end of the incision. The dull prong is positioned on the skin at the caudal margin of the cartilage. The incision is then continued (▶ Fig. 4.8).
- It is advisable to proceed slowly and to reposition the hook frequently.
- When the dome is reached, extra pressure is exerted by the middle finger to expose the ventricle. The incision is continued by carefully following the caudal border of the dome and then turning downward over the medial crus.
- The lateral crus, dome, and the upper part of the medial crus are now supraperichondrially dissected free from the overlying lobular skin with pointed, slightly curved scissors. The vestibular skin remains attached to the cartilage (▶ Fig. 4.9).
- The lobular cartilage can now be delivered by pulling it in a caudal direction by means of a small, round hook that is poked through the skin and cartilage at the inferior margin of the dome (see ▶ Fig. 7.10).

Suturing

The infracartilaginous incision is closed with 5-0 monofilament resorbable sutures.

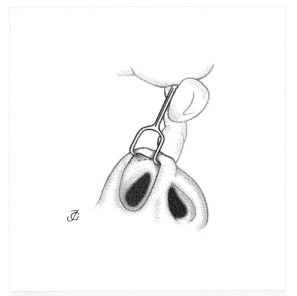

Fig. 4.11 The infradomal incision for inserting a small cartilaginous transplant or crushed cartilage.

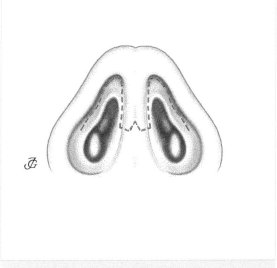

Fig. 4.12 The transcolumellar inverted V incision at the narrowest part of the columella, which is usually just below the middle, and bilateral infracartilaginous incisions as used for the external approach.

Limited Infracartilaginous Incisions

In special cases, a limited infracartilaginous incision is used, for instance when inserting (crushed) cartilage as filler or for reinforcement.

- *Lateral infracartilaginous (or "slot") incision*
  The incision is limited to the lateral part of the lateral crus (▶ Fig. 4.10). This incision may be used as an approach to the lateral wall of the lobule and the cartilaginous vault. It may be used to insert a small transplant or crushed cartilage as an underlay.
- *Infradomal incision*
  The incision is limited to the dome area (▶ Fig. 4.11). It may be used as an approach to the tip and interdomal area when inserting a small cartilaginous transplant.

Access

The infracartilaginous incision may be used to approach the lobular cartilages, as described in Chapter 7 (page 267).

4.2.5 Transcolumellar Inverted V Incision

The transcolumellar incision is a horizontal reversed V-shaped incision that is usually made at about two-thirds of the distance from the columellar base. It is made in combination with an infracartilaginous incision on both sides in the external (or open) approach (▶ Fig. 4.12). This method provides wide and direct access to the lobular cartilages, the cartilaginous dorsum, and the anterior septum (see also Chapter 7, page 264).

Steps

- The line of the incision is outlined on the skin. The columella is lifted and stretched, using the thumb and index finger of the left hand. The skin and subcutis is incised horizontally in a reversed V fashion at the narrowest part of the columella using a No. 15 blade.
- The incision is continued endonasally along the medial crura on both sides. Complete infracartilaginous incisions are then made as described and illustrated above (▶ Fig. 4.12).
- A columellar flap is dissected supraperichondrially from the medial crura in an upward direction, using pointed, slightly curved scissors and/or small angulated scissors (▶ Fig. 4.13).
- The end of this flap is handled with utmost care. Damage to the wound margin will later show as a scar with some retraction of the skin. Therefore, a delicate two-pronged or a small one-pronged retractor (Gillies type) is used (▶ Fig. 4.13).
- Bleeding from the columellar artery and its branches is controlled by bipolar coagulation, avoiding trauma to the adjacent tissues as much as possible.

Suturing

The transcolumellar inverted V incision is closed with 5–0 or 6–0 monofilament sutures.

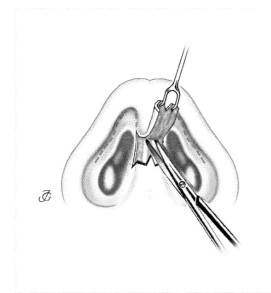

Fig. 4.13 Approach to the lobular cartilages, the septum, and the cartilaginous dorsum by supraperichondrial dissection with pointed, slightly curved scissors and/or small angulated scissors.

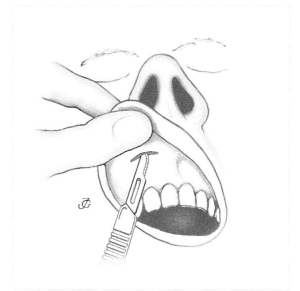

Fig. 4.14 The labiogingival incision may be used as an approach for lateral and transverse osteotomies and for narrowing of the nasal cavity.

Access

The transcolumellar inverted V incision may be used to approach the columella and domes. When combined with a bilateral infracartilaginous incision, it gives wide access ("open approach") to the lobule, the cartilaginous and bony vault, and the septum (see ▶ Fig. 7.14, ▶ Fig. 7.15, ▶ Fig. 7.16, ▶ Fig. 7.17, and ▶ Fig. 7.18).

4.3 Special Incisions—External

4.3.1 Labiogingival Incision

The labiogingival incision is an incision of the mucosa of the labiogingival fold at the floor of the piriform aperture laterally from the philtrum (▶ Fig. 4.14). Depending on its position and length, this incision allows access to the paranasal area, the piriform aperture, and the septum, as well as the floor and lateral wall of the nasal cavity.

For a lateral and transverse osteotomy, a 2-cm incision at the lateral margin of the piriform aperture suffices. The approach should be wider when narrowing the nasal cavity. In that case the incision is continued in a medial direction up to the philtrum (Denker's approach).

Steps

- The upper lip is lifted by holding it between the thumb and the index finger of the left hand.
- An incision is made in the mucosa just below the labiogingival fold using a No. 15 blade. Mucosa and periosteum are cut simultaneously.

- The periosteum is elevated in a cranial direction by means of an elevator. The extent of the periosteal elevation depends on the type of surgery.

Suturing

The labiogingival incision is closed with 4–0 sutures.

4.3.2 Sublabial Incision

A sublabial incision is a cut 4 to 5 cm in length made in the labiogingival fold (▶ Fig. 4.15). It provides a wide approach to the nasal cavity, septum, turbinates, paranasal sinuses, orbit, anterior skull base, and pituitary gland. This incision is mainly used for the transseptal–transsphenoidal approach to the pituitary gland (see Chapter 9, page 346). It is also used in sublabial rhinotomy (or the degloving technique) as an approach to major pathology of the nose, paranasal sinuses, orbit, and skull base.

Steps

- An incision 4 to 5 cm in length is made in the labiogingival fold using a No.15 (or No. 10) blade as described previously.
- The periosteum is elevated in a cranial direction. The floor of the piriform and the anterior nasal spine are exposed.

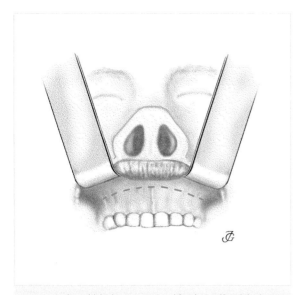

Fig. 4.15 The sublabial incision as used for the midfacial degloving technique and to approach the nasal floor and lateral walls.

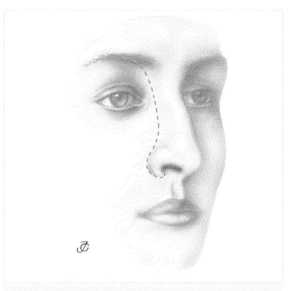

Fig. 4.16 The paranasal incision. This incision may be used as an approach to the nasal cavity (including the septum and turbinates), the maxilla, the paranasal sinuses, the orbit, and the anterior skull base.

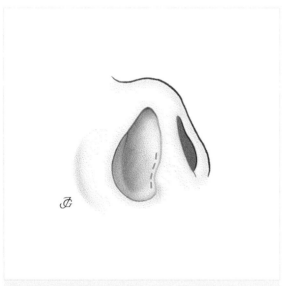

Fig. 4.17 The lateral columellar incision to approach the medial crus of the lobular cartilage.

sinuses, orbit, and anterior skull base. It is the classic approach to all major pathology in these areas (lateral rhinotomy). It has nowadays been replaced more and more by endonasal endoscopic techniques and the degloving technique (see page 346).

Steps

- The incision line is marked on the skin.
- The incision is made up to the periosteum using a No. 20 or a No. 15 blade.
- The periosteum is elevated with a McKenty and a Cottle elevator.

Suturing

The paranasal incision is closed in two layers. The subcutis is joined with 4–0 interrupted or uninterrupted resorbable sutures. The skin is closed with an uninterrupted 5–0 nonresorbable suture.

4.3.3 Paranasal Incision

A paranasal incision is an external nasal incision at the nasal base line (▶ Fig. 4.16). It may be extended downward into an alar-facial and alar-labial incision (including alatomy), and upward into an eyebrow incision. A paranasal incision provides wide access to the nasal cavity (including the septum and turbinates), maxilla, paranasal

4.3.4 Lateral Columellar Incision

The lateral columellar incision is an incision of the skin overlying the medial crus of the lobular cartilage. It is used to expose and modify the medial crus and the columella (▶ Fig. 4.17).

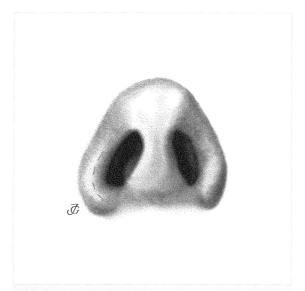

Fig. 4.18 The rim incision to correct deformities of the alar skin and the soft tissues.

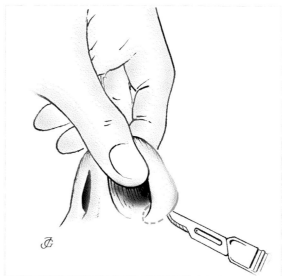

Fig. 4.19 The alar-facial and alar-labial incision (long-arm-U incision).

4.3.5 Rim Incision

The rim incision is an incision of the skin of the alar rim (▶ Fig. 4.18). It may be used to correct deformities of the alar margin or to resect connective tissue from the ala to thin an abnormally thick ala. However, an incision at this place is likely to leave a visible scar with upward retraction of the ala (see Chapter 9, page 363, and ▶ Fig. 9.84). Therefore, a rim incision should be performed only by very experienced surgeons and only in exceptional cases.

4.3.6 Alar-facial Incision (Long-Arm-U Incision; Alatomy)

The alar-facial incision is an incision at the alar-facial fold. It may be continued along the alar-labial fold and the inferior wall of the vestibule into a "long-arm-U incision" (▶ Fig. 4.19). An alar-facial incision may be used as a substitute for a vestibular or labiogingival incision in lateral osteotomies. It may also be used as an approach to the lateral wall of the nasal cavity. A long-arm-U incision is made to separate the ala from its base (alatomy) in cases where the ala is to be shortened (alar wedge resection) or displaced (lateral, medial, and inferior displacement). An alatomy may also be carried out to gain wide access to the nasal cavity, for example when closing a septal perforation or removing a foreign body.

Steps

- The ala is held between the thumb and the index finger and pressed dorsally to make the alar-facial fold more pronounced.

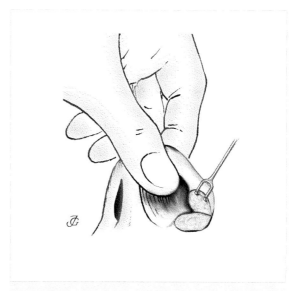

Fig. 4.20 The alar base is cut through.

- The skin and subcutis are cut in a craniocaudal direction with a No. 15 blade (▶ Fig. 4.19).
- If an alatomy is required, the incision is continued following the alar-labial fold into the vestibule. Meanwhile, the ala is lifted somewhat laterally to allow a better view.
- The alar base is cut through (▶ Fig. 4.20). Bleeding from branches of the angular artery is controlled by bipolar coagulation.

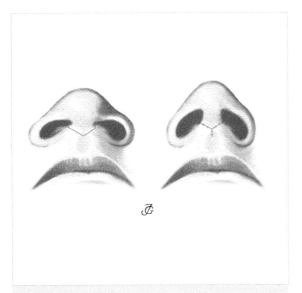

Fig. 4.21 The V–Y incision of the columellar base and upper lip to lengthen the columella.

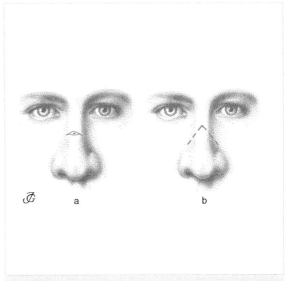

Fig. 4.22 (a) The horizontal dorsal incision of the nasal dorsum with resection of skin for removal of a congenital midline fistula. (b) Reversed V incision of the nasal dorsum for removal of a cyst or small tumor and for a "nose lift" procedure.

Suturing

The soft tissues are aligned with 4–0 resorbable sutures. The skin is closed with 5–0 monofilament nonresorbable sutures.

4.3.7 V Incision of the Columellar Base

A V-shaped incision of the columellar base may be used in a V–Y plasty to elongate a short columella (▶ Fig. 4.21).

Steps

- The incision is outlined on the skin.
- The incision is made with a fresh No.15 blade.
- To elongate the columella, the skin is widely undermined and then closed with 4–0 resorbable (subcutis) and 5–0 nonresorbable (skin) sutures.

4.3.8 Dorsal Incisions—Horizontal Dorsal and Dorsal Reversed V Incision

A horizontal dorsal incision may be used to remove a cyst (dermoid cyst), a tumor (glioma), or a large scar (▶ Fig. 4.22a).

A single reversed V incision on the dorsum may be used to excise a congenital midline fistula, a small cyst, or a scar (▶ Fig. 4.22b). In special cases, a double reversed V incision may be used to resect a wedge from the dorsal skin to shorten the nose and upwardly rotate the tip in patients with an elongated nose and a pendant tip due to laxity of the tissues in old age (▶ Fig. 4.22b). For the "nose lift" technique, see Chapter 7 (page 280).

4.4 Special Incisions—Endonasal

4.4.1 Transfixion

The transfixion is an incision through the membranous septum just in front of the caudal end of the cartilaginous septum (▸ Fig. 4.23). In earlier times, the transfixion was usually made continuous with bilateral intercartilaginous incisions. As a consequence, the lobule was separated from the cartilaginous vault, providing wide access to the septum and the whole pyramid. For many decades, the technique was used as a universal approach in rhinoplasty. Because of its disadvantages (retraction of the membranous septum and columella, drooping of the tip), this approach was later replaced by various separate incisions. The transfixion has been replaced by the hemitransfixion (CSI) as the method of choice to approach the septum. Bilateral intercartilaginous incisions have become the preferred approach to the dorsum. In recent years, the transfixion has regained some popularity, especially in combination with repositioning of the nasal tip with sutures. It is now used in combination with a sublabial incision in the degloving technique as an approach to the nasal cavity, paranasal sinuses, maxilla, orbit, and anterior skull base (see Chapter 9, page 346).

Steps

- The columella is grasped with the columellar clamp and pulled downward.
- The membranous septum is cut through just anterior to the caudal margin of the septum with a No. 15 or a No. 11 blade.
- The incision can be combined with a sublabial incision for a wide approach to the nose and its adjacent structures.

Suturing

The transfixion is closed bilaterally with several 5–0 resorbable sutures.

4.4.2 Transcartilaginous Incision

The transcartilaginous incision is an incision of the vestibular skin and the lateral crus of the lobular cartilage. It provides access to the lobular cartilage and allows modification of the lateral crus and, to a limited extent, the dome. Several surgeons use this "cartilage splitting technique" to narrow the lobule and the tip. It should be noted, however, that by this technique only the cranial part of the nasal tip and lobule can be reduced. One has to also take into account that narrowing of the tip and upward rotation by this method produces a certain connective tissue contraction that is not easily predictable.

Steps

- Since the transcartilaginous incision cuts through the lateral crus, it is advisable first to outline the margins of the lobular cartilages on the outside of the lobule. The line of the incision is then marked a minimum of 4 to 5 mm from the lower margin of the lateral crus. It is prudent to leave more cartilage, as additional resections may be carried out for symmetry. This marking may be done on the vestibular skin.
- A 27-gauge needle may be placed from the outside into the vestibulum at the desired level of the transcartilaginous incision.
- The ala is retracted with a dull four-pronged hook.
- The lateral wall of the vestibule and the lateral crus of the lobular cartilage are exposed by applying pressure with the middle finger (▸ Fig. 4.24).

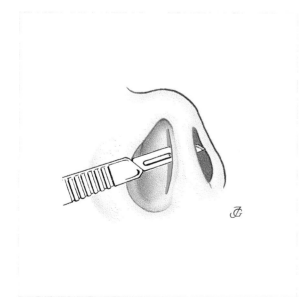

Fig. 4.23 Transfixion: this incision was used as the most common approach to the septum and dorsum in earlier times.

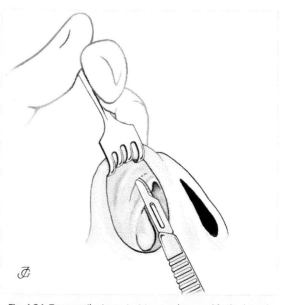

Fig. 4.24 Transcartilaginous incision used to modify the lateral crus and dome of the lobular cartilage (cartilage-splitting technique).

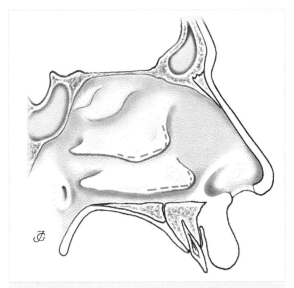

Fig. 4.25 L-shaped incision in the head of the inferior and middle turbinate for turbinate reduction.

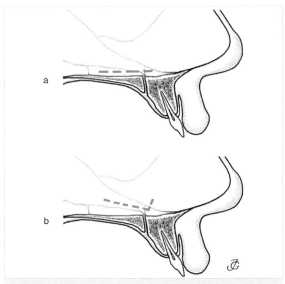

Fig. 4.26 (a) Horizontal basal incision in the septal mucosa to drain a septal hematoma. (b) Vertical incision in the septal mucosa to approach limited pathology of the posterior septum when reopening the anterior septum is risky.

- An incision is made in the vestibular skin and the lateral crus 4 to 5 mm (or more) cranial to the caudal margin of the cartilage using a No. 15 blade.
- The dorsal and lobular skin is undermined. The cartilages can then be modified as required (see cartilage-splitting technique, Chapter 7, page 265).

4.4.3 Incisions in the Turbinate Mucosa

Pathology of the middle and the inferior turbinate is usually addressed through an L-shaped incision in the mucosa of the head and the inferior margin of the turbinate, as shown in ▶ Fig. 4.25. A mucoperiosteal flap may then be elevated on both sides of the turbinate. This provides wide access to the turbinate bone and parenchyma and its pathology while preserving the mucosa.

Steps
- The mucosa of the head of the turbinate is incised in a craniocaudal direction using a No. 64 Beaver knife. The horizontal leg of the L is then cut from posterior to anterior.
- The mucoperiosteum is elevated bilaterally and the turbinate bone is freed (see Chapter 8, page 301).

Suturing

Incisions in the turbinate mucosa are difficult to suture, and suturing will not be necessary when a nasal dressing (gelfoam, Merocel, fingerstalls, or a small anointed dressing) is applied.

4.4.4 Incisions in the Septal Mucosa

Incisions in the septal mucosa are only made in special circumstances. They are generally avoided, as scarring of the mucosa may lead to epithelial metaplasia and interference with nasal mucociliary transport (MCT). This applies in particular to vertical incisions in the nasal mucosa. However, an incision in the septal mucosa may be indicated to drain a posterior septal hematoma (horizontal basal septal incision). In special cases, it may also be used to resect a limited deformity of the posterior septum when reopening of the anterior septum is hazardous.

Horizontal Basal Incision

A posterior septal hematoma may be drained by making a horizontal basal incision in the septal mucosa (▶ Fig. 4.26a). This incision is made in a posterior–anterior direction using a No. 64 Beaver knife or a No. 15 blade on a long handle. Anterior hematomas are usually drained by reopening the CSI and re-elevating an anterior–superior tunnel.

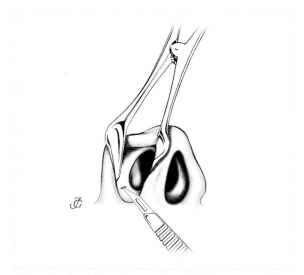

Fig. 4.27 Vestibular stab incision for endonasal lateral osteotomies.

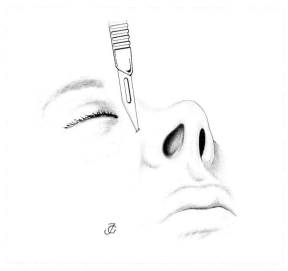

Fig. 4.28 Paranasal stab incision for an external lateral osteotomy.

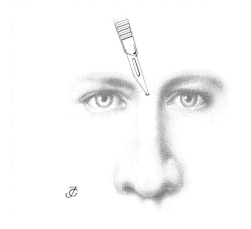

Fig. 4.29 Nasion stab incision for an external transverse osteotomy.

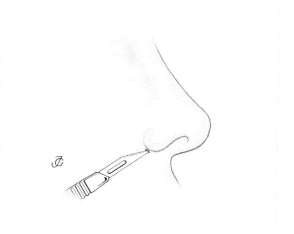

Fig. 4.30 Alar-facial stab incision for narrowing of the lobular base by a buried bunching suture.

Vertical and L-Shaped Incision

A vertical or an L-shaped incision may be made to address a limited deformity of the bony septum (e.g., a vomeral spur) in patients in whom a transseptal operation would be difficult and risky (▶ Fig. 4.26b).

4.5 Stab Incisions

Stab incisions are minor (1- to 2-mm) incisions that are made by poking a No. 15 or a No. 11 blade through the skin.

4.5.1 Vestibular Stab Incision

A horizontal stab 2 to 3 mm in length may be made in the vestibular skin at the base of the bony pyramid (at the level of the nasal base line) with a No. 15 blade. It provides an approach for an endonasal transperiosteal lateral osteotomy with a narrow osteotome (▶ Fig. 4.27). It is a matter of personal preference whether to suture the incision.

4.5.2 Paranasal Stab Incision

A paranasal stab incision may be used for external transperiosteal lateral osteotomies with a narrow (2-mm) osteotome (▶ Fig. 4.28). A paranasal stab is generally closed with a single suture and/or a Steristrip.

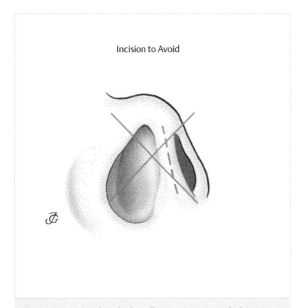

Fig. 4.31 A vertical midcolumellar incision is avoided as it may leave an external retracted scar.

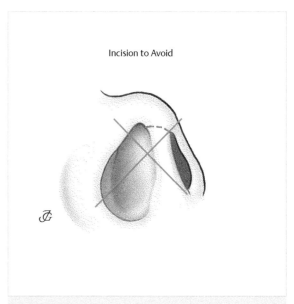

Fig. 4.32 High horizontal transcolumellar incision.

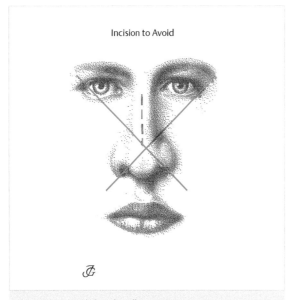

Fig. 4.33 Vertical dorsal midline incision.

4.5.3 Nasion (Glabellar) Stab Incision

A stab incision at the depth of the nasal angle or nasion (sometimes incorrectly called "glabellar incision") may be used for transverse osteotomies using a narrow 2-mm osteotome (▶ Fig. 4.29). It is made in one of the horizontal skin folds that arise when frowning. The incision is closed with one or two sutures.

4.5.4 Alar-facial Stab Incision

A stab may be made at the alar-facial fold to bury a lobular base suture, narrowing a broad lobular base (▶ Fig. 4.30). The stab should not be made too deep to prevent bleeding from a branch of the angular artery.

4.6 Incisions to Avoid

Several books on nasal surgery describe a number of incisions that were once used but have lost their significance because of evident disadvantages. We briefly discuss some of them here for historical as well as for educational reasons.

4.6.1 Vertical Midcolumellar Incision

A vertical midcolumellar incision was a popular approach to the septum and the nasal dorsum for a long time (▶ Fig. 4.31). It was used mainly for inserting dorsal transplants and implants. This approach has been abandoned. The incision does not follow the course of the relaxed skin lines and is made in skin that is not supported by cartilage (intercrural area). Therefore, retraction of the skin at the intercrural area could easily occur (see ▶ Fig. 9.71).

4.6.2 Horizontal Columellar Incision

A high horizontal columellar incision was introduced by Réthi as an approach to the nasal dorsum (▶ Fig. 4.32). It was later applied to "decorticate" the lobular cartilages and the cartilaginous vault (Šerçer). Since this incision does not provide wide access and often leaves a visible external scar, it is no longer used. It has been replaced by the transcolumellar inverted V incision at the midcolumellar level.

4.6.3 Vertical Dorsal Incision

A vertical incision on the nasal dorsum was introduced for corrective nasal surgery by Dieffenbach (1845). Later, it was frequently used to remove a congenital fistula, cyst, glioma, or other tumor (▶ Fig. 4.33). It has been replaced by a slightly curved horizontal dorsal incision. The latter follows the relaxed skin lines and consequently leaves a more acceptable scar.

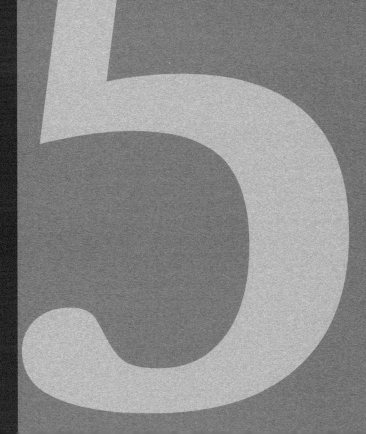

Chapter 5

Septal Surgery

5 Septal Surgery

5.1 Septal Surgery—An Essential Element of Functional Reconstructive Nasal Surgery

Septal pathology contributes to almost all nasal deformities. In a high percentage of all patients seen in rhinological practice, septal deformities are the main cause of functional complaints. In many cases, they are also at the root of aesthetic complaints. A deviated pyramid, saddle nose, narrow prominent pyramid, and most humps, are usually associated with some kind of septal pathology. This applies in particular to deviations of the bony and/or cartilaginous pyramid. In this regard, we may quote Cottle, who said, "As the septum goes, so goes the nose."

Consequently, correction of a septal deformity is one of the basic procedures of functional reconstructive nasal surgery. Repositioning of the bony and the cartilaginous pyramid is impossible without mobilization and repositioning of the septum, especially the anterior cartilaginous septum. In a sense, the septum is the "soul" of the human nose.

5.1.1 Sequence of Surgical Steps in Functional Reconstructive Nasal Surgery

The sequence of surgical steps in functional reconstructive nasal surgery depends primarily on the pathology, the history of the patient, and the surgical goals. A secondary determining factor is whether the surgery is performed by the endonasal or the external approach.

> "As the septum goes, so goes the nose." Cottle

Endonasal Approach

In most cases, the endonasal approach is preferred. For a discussion of the advantages, disadvantages, and indications of both methods, see Chapter 3, page 127.

Steps

- A caudal septal incision (CSI) is made. The septum is approached by elevating the mucoperichondrium and mucoperiosteum. The various septal parts are dissected free and mobilized by chondrotomies, as required.
- Parts of the septum that are irreversibly deformed or need to be removed to allow for repositioning are resected.

- The skin over the bony cartilaginous pyramid and lobule is undermined through bilateral intercartilaginous incisions.
- This is generally followed by correction of the bony and cartilaginous pyramid. If indicated, the dorsum is modified (hump reduction or resection). The cartilaginous pyramid is modified and repositioned, depending on the pathology. Valve surgery is carried out, if indicated.
- The bony pyramid is mobilized by performing osteotomies in combination with unilateral or bilateral wedge resections, if indicated. The pyramid is then repositioned.
- We now return to the septum. The bony and cartilaginous septa are adjusted to the new position of the pyramid. Additional resections of septal cartilage and/or bone may be necessary to allow repositioning of the septum in the midline. The relationship between the cartilaginous pyramid and the bony pyramid is realigned when required. The septum is reconstructed and fixed in its new position.
- Lobular surgery usually follows as the final phase of the operation. The desired modifications are carried out and the lobule is adjusted to the new position of the pyramid. Some surgeons perform the lobular surgery before, not after, repositioning the bony pyramid. This decision depends on the pathology and the surgeon's personal preference.
- The final step consists of fixing the bony and cartilaginous pyramid, lobule, and septum into their new relationships using sutures, dressings, splints, tapes, and stents.

External Approach

When the external approach is used, the sequence of surgical steps will be different.

Steps

- A transcolumellar inverted-V incision and a bilateral infracartilaginous incision are made. The skin is dissected from the medial crura, domes, and the medial parts of the lateral crura.
- The caudal end of the septum and the cartilaginous dorsum are dissected free and exposed.
- From this point on, the sequence of steps is similar to that in the endonasal approach. The septal mucoperichondrium and mucoperiosteum are elevated. The cartilaginous septum is dissected free and mobilized by the necessary chondrotomies.
- Parts of the septum that are irreversibly deformed or need to be removed to allow for septal repositioning are resected.
- The skin over the bony pyramid is undermined to allow for hump reduction or transplantation, if indicated.

- The cartilaginous pyramid is modified and repositioned, depending on the pathology. Valve surgery is carried out, if indicated.
- The bony pyramid is mobilized by performing osteotomies in combination with unilateral or bilateral wedge resections, if indicated. The pyramid is then repositioned.
- The septum is adjusted to the new pyramid, or reconstructed, as required. It is fixed in its new position.
- Lobular modification and reconstruction follow as the final surgical procedure.
- The various structures are fixed in their new position.

5.2 Basics of Septal Surgery—The Six Phases of Septal Surgery

In functional reconstructive septal surgery, six phases may be distinguished:
1. Approach
2. Mobilization
3. Resection
4. Repositioning
5. Reconstruction
6. Fixation

5.2.1 Phase 1: Approach

Caudal Septal Incision (Hemitransfixion)

The septum is approached through a CSI on the right side (▶ Fig. 5.1). This approach provides access to all parts of the septum, including the anterior nasal spine, premaxilla, and nasal floor, as well as the nasal dorsum and tip. As the incision is made just cranial and parallel to the caudal septal margin, a wide approach is obtained at the same time. A right-handed surgeon will make this incision on the right side. There is almost no exception to this rule. Even in patients with a luxation of the caudal septal end into the left vestibule, the approach from the right side is strongly preferred. For a detailed discussion of the technique of the CSI, see section Main Incisions on page 141 in Chapter 4.

Exposure of the Caudal Septal End

The caudal septal end is subperichondrially dissected over its full length, from its ventrocaudal corner to the anterior nasal spine, by means of a sharp knife (Cottle) and sharp, slightly curved scissors. The caudal septal end must be fully exposed to gain full access to the nasal dorsum, anterior nasal spine, premaxilla, nasal floor, and columella. Complete dissection of the caudal end is also essential for correcting a deviated caudal septal end, septal reconstruction, shortening of the nose, and rotation of the tip.

Steps

- The caudal margin of the incision and the columella are retracted to the other side by the assistant using a small, sharp, double-pronged retractor. The surgeon may use a small hook to retract the mucoperichondrial flaps.
- The last perichondrial fibers are scraped aside using a No. 15 knife (▶ Fig. 5.2). A scratching sound will be heard, indicating that the cartilage is reached. Care is taken not to cut into the cartilage, as this may lead to bending toward the opposite side in the healing phase.

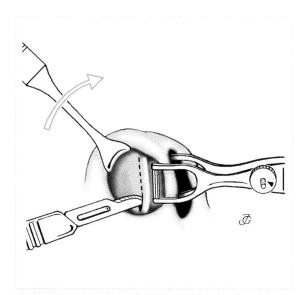

Fig. 5.1 CSI on the right side.

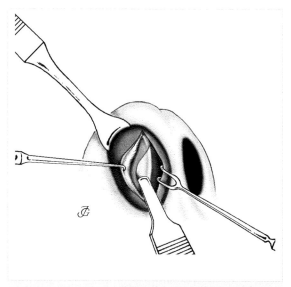

Fig. 5.2 The last perichondrial fibers are scraped away with a Cottle knife to expose the caudal end of the cartilage fully.

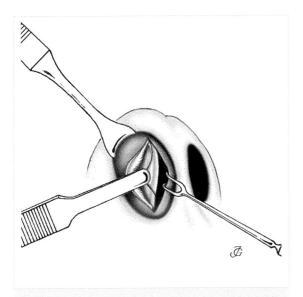

Fig. 5.3 The caudal septal cartilage is exposed by elevating the mucoperichondrium on the right side in a cranial direction.

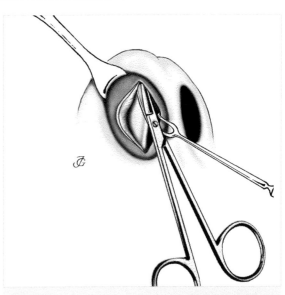

Fig. 5.4 The ventrocaudal corner of the cartilaginous septum is dissected.

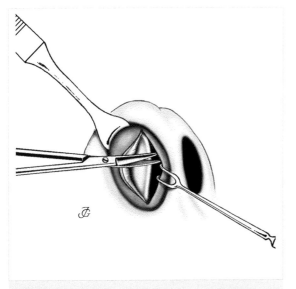

Fig. 5.5 The caudal margin of the cartilaginous septum is exposed and a (limited) columellar pocket created with sharp, slightly curved scissors.

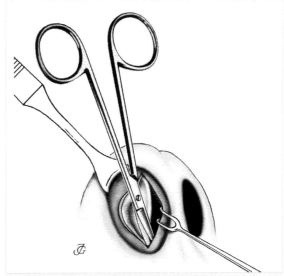

Fig. 5.6 The anterior nasal spine and the chondrospinal junction are exposed.

- The mucoperichondrium is elevated in a cranial direction and in a caudal direction to expose the caudal end of the cartilage (▸ Fig. 5.3).
- The pointed, slightly curved scissors are introduced to:
  - Completely free the caudal border of the cartilage
  - Expose its ventrocaudal corner (▸ Fig. 5.4)
  - Prepare a limited columellar pocket (▸ Fig. 5.5)
    - Expose the anterior nasal spine and premaxilla (▸ Fig. 5.6)
    - Start an anterosuperior tunnel (▸ Fig. 5.7)
- As an alternative, the Cottle knife may be used to scrape away the deepest perichondrial fibers (▸ Fig. 5.8).

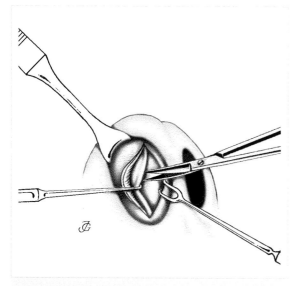

Fig. 5.7 Beginning an anterosuperior tunnel on the left side.

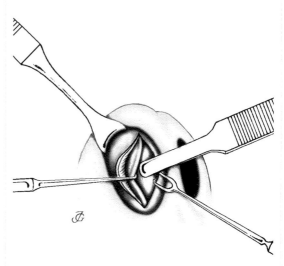

Fig. 5.8 The deepest mucoperichondrial fibers are scraped away on the left side.

How to Be Sure that You Are Working Subperichondrially

1. The color of the septal cartilage is bluish-gray. "If it is not blue, you are not through" (Cottle).
2. Using a knife produces a scratching sound.
3. There is no bleeding, as there are no vessels between perichondrium and cartilage.
4. Elevating the mucoperichondrium proceeds easily.
5. A "white line" is visible where the inner perichondrial layer is separated from the cartilage (connective tissue is stretched, no vessels are present at this level).

The Myth of Hydrodissection of the Septal Mucosa

Some old textbooks proclaim that injecting a local anesthetic–vasoconstrictive solution in the proper mucoperichondrial plane will "hydrodissect" the mucoperichondrium from the septal cartilage. This is very unlikely, as the perichondrium consists of several layers of parallel-running fibers (see ▶ Fig. 1.75). Injecting fluid just under the lowest layer by a needle that is thicker than the whole perichondrium itself is virtually impossible.

5.2.2 Phase 2: Mobilization

The next step is to expose and mobilize the cartilaginous and bony septum. This phase consists of:

- *Elevating the mucoperichondrium* and creating a bilateral (or unilateral) anterosuperior tunnel in combination with a unilateral or bilateral inferior tunnel, if required
- *Mobilizing the cartilaginous septum* by one or more vertical chondrotomies, dissecting its base from its bony pedestal, and creating a so-called swinging door
- *Elevating the mucoperiosteum* from the bony septum by creating posterior tunnels
- *Mobilizing the bony septum* by osteotomies (osteotome) and/or fracturing (forceps)

The Four Septal Tunnels

Four different tunnels are distinguished. Their use depends on the pathology and surgical aims.

We divide the septum into four regions (▶ Fig. 5.9):

- *Anterior and posterior,* with the cartilaginous–perpendicular junction as their border; and
- *Superior and inferior,* with the chondrospinal, chondropremaxillary, and chondromaxillary junction as their boundaries

Based on this septal geography, we distinguish the following tunnels:

- *Anterosuperior tunnel (left and right):*
  - Submucoperichondrial tunnels on the cartilaginous septum
- *Anteroinferior tunnel (left and right):*
  - Submucoperiosteal tunnels caudal to the cartilaginous bony junction

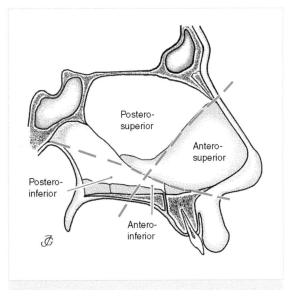

Fig. 5.9 The four septal regions.

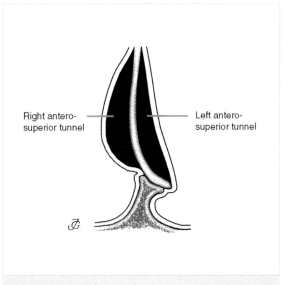

Fig. 5.10 Two-tunnel approach.

- *Posterosuperior tunnel (left and right):*
  ○ Submucoperiosteal tunnels posterior to the chondro-perpendicular junction
- *Posteroinferior tunnel (left and right):*
  ○ Subperiosteal tunnels on the vomer

The border between a superior and an inferior tunnel is more or less arbitrary, as the junction between the perpendicular plate and the vomer is very smooth.

The Different Methods

The combination of tunnels to be made in an individual case will depend on the deformities that we find as well as on our surgical aims. The following approaches are the most common:

1. Two-tunnel approach
2. Three-tunnel approach
3. Four-tunnel approach
4. One-tunnel approach

Two-Tunnel Approach

(Bilateral superior tunnels; ▶ Fig. 5.10.)

Indication

- Moderate septal pathology.

The two-tunnel approach is the most common and the traditional approach to the cartilaginous and bony septum in septo(rhino)plasty. It gives access to the entire cartilaginous and bony septum as well as to the various chondro-osseous junctions. This approach suffices in cartilaginous and bony deviations, fractures, crests, and

spurs. If undertunneling appears hazardous, a two-tunnel approach can easily be extended to a three-tunnel or four-tunnel approach.

Steps

- The mucoperichondrium is elevated (for technique see ▶ Fig. 5.14) on both sides in a posterior direction just beyond the chondroperpendicular junction. In the case of a vertical fracture, it is elevated just up to the fracture line. We do not elevate beyond a vertical fracture. Rather we prefer to make a vertical chondrotomy and then continue the elevation posteriorly on both sides of the cartilage (see ▶ Fig. 5.69 and ▶ Fig. 5.70).
- In a caudal direction (downward), the undertunneling is continued up to the chondrospinal and the chondro (pre)maxillary junction.

Three-Tunnel Approach

(Bilateral superior tunnels combined with a unilateral inferior tunnel on the left or right; ▶ Fig. 5.11.)

Indication

- Severe pathology of the premaxillary area.

An anteroinferior tunnel on the right or left side is joined with bilateral anterosuperior tunnels. This is the classical maxilla–premaxilla (MP) approach as described by Cottle et al (1958). It is used in patients with more severe pathology of the septal base, for example deformities of the premaxilla, a pronounced basal crest, or scar tissue. When special problems are encountered, the three-tunnel approach may be extended to a four-tunnel approach.

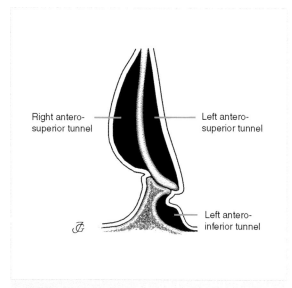

Fig. 5.11 Three-tunnel approach.

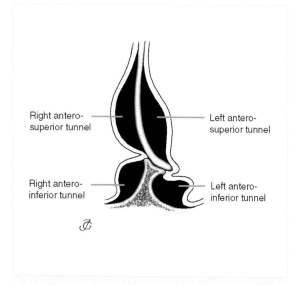

Fig. 5.12 Four-tunnel approach.

Steps

- Anterosuperior tunnels are made on both sides in combination with an inferior tunnel on the side of the deformity.
- The sequence of the different steps depends upon the problems encountered. In general, we start with a left anterior tunnel. This is followed by a right anterior tunnel, and finally by an inferior tunnel on the side of the pathology.
- The inferior tunnel is combined with the anterosuperior tunnel on the same side with a knife or the sharp end of the elevator or osteotome (see ▶ Fig. 5.19).

Four-Tunnel Approach

(Bilateral superior and bilateral inferior tunnels; ▶ Fig. 5.12.)

Indications

1. Severe pathology of the anterior septum due to previous trauma, surgery, and/or infection
2. Missing cartilaginous septum
3. Closure of an anterior septal perforation

Steps

- Anterosuperior and inferior tunnels are created on both sides. The sequence of the steps depends upon the pathology.
- We usually start making one or both superior tunnels, then elevate an inferior tunnel on the side opposite the pathology (crest), and combine this tunnel with both superior tunnels. Finally, the inferior tunnels are elevated while dissecting the pathology.

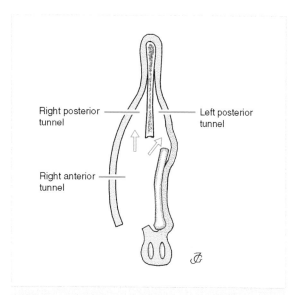

Fig. 5.13 One-tunnel approach. Anterosuperior tunnel is on the right, posterior chondrotomy and posterior tunnels are on both sides (axial view).

One-Tunnel Approach

(Unilateral anterior and bilateral posterior tunnels; ▶ Fig. 5.13.)

Indications

1. Isolated pathology of the bony septum
2. Approach to the sphenoid bone.
3. Transsphenoidal hypophysectomy

Whether the left or the right anterior tunnel is made first depends on the pathology. When a (vertical or horizontal) fracture is present, it is advisable to start elevating on the side of the deviation, then to cut through the fracture line, and from there continue with bilateral undertunneling.

Steps

- An anterosuperior tunnel is elevated on the right or left. The mucosa on the other side remains attached to the cartilage.
- A posterior chondrotomy is made at the chondroperpendicular junction.
- Posterior tunnels are created on both sides.
- If the sphenoid bone is to be opened, the bony septum is temporarily resected.

In severe pathology (scar tissue, missing septal cartilage), we usually decide not to continue elevating the anterior tunnels up to the bony septum. Instead, we first make bilateral inferior tunnels to facilitate dissection of the pathology and separation of the mucosal blades.

How to Create the Different Tunnels

Anterosuperior Tunnel

Steps

- The mucoperichondrium is elevated by means of the blunt end of the elevator (Cottle type). This is done in a sweeping up-and-down movement. Care is taken to avoid pushing forward, as this could easily lead to a perforation of the mucosa, especially in areas with pathology (▶ Fig. 5.14).
- It is of utmost importance to elevate under the inner layers of the perichondrium and to remain in the subperichondrial plane. Undertunneling should not be started before the cartilage is fully exposed. All perichondrial fibers have to be cut first.
- The blunt end of the elevator is used if no scar tissue is present. When a scar is encountered, the sharp end or a Beaver knife No. 64 is used.
- The mucoperichondrium is elevated either under direct view intraseptally or under indirect control through a speculum in the nasal cavity. When elevation is difficult, it may be safer to work under direct vision with the speculum in the intraseptal space.
- The mucoperichondrium is elevated in a downward direction to the chondro-osseous junction. In the case of a basal crest, elevation is continued down to the edge of the crest, but not beyond.

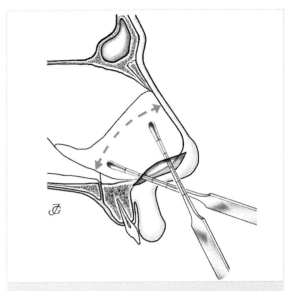

Fig. 5.14 The mucoperichondrium is elevated in a sweeping movement with the blunt end of the elevator.

Posterior Tunnel

Steps

- The cartilaginous septum is detached from the bony septum by a vertical posterior chondrotomy (see ▶ Fig. 5.20). Its base is then dissected from the nasal spine, premaxilla, and maxillary crest (see ▶ Fig. 5.26).
- A medium or long speculum is introduced intraseptally, and the septal cartilage is pushed to one side.
- The bony septum can now be addressed. With the sharp end of the elevator, the mucoperiosteum is elevated on both sides.
- If a spur is present, the mucoperiosteum is first detached on the contralateral side and then on the ipsilateral side, first cranially and finally caudally to the spur (see ▶ Fig. 5.67).

Inferior Tunnel

Inferior tunnels may be elevated (a) from above, or (b) from the anterior by the MP approach (▶ Fig. 5.15).

The first method implies that the chondropremaxillary area is approached from the posterior, whereas in the latter technique, the premaxilla is approached from the anterior. In patients with limited and moderate pathology, we usually choose the posterior approach, as it is less traumatic and generally provides sufficient access. In severe pathology, however, the anterior approach to the premaxilla is the better option.

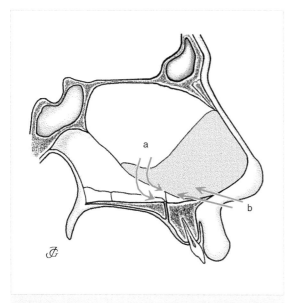

Fig. 5.15 The two approaches to premaxillary pathology: from above and posterior (cranioposteriorly) (**a**); and from anterior (MP approach) (**b**).

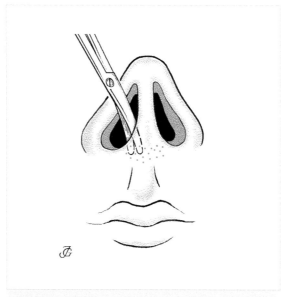

Fig. 5.16 The prespinal area is undermined to allow identification and exposition (if required) of the anterior nasal spine and premaxilla.

Inferior Tunnel from Above: Cranioposterior Approach

Steps

- The anterosuperior subperichondrial tunnel is extended downward (in a caudal direction) behind the premaxilla (i.e., along the lateral surface of maxillary crest and vomer). Elevation of the mucoperiosteum is continued to the nasal floor.
- Whether this is done unilaterally or bilaterally depends upon the nature and extent of the pathology.
- The undertunneling is extended from posterior in an anterior direction by dissecting the premaxillary wing. In the case of pathology (e.g., a crest), we cut though the wing with an osteotome (see ▶ Fig. 5.61**b**).
- The inferior tunnel is extended as far as necessary to expose the pathology, keeping the incisive nerve intact.

Inferior Tunnel from Anterior; MP Approach

Steps

- The lobular base is undermined to obtain sufficiently wide access to the lower part of the nasal cavity. The columella is taken between the thumb and index finger of the left hand and pulled somewhat downward. Blunt, slightly curved scissors is introduced into the lower edge of the CSI. It is gently pushed toward the anterior nasal spine and then spread. The tip of the scissors is now in between the mucosa of the upper lip and the orbicularis oris muscle. When the upper lip is lifted, the point of the scissors is visible under the mucosa just below the attachment of the frenulum (▶ Fig. 5.16).

- The loose connective tissue between the orbicularis muscle and the mucosa of the upper lip is gently spread, first medially then laterally. The plane of undermining is sometimes called the "magic plane."
- A small-bladed speculum is introduced, and the anterior nasal spine is palpated and visualized. The connective tissue fibers lateral to the spine are pushed aside, while the fibers in the midline in front of the spine are left in place.
- The periosteum of the maxilla below the piriform aperture is pushed laterally by means of a straight (McKenty) elevator (▶ Fig. 5.17). The medial part of the piriform crest is visualized.
- The fully curved end of a curved McKenty elevator is introduced and guided subperiosteally over the medial side of the piriform crest. Some force may be needed to insert the instrument underneath the periosteum and over the piriform crest, especially in Caucasians with a high crest. Perforation of the mucoperiosteum is prevented by keeping the end of the elevator in constant contact with the bone. This is done by exerting pressure with the thumb of the left hand (▶ Fig. 5.18).
- The slightly curved end of the McKenty elevator is introduced. A submucoperiosteal tunnel is elevated underneath the premaxillary wing and the medial part of the nasal floor. This may be done under indirect view through a speculum in the nasal cavity.
- The tunnel is extended upward to the chondropremaxillary and chondromaxillary junction using the sharp end of a septal elevator.

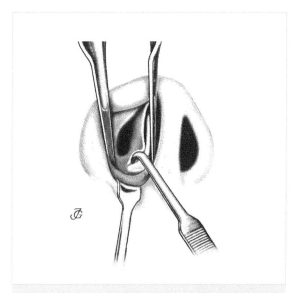

Fig. 5.17 The mucoperiosteum of the maxilla is pushed aside with a straight elevator to expose the piriform crest.

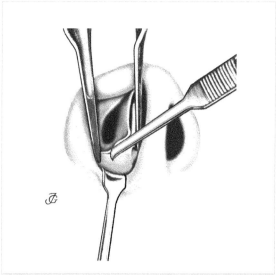

Fig. 5.18 Beginning an inferior tunnel by elevating the mucoperiosteum with a curved elevator.

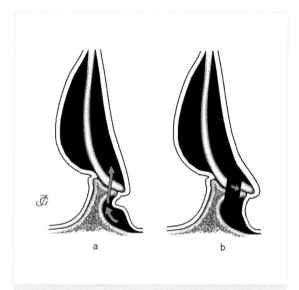

Fig. 5.19 a, b Connecting an inferior with a superior tunnel. (a) Cutting through the pathology from below. (b) The lateral part of the basal crest is temporarily left attached to the mucosa and resected at a later stage.

When elevating the mucoperiosteum of the nasal floor in making an inferior tunnel, the incisive nerve and vessels will be cut. This may cause temporary loss of sensitivity in a small triangular area of the palatal mucosa just behind the incisor teeth (see also ▶ Fig. 1.59; page 27).

Connecting an Inferior with a Superior Tunnel

Steps

- An inferior tunnel is connected with a superior tunnel by dissecting through the connective (and scar) tissue lateral to the chondro-osseous junction using semi-sharp or sharp instruments (sharp end of the elevator, Beaver No. 64 knife, Cottle knife, or No. 15 blade). Dissection is best carried out in an upward direction, as this offers the best overview (▶ Fig. 5.19 a).
- A crest, loose fragments of cartilage or bone, and extensive scar formations may be resected during the dissection.
- The cartilaginous septum is disconnected from its base (▶ Fig. 5.19 b).

Chondrotomies

The cartilaginous septum may be cut in a vertical, horizontal, or oblique direction to mobilize and resect parts of the cartilage and to allow its repositioning.

Posterior Vertical Chondrotomy

The cartilaginous septum is disconnected posteriorly by a vertical incision at the chondroperpendicular junction (▶ Fig. 5.20). This is usually followed by dissecting the septum from its base to create a "swinging door."

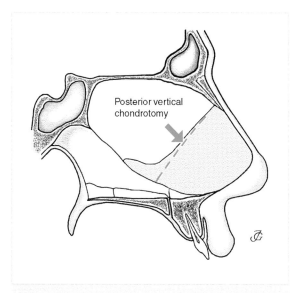

Fig. 5.20 Posterior chondrotomy at the chondroperpendicular junction. The upper 1 to 1.5 cm of the cartilaginous septum is left attached to the bony septum and bony pyramid to avoid endorotation of the cartilaginous septal plate with sagging of the dorsum and retraction of the columella.

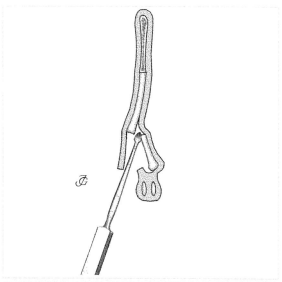

Fig. 5.21 Vertical chondrotomy with a Cottle elevator.

Steps

- A vertical cut is made at the junction between the cartilaginous and bony septum (or 1 to 2 mm anterior) with the sharp end of a Cottle elevator, a Masing Ritzmesser, or a Beaver knife (▶ Fig. 5.21).
- It may be helpful at this stage to resect a small triangular vertical strip of cartilage to facilitate mobilization of the cartilaginous septum.

Vertical Chondrotomy at a Fracture Line

The cartilaginous septum is cut at, or just in front of, a vertical fracture to allow mobilization, resection, and repositioning of deviated and fractured parts (▶ Fig. 5.22).

Steps

- The cartilage is cut with a knife just in front of the fracture line, working from above and cutting downward. Care is taken to keep the mucoperichondrium of the opposite side intact.
- The cartilage is left attached to its posterior part and to the triangular cartilages, unless the pathology dictates otherwise.
- The deformity may be such that separating the septum from one or both triangular cartilages is necessary to straighten the cartilaginous pyramid and the septum. The septal plate will then become detached from all other structures. It will thus have to be fixed in its new position by sutures (and splints) in the reconstruction and fixation phase.

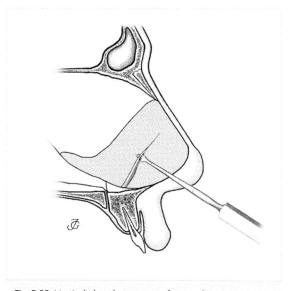

Fig. 5.22 Vertical chondrotomy at a fracture line.

Double Vertical Chondrotomy

Sometimes two vertical chondrotomies behind each other (double vertical chondrotomy) are required for repositioning. This technique may be applied for correcting a double vertical fracture ("harmonica septum") or a convexity (▶ Fig. 5.23).

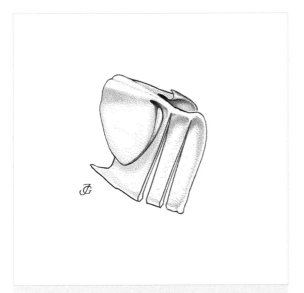

Fig. 5.23 Double vertical chondrotomy.

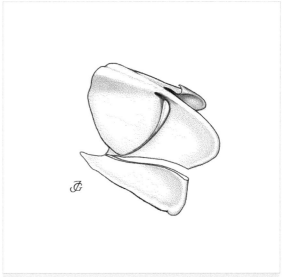

Fig. 5.24 Chondrotomy at a horizontal fracture line.

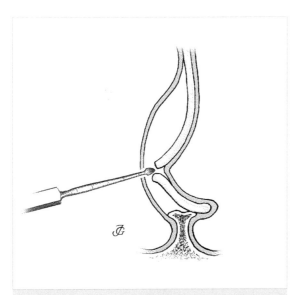

Fig. 5.25 Horizontal chondrotomy using the sharp end of a Cottle elevator.

Horizontal Chondrotomy

The cartilage is cut in a horizontal direction (▶ Fig. 5.24 and ▶ Fig. 5.25). This may be required at a horizontal fracture (see page 101 and ▶ Fig. 2.109) or just above a crest to allow mobilization, resections, and repositioning. In general, we try to refrain from making horizontal cuts in the cartilaginous septum, as they deprive the cartilaginous pyramid of its support. Horizontal chondrotomies are particularly risky if they are followed by resection of a horizontal strip or crest, leaving a horizontal defect. This may lead to sagging of the cartilaginous dorsum, unless the anterior septum still rests on the anterior nasal spine.

Dissecting the Cartilaginous Septum from Its Base ("Swinging Door" Technique)

After disconnecting the cartilaginous septum from the bony septum by one or more vertical chondrotomies, its base will have to be dissected and dislocated from the premaxilla and anterior nasal spine to create a "swinging door" and provide wide access to the posterior septum.

Steps

- The cartilaginous septum is dissected from its base from posterior to anterior at the chondro-osseous junction with the sharp end of the elevator (▶ Fig. 5.26).
- The septal plate is now mobile and can be displaced laterally by means of a broad-bladed speculum (▶ Fig. 5.27). A right-handed surgeon standing on the right side of the patient will generally choose to move the cartilaginous plate to the left. This will provide the best approach to the posterior septum.

Steps

- The first vertical chondrotomy is made just anterior to the first fracture line. A small vertical strip of cartilage is removed.
- A second vertical chondrotomy is made either at the second fracture line or at the cartilaginous–osseous junction, depending on the deformity. A second vertical strip may be resected here (see ▶ Fig. 5.28).

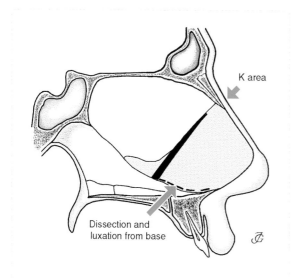

Fig. 5.26 The cartilaginous septum is dissected from its base: a "swinging door" is created.

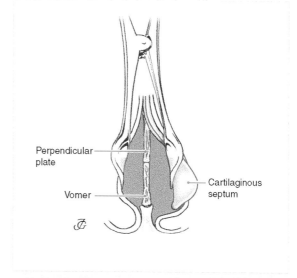

Fig. 5.27 The "swinging door" technique. The cartilaginous septum has been mobilized and is dislocated to the left with a speculum to obtain wide access to the bony septum, vomer, and perpendicular plate.

- A triangular strip may be resected at the posterior chondrotomy (▶ Fig. 5.28) and from the septal base to obtain greater mobility of the cartilaginous plate. However, no cartilage is resected underneath the K area or from the septal base in the region of the anterior nasal spine. Resections in these areas may lead to endorotation of the septal cartilage, which in turn will result in postoperative sagging of the dorsum and retraction of the columella.
- A cartilaginous and bony crest may impede an attempt to dissect the septal base from the premaxilla and maxillary crest. A horizontal cut is then made in the cartilage just above the crest. The septal cartilage is dissected first, then the crest is resected. First, its cartilaginous part is dissected and removed, then its bony part is resected with a chisel or a biting forceps (for further details, see ▶ Fig. 5.60, ▶ Fig. 5.61, and ▶ Fig. 5.62).

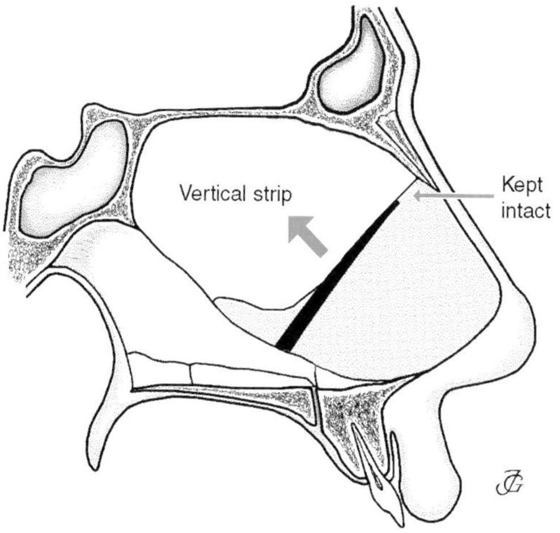

5.2.3 Phase 3: Resection

Resection of parts of the cartilaginous and bony septum will only be carried out where necessary for repositioning, and when they are irreversibly deformed.

Vertical Strips

Vertical Strip at the Chondro-Osseous Junction

A narrow, triangular, vertical strip may be resected at the chondroperpendicular junction to facilitate mobilization

Fig. 5.28 Resection of a triangular vertical strip of cartilage at the chondroperpendicular junction to mobilize the cartilaginous septum.

of the cartilaginous septum. Care is taken to keep the upper 1 to 1.5 cm of the cartilage attached to the nasal pyramid to avoid endorotation of the septum with subsequent sagging of the dorsum and retraction of the columella (▶ Fig. 5.28).

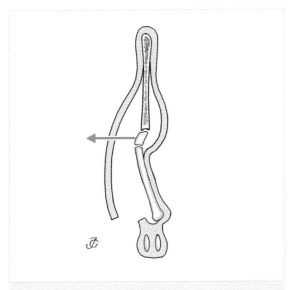

Fig. 5.29 Resection of a vertical strip at a vertical fracture line.

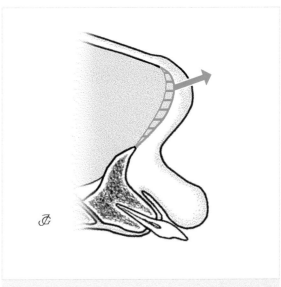

Fig. 5.30 Resection of a vertical strip at the caudal septal end.

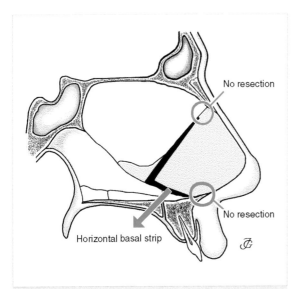

Fig. 5.31 Resection of a horizontal basal strip to obtain greater mobility of the septum. Note the two areas where no cartilage is resected to avoid endorotation of the septal plate.

Vertical Strip at a Vertical Fracture

A triangular or parallel strip may be resected at a vertical fracture line or a bend to remove superfluous cartilage and to enable repositioning of the dislocated parts into the midline (▶ Fig. 5.29). See also the discussion on Vertical Fracture, page 185.

Vertical Strip at the Caudal Septal End

A vertical strip may be resected at the caudal end of the septum to shorten the septum (▶ Fig. 5.30). This strip may be rectangular or triangular, depending on the surgical goals (for details, see ▶ Fig. 5.48; page 177).

Horizontal Strips

Horizontal Basal Strip

A horizontal basal strip may be resected to obtain greater mobility of the septal plate, facilitate its repositioning, and obtain wide access to the bony septum. The resected strip should be narrow (2 to 3 mm) and triangular in shape to avoid loss of support and endorotation of the septum, resulting in sagging of the dorsum and retraction of the columella (▶ Fig. 5.31). See also Chapter 9, page 358.

Horizontal Strip at a Horizontal Fracture

A horizontal strip will usually have to be resected at the level of a horizontal fracture to allow repositioning of the deviated parts. This too is done in a conservative way to avoid creating a gap that may lead to loss of support of the dorsum. (For further details, see page 186; ▶ Fig. 5.72, ▶ Fig. 5.73, and ▶ Fig. 5.74).

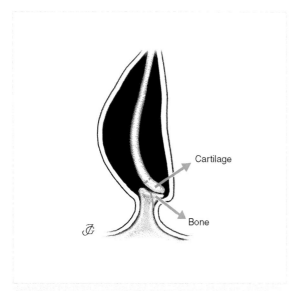

Fig. 5.32 Resection of a bony and cartilaginous crest from above.

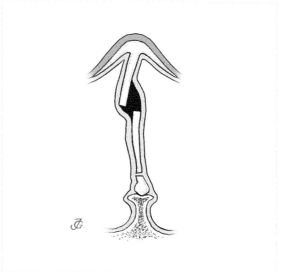

Fig. 5.33 Persistent high bony deviation with "tenting" effect.

Bony and Cartilaginous Crest

A bony and cartilaginous (basal) crest has usually to be removed. In most cases, this can be done from above. A horizontal chondrotomy is made just above the crest, allowing the cartilaginous part of the crest to be dissected and removed. Its bony part is then cut off with an osteotome while still attached to the mucosa, and carefully freed from the mucoperiosteum and resected (▶ Fig. 5.32). In severe pathology, however, a three-tunnel approach is the method of choice. The technique is presented in detail on page 182 and in ▶ Fig. 5.60, ▶ Fig. 5.61, and ▶ Fig. 5.62.

Bony and Cartilaginous Deviation

A bony and cartilaginous deviation is either resected or fractured into the midline with a strong forceps (Craig type). Resection is carried out by means of a forceps, bone scissors, or osteotome, depending on the deformity and the thickness of the bone. The resected area is later reconstructed by reimplanting plates of removed bone or cartilage. The procedure is described in detail on page 182 and in ▶ Fig. 5.63, ▶ Fig. 5.64, and ▶ Fig. 5.65.

Bony Spur

A posterior bony spur can only be corrected by resection. A spur is dissected and mobilized using an elevator and an osteotome, and removed with a forceps. The technique is described in detail on page 183 and in ▶ Fig. 5.66, ▶ Fig. 5.67, and ▶ Fig. 5.68.

5.2.4 Phase 4: Repositioning

If the septum has been mobilized by adequate undertunneling, chondrotomies, and resections, it should be easy to reposition the remaining parts. If certain parts still tend to deviate, the mucoperichondrium and mucoperiosteum may have to be further elevated. A resistant cartilaginous deviation may require an additional vertical or horizontal chondrotomy, or resection of a somewhat larger or additional strip.

Sometimes, the cartilaginous septum can only be straightened by separating it from the triangular cartilages. It is temporarily removed, modified outside the nose, and reimplanted and fixed (see ▶ Fig. 5.81).

A residual bony deviation requires additional fracturing or resection. If the pyramid is deviated, separating the perpendicular plate from the bony pyramid by osteotomies may also be necessary to straighten a persisting high bony deviation (▶ Fig. 5.33). For details, see ▶ Fig. 5.63, ▶ Fig. 5.64, and ▶ Fig. 5.65. One should never rely on "repositioning" the septum using pressure of some kind of endonasal tamponade.

5.2.5 Phase 5: Reconstruction

Reconstruction of the septum is an essential element of septal surgery. All defective parts of the septal skeleton are repaired by inserting plates of bone or cartilage. Rebuilding the septum serves various purposes:
- Maintaining and restoring the support and projection of the cartilaginous pyramid and lobule
- Restoring the normal stiffness and thickness of the septum, thus preventing well known sequelae of submucous resection, such as late perforations, mucosal atrophy, and mucosal fluttering during breathing
- Facilitating revision surgery

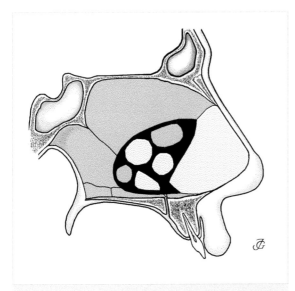

Fig. 5.34 Reconstruction of a defect of the posterior septum with small plates of (slightly crushed) bone and/or cartilage.

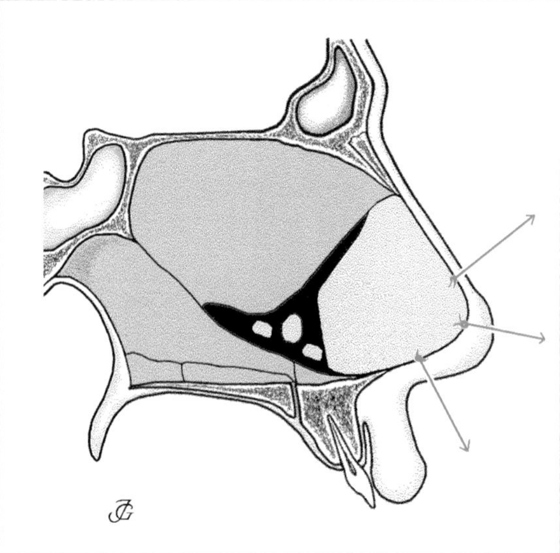

Fig. 5.35 Repositioning of the anterior septum by transdorsal, interdomal, and transcolumellar (intercrural) guide sutures.

> "If you meet a problem, divide it into two. Then solve the easier problem first."

Reconstruction of the Posterior Septum

The bony septum does not have a supporting function. Inserting small plates of bone and cartilage, made by cutting or slightly crushing resected parts, therefore suffices. Reconstruction of the posterior septum is the penultimate phase of septal surgery (▶ Fig. 5.34).

Steps

- Internal dressings (commonly called "packings") are applied bilaterally.
- A long speculum is placed into the septal space, and remnants of blood are removed by suction to avoid a septal hematoma.
- Small plates of bone (or cartilage, if insufficient bone is available) are inserted into the posterior septal space using a long bayonet forceps.
- These small plates are made from the resected bony and cartilaginous septum, either by cutting or using a crusher.
- The pieces of bone and/or cartilage are placed mosaic-fashion on the inside of the left mucosal flap. Care is taken to avoid overlap.
- Immediately afterwards, the septal space is closed. The mucosal flaps are brought together by adjusting the internal dressings intranasally.

Reconstruction of the Anterior Septum

The anterior septum is a supporting structure of the cartilaginous pyramid and lobule. When defective, it must therefore be reconstructed by one or more large plates of cartilage or bone (▶ Fig. 5.35). The surgical technique is described on page 180 and page 188.

5.2.6 Phase 6: Fixation

Fixation of the septum and of the reimplanted (or transplanted) bony or cartilaginous plates is the final phase of septal surgery. Proper fixation of the various parts is of utmost importance. It is a precondition of a good functional and aesthetic result, and it can prevent complications such as postoperative bleeding, hematomas, ecchymosis, and edema. Various methods may be used, such as internal dressings, special sutures, or internal and external splinting. The choice depends upon the type of surgery performed and the personal preference of the surgeon.

Internal Dressings

Internal dressings are used to keep the reconstructed septum in the midline and prevent a septal hematoma. They may also serve to support the nasal bones and cartilaginous pyramid in their new position.

These internal dressings are more commonly called "packings," a term that should be preferred less as dressings should not be packed but gently applied.

Following septal surgery, most surgeons nowadays only insert a strip of a self-expanding material in the inferior meatus on both sides to close the septal space, keep the septum in position and control bleeding (▶ Fig. 5.36). It is usually removed on the first postoperative day.

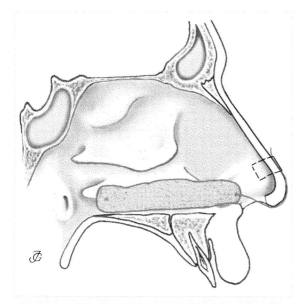

Fig. 5.36 Internal dressing to close the septal space, stabilize the septum in the midline, and prevent bleeding.

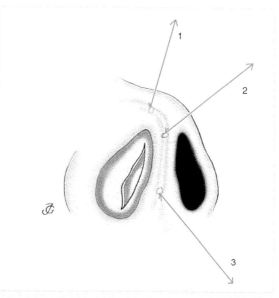

Fig. 5.37 Positioning of the anterior septum with transdorsal and transcolumellar guide sutures.

Other options are gauze strips with ointment. Experience has shown that it is not the material that counts but the care with which these internal dressings are applied.

Steps

- The nasal cavity is cleansed of blood and secretions.
- The intraseptal space is reinspected and blood is removed by suction.
- A slightly humidified strip of a self-expanding material is applied in the inferior meatus on both sides (▸ Fig. 5.36). These dressings consist of a polyvinyl acetate sponge impregnated with oxidized cellulose. The material is biocompatible and hemostatic.
- The septal space is closed by bringing the two mucosal flaps gently together with the internal dressings, using the blunt end of the elevator.
- After the internal dressings are positioned, they are humidified by dripping some isotonic saline into the nose to cause them to expand.
- A posterior septal defect is repaired by inserting plates of bone or cartilage with a long (14 cm) bayonet forceps (see Phase 5: Reconstruction).
- Many surgeons apply the internal dressings at the very end of the operation, after closing all incisions. Others prefer to apply the self-expanding internal dressings first, close the septal space, reconstruct the posterior septum, and then finally fixate the anterior septum in place and suture the various incisions.
- The internal dressing is fixed to the nasal dorsum to prevent it from slipping into the nasopharynx.

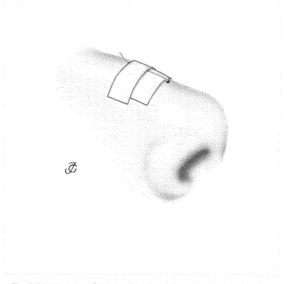

Fig. 5.38 Fixation of a transdorsal guide suture by tapes.

Sutures and Splints

Guide Sutures

Guide sutures are used to maneuver the cartilaginous and bony plates into position. Slowly resorbable 3–0 sutures are fixed to the plate(s) and guided transdorsally, interdomally, and/or through the columella (▸ Fig. 5.37). After the plates have been fixed in place and the operation is over, these guide sutures may be cut off flush to the skin, attached to the skin by tape (▸ Fig. 5.38), or fixed to a Hexalite splint according to Hellmich's method.

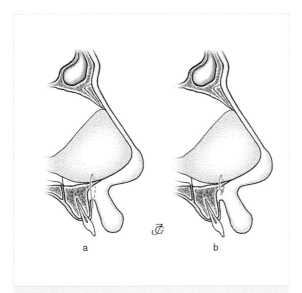

Fig. 5.39 a, b Septospinal suture: fixation of the septal base around the nasal spine.

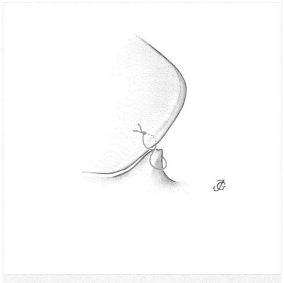

Fig. 5.40 Septopremaxillary figure of eight suture.

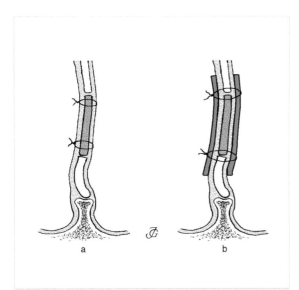

Fig. 5.41 The reconstructed septum is fixated by transseptal sutures without (a) or with (b) Silastic splints.

Septospinal Suture

If the septal base has the tendency to slip off the anterior nasal spine and premaxilla, the septal plate may be held in place by a septospinal suture. A slowly resorbable 3–0 suture is passed through the septal base, downward through the connective tissue fibers and the buccal mucosa on the left side of the anterior nasal spine and the frenulum of the upper lip, and then back through the mucosa and the connective tissue on the right side of the nasal spine. It is then closed intraseptally (▶ Fig. 5.39).

Just before closing, a small cut is made into the frenulum to bury the suture deep to the mucosa.

Septopremaxillary Figure of Eight Suture

Another way to attach the septal base in the midline to its pedestal is to apply a septopremaxillary figure of eight suture. A slowly resorbable 3–0 or 4–0 suture is brought:
1. From right to left through the septal base
2. Back through the gap between the septum and premaxilla
3. Through the prespinal and paraspinal connective tissue fibers
4. Back through the gap, after which it is closed intraseptally (▶ Fig. 5.40)

Transseptal Sutures with or without Splints

In reconstructing the septum, transseptal fixation sutures and septal splints may be of great help. Cartilaginous plates are transseptally fixated by applying two or three catgut or slowly resorbable sutures with or without the help of bilateral intranasal splints (made from Silastic or simple plastic sheets) (▶ Fig. 5.41). The splints should not touch the mucosa of the floor or the roof of the nasal cavity. Any contact may lead to pain, granulations, and bleeding. Generally, splints are removed after some days. In special cases, they are left in place for a longer period of time, for example to prevent recurrence of synechiae.

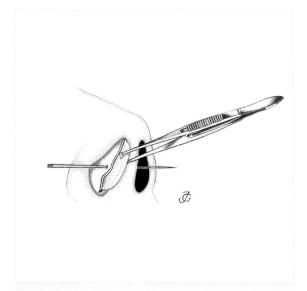

Fig. 5.42 The cartilaginous septum is temporarily fixated into the desired position with a straight needle.

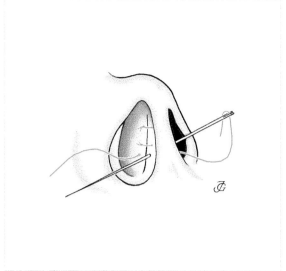

Fig. 5.43 The cartilaginous septum is fixated by two to three septocolumellar sutures, and the caudal septal incision simultaneously closed.

Septocolumellar Sutures

Septocolumellar (SC) sutures are applied to stabilize the anterior septum in the midline. At the same time, they serve to close the CSI.

Steps

- The cartilaginous septum is grasped with a forceps (e.g., von Graefe forceps). It is lifted upward and exorotated until the cartilaginous dorsum has reached the desired level.
- In this position, it is fixed by a straight needle to both mucosal flaps (▶ Fig. 5.42).
- This temporary fixation needle is left in place while the caudal margin of the septum is fixed by two or three horizontal mattress sutures:
  - From right to left: mucosa–cartilage–mucosa
  - From left to right: skin–columellar connective tissue (or medial crura)–skin
- The CSI is closed simultaneously (▶ Fig. 5.43).

Fixation of the Septal Base in a Groove in the Premaxilla

To stabilize the septum, a groove may be cut in the middle of the premaxilla with a 4-mm or 7-mm chisel. The septal base is positioned into this groove. Obviously, this method is only effective when the septal cartilage is large enough (▶ Fig. 5.44).

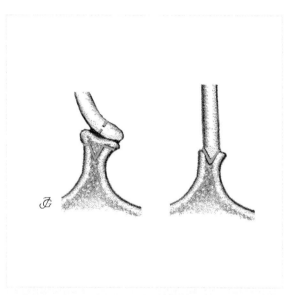

Fig. 5.44 The septum is repositioned in a V-shaped groove in the premaxilla.

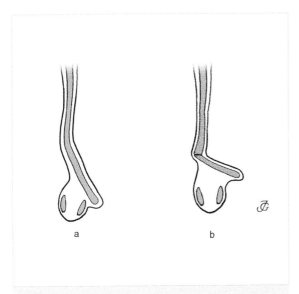

Fig. 5.45 Dislocation of the caudal septal end with obstruction of the nostril and narrowing of the valve area on the opposite side due to a bend (**a**), or a vertical fracture (**b**) of the cartilaginous septum.

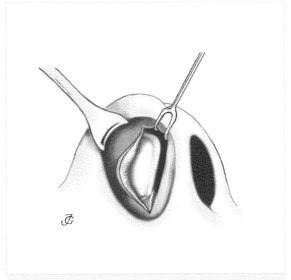

Fig. 5.46 The caudal septal end is dissected completely free from its ventrocaudal corner to the anterior nasal spine.

5.3 Special Problems of Septal Surgery

In this section, we shall discuss the 11 most common special problems that may be encountered in septal surgery:
1. Dislocated (fractured) caudal end
2. Missing (or irreversibly deformed) caudal end
3. Convexity of the caudal end
4. Convexity of the (whole) cartilaginous septum
5. Basal crest
6. High deviation
7. Vomeral spur
8. Vertical fracture of the caudal end
9. Horizontal fracture
10. Anterior convexity
11. Missing septum: (sub)total septal reconstruction

5.3.1 Dislocated (Fractured) Caudal End

The anterior part of the septal cartilage is vertically fractured. It obstructs the valve area on the side of the fracture, and its caudal end protrudes into the vestibule (▶ Fig. 5.45). This common type of pathology is usually the result of laterobasal trauma. It leads to breathing obstruction on inspiration and sometimes also to cosmetic complaints because of the visible protrusion of the caudal septal end into the nostril. See also ▶ Fig. 5.96.

Steps
• The caudal septal end is exposed through a CSI and completely dissected free with slightly curved, pointed scissors. Its ventrocaudal corner, caudal margin, and base, as well as the anterior nasal spine, are all fully exposed (▶ Fig. 5.46).
• Anterosuperior tunnels are elevated bilaterally and the premaxilla is visualized.
• A vertical chondrotomy is made at the bend (fracture line) on the opposite side, and the septal base is disconnected from the anterior nasal spine and premaxilla. Sharp dissection is often necessary. In cases with severe scarring, a unilateral or bilateral inferior tunnel may also be required (three-tunnel or four-tunnel approach). The dislocated anterior part is now mobile. It only remains attached to the posterior part of the septum underneath the nasal dorsum.
• To allow repositioning of the dislocated part, resection of a small horizontal basal and a triangular vertical strip (at the vertical chondrotomy) is usually necessary (▶ Fig. 5.47**a**). In spite of these resections, the anterior septum may tend to return to its dislocated position. This is usually due to tension at its attachment to the posterior septum. The vertical chondrotomy is then extended further upward to the nasal dorsum (▶ Fig. 5.47 **b**).
• If the septum is too long, its caudal border is shortened by resection of a parallel or a triangular strip, depending on the surgical goals (▶ Fig. 5.48).
(a) A parallel strip is resected to shorten the pyramid and to position the columella more cranially.

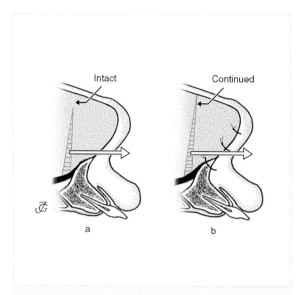

Fig. 5.47 Resection of a triangular vertical strip and a horizontal basal strip to allow repositioning of a dislocated caudal septal end. **(a)** Incomplete vertical strip. **(b)** Complete vertical strip. Fixation of the caudal septal end by septocolumellar sutures and a septospinal suture.

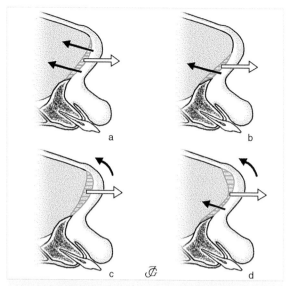

Fig. 5.48 Resection of a strip or triangle from the caudal septal end. **(a)** Parallel strip: entire columella higher. **(b)** Triangular strip with its base dorsally: columellar base higher. **(c)** Triangular strip with its base ventrally: upward rotation of tip. **(d)** Double triangular strip: columellar break.

(b) A triangular strip with its base located dorsally is resected to shorten the height of the pyramid and to bring the columellar base up.

(c) A triangular strip with its base located ventrally is removed to shorten the length of the pyramid with upward rotation of the tip.

(d) A double triangular strip is removed to shorten the pyramid and to create a "break" of the columella.

- A columellar pocket is made using fully curved scissors. The new caudal end is fixed by two or three septocolumellar sutures and, if desired, a septopremaxillary suture (▶ Fig. 5.49). Alternatively, a small groove may be cut into the premaxilla with a 4-mm or 7-mm chisel, in which the septal base is positioned for stabilization (see ▶ Fig. 5.44).

5.3.2 Missing (or Irreversibly Deformed) Caudal End

The caudal septal end is missing or irreversibly deformed (e.g., curled or severely damaged by multiple fractures or previous surgery). The membranous septum is usually more or less scarred, the columella is retracted, and the tip lacks its normal support (▶ Fig. 5.50a, b). See also ▶ Fig. 2.91.

In this case, the caudal end is resected and reconstructed by a cartilaginous graft (preferably autogeneic septal cartilage or auricular cartilage) that is positioned on the anterior nasal spine and premaxilla, and sutured to the intact posterior part of the septum. This graft corrects the retracted columella and the underprojected tip, and is called a *septal extension graft* (▶ Fig. 5.51 and ▶ Fig. 5.52). Such a graft is usually 20 to 25 mm long, somewhat longer than the height of the still intact more posterior part of the septum. The graft is preferably harvested from the posterior cartilaginous septum. If no septal cartilage is available, auricular cartilage is the second choice (see page 244 and page 350). See also the technique described in Convexity of the Caudal End.

Steps

- An incision (here, the term *hemitransfixion* would be correct!) is made into the membranous septum on the right using a No. 15 blade.
- A columellar pocket is created in the membranous septum using small, sharp and blunt curved scissors. Care is taken not to extend the pocket superiorly to the upper (ventral) end of the nostril.
- The remaining caudal septum is carefully dissected up to its ventrocaudal corner, and then cranially up to the remaining septal cartilage. When this point is reached, anterosuperior tunnels can be elevated.
- A posterior chondrotomy is made, and the cartilaginous septum is mobilized.
- A rectangular piece of cartilage of sufficient size is now resected from the posterior part of the cartilaginous septum. Its length should be 20 to 25 mm, the distance between the anterior nasal spine and premaxilla and the domes. Its width depends on the size of the defect (▶ Fig. 5.51). The graft should not be too thick to avoid broadening of the columella and narrowing of the valve area.

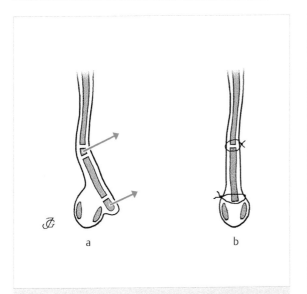

Fig. 5.49 Resection of a small strip at the vertical chondrotomy, and of the caudal septal end (a). Fixation of the anterior septum to the columella by septocolumellar sutures (b).

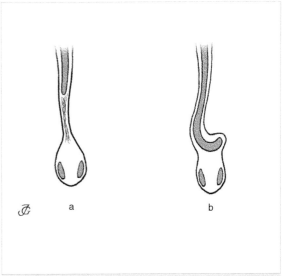

Fig. 5.50 Pathology of the anterior septum requiring reconstruction by a transplant. (a) Missing caudal septal end with scarring and retraction of the columella. (b) Curled caudal end.

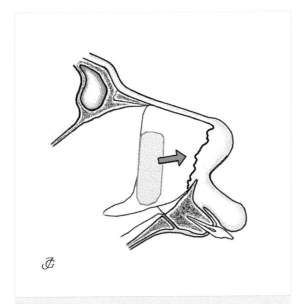

Fig. 5.51 A rectangular graft some 20 to 25 mm long (height) is taken from the posterior part of the cartilaginous septum.

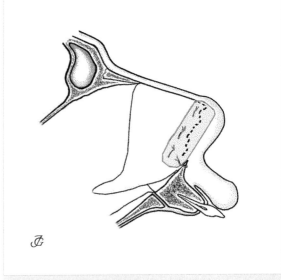

Fig. 5.52 The graft is sutured to the remaining caudal part of the septum with both ends slightly overlapping to lengthen and reconstruct the caudal septal end.

- The strut is then sutured by mean of three to four resorbable or 4–0 vicryl mattress sutures to the remaining part of the septum, with both ends slightly overlapping to lengthen and reconstruct the caudal septal end (▶ Fig. 5.52).

5.3.3 Convexity of the Caudal End

A convexity of the caudal septum end is a common deformity that is difficult to correct. When the convexity concerns the nasal valve area and inspiratory breathing is impaired, its correction is of utmost importance. A caudal convexity usually results from frontobasal trauma, and is often combined with asymmetry of the lobule.

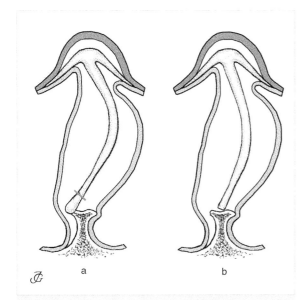

Fig. 5.53 a, b The caudal septal end is corrected by a vertical batten. The cartilaginous septum is exposed and dislocated from its base and a small basal strip is resected. This usually leads to a certain straightening of the cartilage.

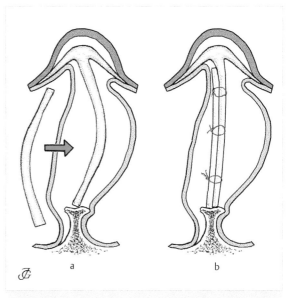

Fig. 5.54 a, b A vertical batten taken from the posterior part of the cartilaginous septum is then sutured to the septum by at least three transcartilaginous sutures, its concave side facing the concave septum.

Sometimes such a cartilaginous convexity straightens out when the mucoperichondrium on both sides is elevated. In most cases, the cartilage is irreversibly bent, however. Various methods have been advocated to correct such a convexity.

- *Gridding* or so-called cross-hatching of its concave side to break the elastic forces of the cartilage is often advocated. In our experience, the results of this technique are unpredictable and frequently inadequate (see also ▶ Fig. 5.88 in Septal Surgery in Children). In combination with a batten graft (see below), some gridding of the concave side may be helpful.
- *Morcellation* is more effective than gridding. However, it weakens the cartilage and may thus cause sagging of the dorsum and retraction of the columella. It is therefore not advisable.
- A *batten graft* sutured to the concave side is more reliable and is therefore the method of choice. If required it may be combined with *limited* gridding of the concave side. The gridding weakens the cartilaginous forces and the batten straightens and reinforces the septum end keeping it in position (▶ Fig. 5.53 and ▶ Fig. 5.54).
- *Resection and Reconstruction.* When, after complete exposure of the septal pathology, the convexity does not straighten out by itself, resection of the convexity followed by reconstruction of the defect by a cartilaginous plate may also be an option (▶ Fig. 5.55).

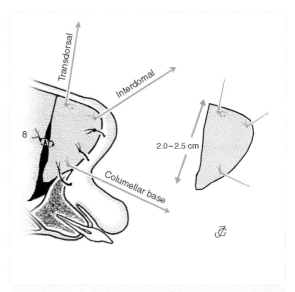

Fig. 5.55 The transplant is fixated by a transdorsal, interdomal, and intercrural guide suture at the level of the columellar base, to reconstruct a missing anterior septum.

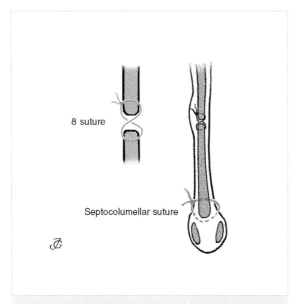

Fig. 5.56 The transplant is fixated with septocolumellar and transseptal figure of eight sutures.

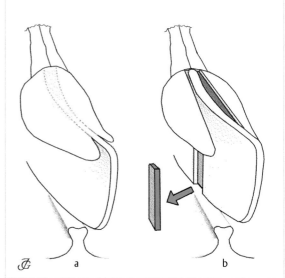

Fig. 5.57 a, b A rectangular graft is resected from the cartilaginous septum.

Batten Graft

Steps

- Anterosuperior tunnels are made on both sides to completely expose the septal pathology.
- The cartilaginous septum is dislocated from its base and a small basal strip is resected (▶ Fig. 5.53).
- If the convexity does not straighten out by itself, a vertical chondrotomy is performed at the area of the maximal bending.
- A rectangular cartilaginous batten of the desired size is then harvested from the posterior part of the cartilaginous septum.
- The graft is positioned in alignment with the caudal septum. It should bridge the distance between the anterior nasal spine and the nasal dorsum.
- The batten is fixed side to side to the concave side of the septum and to the anterior nasal spine and/or paraspinal connective fibers by 4–0 vicryl mattress sutures (▶ Fig. 5.54).

Resection and Reconstruction

Steps

- Anterosuperior tunnels are made on both sides to completely expose the septal pathology.
- If the convexity does not straighten out by itself, a vertical chondrotomy is performed just posterior to the concavity.
- The convex part is intraseptally separated from the triangular cartilages and then resected. We use a No. 64 Beaver knife.

- The removed cartilage is extracorporally modified to a flat plate by conservative gridding, cross-hatching, or slight morcellation. The use of a burr may also be helpful.
- The plate should have a height of 2 to 2.5 cm, the average distance between the premaxilla and the domes.
- Two or three guide sutures (3–0 resorbable vicryl) are fixed to the transplant: one at its future ventrocaudal corner; one just above its inferior caudal corner; and one through its dorsal margin. They are passed through the interdomal, columellar base, and dorsal skin, respectively (▶ Fig. 5.55).
- While the assistant is pulling the three guide sutures, the surgeon fixes the plate with two or three transseptal sutures. One may also fix it by a figure of eight suture or overlapping the remaining posterior septum (▶ Fig. 5.56).
- Positioning and fixing the autotransplant in its proper position is of utmost importance to avoid postoperative sagging of the cartilaginous dorsum. In case of doubt, a batten graft may be added for reinforcement.

5.3.4 Convexity of the Whole Cartilaginous Septum

The cartilaginous septum is always involved in the C-shape and the S-shape deformity of the nasal pyramid (▶ Fig. 2.3, ▶ Fig. 2.4, ▶ Fig. 2.5, ▶ Fig. 2.6, ▶ Fig. 2.7, and ▶ Fig. 2.8). Although osteotomies may align the bony pyramid, the cartilaginous part will remain curved. To deal with this pathology, the same principle as the batten graft is used, and unilateral or bilateral battens (▶ Fig. 5.57 and ▶ Fig. 5.58) or spreader grafts are applied.

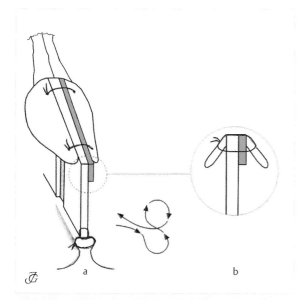

Fig. 5.58 **a, b** The graft is fixed in place to the septum and the triangular cartilages by two figure of eight sutures.

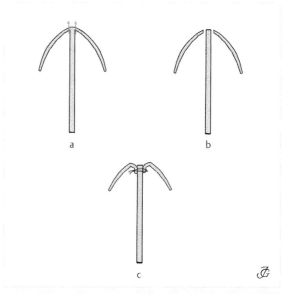

Fig. 5.59 Autospreader maneuver. (**a, b**) The triangular cartilages are separated from the septum. (**c**) The medial ends of the triangular cartilages are rotated inwards and fixed to the septum.

An oblong graft is unilaterally or bilaterally inserted in between the triangular cartilage(s) and the septum. To this end, the septum and the triangular cartilage(s) have to be separated. Disconnecting this morphological and functional unit may easily lead to collapse of the cartilaginous vault. The so-called *autospreader maneuver* may then be applied (▶ Fig. 5.59).

Unilateral (or Bilateral) Horizontal Batten Grafts and Spreader Grafts

Steps

- The pathology is approached using the open approach technique (see page 264). An endonasal approach can also be used but may be more complicated.
- The nasal dorsum is exposed by upward retraction of the dorsal skin.
- Septal tunnels are made bilaterally up to the nasal dorsum.
- A piece of cartilage is harvested from the posterior part of the cartilaginous septum (▶ Fig. 5.57).
- The triangular cartilage is separated from the septum, and a small space is created between septum and triangular cartilage. This can be done from above or from below (intraseptally).
- A batten about 25 mm in length is cut from the harvested cartilage and inserted in between the septum and triangular cartilage. If the batten is slightly bent, then the concave side should face the concave side of the septum. The (thicker) end of the graft is positioned underneath the nasal bones to avoid a step on the dorsum (▶ Fig. 5.58).

- If the straightening effect of the batten seems to be insufficient, a similar batten is inserted on the other side.
- The graft(s) are fixed by resorbable transcartilaginous sutures to the septum, and by two figure of eight sutures to the triangular cartilages.
- Care is taken to align the grafts, the septum and the triangular cartilages precisely, to avoid any visible or palpable irregularities of the dorsum.
- Finally, the battens are caudally shortened to the required length to avoid projecting too much.

Autospreader Maneuver

As an alternative to the batten technique, described above, the medial margins of the triangular cartilages may be inverted and fixed to the septum (▶ Fig. 5.59). This so-called autospreader maneuver is especially suitable in cases with a cartilaginous hump, where the surplus of cartilage can be used to straighten the septum and the dorsum. This method has the advantage that the spring of the cartilaginous vault is kept intact. The autospreader maneuver can be combined with the batten (spreader) technique. The technique leads to a widening of the nasal valve area. However, the valve angle may become smaller due to inversion of the medial ends of the triangular cartilages. The surgeon should take both effects into account when applying the autospreader maneuver.

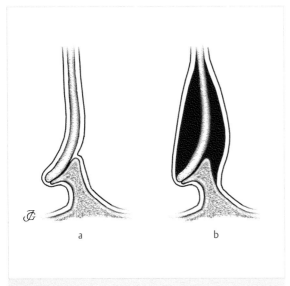

Fig. 5.60 Correction of a basal crest. (a) Basal crest consisting of a cartilaginous and bony part. (b) Exposure of the pathology by a two-tunnel approach.

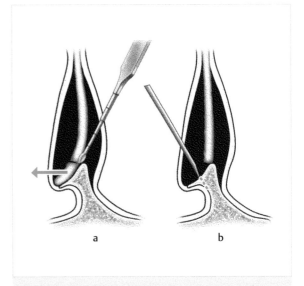

Fig. 5.61 Correction of a basal crest. (a) Dissection and resection of the cartilaginous part. (b) Resection of the bony part using a chisel.

Steps

- The external approach is used.
- The triangular cartilages are separated from the septum. This can be done from above or intraseptally (▶ Fig. 5.59**a, b**).
- The medial ends of the triangular cartilages and the ventral end of the septum are adjusted (by minute resections) in order to achieve a symmetrical and straight cartilaginous dorsum.
- The medial ends of the triangular cartilages are then rotated inwards and fixed to the septum (▶ Fig. 5.59**c**).

5.3.5 Basal Crest

A basal crest is one of the most common types of septal deformity. As a result of a laterofrontal trauma (in youth), the septal base is luxated from its bony base to the opposite side. During growth, the base of the dislocated septum shows excessive growth. The result is a basal cartilaginous and bony crest, an asymmetrical deviated premaxilla and maxillary crest, and usually a high bony and cartilaginous deviation to the opposite side (▶ Fig. 5.60**a**).

Steps

- Anterosuperior tunnels are elevated bilaterally in the standard way (two-tunnel approach). The tunnel on the side of the crest is continued down to its very edge. No attempt should be made to elevate the mucoperichondrium over the crest, as this almost invariably leads to a mucosal tear (▶ Fig. 5.60**b**).

- The septal cartilage is then horizontally cut just superior to the crest. The cartilaginous part of the crest is dissected out with the sharp end of the elevator (▶ Fig. 5.61**a**).
- The anterosuperior tunnel on the noncrest side is continued downward. An inferior tunnel posterior to the maxilla is created from above. The bony part of the crest is now chiseled off vertically (4-mm or 7-mm chisel) while still attached to the mucoperiosteum (▶ Fig. 5.61**b**).
- The mobilized bony piece is dissected from the mucoperiosteum.
- The remaining part of the premaxilla and maxillary crest is fractured to the midline, if necessary, by a strong forceps (Craig type, ▶ Fig. 5.62).

Care is taken to avoid creating a gap between the base of the cartilaginous septum and the remnants of the premaxilla and the maxillary crest, as this may cause sagging of the cartilaginous dorsum and retraction of the columellar base.

5.3.6 High Deviation

A high deviation usually consists of the posterior part of the cartilaginous septum and the anterior part of the perpendicular plate. This deformity is often combined with asymmetry of the bony and cartilaginous pyramid (▶ Fig. 5.63**a**). It may cause both functional and cosmetic complaints. Vague pain and pressure sensations may occur. See also ▶ Fig. 2.111.

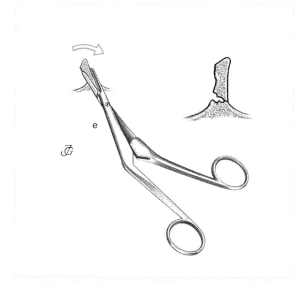

Fig. 5.62 Correction of a basal crest. Fracturing of the deviated premaxilla and maxillary crest to the midline using a strong forceps (Craig type).

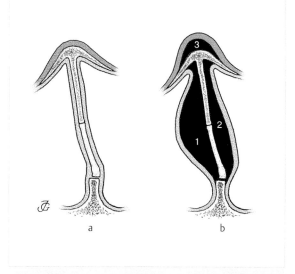

Fig. 5.63 Correction of a high deviation. **(a)** Deviation of the perpendicular plate, vomer, and bony pyramid. **(b)** Exposure of the pathology by a two-tunnel approach (1, 2) and undermining of the dorsal skin (3).

Steps

- Bilateral anterosuperior tunnels are made in the usual way (▶ Fig. 5.63 **b**).
- A posterior chondrotomy is made just in front of the cartilaginous part of the deviation. The cartilaginous septum is dislocated from its base, and a "swinging door" is created.
- Posterosuperior tunnels are elevated on both sides. The cartilaginous and bony deviation is now fully exposed.
- The major part of the deviation is resected or fractured into the midline with a strong biting forceps (Craig type), bone scissors (Koffler type), or a straight 7-mm chisel (▶ Fig. 5.64**a**).
- The removed parts are preserved in isotonic saline.
- The cartilaginous and bony pyramids are then dealt with. The skin over the cartilaginous and bony pyramid is undermined through bilateral intercartilaginous incisions. Osteotomies are performed and the pyramid is repositioned (▶ Fig. 5.64**b**).
- The septum is then reinspected. If the upper part of the septum is still deviating, it is resected or fractured toward the midline. Otherwise, a "tenting effect" may occur. The persisting deviation will prevent positioning of the mucosal flaps in the midline (see also ▶ Fig. 5.33).
- The septal defect is carefully reconstructed by reimplantation of small plates of bone and cartilage from the resected deviated parts. They are inserted to prevent dislocation after the internal dressings have been applied (▶ Fig. 5.65).
- The skin over the K area may be reinforced by an underlay of thoroughly crushed septal cartilage, which is inserted through the intercartilaginous incisions.

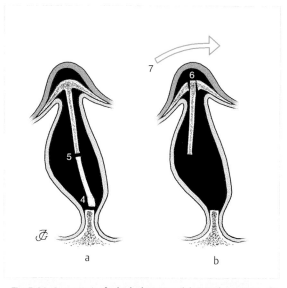

Fig. 5.64 Correction of a high deviation. **(a)** Partial resection of the lower part of the deviation (4, 5). **(b)** Paramedial osteotomies (6) and fracturing of the upper part to the midline (7).

5.3.7 Vomeral Spur

A septal spur or spine is one of the most frequent septal deformities. The most common type is the vomeral spur impacting into the posterior half of the inferior turbinate (▶ Fig. 5.66). It develops after trauma or disturbed growth at the point where the perpendicular plate, vomer, and cartilaginous septum (sphenoidal process) meet.

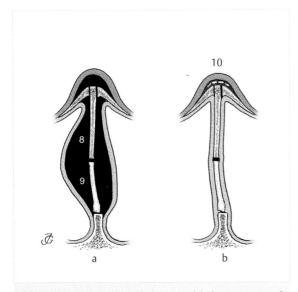

Fig. 5.65 Correction of a high deviation. (a) The upper part of the deviation is positioned (fractured) into the midline (8) and the defect is reconstructed by reimplantation of bone or cartilage (9). (b) Fixation of the implanted plate by careful adjustment of the mucosal flaps by inner dressings (and septal splints). Insertion of crushed cartilage under the dorsal skin (10).

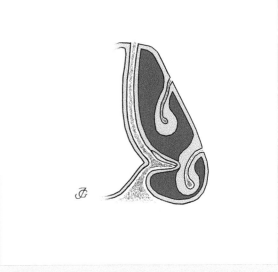

Fig. 5.66 Correction of a vomeral spur. Vomeral spur with sphenoidal process of the septal cartilage impacting in the inferior turbinate.

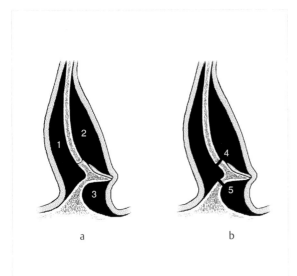

Fig. 5.67 Correction of a vomeral spur. a Exposure of the pathology by a posterior tunnel on the opposite side (1), a posterior tunnel cranial to the spur (2), and a posterior tunnel caudal to the spur (3). b Mobilization of the pathology: horizontal osteotomy above (4) and below (5) the spur.

If a vomeral spur is the only septal deformity, it will not be removed unless it causes symptoms like unilateral headache or hyperreactive complaints. An asymptomatic spur is usually left untouched. If it is part of more extensive septal pathology, it is always resected and the defect repaired.

Steps

- Bilateral anterosuperior tunnels are made and a "swinging door" is created, providing access to the bony septum.
- A posterior tunnel is made, first on the side opposite the spur, then above and below the spur (▶ Fig. 5.67a).
- With a straight 7-mm chisel (or bone scissors), the bony septum is cut horizontally, first above and then below the spur (▶ Fig. 5.67b).
- The isolated bony block is fractured toward the opposite side with the sharp end of the Cottle elevator while dissecting it from the mucoperiosteum. It is then taken out in one or more pieces with a Blakesley forceps (▶ Fig. 5.68a).
- The resulting defect is reconstructed by reimplantation of small plates of bone that are fixed by internal dressings (▶ Fig. 5.68).

One should not try to elevate the (usually very thin) mucoperiosteum that is overlying the spur. This almost always leads to a tear.

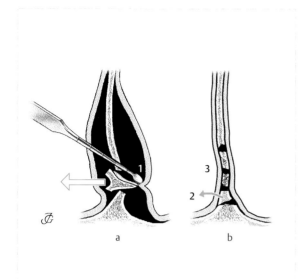

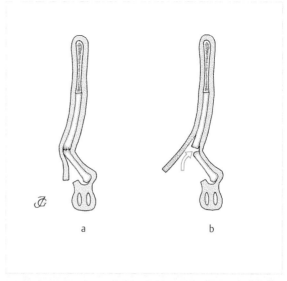

Fig. 5.68 Correction of a vomeral spur.**a** Mobilization of the bony and cartilaginous block to the opposite side with an elevator by dissecting the bone from the mucosa (1).**b** Fracturing of the deviated lower part of the vomer to the midline (2), and reconstruction of the defect by reimplantation of a plate of bone (3).

Fig. 5.69 Correction of a vertical fracture. **(a)** Approach through a CSI and an anterosuperior tunnel on the side of the fracture. **(b)** Vertical chondrotomy through the fracture line.

5.3.8 Vertical Fracture

A vertical fracture of the septal cartilage is most commonly located at the level of, or immediately behind, the nasal valve area. The caudal septal end usually protrudes into the vestibule of the opposite side (▶ Fig. 5.69a). See also ▶ Fig. 2.107 and ▶ Fig. 2.108.

In most cases, breathing is severely obstructed in area 2 at the level of the fracture, and usually also in area 1 on the opposite side due to dislocation of the caudal septal end.

Steps

- The pathology is approached through a right CSI. An anterosuperior tunnel is elevated on the side of the fracture up to the fracture line. No attempt is made to elevate over the fracture, as this would easily cause a mucosal laceration (▶ Fig. 5.69a).
- Instead of trying to get behind the fracture, the cartilage is incised at (or just in front of) the fracture (▶ Fig. 5.69b).
- Subperichondrial tunneling is continued on both sides of the cartilage (▶ Fig. 5.70a).
- A posterior chondrotomy is carried out, and the septum is detached from its base. The deflected caudal part is freed from the mucoperichondrium and columella. Now there are two mobile cartilaginous plates that are still connected to the triangular cartilages (▶ Fig. 5.70b).

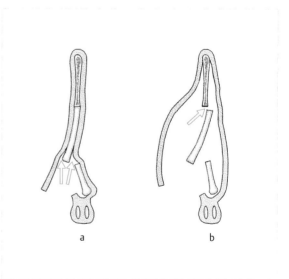

Fig. 5.70 Correction of a vertical fracture. **(a)** Bilateral elevation of the mucoperichondrium of the posterior part, and dislocation of the anterior part. **(b)** Posterior chondrotomy, bilateral posterior tunnels, and mobilization of the two parts of the cartilaginous septum.

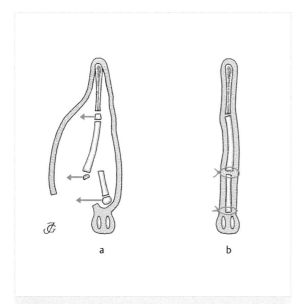

Fig. 5.71 Correction of a vertical fracture. (a) Resection of small vertical strips to allow repositioning of the septum in the midline. (b) Fixation by transseptal and septocolumellar sutures.

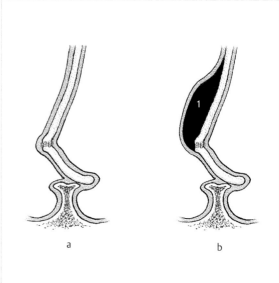

Fig. 5.72 Correction of a horizontal fracture. (a) Horizontal fracture. (b) Anterosuperior tunnel above the fracture (1).

- Vertical strips are resected at the fracture line and the cartilaginous–osseous junction (▶ Fig. 5.71a). A basal horizontal strip is removed to allow repositioning of the two cartilage plates without overlap. As the caudal septal end is usually too long, it has to be shortened. The different modes to correct the caudal septal end are discussed earlier in this chapter on page 177 and shown in ▶ Fig. 5.48.
- In some cases, the anterior or posterior part of the cartilaginous septum may still tend to deviate. This is usually due to distortion of the triangular cartilages. The septum is then separated intraseptally from the triangular cartilages on both sides with a No. 64 Beaver blade. Care is taken to avoid injury to the mucosa. The anterior septal plate is now completely loose. The posterior part is still connected superior to the bony septum. The loose anterior plate is taken out, inspected, and corrected outside the nose. It is then replaced and fixed in position in the usual way (see ▶ Fig. 5.71b).

5.3.9 Horizontal Fracture

A horizontal fracture of the cartilaginous septum is most commonly located in its lower half. It is usually the result of frontolateral trauma. The septum shows a ridge, crest, or convexity on one side, in combination with a concavity and a basal crest on the other side (▶ Fig. 5.72a). See also ▶ Fig. 2.109.

The condition usually occurs along with deviation of both the bony and the cartilaginous pyramid. The patient may have both breathing and cosmetic complaints. Homolateral pain and pressure sensations may also be present, especially when the horizontal crest impacts on the inferior or middle turbinate.

Steps

- The septum is approached in the usual way through a CSI on the right. An anterosuperior tunnel is elevated on the side of the fracture, cranial to the fracture line. No attempt is made to elevate the mucoperichondrium over a sharp ridge or crest, as this almost invariably leads to a mucosal tear (▶ Fig. 5.72b).
- A horizontal chondrotomy is made at, or just above, the fracture line. Undertunneling is continued downward on the opposite side (▶ Fig. 5.73a).
- The superior tunnels are then bilaterally completed. Sometimes an inferior tunnel on the side of the basal crest has to be made to expose the pathology at the septal base (▶ Fig. 5.73b).
- A posterior chondrotomy is performed. Horizontal strips are resected at the fracture line to allow repositioning without overlapping of the two plates. The basal crest is dealt with as described on page 182 (▶ Fig. 5.60, ▶ Fig. 5.61, and ▶ Fig. 5.62).
- Sometimes an extra horizontal chondrotomy is required (▶ Fig. 5.74a). A strip or part of the deviation is then resected to allow repositioning without tension.
- Large defects are reconstructed by reimplantation of a plate of cartilage that is fixed by transseptal sutures. The anterior septum is fixed to the columella by two or three septocolumellar sutures (▶ Fig. 5.74b).

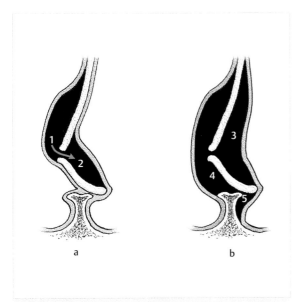

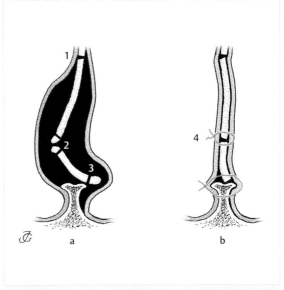

Fig. 5.73 Correction of a horizontal fracture. **(a)** Horizontal chondrotomy through the fracture line (1), and continuation of the undertunneling of the lower part of the septum on the opposite side (2). **(b)** Superior undertunneling is completed (3, 4), and an inferior tunnel is made on the left (5) to expose the crest, if necessary.

Fig. 5.74 Correction of a horizontal fracture. **(a)** Second horizontal chondrotomy (1), if required, and resection of horizontal strips (2, 3) to allow repositioning of the various parts in the midline. **(b)** Transseptal (4) and septocolumellar sutures for fixation.

5.3.10 Anterior Convexity

A convexity of the anterior septum is one of the most troublesome septal deformities. It is particularly bothersome if present at the valve area, where a minimal bend may produce inspiratory obstruction. An anterior convexity is usually the result of frontobasal trauma. Often it is combined with asymmetry of the cartilaginous pyramid (▶ Fig. 5.75a). See also ▶ Fig. 2.112.

Sometimes a cartilaginous convexity straightens out after the mucoperichondrium has been elevated on both sides. However, in most long-standing convexities, the cartilage is irreversibly bent. Different methods have been advocated to correct such an irreversible cartilaginous convexity.

Gridding of the concave side to break the elastic forces is often advocated as the method of choice. In our experience, however, the results of this technique are unpredictable and frequently inadequate.

Morcellation in situ is more effective than gridding. However, it tends to weaken the cartilage and may cause sagging of the dorsum.

Resection of the convex area and reconstruction of the defect appears to be the best option.

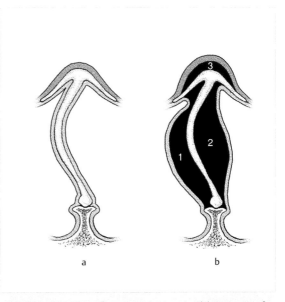

Fig. 5.75 Correction of an anterior convexity. **(a)** Convexity of the cartilaginous septum at the valve area. **(b)** Exposure of the pathology: two-tunnel approach (1, 2) and undermining of the skin of the nasal dorsum (3).

Steps

• Bilateral anterosuperior tunnels are made in the usual way, and the convexity is completely exposed. If it does not straighten by itself after being freed from its perichondrium, it is resected and the defect is repaired.

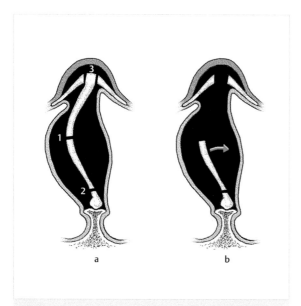

Fig. 5.76 Correction of an anterior convexity. **(a)** Horizontal chondrotomies (1, 2) and separation of the septum from the triangular cartilages (3). **(b)** Resection of the irreversibly deformed part.

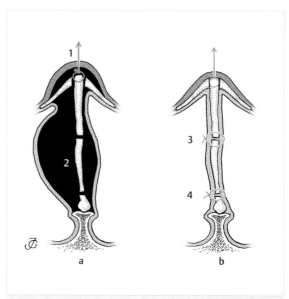

Fig. 5.77 Correction of an anterior convexity. **(a)** Reimplantation of the remodeled part by a transdorsal guide suture (1) and repositioning of other parts of the septum (2). **(b)** Fixation by transseptal sutures with or without intranasal splints (3, 4).

- To this end, the cartilaginous pyramid is exposed by undermining the dorsal skin via intercartilaginous incisions (▶ Fig. 5.75**b**).
- The convex part of the septal cartilage is intraseptally separated from the triangular cartilages and resected with a straight No. 64 Beaver knife or an angulated No. 66 Beaver knife (▶ Fig. 5.76).
- The removed cartilage is modified extracorporally to a flat plate. This may be achieved by limited gridding or slight morcellation. The use of a burr may be helpful. Sometimes, it suffices to reinsert the plate after rotating it 90°.
- This plate is then reinserted into the defect with the help of a transdorsal guide suture (▶ Fig. 5.77**a**). While the assistant keeps the plate in place, the surgeon fixes it in position with one or two transseptal sutures (▶ Fig. 5.77**b**).

5.3.11 Missing Septum: (Sub) Total Septal Reconstruction

A "missing" or defective septum is usually the result of a septal abscess, multiple traumas, or previous surgery. An anterior cartilaginous defect is the most common deformity. Sometimes, however, the whole septal skeleton is missing. It may be so irreversibly deformed that all cartilaginous and bony remnants have to be removed and a new septum has to be built up.

These patients show a low-wide pyramid syndrome. The bony pyramid is broad and flat. It may show a relative hump or pseudohump, especially when the septal trauma or infection occurred before completion of nasal growth. The cartilaginous pyramid is saddling and lacks support, the lobule is broad and ballooning, and the nostrils are more or less round. The tip is depressed; the columella is retracted and short. The vestibule is broad; the valve area is low and wide. On palpation, the septum feels membranous and flaccid (see Chapter 2, ▶ Fig. 2.113, ▶ Fig. 2.114, ▶ Fig. 2.115, ▶ Fig. 2.116, ▶ Fig. 2.117).

The missing septum is reconstructed anteriorly by one to three plates, and posteriorly by implanting small pieces of cartilage and bone. The anterior plate-type reconstruction helps to lift and support the cartilaginous dorsum, valve area, and lobule, thereby improving both function and aesthetics. The posterior mosaic-type reconstruction gives the posterior septum more stiffness and reduces mucosal atrophy.

Approach

In most patients, a missing anterior septum can be best repaired by the endonasal approach. In the following paragraphs, we concentrate on endonasal reconstruction of this type of pathology. However, in complicated cases, the external approach is a very good alternative, as shown clearly by Rettinger. The open approach allows repairing the septum, reinforcing the columella and the domes, augmenting the tip, and inserting a dorsal graft in one procedure.

Methods

As a matter of principle, we try to repair septal defects using the original tissues. Autogeneic septal cartilage is used for the anterior part and autogeneic septal bone for the posterior part of the septum. However, we can only follow this rule in a minority of cases. Generally, there is not enough usable autogeneic material available. We then have to use special methods and other tissues such as:

- *Transposition of autogeneic perpendicular plate and vomer* to reconstruct a missing anterior septum ("exchange technique")
- *Assembling a composite graft* by suturing and/or gluing remnants of autogeneic septal cartilage and bone together
- *Sculpting plates* from autogeneic rib cartilage, or sculpting or assembling a plate from autogeneic conchal cartilage

Materials

Plates of Autogeneic Septal Cartilage

The first choice of material to reconstruct a missing anterior septum is autogeneic septal cartilage. In Caucasians, the dimensions of the plate must be approximately 2.5 by 1.0 to 1.5 cm. Frequently, a plate of this size is not available. Sometimes, however, one can be harvested from parts that cannot be repositioned or are irreversibly deformed. These parts are then resected, temporarily preserved in isotonic saline, and later cut to measure for reconstruction.

Notes

1. Morcellation may be attempted if the septal cartilage is irreversibly bent. This will unavoidably lead to some loss of stiffness and support, however.
2. Limited convexity of a plate used for reconstruction may be acceptable when rebuilding the septum in areas 4 and 5. However, it is never allowed for reconstruction in areas 1 and 2.

Plates of Autogeneic Septal Bone

The second choice of material to reconstruct the anterior septum is autogeneic septal bone. Many patients in whom the cartilaginous septum has been destroyed have a bony septum that is more or less intact. A bony plate can then be cut from the perpendicular plate and vomer, and transpositioned anteriorly ("exchange technique"). The posterior defect is reconstructed by reimplantation of small pieces of cartilaginous and bony remnants.

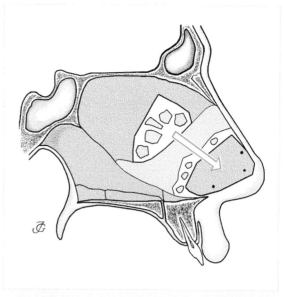

Fig. 5.78 Missing anterior septum: anterior plate reconstruction ("exchange technique").

Steps

- The perpendicular plate is cut parallel to the bony dorsum with bone scissors (Koffler type), taking care not to fracture the cribriform plate. The vomer is cut horizontally at its base. Scissors are superior to a chisel, as they allow a more controlled cut.
- Posteriorly, the bone can best be cut with a curved chisel.
- The removed piece is cut to the desired length and width, avoiding a sharp ventrocaudal corner.
- Usually, two holes are drilled into its caudal margin and one into its ventral border to fix guide sutures (▶ Fig. 5.78).

Plates Assembled from Remnants of Autogeneic Septal Cartilage and Bone (Composite Graft or Cartilage–Bone Assembly)

Composite grafts are probably the best alternative if insufficient material is available to cut single plates of the required size. The better quality pieces of cartilage and bone that were removed during surgery are assembled by means of sutures and tissue glue to form a graft of the desired dimensions (▶ Fig. 5.79).

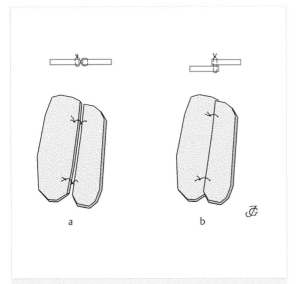

Fig. 5.79 Composite grafts. (a) Two plates fixated with figure of eight sutures. (b) Two overlapping plates fixated with sutures (and glue).

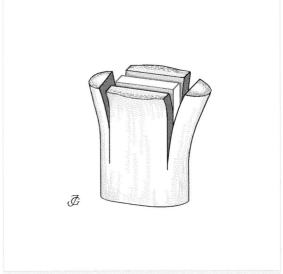

Fig. 5.80 Plate of rib cartilage cut from the center of the rib.

Plates from Autogeneic Rib Cartilage

Plates cut from rib cartilage are likely to be the best alternative if no sufficient autogeneic septal material is available. They are cut from the very center of the rib to avoid bending of the plate (▶ Fig. 5.80). The early results are usually very good. Due to resorption of the donor cartilage, some retraction of the dorsum and columella often occurs after 1 to 3 years. In most cases, sufficient stiffness remains, however. In some patients, reoperation may be required.

Several factors are likely to play a role in the resorption process. The heterotopic cartilage has a different structure to septal cartilage. It is in contact with the large surface of an immunologically active (sub)mucosa. No perichondrium is attached, since the plate is cut from the center of the rib. Also, an anterior septal transplant is under continuous mechanical stress.

For a discussion of the technique of harvesting rib cartilage, see Chapter 6 (page 246).

Autogeneic Conchal Cartilage

Conchal cartilage has also been advocated as a substitute material. The perichondrium is left attached on one side. The harvesting technique of auricular cartilage is discussed in Chapter 6 (see ▶ Fig. 6.81, ▶ Fig. 6.82, and ▶ Fig. 6.83).

When choosing auricular cartilage, we should realize that this material has two limitations. First, conchal cartilage is less stiff than septal cartilage. Second, its convexities and concavities make it very difficult to construct a straight plate.

Nonbiological Materials

Nonbiological materials such as Proplast, Teflon, and Silastic have also been used. In the septum, these materials are not tolerated, however. They become extruded (see also Chapter 9 and ▶ Fig. 9.91, ▶ Fig. 9.92, ▶ Fig. 9.93, and ▶ Fig. 9.94).

Tissue Engineering

A promising option for the future is tissue engineering—that is, in vitro production of cartilage and bone from cells taken from the septum of the patient.

Surgical Techniques

Boomerang-Type Plate Reconstruction of the Anterior Septum

The caudal part of the anterior cartilaginous septum is reconstructed by a boomerang-type plate. Previously, L-type constructions were often used. These prove to have serious drawbacks since they provide less support, are more easily dislocated, and may fracture.

Steps

- A boomerang-type plate is cut from cartilage or bone. In Caucasians, the height of a boomerang-type plate must be about 22 to 25 mm in males and 20 to 22 mm in females.
- The caudal end should have two obtuse angles: a ventrocaudal one of about 110° and a dorsocaudal one of about 90°.

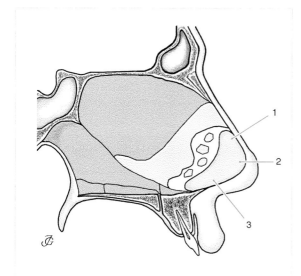

Fig. 5.81 Missing anterior septum: reconstruction by an anterior boomerang-shaped plate using a transdorsal (1), interdomal (2), and an intercrural guide suture at the columellar base (3). Fixation with two or three septocolumellar sutures and by fixating the transdorsal guide suture with tape or to a Hexalite stent.

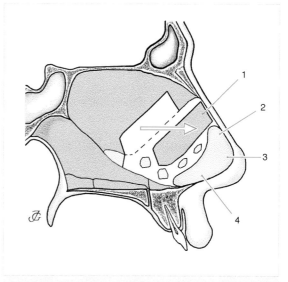

Fig. 5.82 Two-plate reconstruction of the anterior septum. The transplants are maneuvered into position with transdorsal guide sutures (1, 2), an interdomal guide suture (3), and a columellar base guide suture (4).

- Care is taken to round off the new ventrocaudal corner so that it is not visible or palpable between the two domes.
- Three guide sutures are fixed to the transplant and led transdorsally, intradomally, and intracrurally through the columellar base. When a bony transplant is used, holes will have to be drilled to fix these sutures (▶ Fig. 5.81).
- A columellar pocket is created to accommodate the caudal margin of the transplant.
- Before the anterior plate is definitively fixed, any posterior defect is reconstructed. This is done by mosaic-type reimplantation of platelets of bone or cartilage (see ▶ Fig. 5.34).
- While the assistant is pulling the guide sutures to keep the transplant in the desired position, the surgeon fixes it with two or three septocolumellar sutures. These sutures usually pass through the medial crura for better fixation and support.
- The dorsal guide suture is fixed to dorsal tapes or to a Hexalite stent.
- A septospinal or a septopremaxillary suture and/or a septal splint may also be helpful for stabilization (see ▶ Fig. 5.39 and ▶ Fig. 5.40).

Reconstruction by Two or Three Rectangular Plates

In some cases, the whole cartilaginous septum is defective or has to be completely resected. At least two plates, sometimes three, are then required for proper functional and aesthetic reconstruction (▶ Fig. 5.82 and ▶ Fig. 5.83).

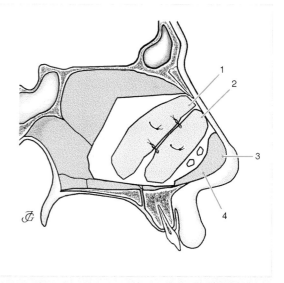

Fig. 5.83 Three-plate reconstruction of the anterior and posterior septum. The posterior plates are brought in place with transdorsal guide sutures (1, 2) and fixed by transseptal sutures and a septal splint. The anterior boomerang-type plate is maneuvered into position with an interdomal and a transcolumellar guide suture (3, 4).

Steps

- Two or three plates are cut or assembled. The posterior ones should be as long as possible and more or less trapezoid shaped. The caudal one is cut like a boomerang, as previously described.
- The posterior plate is introduced first by means of one transdorsal guide suture. Care is taken that its upper margin just underlies the K area to avoid a postoperative step at this critical area.
- The posterior plates (in case of a three-plate reconstruction) are introduced with transdorsal guide sutures. Marks on the skin where these sutures should pass may be of great help in positioning the plates.
- Both the posterior and the middle plate are separately fixed by one to two transseptal sutures. Care is taken that their margins do not overlap. If this does occur, one of the plates is intraseptally narrowed with a sharp knife (e.g., an angulated No. 66 Beaver knife).
- The anterior plate is introduced and fixed according to the technique described above (▶ Fig. 5.81).
- Any remaining defects are reconstructed by inserting remnants of cartilage and/or bone before the anterior plate is fixed.
- Septal splints are used to stabilize the construction.
- The guide sutures may be fixed to external tapes (see ▶ Fig. 5.38) or tied to a Hexalite stent to prevent sagging of the plates.

5.4 Septal Surgery in Children

Septal surgery in children has been taboo for a long time. After submucous septal resection was introduced around 1890 to 1910, this operation was also performed in children. It soon became evident, however, that resection of a major part of the cartilaginous septum in childhood does not only cause saddling of the dorsum and retraction of the columella, but also retards nasal growth (e.g., Ombrédanne 1942). Septal resection before puberty was therefore condemned. Parents were told that nasal surgery in their child had to be postponed until the age of 16 to 18 years. That advice has now been revised thanks to the development of more conservative and reconstructive surgical techniques. Short-term and long-term follow-up studies in children have shown that damage to nasal growth can mostly be avoided if septal surgery is limited to repositioning the deviated cartilaginous septum using as few incisions and resections as possible. In some cases, nasal growth may even benefit from early repositioning of the septum (Huizing 1966, 1979; Pirsig 1974, 1977).

5.4.1 Indications

Septal surgery in children may be carried out in the following conditions:
1. Septal deformity causing impaired nasal breathing
2. Septal deformity disturbing nasal growth
3. Acute nasal trauma
4. Septal hematoma or abscess

Impaired Nasal Breathing

If nasal respiration is impaired to such an extent that mouth breathing is necessary even at rest, there may be an indication for surgery, regardless of the age of the child. The improvement in health that may be achieved by restoring nasal breathing is generally so significant that the disadvantages of early surgery are fully acceptable. When nasal breathing is sufficient at rest but fails during exercise and sports, the choice between surgery and a wait-and-see policy is more difficult. The advantages and disadvantages of both options should be carefully weighed. Various factors should be taken into account: the age of the child (see following text); the presence of other complaints such as sniffing, crusting, or bleeding; and the degree of growth disturbance. In case of doubt, surgery is postponed. Standard photographs and function tests are made for documentation. Arrangements are made for follow-up every 1 or 2 years.

Disturbance of Nasal Growth

Disturbance of nasal growth due to a septal deformity may be another (usually additional) reason for surgery. It is well known that septal deformities may lead to disturbed nasal growth. Septal growth is the main determining factor of the outgrowth of the bony and cartilaginous pyramid, lobule, and midface. This is illustrated by various characteristic types of nasal pathology. The most well known is the severe retardation of the growth of the nose and midface after destruction of the cartilaginous septum by a septal abscess or severe trauma at a young age. Another example is the gradually increasing deviation of the external pyramid and septum during childhood and pubertal growth following traumatic dislocation of the anterior septum from its base. Experience has shown that these growth deformities may be partially prevented by early repositioning of the septum. This is particularly true in cases of a deviated or twisted nose.

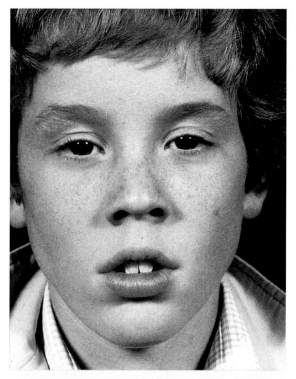

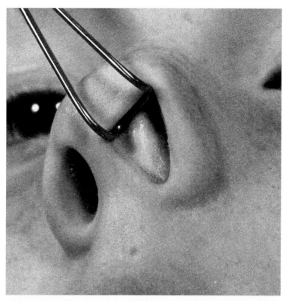

Fig. 5.85 Severe dislocation of the caudal end of the septum to the left, causing vestibular obstruction associated with a vertical fracture of the cartilaginous septum to the right.

Fig. 5.84 Deviation of the cartilaginous pyramid to the left associated with a vertical fracture of the cartilaginous septum to the right, causing impaired nasal breathing in a young boy.

Acute Nasal Trauma

Acute nasal trauma is one of the most important reasons to perform nasal surgery in children. In cases of fresh septal fracture, the best end results are obtained when the dislocated parts are repositioned and fixed in the acute stage (i.e., within about 5 days). The same applies to children with a freshly dislocated bony pyramid, and those with a depressed cartilaginous or bony pyramid (see Chapter 9, page 321).

Septal Hematoma and Abscess

A septal hematoma must be drained as soon as possible to avoid infection and necrosis of the cartilaginous septum. A septal abscess should be treated as an emergency. It must be drained the same day, and the defect should be reconstructed immediately (see page 198).

5.4.2 Age Factor

There is no minimum age for septal surgery in children. Decision-making is a tradeoff procedure in which the degree of breathing obstruction and the deformity are weighed against age and the possible negative effects of surgery on nasal growth and the psyche of the child. The younger the child, the greater the risk that surgery will have a negative influence on nasal growth. Especially critical is surgery in the first 3 years of life, when most of

the septal cartilage shows rapid development (Pirsig 1984) (▶ Fig. 1.113). On the contrary, the longer the intervention is postponed, the longer the child has to endure nasal obstruction and the more serious the negative effects on nasal growth.

5.4.3 Most Common Deformities

The most common septal deformities in children are vertical fracture, horizontal fracture, and defective anterior septum.

Vertical Fracture

A vertical fracture is usually the result of frontobasal trauma. As a result, the cartilaginous septum fractures or bends at the level of the piriform aperture, sometimes in combination with a fracture of the premaxilla and damage to the frontal teeth. The most common causes are falling, with the nose hitting the street or a table edge, or getting hit by a ball or swing, etc. The valve area is obstructed on the side of the fracture, while the nostril on the opposite side is (usually partially) obstructed by the dislocated caudal septal end. The cartilaginous pyramid is twisted to the side of the dislocated caudal end (▶ Fig. 5.84 and ▶ Fig. 5.85). Early repositioning of the fractured and dislocated parts mostly restores nasal function and prevents a gradually increasing deviation of the pyramid. In general, the long-term results obtained by early surgery of vertical fractures are less satisfying than those in horizontal fractures.

Horizontal Fracture

A horizontal fracture is most frequently caused by fronto-lateral trauma. The cartilaginous septum is fractured (or bent) horizontally at its lower part, or luxated at its base from its pedestal. This results in deviation of the lower part of the septum with a basal crest to the contralateral side and a high deviation to the homolateral side. Breathing complaints may be bilateral or unilateral. Both the bony and the cartilaginous pyramid are usually involved and lean to the opposite side. Early repositioning of the fractured and dislocated parts will restore nasal function and may prevent the deviation of the pyramid from progressing during further growth (▶ Fig. 5.86).

Defective Anterior Septum

A missing or destroyed anterior septum is usually the result of a septal abscess or recurrent trauma and/or surgery. The pyramid and lobule are broad and low, with saddling of the dorsum and lack of support by the septum. The valve angle is wide. Breathing complaints are common.

In such cases, we try to reconstruct the anterior septum with a transplant taken preferably from the auricle (see page 177). Reconstructing the septum will improve the configuration of the valve area and thereby improve breathing. At the same time, the projection of the cartilaginous pyramid and the lobule will be improved. Transplants used for septal reconstruction do not grow with age and may show signs of calcification (▶ Fig. 5.87). Since they may also become partially resorbed, revision surgery may be required later.

5.4.4 Surgical Techniques

In the majority of children, mobilization and repositioning of the septum suffices to restore nasal breathing and limit disturbance of further nasal growth. Only in cases with pronounced deviation of the bony pyramid will the bony pyramid also have to be repositioned (see Chapter 9, page 321). In children with a defective septum, the septum is reconstructed with autogeneic cartilage. In these patients, secondary surgery after puberty is required in the majority of cases.

The *cartilaginous septum* is approached, mobilized, repositioned, and fixed into its new position according to the methods described on page 171. Incisions are made at fracture lines and bends to mobilize the septum. Vertical fractures are dealt with as described on page 185, horizontal fractures as shown on page 186. Resections

are only carried out where needed to reposition the deviated parts. If necessary, defects are reconstructed with autogeneic transplants taken from the auricle or the rib. Parts of the septum itself are not used for this purpose, as resections will interfere with growth. Gridding, cross-hatching, and morcellation of the septal cartilage to straighten a convexity are avoided. Clinical follow-up studies have clearly shown that these techniques impair healing and further growth (Pirsig 1992) (▶ Fig. 5.88).

The *bony septum* can usually be left largely untouched. Breathing impairment and growth disturbance are almost always caused by deformities of the cartilaginous septum. Resection of pathology of the bony septum is avoided. Vomeral spurs are usually left in place to avoid unnecessary interference with growth, since they rarely cause symptoms at a young age. However, deviations of the perpendicular plate are corrected by fracturing the deviated part toward the midline.

The *cartilaginous pyramid* should in general remain untouched.

The *bony pyramid* is only corrected in children with a pronounced bony deviation. Osteotomies can be performed without harming further nasal outgrowth. Nevertheless, limited pathology of the bony pyramid is usually approached by a watchful waiting policy, as osteotomies can always be performed at a later stage, if required.

Limitations to be Observed in Surgery of a Growing Septum

As discussed above, septal surgery in a growing nose carries considerable risks. Research in animals by Verwoerd et al and long-term clinical observations by Pirsig have led to the following conclusions and recommendations:

- Avoid separating the cartilaginous septum from the perpendicular plate, as enchondral ossification of the septal cartilage takes place at its posterior margin.
- Avoid complete vertical cuts through the septal cartilage, especially in its thick sphenodorsal part, as this area is essential for the growth of the nasal dorsum.
- If the resection of a small, deviated basal rim of the septal cartilage is required, it should be performed posterior to the incisive canal. The septospinal ligament should thereby be kept intact to prevent anterior growth inhibition of the maxilla.
- In cases with a luxated caudal septum, a complete separation of the anterior septal base from the premaxilla has to be performed. After repositioning of the caudal septum in the midline, it should, however, be fixed by a permanent suture to the anterior nasal spine between the feet of the medial crura.
- Cross-hatching (gridding, morcellation) of a growing septal cartilage to straighten a bend is to be avoided.
- It is better to use cartilaginous plates instead of crushed cartilage for the reconstruction of the septum.

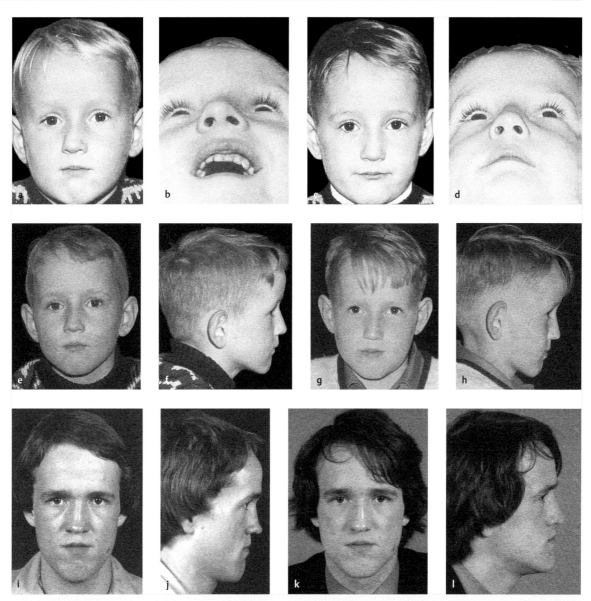

Fig. 5.86 A 16-year follow-up after septal surgery (septal mobilization and reposition) in a 3-year-old boy with a horizontal septal fracture and a deviation of the cartilaginous pyramid to the right, accompanied by bilateral breathing impairment.

a, b Age 3 years, before surgery. Impaired nasal breathing (open mouth), horizontal basal fracture of the septum to the right, deviation of the cartilaginous pyramid and lobule to the right.

c, d Age 3 years, 3 months after conservative septal surgery. Septum and pyramid are straightened, breathing is restored.

e, f Age 7 years. Normal nasal development, no sagging of the dorsum.

g, h Age 10 years. Normal nasal growth.

i, j Age 16 years. Slight sagging of the cartilaginous dorsum, retraction of the columella, and a somewhat underdeveloped lobule. Normal nasal breathing.

k, l Age 19 years. Same findings, possibly less distinct. Additional aesthetic surgery was offered but declined, as function was normal.

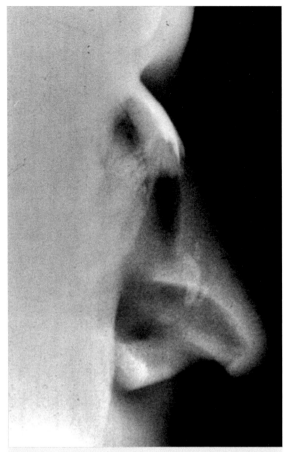

Fig. 5.87 Calcification of an autotransplant (transposition technique) performed 16 years earlier in a boy aged 10 years. (Photo courtesy Prof. Pirsig.)

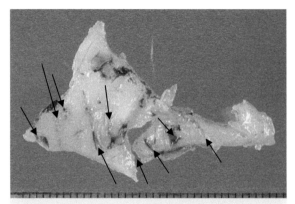

Fig. 5.88 Ingrowth of scar tissue into gridded cartilage. (Photo courtesy Prof. Pirsig.)

5.4.5 Long-Term Effects

In general, the long-term results of septal surgery may be considered satisfactory. Yet it is evident that the more conservative the surgery, the better the ultimate outcome. Improvement of breathing is achieved in many cases. The extent to which growth deformities (e.g., in a child with a deviated cartilaginous pyramid) can be prevented by medianizing the septum is hard to predict. It is equally hard to estimate the extent to which nasal growth may be impaired by early septal surgery. The outcome depends mainly on the amount of damage to the growing cartilage, the age at which the damage occurred, and the direction of the force hitting the nose. Follow-up of individual cases until after puberty is therefore required. An example of such a long-term follow-up is presented in ▶ Fig. 5.86.

Most children need no further surgery. In others, additional intervention after puberty may be required for functional and/or aesthetic reasons. In general, revision surgery of the septum would then be combined with osteotomies and lobular surgery, where feasible.

5.5 Septal Hematoma and Abscess

Septal hematomas and abscesses are among the most feared nasal diseases. They may have grave consequences for nasal form and function, especially when occurring in childhood. If a septal hematoma or a septal abscess is not recognized and treated in time, the cartilaginous septum will be destroyed. In long-standing cases, the triangular cartilages will be destroyed, too. A saddle nose with impairment of breathing will result within a few months (▶ Fig. 5.89). Further outgrowth of the nasal pyramid will be severely disturbed, leading to a low-wide pyramid syndrome. The younger the child, the more serious these consequences will be. An example of such a growth disturbance in the case of identical twins is shown in Chapter 1 (▶ Fig. 1.118). One of the boys suffered from nasal trauma and a septal infection at age 8 years, which resulted in severely retarded nasal growth. In his twin brother, nasal growth was normal.

The grave consequences of a fall on the nose in a young child have been recognized for centuries. This is illustrated by the historical use of so-called fall hats or bonnets (▶ Fig. 5.90).

5.5.1 Septal Hematoma

Septal hematomas are well-known complications of nasal trauma and septal surgery. Prompt diagnosis and treatment is imperative, as they may progress into a septal abscess and lead to destruction of the septal cartilage within hours. As the result of trauma or surgery, blood accumulates between the cartilage and the perichondrium, usually on both sides. Unlike subcutaneous hematomas and ecchymoses, subperichondral blood is not easily reabsorbed. Since bacteria (in particular, staphylococci and streptococci) are usually abundantly present in the nasal vestibule and nasal cavity, especially in

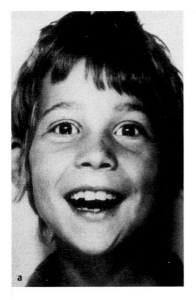

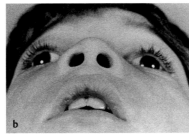

Fig. 5.89 A 13-year-old boy before and after a septal abscess that was treated only by drainage and antibiotics. No septal reconstruction.

a, b Three months before the abscess. Normal nasal development.

c, d Four months after. Severe broadening and saddling of the bony and cartilaginous pyramid. Widening and loss of prominence of the lobule with depression of the valve area and impaired breathing. Note open mouth.

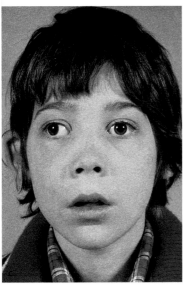

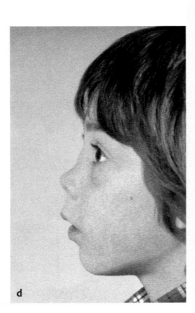

youngsters, a septal hematoma can easily develop into an abscess. The cartilaginous septum will be destroyed quickly—in a matter of hours to a few days—with disastrous consequences for nasal form and function.

Posttraumatic hematomas are chiefly seen in young and school-age children. Since they are due to a fracture or dislocation of the cartilaginous septum, they mostly occur in the anterior septum.

Postoperative hematomas usually develop more posteriorly because of the recumbent position of the patient during and after surgery. They are usually caused by insufficient cleaning and closing of the intraseptal space at the final stage of septal surgery. Persistent bleeding from a small artery of the premaxilla or maxillary crest, or oozing from the perichondrium and periosteum may also play a role.

Symptoms

In a traumatic hematoma, the anterior and caudal part of the septum is severely swollen and is bluish red in color. The hematoma protrudes into the vestibules and completely obstructs the nasal entrance on both sides.

Diagnosis

An anterior traumatic hematoma is easily diagnosed on inspection and gentle palpation of the swelling with a cotton wool applicator. Diagnosing a posterior hematoma usually requires decongestion and anesthesia of the mucosa. The swelling is then palpated with a blunt instrument. If there is any doubt, a small exploratory incision (using a No. 64 Beaver knife) may be considered. Puncturing with a thick needle is generally not conclusive.

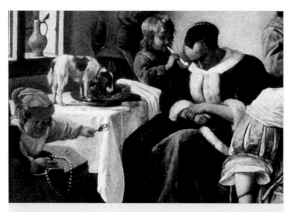

Fig. 5.90 Child with a so-called fall hat. Detail from Jan Steen's painting "Wrong World." During the 17th and 18th centuries in The Netherlands, Northern Germany, and Denmark, it was common for toddlers to wear a bonnet (in German "Fallhut," literally "fall hat") to prevent damage to the nose, face, and skull when they were learning to walk. These bonnets have often been depicted by Dutch painters from that era, among them Jan Steen, Rembrandt, and Nicolaas Maes. (Pirsig 1987.)

Prevention

A postoperative septal hematoma can almost always be avoided by taking the following precautions (see also Chapter 5, page 172):
- Coagulation of bleeding arterioles in the septal framework (premaxilla, maxillary crest)
- Careful cleansing of the intraseptal space at the end of surgery
- Closing the septal space by conscientiously adjusting the mucosal blades with an internal dressing or splint

In our experience, there is no indication to routinely incise the mucosa for drainage, although many surgeons say that they feel "safer" doing so.

Treatment

Hematomas should be drained as soon as possible by opening the area and cleansing. Puncturing and aspiration is usually ineffective, as the blood clot cannot be removed through a needle. Depending on its cause and the pathology, the hematoma is opened either through a CSI or via a horizontal basal mucosal incision. Antibiotics are administered systemically to prevent a septal abscess.

Approach through a Caudal Septal Incision

Steps

- In general, large posttraumatic and postoperative hematomas can best be drained by a CSI.
- The mucoperichondrium and mucoperiosteum are carefully elevated. Blood coagula are aspirated, and the septum is explored in the normal way.

- Internal dressings are applied. The intraseptal space is then closed by carefully pressing the mucosal blades together to prevent recurrence.

Approach through a Horizontal Basal Incision of the Mucosa

In old (noninfected) hematomas without septal fractures or dislocation, an approach through a horizontal basal incision of the septal mucosa may be considered. This cut is made parallel to the nasal floor in the lower half of the hematoma (see ▶ Fig. 4.26a). Vertical mucosal incisions are avoided as they leave a vertical scar that may interrupt mucociliary transport (MCT).

5.5.2 Septal Abscess

A septal abscess is almost invariably an infected septal hematoma. It is seen most frequently in young children some days after nasal trauma resulting in a septal fracture and hematoma that have not been properly diagnosed and treated. *Streptococcus pyogenes* and *Staphylococcus aureus* are the most commonly cultured bacteria. A septal abscess results in necrosis of the cartilaginous septum within hours due to the toxic effects of the infection. The hematoma and abscess elevate the perichondrium from the cartilage, depriving it of its nutrition and defense. If no immediate treatment is given, the bony septum and the triangular cartilages will also become involved. A septal perforation may finally occur. Ultimately, a more or less severe saddling of the cartilaginous pyramid and retraction of the columella will result. One reason for this disastrous outcome is the loss of support of the cartilaginous pyramid due to necrosis of the septum. An equally important factor is scarring of the mucoperichondrium occurring in the healing phase.

Symptoms

The patient has a high temperature, severe local pain, and headache. The nose is completely blocked. The nasal mucosa is severely swollen and red. The abscess usually protrudes into the vestibules on both sides (▶ Fig. 5.91). The skin of the nose and face is swollen. Septicemia and meningitis may ultimately set in.

Diagnosis

Diagnosing a septal abscess is relatively simple for the expert. Unfortunately, many family physicians fail to recognize this grave condition, while few are aware of the serious consequences of a septal abscess on nasal form and function.

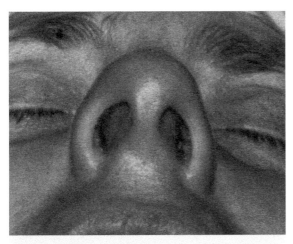

Fig. 5.91 Septal abscess following an untreated traumatic septal fracture and hematoma.

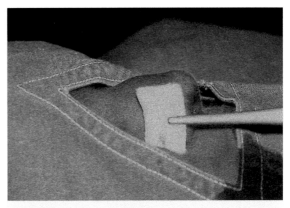

Fig. 5.92 Preserved rib cartilage transplant from the tissue bank is used to reconstruct the septal defect. (Photo courtesy Prof. Hellmich.)

Prevention

A septal abscess should be prevented by recognizing and treating a septal hematoma at an early stage. It is for this reason that the septum should be inspected and palpated (after decongestion and anesthesia of the mucosa) in patients with a fresh nasal injury, especially children. The same applies to patients who have undergone septal surgery and cannot breathe through the nose after removal of the inner nasal dressings.

Treatment

For centuries, drainage was the only way to treat a septal hematoma and abscess. Later, sulfonamides and other antibiotics were also administered, greatly reducing the number of general complications such as septicemia and meningitis. The local effects on nasal form, function, and growth remained the same, however. In the 1960s, it was proven that these sequelae can largely be prevented by repairing the septal defect in the (sub)acute stage of the abscess (Cottle 1961, Masing 1965, Huizing 1966). Follow-up studies have demonstrated that the feared consequences on nasal form and function, as well as the long-term effects on nasal growth, can thereby be largely prevented (Huizing 1984).

Patients with a septal abscess must be considered emergency cases. They should be treated as follows:
1. Immediate intravenous administration of a broad-spectrum penicillin
2. Drainage of the abscess and reconstruction of the septal defect by a transplant the same day

Steps
- General anesthesia is given.
- The nasal mucous membranes are decongested and anesthetized.
- A CSI is made, and the septal abscess is opened. A bacteriological culture is taken.
- Pus and detritus are removed by aspiration.
- The septum is explored by carefully elevating the swollen mucosal blades.
- The septal defect is measured. A bony or cartilaginous transplant of the same proportions is prepared. The graft may be taken from the bony septum, rib, auricle, or the tissue bank (▶ Fig. 5.92).
- A transplant from the bony septum is the first choice. However, in a young child, one would hesitate to resect part of the bony septum. A plate cut from preserved allogeneic rib cartilage could then be the best choice. Satisfactory long-term results after such transplantations have been reported. Other options are autogeneic auricular cartilage or rib cartilage.
- Internal dressings with an antibiotic ointment (e.g., Terracortril) are loosely applied intranasally.
- The transplant is inserted into the defect. No special fixation is required.
- The septal space is carefully closed by gentle pressure with intranasal dressings.
- The upper half of the incision may be closed. The lower half is usually left open. A small strip of Silastic sheet or gauze may be introduced to assure drainage.
- The area is reinspected and cleaned daily.
- The internal dressings and drain can be removed after 3 days. The transplant is almost always accepted in spite of the acute infection. We have never observed extrusion.

Long-Term Results

Follow-up studies have demonstrated that the short-term effects of saddling and broadening of the pyramid and lobule can be almost entirely prevented by reconstructing the septal defect in the (sub)acute phase of the abscess.

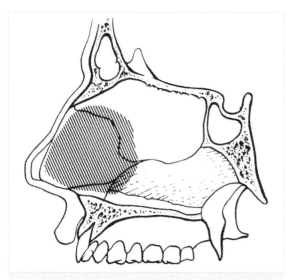

Fig. 5.93 Septal defect found at surgery in an 8-year-old boy with a septal abscess. For a 19 year follow-up, see ▶ Fig. 5.94.

Negative sequelae on nasal growth can usually not be prevented completely, but they may be avoided to a considerable degree, as illustrated in ▶ Fig. 5.93 and ▶ Fig. 5.94.

Reconstructing the septal defect in a patient with a septal abscess in the acute phase will prevent short-term damage to nasal form and function almost completely, while the long-term effects on nasal growth and function are largely limited.

5.6 Septal Perforation

Perforations of the septum are among the more frequent and serious rhinological disorders. They may cause a variety of complaints such as crusting, blood loss, a whistling sound at inspiration, and a sensation of nasal obstruction and pain. Whether or not these symptoms are present depends upon various factors, in particular pathogenesis, location, size, shape, and the condition of the margins.

When considering the therapeutic options, all these aspects should be taken into account. Surgical closure is definitely the best treatment, though it is not always possible or necessary. Whether a perforation can be closed depends on more than the surgical method and the skill of the surgeon. The above-mentioned parameters of the defect also play an important role. Therefore, septal perforations should be classified according to these parameters.

5.6.1 Classification

Septal perforations may be classified according to the following parameters: (1) cause; (2) symptoms; (3) location; (4) size; (5) shape; (6) condition of the margins; and (7) presence or absence of cartilage (or bone) around the defect.

Cause

Unfortunately, septal surgery is still the most frequent cause of septal perforation. Other well known causes are nose-picking, repeated bilateral coagulation for epistaxis (e.g., in patients with hereditary telangiectasias), trauma, cocaine abuse, industrial dusts, septal abscess, granulomatous diseases, and tumor surgery. In patients with a caustic perforation, we should be aware of the poor quality of the mucosa around the defect. In a postoperative perforation, the cartilage (bone) around the defect is usually missing, whereas it is generally present in a perforation caused by nose-picking.

Symptoms

The complaints of patients with a septal perforation vary from no complaints at all to distressing symptoms such as severe crusting, daily bleeding, and a permanent whistling sound on inspiration. Perforations of the anterior part of the septum usually lead to greater distress than those located more posteriorly, while smaller defects often produce more severe symptoms than larger ones.

Location

A distinction may be made between anterior (in areas 1 and 2), central (areas 3 and 4), and posterior (area 5) perforations, as well as between cranial, central, and basal (caudal) perforations (▶ Fig. 5.95). The location of the defect plays a major role in its symptomatology. It is also one of the main parameters to consider when choosing treatment. Anterior and central perforations generally produce more symptoms than posterior and cranial ones, as they cause abnormal turbulence of the inspiratory air. Posterior and basal defects are usually more difficult to close.

Size

The size of a perforation is of paramount importance, both for the symptomatology and the chances of success of surgery. Small perforations, especially when located anteriorly, cause more complaints than larger ones. An inspiratory whistling noise and crusting are both typical symptoms of a small (anterior) perforation. Obviously, the size of the defect is a critical factor when attempting a surgical closure. The height of the defect should not be larger than half the height of the remaining cartilaginous septum.

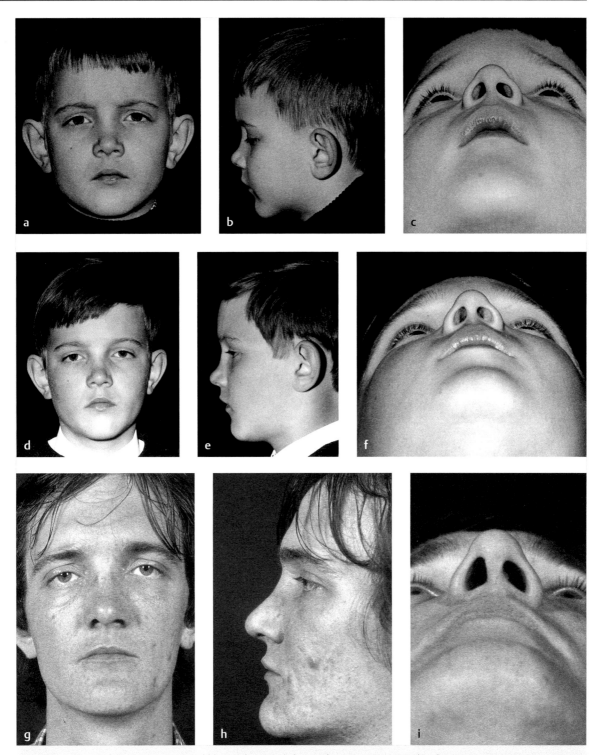

Fig. 5.94 A 19 year follow-up in a 8-year-old boy with a septal abscess that was reconstructed in the acute stage.
a–c Five months after septal reconstruction, there is slight sagging of the cartilaginous dorsum.
d–f Four and a half years after surgery at the age of 13 years. Some underdevelopment of the bony and cartilaginous pyramid, normal development of the lobule, normal breathing.
g–i Nineteen years after surgery, at the age of 27 years. Normal length, prominence and width of the external nasal pyramid is seen. There is slight sagging of the dorsum, and normal adult configuration of the lobule with normal length of slightly deviated columella. Adult-type nostrils and valve area and normal nasal function are also observed. No further surgery was required.

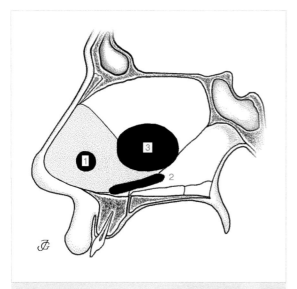

Fig. 5.95 Most frequent location and shape of septal perforations. Round or ovaloid perforation centrally located in the cartilaginous septum (1); oblong basal perforation at the region of the premaxilla and maxillary crest (2); large central perforation (3).

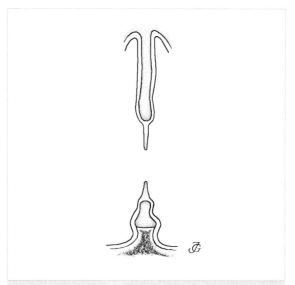

Fig. 5.96 In many cases, the mucosa around a septal perforation is atrophic and infected, while the cartilage or bone around the defect is partially missing. In surgery, the perforation often turns out to be larger than expected.

Shape

Slitlike perforations usually produce fewer symptoms and are easier to close than round and ovaloid defects.

Condition of the Mucosal Margins

The condition of the mucosa along the margins of the defect is another highly important factor determining the symptomatology and the chances of success of surgery. Infection, crusting, and bleeding are signs of a poor quality mucosa that is likely to tear when mucosal flaps are mobilized and sutured. Many surgeons, therefore, start with conservative treatment to improve the condition of the mucosa before attempting surgery (▶ Fig. 5.96).

Presence of Cartilage or Bone around the Defect

The presence or absence of cartilage or bone around the defect is another important parameter when considering surgical closure. If the margins of the perforation are membranous, it will be much more difficult to separate, mobilize, and suture the two mucosal membranes together. Besides, the defect to be closed may also turn out to be larger than expected.

5.6.2 Prevention

Septal perforation is one of the most distressing complications of septal surgery, both for the patient and for the surgeon. Therefore, we should make every effort to prevent this from happening.

In the era of the Killian-Freer submucous septal resection, a postoperative septal perforation was observed in 5 to 24% of the cases. In modern conservative reconstructive septal surgery, that percentage has been greatly reduced. This is the result of several improvements. First of all, the general conditions during nasal surgery and the quality of intranasal illumination and surgical instruments are much better than before. A second and even more important factor is the surgical technique of repositioning and reconstructing the septum instead of resecting the deviated parts. When the new methods are applied in the proper way, postoperative septal perforations are rare. Nowadays, (training) clinics report an incidence of 0.5 to 1%. Nonetheless, a postoperative perforation may occur in the hands of even the most experienced and careful surgeon.

Guidelines

Knowing how to prevent a perforation is more important than mastering the complicated techniques for surgical closure. The following guidelines may prove helpful in preventing a postoperative septal perforation.

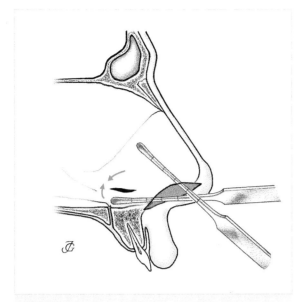

Fig. 5.97 If a tear has been made inadvertently in the mucosa, the laceration is immediately isolated by elevating the neighboring mucoperichondrium (mucoperiosteum) to release tension on its margins.

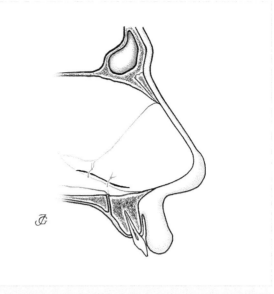

Fig. 5.98 A large mucosal tear is closed immediately with two or three 4–0 resorbable sutures (with a round atraumatic needle) that are knotted intranasally.

1. Ensure good illumination, sufficient surgical exposure, and a bloodless surgical field. Good illumination, sufficient exposure, and a bloodless surgical field are critical factors. For ways to ensure a bloodless surgical field in nasal surgery, we refer to Chapter 3, page 132.
2. Elevate (dissect) the septal mucosa in the proper plane, using the right instrument and the correct movements. The septal mucosa is elevated subperichondrially and subperiosteally using the proper instruments in the correct way:
   - In elevating the mucoperichondrium from cartilage, the blunt end of the elevator is used in an upward and downward sweeping movement (like windscreen wipers). Pushing the instrument should be avoided.
   - In elevating the mucoperiosteum from bone, the semi-sharp end of the elevator is preferred. While dissecting, care is taken that the instrument stays in continuous contact with the bone.
   - Scar tissue is cut by a sharp instrument (e.g., a No. 64 Beaver knife or small, sharp scissors). Cutting is preferably done from inferior to superior under direct view.
3. Safeguard a mucosal laceration immediately. If the mucosa is accidentally lacerated, the lesion should be immediately isolated and safeguarded. Dissection of the mucoperichondrium or periosteum is only continued above and below the defect. We will then try to circumvent and isolate the perforation. An extra inferior tunnel may be required to achieve this (► Fig. 5.97). As soon as the tension of the mucosa around the defect has been released, the perforation is safeguarded from further tearing.

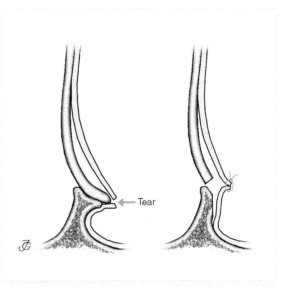

Fig. 5.99 A mucosal tear at a basal crest is closed immediately after resection of the crest.

4. Close a tear as soon as possible. Tears of the septal mucosa larger than 1 cm should be closed as soon as possible. The area of the lesion is first mobilized as described above. Its margins are then sutured together with 4–0 resorbable sutures using a round atraumatic needle. It is essential to evert the mucosal margins toward the nasal cavity and to knot the sutures intranasally (► Fig. 5.98 and ► Fig. 5.99).

5. Carefully adjust the margins of a mucosal defect at the end of the operation. Careful adjustment of the margins of a mucosal defect if they have not been sutured together is one of the most important measures in avoiding a permanent perforation. We take the following steps:

   • Intranasal dressings are applied on both sides.
   • The septal space is reinspected and cleaned of blood. The margins of the defect are optimally adjusted to each other using the blunt end of the elevator. Care is taken that the internal dressing does not protrude between the mucosal margins into the septal space.

6. Reconstruct the septum by inserting a plate or several small plates of cartilage or bone, particularly in the area of the defect. Reconstruction of the cartilaginous or bony defect of the septum in the area of the mucosal laceration is the last important means to prevent a perforation. Small plates of bone or cartilage are inserted into the septal space after the internal dressings have been applied and the inside of the mucosal laceration has been checked again (see point 5). The right-handed surgeon will usually position the plates mosaic-style on the inside of the left mucosal blade. The lacerated area is covered by the largest plate available. If there is not enough bone or cartilage left, preserved allogeneic dura or fascia may be used as an "interlay." Inserting a plate of compressed gelfoam or thick gelfilm in between the mucosal flaps and the internal dressing may facilitate later removal of the dressings.

5.6.3 Treatment Options

How to best treat a septal perforation has been a matter of debate for decades. There are four modalities:

No Treatment

No treatment is given when there are no complaints. This may seem self-evident. However, sometimes patients without complaints are advised to have their perforation surgically closed. This is a risky course of action because if it fails, the patient's condition may worsen.

Conservative Treatment

Applying some ointment once or twice daily in and around the perforation with a cotton wool applicator may provide relief for some patients. Sometimes an ointment, such as lanolin–glycerin–Vaseline in equal parts, is sufficiently effective in diminishing crusting, bleeding, and pain. In addition, nasal washings with isotonic or slightly hypertonic saline may be advised in patients with extensive crusting. In cases with infected perforations, an antibiotic–corticosteroid ointment (e.g., Terracortril) might be given first. This is always done some weeks prior to surgery.

Surgical Closure

Surgical closure of a perforation is without any doubt the best therapeutic option. With some rare exceptions, surgical closure yields permanent relief from almost all symptoms. Whether or not surgical closure is attempted depends upon the patient's complaints and the likelihood that the attempt will be successful. Since the 1930s, a great variety of techniques has been proposed. Several of them were abandoned, others were improved step by step to become more or less reliable methods. Unfortunately, the success rate of the various techniques is almost always presented in relation to the diameter of the perforation. The size of the defect is only one of the parameters that determines surgical success, however. As previously discussed, the location and the shape of the perforation, the quality of its margins, and the presence or absence of cartilage (bone) around the defect are also important.

Prosthesis (Septal Button, Obturator)

A septal prosthesis has proven an effective means of treatment in many patients. Firstly, it is the only option when surgical closure is out of the question or has failed in patients who do not get sufficient relief from conservative measures. Secondly, a prosthesis might be a good substitute when the outcome of surgery is questionable. Several authors recommend first placing a button and evaluating its effects before deciding to go ahead with surgery. The results obtained with a prosthesis give some indication of the effect of surgical closure on the patient's complaints. Sometimes the symptoms are alleviated to such a degree that surgery can be cancelled, but sometimes the defect is also enlarged by the prosthesis.

Surgical Closure

Surgical closure is clearly the best treatment for a septal perforation. Unfortunately, however, surgical attempts are often unsuccessful and the condition of some patients worsens. Many factors play a role in closing a septal perforation: the technique, the skill of the surgeon, and, above all, the characteristics of the perforation. Closure of a posterior perforation is usually more difficult than that of an anterior one. Closure of a perforation caused by chemocautery has a limited chance of success as the mucosal margins are in poor condition. It is more difficult to close an irregularly shaped defect resulting from a septal resection than a round central defect caused by nasal picking. A crucial step for successful closure of a perforation is the interposition of a plate of autogeneic cartilage or bone between both sutured mucoperichondrial/mucoperiosteal flaps.

Sometimes, a septal perforation is combined with a marked deformation of the bony pyramid and the nasal lobule. In such cases, it is recommended to close the perforation in a first stage and to correct the nasal deformity in a second stage after 9 to 12 months.

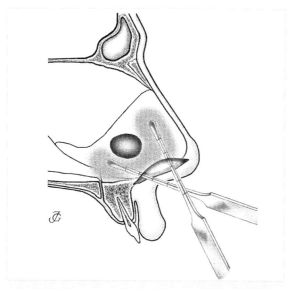

Fig. 5.100 The mucoperichondrium and mucoperiosteum are elevated anterior, superior, and inferior to the perforation.

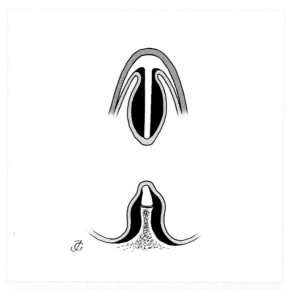

Fig. 5.101 The mucosal edges of the perforation are left intact.

In our hands, the following four techniques of closing a septal perforation have proven to be successful:

1. *Direct closure* Direct closure is chosen in cases with a small perforation and a remaining septal deformity. By widely mobilizing the mucosa and straightening the septum, sufficient mucosa is gained to close the defect.
2. *Rotation-flap technique* The rotation-flap technique is used for anterior perforations up to 2 cm in diameter, with margins of reasonable quality, and cartilage or bone around the defect.
3. *Bridge-flap technique* The bridge-flap technique is applied for larger anterior (2 to 3 cm in diameter) and posterior perforations. This method may be technically more complicated, but it is certainly one of the most reliable and can be successful in the great majority of cases.

Dissecting the Perforation

Before mucosal flaps can be created, the mucoperichondrium (mucoperiosteum) has to be elevated bilaterally. This must be performed with utmost care to avoid damage to the margins of the defect. Meticulous preparation is required to avoid tearing of the tissues, which are usually thin and delicate. The use of magnifying glasses or a microscope will hereby be of great help.

Steps

- A CSI and bilateral anterosuperior tunnels are made in the usual way. The undertunneling proceeds up to the anterior edge of the perforation. At this stage, the margins of the defect are kept intact (▸ Fig. 5.100 and ▸ Fig. 5.101).
- Inferior tunnels are elevated bilaterally and connected with the superior tunnels.
- The inferior tunnels are extended over the nasal floor and the lateral nasal wall, depending on the technique to be used (e.g., rotation-flap or bridge-flap technique). Damage to the incisive nerves and arteries is unavoidable and should be mentioned in the informed consent.
- The edges of the perforation are incised using a No. 15 blade or a No. 64 Beaver knife. Depending on the pathology, the anterior, superior, and inferior edges are usually incised through one of the anterior tunnels (▸ Fig. 5.102, ▸ Fig. 5.103, and ▸ Fig. 5.104), whereas the posterior edge is incised through the nasal cavity (▸ Fig. 5.105).
- The mucoperichondrium and mucoperiosteum are further elevated as widely as possible (i.e., from underneath the nasal dorsum down to the nasal floor) to achieve maximum mobility of the mucosa (▸ Fig. 5.106). The mucosa is now completely detached from the septal skeleton (▸ Fig. 5.107).
- After widely mobilizing the mucosal layers, we choose the technique that appears the most likely to successfully close the defect.

Direct Closure

Direct closure is sometimes possible in patients with a small perforation (< 5 mm) in whom the septum is still deviated. In straightening the septum, the mucosa is bilaterally mobilized. As a certain amount of mucosa is gained, primary closure becomes possible.

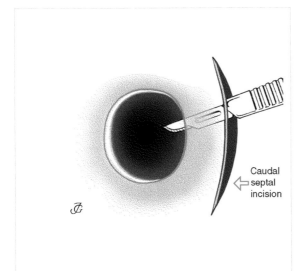

Fig. 5.102 The edges of the perforation are incised using a No. 15 blade or a No. 64 Beaver knife. The anterior edge is incised via the anterior tunnel.

Caudal septal incision

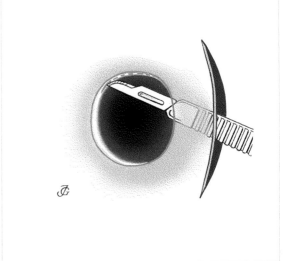

Fig. 5.103 The edges of the perforation are incised using a No. 15 blade or a No. 64 Beaver knife. The superior edge is incised via the anterior tunnel.

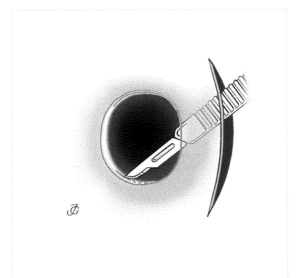

Fig. 5.104 The edges of the perforation are incised using a No. 15 blade or a No. 64 Beaver knife. The inferior edge is incised via the anterior tunnel.

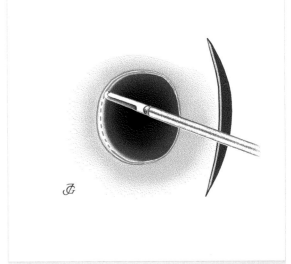

Fig. 5.105 The edges of the perforation are incised using a No. 15 blade or a No. 64 Beaver knife. The posterior edge is incised through the nasal cavity.

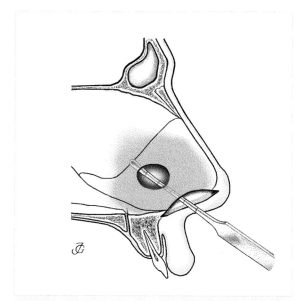

Fig. 5.106 After incising all the margins of the perforation, the mucoperichondrium and mucoperiosteum are further elevated in posterior, superior, and inferior directions.

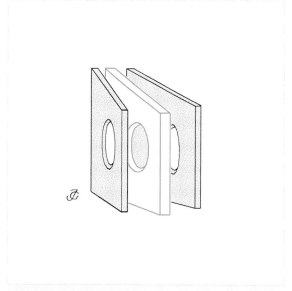

Fig. 5.107 The mucosa is completely detached from the septal skeleton.

Steps

- The mucosa is bilaterally elevated (see ▶ Fig. 5.100, ▶ Fig. 5.101, ▶ Fig. 5.102, ▶ Fig. 5.103, ▶ Fig. 5.104, ▶ Fig. 5.105, ▶ Fig. 5.106, and ▶ Fig. 5.107).
- The remaining septal deviation is corrected by resection and repositioning as usual.
- The excess mucoperichondrium that is obtained is used to close the defect.
- It may be necessary to further mobilize the mucosa and to cut one or two pedicled flaps on one or both sides as described later.

Rotation-Flap Technique

The rotation-flap technique is a reliable method in perforations of the anterior septum with a diameter of up to 20 mm, provided that the septal cartilage around the defect is partially preserved and the quality of the mucosal margins is fair (▶ Fig. 5.108 and ▶ Fig. 5.109). Two pedicled mucosal flaps are created: an upper septal flap on one side and a lower one from the nasal floor on the opposite side. The septal flap has its base cranioposteriorly and receives its blood supply from the anterior and posterior ethmoidal artery. The lower flap is pedicled caudoposteriorly and is supplied by the palatine artery (see ▶ Fig. 1.53). As the two flaps are cut from different areas, the septal cartilage will not become denuded at opposite regions. The method is reliable and technically not too difficult. It can only be used for anterior perforations of moderate size.

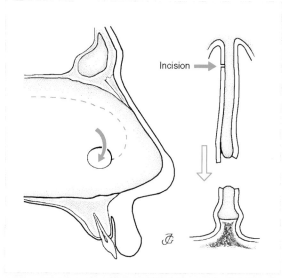

Fig. 5.108 Rotation-flap technique. Step 1: The superior flap is cut from the septal mucoperichondrium cranial to the defect.

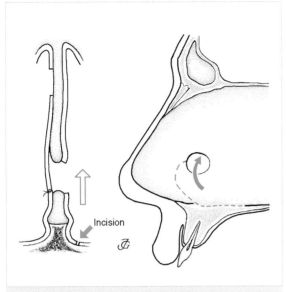

Fig. 5.109 Rotation-flap technique. Step 2: The inferior flap is cut from the mucoperichondrium caudal to the defect and mucoperiosteum of the nasal floor.

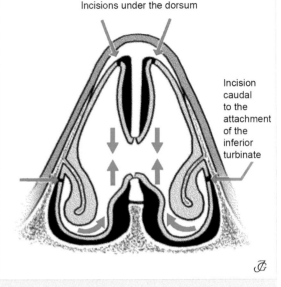

Fig. 5.110 Bilateral bridge-flap (advancement) technique. Bilateral superior flaps from the septum and inferior flaps from the septum and nasal floor are created and advanced to close the defect.

Steps

- The mucosa is bilaterally elevated by creating superior and inferior septal tunnels (see ▶ Fig. 5.100, ▶ Fig. 5.101, ▶ Fig. 5.102, ▶ Fig. 5.103, ▶ Fig. 5.104, ▶ Fig. 5.105, ▶ Fig. 5.106, and ▶ Fig. 5.107).
- The inferior tunnel is extended on one side over the nasal floor up to the lateral nasal wall.
- A posteriorly pedicled flap is cut cranially to the perforation with an angulated No. 66 Beaver knife and pointed, slightly curved scissors. The flap is mobilized and rotated into the defect from above (▶ Fig. 5.108).
- A similar flap is cut inferior to the perforation on the opposite side and rotated into the defect from below (▶ Fig. 5.109).
- The two flaps are sutured to the margins of the perforation from posterior to anterior with interrupted 4–0 resorbable sutures (with a round atraumatic needle) that are knotted intranasally.
- Finally, a plate of autogeneic septal cartilage or bone is inserted between the two septal flaps. Two triangular mucosal defects will result: one above the upper flap, one lateral to the inferior flap. They usually heal without problems in 2 to 4 weeks.

Bridge-Flap (Advancement) Technique

Bilateral advancement or bridge flaps allow the closure of perforations up to 30 mm in diameter. This method is more traumatic than the rotation-flap technique, but it is certainly the best for closing larger defects.

Steps

- The septum is approached either by the "four-tunnel approach" through a CSI (see ▶ Fig. 5.100, ▶ Fig. 5.101, ▶ Fig. 5.102, ▶ Fig. 5.103, ▶ Fig. 5.104, ▶ Fig. 5.105, ▶ Fig. 5.106, and ▶ Fig. 5.107), or by means of the external approach.
- Ventrally, the superior tunnels are extended up to the roof of the cartilaginous and bony pyramid.
- Caudally, the inferior tunnels are continued over the nasal floor and the lateral nasal wall up to the attachment of the inferior turbinates. The incisive nerve will thereby be severed (see ▶ Fig. 1.57, ▶ Fig. 1.58, and ▶ Fig. 5.17).
- Longitudinal incisions are made in the mucosa at the nasal roof. The two superior septal flaps are now advanced downward toward the defect (▶ Fig. 5.110).
- Longitudinal incisions are made just below the attachment of the inferior turbinates. The inferior mucosal flaps are then advanced medially and cranially toward the defect (▶ Fig. 5.110).
- The flaps are sutured together by everted mattress sutures from posterior to anterior with interrupted 4–0 resorbable sutures (with a round atraumatic needle) that are knotted intranasally.
- Finally, a plate of autogeneic cartilage or bone is inserted between the two septal flaps (▶ Fig. 5.111).

Additional Procedures

External Approach for Wide Access

In large and posterior perforations, it may be of great help to have a wide surgical field. The external approach (see ▶ Fig. 4.12 and ▶ Fig. 4.13) may then be the method of choice, particularly when the bridge-flap technique is used.

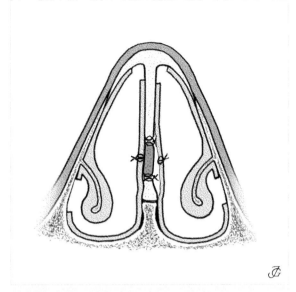

Fig. 5.111 Bilateral bridge-flap (advancement) technique. Bilateral closure of the mucosal defect and interposition and fixation of a cartilaginous graft.

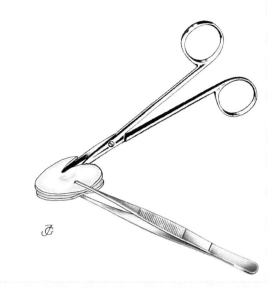

Fig. 5.112 A commercially available Silastic prosthesis is cut to the required size and shape, avoiding sharp edges.

Antibiotics

A broad-spectrum antibiotic will be administered systemically to diminish the chances of infection that would compromise the healing process. We advise starting antibiotics some days before surgery to "sterilize" the surgical field as much as possible.

Dressings and Fixation

It is advisable to insert a plate of compressed gelfoam or another type of sheet between the freshly sutured mucosal margins and the internal dressings. This prevents damage to the vulnerable area when the internal dressings are removed.

Aftercare

The internal dressing is removed after 3 to 4 days. Careful cleaning of the nasal cavity is advised to avoid infection and reduce crusting. Some of us use the "moist chamber" treatment: after removal of the dressings the patient is asked to put a Vaseline-coated cotton wool ball into one nasal vestibule for 2 to 3 hours, then remove it, do the same on the other side, and so on. This results in a "moist nasal cavity" on one side which facilitates healing.

Nicotine avoidance for 10 to 14 days postoperatively is also highly recommended, as nicotine causes permanent vasoconstriction.

Prosthesis (Septal Button, Obturator)

For patients in whom surgical closure is impossible because of the size and location of the defect and for patients in whom surgical closure was unsuccessful, placement of an obturating prosthesis or button may be an alternative.

The idea of closing septal perforations by inserting a disk of nonbiological material is not new. The method only became popular after the introduction of inert artificial materials. Nowadays, Silastic is the preferred material.

In most cases, a septal prosthesis can be fitted under local anesthesia as an office procedure. Buttons have to be renewed after 5 to 10 years, depending on the patient's complaints. The formation of biofilms on the obturator has recently been reported.

Steps

- The width and height of the perforation is measured by a calibrated elevator or, in special cases, by sagittal CT scanning.
- The nasal mucosa is anesthetized and decongested.
- A commercially available prosthesis is cut to the proper shape and size (i.e., about 3 to 4 mm larger than the dimensions of the perforation) (▶ Fig. 5.112).
- To facilitate insertion of the button, both the prosthesis and the left anterior nasal cavity are greased with some ointment. When a large prosthesis is to be introduced, one flange is sutured together (▶ Fig. 5.113).

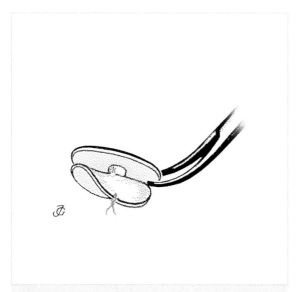

Fig. 5.113 Insertion of a Silastic prosthesis is facilitated by suturing one flange together.

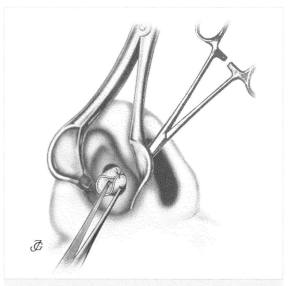

Fig. 5.114 A Silastic prosthesis is introduced through the left nostril. The flange that is sutured together is picked up with a forceps in the right nasal cavity. The suture is cut, and the prosthesis is rotated into position.

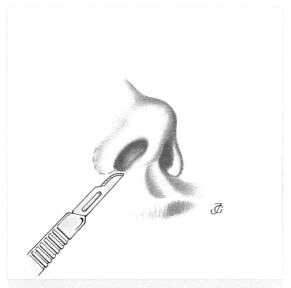

Fig. 5.115 Lateral alatomy. The alar base is incised at the alar-labial fold.

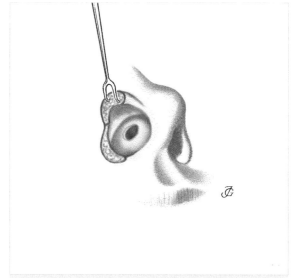

Fig. 5.116 Lateral alatomy. The ala is cut from its base to enlarge the access to the perforation.

- The button can be best introduced through the left nostril. The posterior end of the medial flange is pushed through the perforation. It is picked up on the right side and pulled through by means of a forceps. The prosthesis is then rotated into the desired position (▶ Fig. 5.114).
- Contact between the flanges of the button and the mucosa of the floor or the roof of the nasal cavity should be avoided. Any contact may cause irritation of the mucosa, formation of granulations, bleeding, crusting, and pain.

- In very large perforations, the standard prosthesis may be not large enough. A custom-made prosthesis with dimensions as measured by sagittal CT scanning is then manufactured. An alatomy may be required for sufficient access (▶ Fig. 5.115 and ▶ Fig. 5.116).

Results

The results of a septal prosthesis are generally good. In our experience, a positive outcome is seen in about two-thirds of patients. Pallanch, Facer, Kern, and Westwood reported 73% success in a consecutive series of 171 cases. Whistling, bleeding, and pain almost always disappear. In most cases, crusting is abolished as well, and some patients also find that their breathing improves. Small buttons may be blown out by sneezing or nose-blowing. Application of ointment or nasal washings may be needed for cleaning. In most patients, buttons have to be renewed every 3 to 5 years.

Few patients are unable to tolerate a septal prosthesis. Much depends on the quality of the fit, however. We should not hesitate to remove the button and make adjustments until an optimal fit is achieved.

Obsolete Measures

Over the past decades some other techniques have been advocated that, in our opinion, should no longer be used.

Buccogingival-Flap Technique

Bilateral oblong flaps are cut from the oral gingival mucosa and submucosa with their base medially. They are rotated through a small paraspinal tunnel into the septal defect.

Only anterior perforations with a diameter up to 20 to 25 mm can be successfully closed by this method. Normally the length of a pedicled random-pattern (skin) flap should not exceed 1.5 times its width to avoid necrosis of its end. Because of the rich capillary vascularization of the oral mucosa, pedicled mucosal flaps may be longer. Sometimes, a minor secondary intervention under local anesthesia is required at a later stage to close the paraseptal tunnel.

The method yields reliable results in anterior perforations of 10 to 25 mm. However, it is a somewhat complicated procedure. Its main risks are postoperative asymmetry of the upper lip, stenosis of the nasal entrance, and loss of sensitivity in part of the upper lip. Sometimes oronasal fistulas may result, which are easy to close by excision of the oral opening of the fistula. The method should not be used in patients who play a wind instrument, or in actors or actresses.

Other Obsolete Measures

- *Free grafts* of fascia or skin and composite cartilage–skin grafts were recommended in the 1960s and 1970s. Since they have a high failure rate, their use is no longer advised.
- *Inferior turbinate flaps* have also been recommended. We do not advise this method, however. It is a rather cumbersome two-stage technique, with poor end results. Moreover, it causes permanent damage to the functional anterior part of the inferior turbinate.

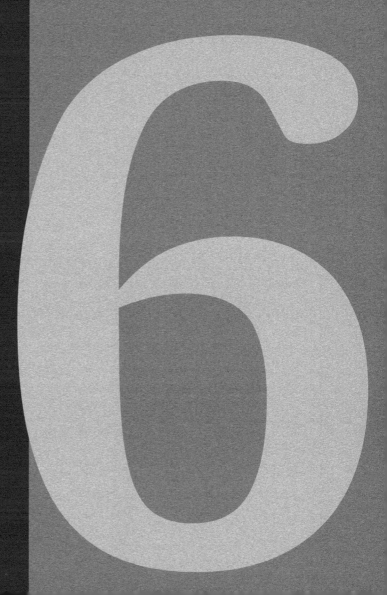

Chapter 6

Pyramid Surgery

6 Pyramid Surgery

6.1 Osteotomies—Mobilizing and Repositioning the Bony Pyramid

Modifying the bony pyramid is one of the basic procedures in functional reconstructive nasal surgery. It may involve repositioning, reduction, or augmentation. Repositioning requires complete mobilization of the bony vault.

6.1.1 Mobilizing the Bony Pyramid

To allow repositioning of the pyramid, the bony pyramid is detached from the frontal bone and the maxillary bones. This is accomplished through a combination of interconnecting osteotomies. Usually, bilateral paramedian, lateral, and transverse osteotomies are performed. Generally, mobilization and repositioning of the pyramid also require mobilization and correction of the septum.

There may be exceptions to this standard procedure, depending upon the pathology and the surgical goals. For example, in aesthetic surgery, a limited amount of narrowing of the pyramid may be sufficient. Two oblique osteotomies instead of lateral and transverse osteotomies may then suffice. In a severely deformed and broad pyramid, on the other hand, extra osteotomies may be required. Instead of the standard osteotomies, one or two intermediate osteotomies may be added. The sequence of steps for mobilizing the bony pyramid is as follows:

Steps

- *Mobilizing and Correcting the Septum*
  As a first step, the cartilaginous and bony septum are mobilized by horizontal and/or vertical chondrotomies and resection of strips where required (see page 169).
- *Outlining the Osteotomies*
  The points and lines of reference and the planned osteotomies are drawn on the skin. The following anatomical and clinical landmarks are indicated: depth of frontonasal angle (nasion), K area (rhinion), the two domes, tip, and nasal base line (NBL) on either side (▶ Fig. 6.1). The planned osteotomies and the hump to be resected are then marked in relation to these landmarks (▶ Fig. 6.2).
- *Undermining the Skin over the Pyramid (Dorsal Tunnel)*
  The skin over the pyramid and the cranial part of the lobule is undermined through bilateral intercartilaginous (IC) incisions and via the caudal septal incision (CSI) using blunt, slightly curved scissors (▶ Fig. 6.3). This is performed in the plane between the subcutis and the perichondrium and periosteum. In other words, the skin is undermined supraperichondrially and

supraperiosteally. Detaching the skin from the bony and cartilaginous pyramid is essential to allow repositioning of the pyramid. If incomplete, a deviation of the pyramid may recur due to contraction of the skin in the healing phase.

- *Bilateral Paramedian Osteotomies*
  Bilateral paramedian osteotomies are made first using the intraseptal approach (▶ Fig. 6.4).
- *Bilateral Lateral Osteotomies*
  Then bilateral lateral osteotomies (with unilateral or bilateral wedge resections, if required) are performed. They are usually carried out by the endonasal route. Some surgeons prefer the external transcutaneous approach, while in special cases, the sublabial approach may be used.
- *Bilateral Transverse Osteotomies*
  Bilateral transverse osteotomies complete the osteotomies. They are made using the approach for the lateral osteotomy or by the external transcutaneous approach.
- *Mobilizing the Bony Pyramid*
  When all required osteotomies have been performed, the pyramid will be mobile. Its walls can be moved in all directions and adjusted as required. If not, one or two of the osteotomies (usually the transverse ones) are incomplete and should be redone.
- *Repositioning and Fixation of the Bony Pyramid*
  The bony pyramid is remodeled and repositioned as required. As the next step, the cartilaginous pyramid and the septum are adjusted to the new bony pyramid. As the last step, the septum and pyramid are fixed in their new position.

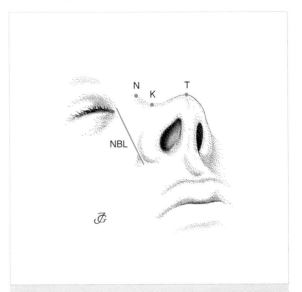

Fig. 6.1 Outlining the osteotomy. The main landmarks are marked on the skin for reference: nasion (N), K area (K), tip (T), and nasal base line (NBL).

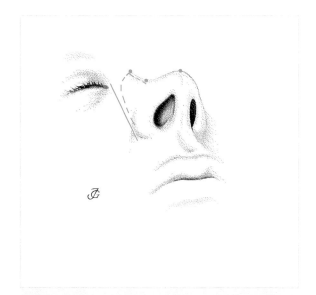

Fig. 6.2 Outlining the osteotomy. The planned osteotomies are marked on the skin.

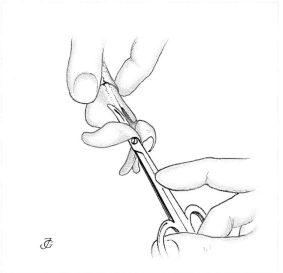

Fig. 6.3 Undermining the skin of the pyramid (dorsal tunnel) by bilateral IC incisions.

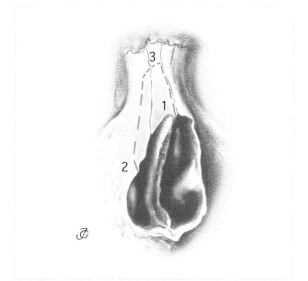

Fig. 6.4 Paramedian (1), lateral (2), and transverse (3) osteotomy.

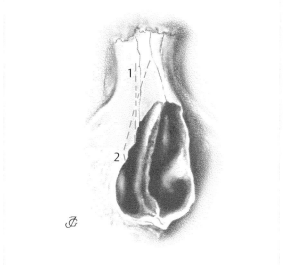

Fig. 6.5 Intermediate (1) and oblique (2) osteotomy.

6.1.2 Types of Osteotomy

Mobilizing and repositioning of the pyramid requires complete mobilization of the septum (see Chapter 5, page 161) and of the bony pyramid by a series of osteotomies. The following types of osteotomy may be distinguished (► Fig. 6.4 and ► Fig. 6.5):
1. Paramedian (or "medial") osteotomy
2. Lateral osteotomy
3. Transverse osteotomy
4. Intermediate osteotomy
5. Oblique osteotomy

The choice of osteotomies to be applied in a certain case depends on the pathology and the goals of the operation. The most common procedure is to combine two (intraseptal) paramedian osteotomies with two (endonasal) lateral osteotomies and transverse osteotomies.

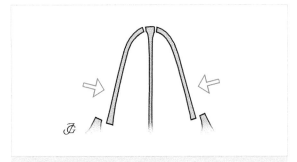

Fig. 6.6 Bilateral infracture.

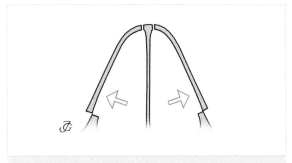

Fig. 6.7 Bilateral outfracture.

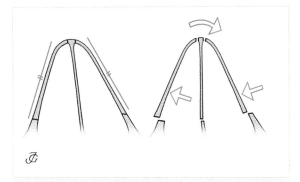

Fig. 6.8 Rotation by unilateral infracture, and outfracture on the opposite side. The lateral osteotomy on the long, shallow side of the bony pyramid is made somewhat higher than the one on the short, steep side.

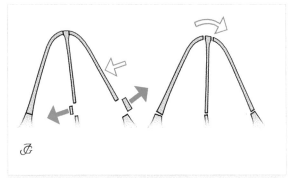

Fig. 6.9 Rotation following osteotomies and resection of a bony wedge at the base of the long side of the pyramid.

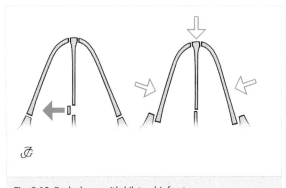

Fig. 6.10 Push-down with bilateral infracture.

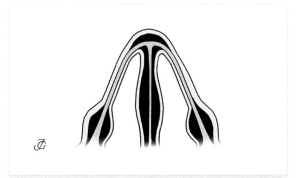

Fig. 6.11 Septal tunnels for intraseptal paramedian osteotomies; external and internal subperiosteal tunnels for wedge resections; undermining of the skin over the dorsum to allow repositioning.

6.1.3 Repositioning the Bony Pyramid

After the bony pyramid and the septum have been mobilized, the bony pyramid is repositioned. The following maneuvers may be carried out (▶ Fig. 6.6, ▶ Fig. 6.7, ▶ Fig. 6.8, ▶ Fig. 6.9, ▶ Fig. 6.10, ▶ Fig. 6.11, ▶ Fig. 6.12, and ▶ Fig. 6.13):

1. Bilateral infracture
2. Bilateral outfracture
3. Rotation by unilateral infracture and outfracture on the opposite side
4. Rotation following unilateral wedge resection
5. Push-down with bilateral infracture
6. Let-down following bilateral wedge resection
7. Push-up

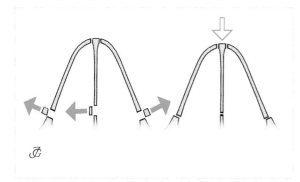

Fig. 6.12 Let-down following osteotomies and bilateral wedge resection.

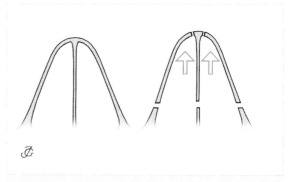

Fig. 6.13 Push-up of the bony pyramid.

Bilateral Infracture

Both lateral walls of the bony pyramid are moved inward (medially). The pyramid is thereby narrowed (▶ Fig. 6.6). Since the triangular cartilages are firmly attached to the nasal bones, the cartilaginous pyramid, and with it the valve area, will be narrowed as well.

Bilateral infracture requires paramedian, lateral (or oblique), and transverse osteotomies on both sides.

The level of the lateral osteotomies is very important. They are generally performed about 1 to 2 mm above the NBL. In patients with a broad and low pyramid, they are usually somewhat lower. When a lateral osteotomy is done too high (too ventral), a visible and palpable "step" in the lateral bony wall may result.

When much infracture is required, the mucoperichondrium on the inside of the bony pyramid may be elevated (inner tunnel) to allow more inward displacement of the bone (see ▶ Fig. 6.11).

An external stent is applied with some pressure to keep the nasal bones in their new position. Endonasally, a limited amount of internal dressing is applied to avoid outward movement of the infractured bones by postoperative swelling.

Bilateral Outfracture

The lateral walls of the bony pyramid are moved outward (laterally), thus widening the pyramid and the valve area (▶ Fig. 6.7). Bilateral outfracturing requires complete paramedian, lateral, and transverse osteotomies on both sides. It may be performed to widen a narrow pyramid. Generally, however, the let-down procedure (see following text) is preferred in these cases. As previously noted, the lateral osteotomy should be done low to avoid a postoperative "step." The bony pyramid is carefully stabilized in its new position by internal dressings. An external stent is applied without pressure.

Rotation by Unilateral Infracture and Outfracture on the Opposite Side

The bony wall is infractured on one side and outfractured on the opposite side (▶ Fig. 6.8). The bony pyramid is thereby rotated. This can only be accomplished successfully when the pyramid is fully mobilized by performing bilateral paramedian, lateral, and transverse osteotomies, and mobilizing the septum. The pyramid is rotated in cases with an asymmetrically deviated pyramid. The long, shallow side is infractured, whereas the short, steep side is moved outward. The lateral osteotomy on the longer side is performed somewhat higher than on the short side. The distance between both osteotomies and the dorsum should be symmetrical so that the new lateral walls are equally high. To preserve the result, it is crucial to fix the bony walls and the septum in their new position.

Rotation by Unilateral Wedge Resection

Following mobilization of the bony pyramid and the septum, a wedge of bone is resected at the base of the long side of the bony pyramid. The pyramid is then rotated toward this side (▶ Fig. 6.9). This method is used in patients with a severely deviated bony pyramid. It was described as early as 1907 by Joseph. The technique of wedge resection is discussed on page 227 and illustrated in ▶ Fig. 6.40, ▶ Fig. 6.41, ▶ Fig. 6.42, ▶ Fig. 6.43, ▶ Fig. 6.44, ▶ Fig. 6.45, ▶ Fig. 6.46, ▶ Fig. 6.47, ▶ Fig. 6.48, ▶ Fig. 6.49, ▶ Fig. 6.50, ▶ Fig. 6.51, and ▶ Fig. 6.52. To stabilize the bony pyramid and the septum in their new position, internal dressings, external taping, and splinting are applied with special care.

Push-Down with Bilateral Infracture

The bony pyramid is pushed down and bilaterally infractured. The projection of the nasal dorsum is reduced, and the pyramid is narrowed (▶ Fig. 6.10). The technique requires resection of a basal horizontal and a posterior vertical strip from the septum in combination with bilateral paramedian, lateral, and transverse osteotomies. We recommend elevating the mucoperiosteum on the inner side of the nasal bones (internal tunnel) to accommodate the infractured and pushed-down nasal bones (▶ Fig. 6.11). This method, introduced by Cottle (1954), may be used in patients with a prominent pyramid and a slight bony hump. Although elegant and conservative in comparison with other methods of hump removal, the technique has two disadvantages. First, it leads to narrowing of the pyramid and the valve area. In patients with a prominent pyramid, this is usually contraindicated, as their external nose and valve area are already narrow. Second, the ultimate effect of a push-down is usually less than expected. In patients with a prominent, narrow nasal pyramid and hump, bilateral wedge resection followed by let-down of the pyramid is usually the best choice.

Let-Down following Bilateral Wedge Resection

The bony pyramid is let down after performing osteotomies and bilateral resection of a wedge at its base (▶ Fig. 6.12). The let-down technique requires resection of both a basal horizontal and a posterior vertical strip from the septum. For a detailed description of the technique, see page 227. This method allows lowering of the bony pyramid without concomitant narrowing. It is therefore the technique of choice in patients with a narrow and prominent nasal pyramid with or without a bony and/or cartilaginous hump. The method was described by us in 1975.

Push-Up

In patients with a low pyramid or saddle nose, a push-up of the bony pyramid may be attempted (▶ Fig. 6.13). However, it is difficult to bring the nasal bones upward and keep them in a more ventral position. External fixation is the only effective means to preserve a push-up of the pyramid.

6.1.4 Instruments Used for Osteotomies

Over the last century, diverse instruments have been developed to perform osteotomies. At first, a saw was used, followed by various types of chisels and osteotomes. Nowadays, most surgeons prefer to use chisels. There is no consensus on which type of chisel is the best; choice is based largely on personal preference.

Saw

In the early era of nasal surgery, lateral osteotomies were performed with a saw. For many decades, the Joseph saw was the most commonly used instrument. In the 1950s, Cottle introduced a greatly improved design with a hand grip and a changeable band saw (see Chapter 10).

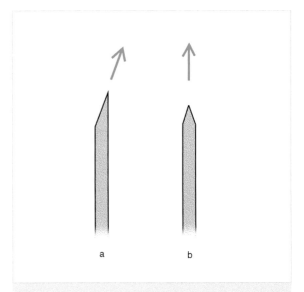

Fig. 6.14 Chisel and osteotome. (a) A chisel has a sloping side or bevel, and a flat side. It deviates slightly toward the flat side while proceeding. (b) An osteotome has two equally sloping sides. It proceeds forward in a straight line.

However, there are several disadvantages to using a saw. The main ones are laceration of the endonasal mucoperiosteum, and production of bone dust. The saw has therefore generally been abandoned in favor of the chisel.

Osteotome

An osteotome has two identically sloping sides. It therefore proceeds forward in a straight line (▶ Fig. 6.14). For this reason, an osteotome may be preferred for certain purposes.

Chisel-Osteotome

A chisel-osteotome combines the features of both the chisel and the osteotome (▶ Fig. 6.14).

Chisel

The chisel is nowadays the preferred instrument for performing osteotomies. It is a reliable and precise tool that can be used for all types of bone cut. Another advantage is that a chisel can easily be sharpened. It is used in septal surgery as well as for osteotomies of the bony pyramid. A chisel has a sloping side (the bevel) and a flat side. Accordingly, the two sides meet a different amount of resistance while proceeding. A chisel will therefore deviate slightly toward its flat side (▶ Fig. 6.14). Consequently, all types of straight and curved bone cut can be made. When the bevel is facing up, the bone cut will be convex; when the bevel is facing down, it will be convex.

Various types of chisel have been developed. They vary in width, curvature, and thickness. Some have sharp edges, while others have rounded or protected edges. Nowadays,

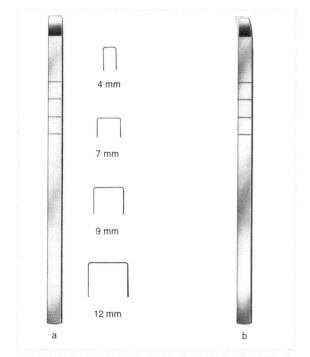

Fig. 6.15 Chisels according to Cottle: 4-mm, 7-mm, 9-mm, and 12-mm straight chisels **(a)** and 6-mm curved chisel **(b)**.

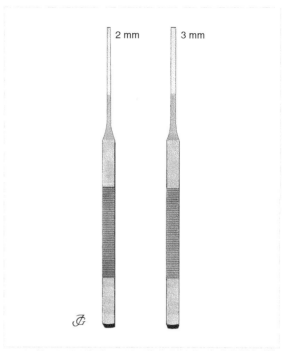

Fig. 6.16 Micro-osteotomes according to Tardy.

Cottle chisels and Tardy micro-osteotomes are the most popular. For beginners, the guided chisel, as advocated by Masing, may be a good alternative for performing lateral osteotomies.

Cottle chisels are available as 4-mm, 7-mm, 9-mm, and 12-mm straight chisels, and as a 7-mm curved chisel (► Fig. 6.15). We have a preference for these chisels, as they are universal and can be used intraseptally as well as for osteotomies and hump resection.

The 4-mm and the 7-mm chisel are used for resecting crests and spurs, as well as for making cuts into the vomer and the perpendicular plate. The curved 6-mm chisel is used to make a vertical cut into the perpendicular plate to resect a bony plate for transplantation.

The 7-mm straight chisel is the instrument of choice for paramedian and lateral osteotomies, as well as for wedge resections. By choosing between "bevel up" and "bevel down," the bone cut can be made along the required course.

The curved 6-mm chisel is used for transverse osteotomies, while the 9-mm and 12-mm chisels are taken for hump resection. It is advisable to sharpen the chisels from time to time on a whetstone.

A disadvantage of Cottle chisels is that beginners may find them somewhat difficult to guide. Their sharp edges may be another drawback for the beginner.

Micro-osteotomes, as introduced by Tardy (1984), are excellent instruments for performing transcutaneous lateral and transverse osteotomies (► Fig. 6.16). They are heavier than other chisels. In experienced hands, they are safe and effective for performing endonasal and external lateral osteotomies, and external transverse osteotomies. It has been claimed that micro-osteotomes produce less trauma to the soft tissues. Indeed, compared with the wider Cottle chisels, they require a smaller incision or, according to some, no incision at all. However, they cut through the periosteum as no subperiosteal tunnels are made. Moreover, when used externally, they leave a small visible scar.

Curved (guided) protected chisels can only be used for lateral osteotomies. One is needed for the left side and one for the right side (► Fig. 6.17**a**, **b**). These chisels are not our choice as they produce a "programmed" bone cut.

Double-protected osteotomes have been advocated for hump removal. Supposedly, they are less risky to the dorsal skin than chisels with sharp edges, such as the Cottle chisels (► Fig. 6.17**c**). However, since the skin over the dorsum is widely undermined, there is, in our opinion, no need for a special osteotome.

Mallet—The Technique of Tapping

The important role of the type of mallet and the tapping technique in performing osteotomies is often ignored. The mallet should be heavy and flat. We suggest using a Cottle-type mallet with a flat and a rounded side. The flat end is used for performing bone cuts; the rounded end to crush bone and cartilage in a crusher. The impetus of the tap should not come from the hand or forearm of the assistant, but the weight of the mallet. Ideally, the impact is made by a movement of the wrist (► Fig. 6.18). The

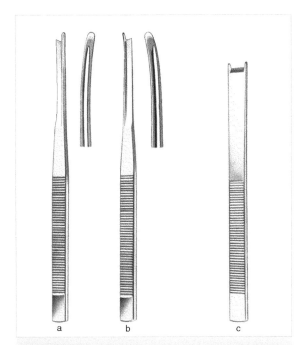

Fig. 6.17 Guided, unilaterally protected chisels for a left (a) and a right (b) lateral osteotomy. Double-protected osteotome for hump removal (c).

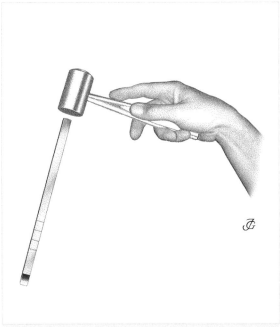

Fig. 6.18 The back of the chisel is hit at a perpendicular angle with a loose wrist using the double-tap technique.

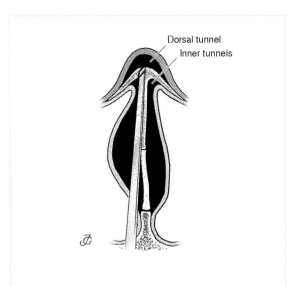

Dorsal tunnel
Inner tunnels

Fig. 6.19 Intraseptal paramedian osteotomy. The skin over the dorsum is undermined (dorsal tunnel); bilateral superior septal tunnels are elevated and extended up to the undersurface of the nasal bones (inner tunnels). A 7-mm straight chisel is introduced intraseptally with the bevel laterally and the flat side against the septal cartilage.

back end of the chisel should be struck at a perpendicular angle. A Teflon coating on the flat end of the mallet may help prevent slipping. A double-tap technique is used in an osteotomy. First, a light tap is made for listening. The sound tells whether the end of the chisel is in thick or thin bone, or in soft tissue. The second tap is somewhat heavier and is intended for "working." The assistant should wait for an okay from the surgeon before delivering the next sequence of two taps.

6.1.5 Techniques of Osteotomy

Paramedian ("Medial") Osteotomy

Paramedian (or "medial") osteotomies separate the nasal bones from each other as well as from the septum. Usually, two paramedian osteotomies are made, one on each side of the septum. These two cuts are thus not exactly in the midline but somewhat paramedian, hence the name. In daily practice, however, the term *medial osteotomy* is more common. The nasal bones are separated at the internasal suture. In a sense, paramedian osteotomies are therefore fibrotomies rather than osteotomies.

Steps

• The skin overlying the pyramid is undermined. Septal tunnels are bilaterally extended up to the undersurface of the nasal bones with the blunt end of a Cottle elevator.
• A straight 7-mm chisel is introduced intraseptally with the flat side on the septum and the bevel laterally (▶ Fig. 6.19).

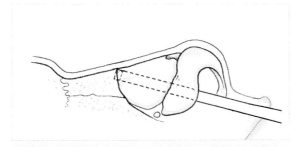

Fig. 6.20 Paramedian ("medial") osteotomy; intraseptal approach. The upper edge of a 7-mm straight Cottle chisel is positioned intraseptally underneath the lower margin of the nasal bones, while its end is pressed against the upper lip. The flat side of the chisel is directed toward the septum; its bevel is directed laterally.

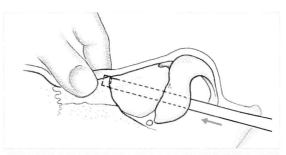

Fig. 6.21 Paramedian ("medial") osteotomy; intraseptal approach. When the mallet hits the chisel, the skin of the dorsum is lifted by the thumb and index finger of the left hand.

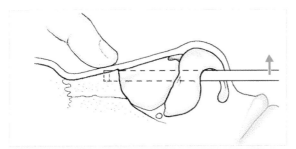

Fig. 6.22 Paramedian ("medial") osteotomy; intraseptal approach. As soon as the edge of the chisel has gone through the bone and can be palpated through the skin, the handle is moved upward.

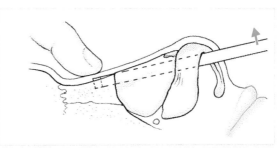

Fig. 6.23 Paramedian ("medial") osteotomy; intraseptal approach. The osteotomy is continued, with the chisel parallel to the bony dorsum. Care is taken to keep about 2 mm of the chisel outside the bony pyramid.

- The upper edge of the chisel is positioned at the caudal margin of the bony pyramid or slightly more cranial to preserve the K area. The lower end of the chisel is pressed down on the upper lip (▶ Fig. 6.20). The osteotomy is now started using the double-tap technique described above.
- While the assistant taps, the surgeon lifts the skin of the dorsum with the thumb and index finger of the left hand to protect it from damage (▶ Fig. 6.21).
- During the pause between each double tap, the position of the upper edge of the chisel is checked. As soon as the upper edge of the chisel can be palpated through the skin, the lower end of the chisel is lifted upward (▶ Fig. 6.22).
- The osteotomy is then continued with the chisel parallel to the nasal dorsum with its upper edge 1 to 2 mm above the level of the bone (▶ Fig. 6.23).
- The osteotomy is continued up above the line marking the planned transverse osteotomies to ensure complete mobilization (▶ Fig. 6.24). It has often been advised to terminate the paramedian osteotomy as soon as a change to a higher pitch is heard when the chisel is hit. The higher pitch indicates that the chisel has entered the more solid bone of the nasal spine of the frontal

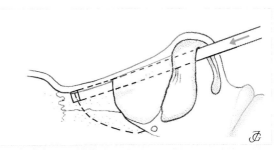

Fig. 6.24 Paramedian ("medial") osteotomy; intraseptal approach. The osteotomy is continued just beyond the marks for the transverse osteotomies.

bone. This characteristic change of pitch usually comes "too early." We therefore suggest using the marks for the transverse osteotomies on the skin as guide.
- After the osteotomy has been completed, the chisel is moved somewhat laterally to open up the cut, and can then be removed easily.
- The same procedure is repeated on the other side. It should be kept in mind that the chisel tends to follow the previous cut. The second paramedian osteotomy should therefore be performed with less force.

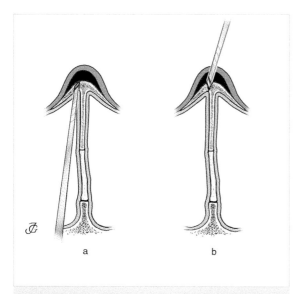

Fig. 6.25 Paramedian osteotomy—alternative approaches. (a) Endonasal–transmucosal route. (b) From above through an IC incision.

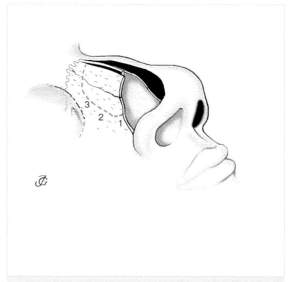

Fig. 6.26 Lateral osteotomy. In the first millimeters (1), the chisel is directed somewhat downward to avoid too much narrowing of the valve area when the bony pyramid is infractured. The second, more horizontal part (2) of the osteotomy is performed with the bevel of the chisel up to make a relatively low bone cut. Halfway through the osteotomy, the chisel is turned 180° with the bevel down to guide it slightly upward (3).

Alternative Approaches

In special cases, the paramedian osteotomies may be made using a different approach: endonasally–transmucosally, or from above through an IC incision.

These techniques are suitable when no surgery of the septum is performed. This may be the case when the septum is normal or when reopening the septum is hazardous. Paramedian osteotomies may then be performed endonasally through the mucosa of the roof of the nasal cavity (▶ Fig. 6.25a). Another option is to separate the nasal bones from above through an IC incision (▶ Fig. 6.25b). In both techniques, the inner mucoperiosteal lining of the nasal pyramid is cut through.

Lateral Osteotomy

A lateral osteotomy separates the lateral bony walls of the pyramid from the nasal process of the maxilla. A cut is made into the bone above and more or less parallel to the NBL. The level of the osteotomy above the NBL depends upon the pathology and the surgical goals. Lateral osteotomies are almost always carried out bilaterally. An exception may be made in patients with an impression of one bony wall due to a recent injury. A unilateral lateral osteotomy may then suffice.

There are several ways to perform a lateral osteotomy. The most commonly used techniques are:
1. Endonasal subperiosteal through a vestibular incision
2. Endonasal transperiosteal through a vestibular incision
3. External transcutaneous
4. Sublabial

We prefer the endonasal–subperiosteal approach, as it avoids periosteal (and mucosal) damage and allows wedge resection under direct view (▶ Fig. 6.26).

Endonasal Subperiosteal Technique

Steps

• A vestibular incision is made with a No. 15 blade. Only the skin is incised to avoid bleeding from a superficially running branch of the angular artery. The incision should be long enough to accommodate the chisel to be used.
• The loose subcutaneous tissue is gently spread in the direction of the incision with blunt, slightly curved scissors. The lower margin of the bony pyramid is palpated.
• An external subperiosteal tunnel is now elevated with the long end of a McKenty elevator. The tunnel is continued up to the marks for the transverse osteotomy. Care is taken not to damage the medial canthal ligament. The tunnel is made wide enough to accommodate the chisel.

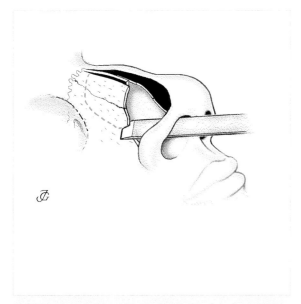

Fig. 6.27 Lateral osteotomy. The beginning of the bone cut is directed downward. The bevel of the chisel is up.

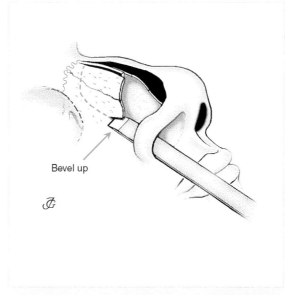

Fig. 6.28 Lateral osteotomy. The osteotomy is continued more or less parallel to the NBL. The bevel of the chisel is up.

- An internal submucoperiosteal tunnel may be elevated as well. This will prevent the inner mucoperichondrium from laceration, and help accommodate the bony wall when it is fractured inward. Moreover, an internal tunnel is mandatory to allow wedge resection.
- A straight 7-mm chisel is introduced using the McKenty elevator as a guide.
- The chisel is positioned with the bevel facing up at the caudal margin of the bony pyramid. The osteotomy is started relatively high. In particular, this is necessary in patients with a prominent-narrow pyramid, as a low osteotomy followed by infracture may narrow the valve area too much (▶ Fig. 6.27).
- The osteotomy is performed using the double-tap technique. The right hand directs the chisel, while the tip of the index finger of the left hand checks its position in relation to the line marked on the skin.
- The first part of the lateral osteotomy is usually carried out with the bevel of the chisel facing up to force the chisel down (▶ Fig. 6.28 and ▶ Fig. 6.29). The second part is started with the bevel up. Halfway, the chisel is turned 180°. With the bevel down, the chisel will turn slightly upward while making the cut (▶ Fig. 6.30).
- Some 3 to 4 mm of the width of the chisel is kept outside the bone to prevent damage to the inner mucosa as much as possible.
- The osteotomy is continued to the level where the transverse osteotomy should start (▶ Fig. 6.31).
- The lateral wall of the bony pyramid is now fractured slightly inward to facilitate correct positioning of the curved chisel for the transverse osteotomy.

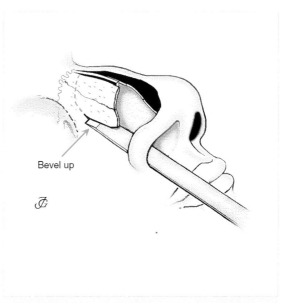

Fig. 6.29 Lateral osteotomy. The bone cut is continued with the bevel up.

Endonasal Transperiosteal Technique

The osteotomy is carried out endonasally by a micro-osteotome. A 2-mm (or stab) incision is made in the vestibular skin at the caudal margin of the piriform aperture. There is no need to spread the tissues nor to elevate the periosteum. The bone is cut together with the periosteum (▶ Fig. 6.32).

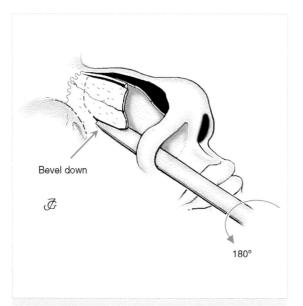

Fig. 6.30 Lateral osteotomy. The chisel is rotated with the bevel down to make a bone cut that is curved slightly upwards.

Bevel down

180°

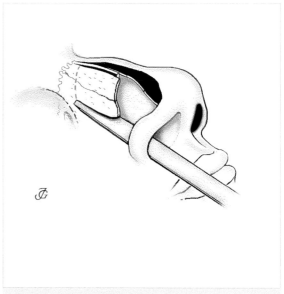

Fig. 6.31 Lateral osteotomy completed.

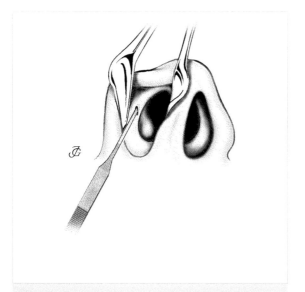

Fig. 6.32 Endonasal transperiosteal lateral osteotomy.

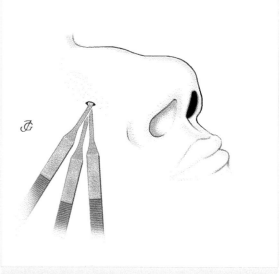

Fig. 6.33 External transcutaneous lateral osteotomy using a micro-osteotome.

External Transcutaneous Technique

The osteotomy is made through the skin and the periosteum with a micro-osteotome through a small (stab) incision (▶ Fig. 6.33 and ▶ Fig. 6.34).

Sublabial Approach

The bony pyramid is approached by the sublabial route through a 1 cm labiogingival incision (▶ Fig. 6.35) (see also Chapter 4, page 147). The periosteum is elevated,

and the osteotomy is performed as described. We take this approach when the lateral osteotomies have to be made very low, for example in patients with a very broad and low pyramid. The method may also be used when there is a risk of too much scarring and stenosis of the vestibule.

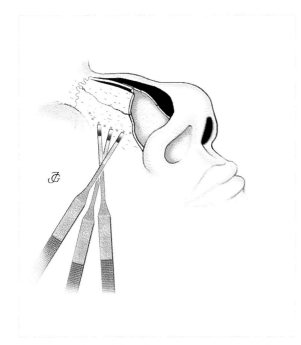

Fig. 6.34 Multiple bone punctures are made transcutaneously.

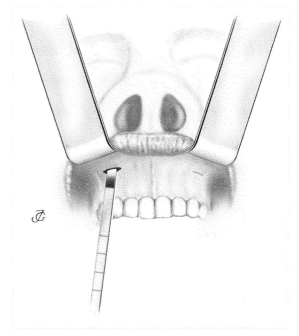

Fig. 6.35 Lateral (and transverse) osteotomy through the sublabial approach.

Transverse Osteotomy

A transverse osteotomy separates the bony pyramid from the frontal bone and the nasal spine of the frontal bone. This osteotomy is usually made at a level just below the nasion (depth of nasofrontal angle). It is technically the most difficult of the three main osteotomies, as the massive frontal nasal spine has to be completely cut through to obtain full mobilization of the bony pyramid.

Two different methods are used:
1. Endonasal subperiosteal technique
2. External transcutaneous technique

Endonasal Subperiosteal Technique

Steps

- This method uses the approach made for the endonasal subperiosteal lateral osteotomy through a vestibular incision and a subperiosteal paranasal tunnel.
- After the lateral osteotomy has been completed, a 6-mm curved chisel is introduced (▶ Fig. 6.36).
- The lower edge of the curved chisel is positioned at the upper end of the lateral osteotomy. The handle of the chisel is then moved as far laterally as possible (▶ Fig. 6.37).
- While the assistant hits the chisel, the surgeon combines two movements—a dorsal–ventral and a lateral–medial maneuver—to obtain a transverse–oblique cut through the root of the bony pyramid.
- The chisel is directed by the right hand while the thumb of the left hand keeps the end of the chisel in its position (▶ Fig. 6.38).

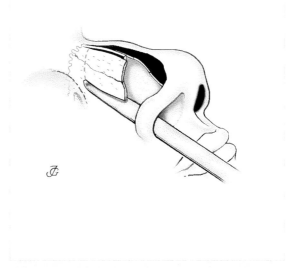

Fig. 6.36 Transverse osteotomy using a curved 6-mm chisel.

- It is better to not complete the first transverse osteotomy until the lateral osteotomy on the other side has been made. In this way, an undesired fracture line on the opposite side is avoided.
- Complete mobility of the bony pyramid is required for effective repositioning. The transverse osteotomy may have to be redone before the strong connection with the frontal bone is completely cut through.

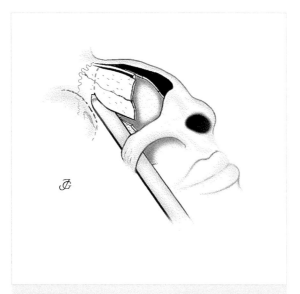

Fig. 6.37 The chisel is moved as far laterally as possible to cut from below and laterally.

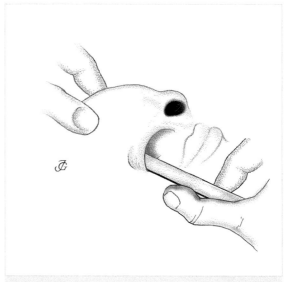

Fig. 6.38 The thumb of the left hand keeps the chisel in position.

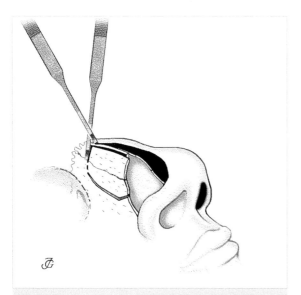

Fig. 6.39 External transcutaneous transverse osteotomy from above with a 2-mm micro-osteotome.

External Transcutaneous Technique

Steps

- A stab incision is made in the skin at a horizontal wrinkle in the depth of the frontonasal angle.
- Transverse osteotomies are performed from above with a micro-osteotome on the left and right side. The procedure is repeated until complete mobility of the bony pyramid is obtained (▶ Fig. 6.39).

Subperiosteal or Transperiosteal Osteotomies?

There are two schools of thought regarding how to perform lateral and transverse osteotomies.

The "subperiosteal school" chooses to not damage the periosteum. Its exponents claim that a subperiosteal osteotomy causes less bleeding, less chance of postoperative neuralgia, and less callus formation and new growth of bone.

The "transperiosteal school," on the other hand, argues that a transperiosteal bone cut involves less trauma to the adjacent soft tissues, as it is performed with a micro-osteotome. This technique does not require a "wide" incision, spreading of soft tissues, or subperiosteal undertunneling. In this way, bleeding and postoperative swelling will be less.

We find it difficult to take an explicit stand in this matter. We regard it as a matter of personal preference, since both methods yield excellent results when performed with care. It might be argued, however, that the transperiosteal technique is preferred for modeling the pyramid in patients with minimal deformities and those requiring cosmetic surgery. The transperiosteal technique, on the other hand, might be the better choice in cases with more severe deformities.

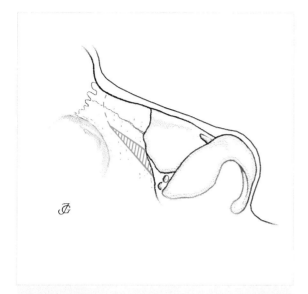

Fig. 6.40 Resection of a wedge at the base of the bony pyramid to rotate the pyramid (unilateral wedge resection), or let-down of the pyramid (bilateral wedge resection).

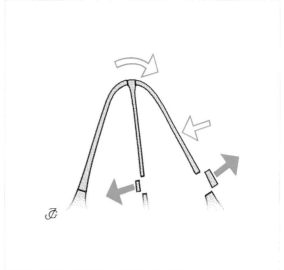

Fig. 6.41 Unilateral wedge resection and resection of septal strips to rotate the pyramid in cases with a severe deviation.

6.2 Wedge Resection

6.2.1 Principles

Resecting a unilateral or bilateral wedge of bone at the base of the bony pyramid is one of the basic procedures in modifying the nasal pyramid. Unilateral wedge resection at the base of the long side of a deviated pyramid allows rotation of the pyramid (▶ Fig. 6.40 and ▶ Fig. 6.41). Bilateral wedge resection is an effective method to lower or "let down" a prominent nasal pyramid (▶ Fig. 6.42). Both modifying procedures require complete osteotomies at the same time. They will also only be effective after complete mobilization of the septum with resection of a vertical and a horizontal septal strip (▶ Fig. 6.41 and ▶ Fig. 6.42).

Unilateral wedge resection may be performed to correct a severely deviated pyramid. The resection is carried out at the long, shallow side of the pyramid and is combined with a lateral osteotomy on the other side, bilateral paramedian and transverse osteotomies, and resection of strips from the septum. This allows rotation and medianization of a severely deviated pyramid. The method was described by Joseph as early as 1907. In spite of its logic, it was not often practiced. Reports have been scarce (e.g., Lautenschläger 1929, Fomon 1936, Huffmann and Lierle 1954, Sulsenti 1972). Nowadays, however, the technique is accepted as an effective means to address severe asymmetry of the bony pyramid (▶ Fig. 6.40 and ▶ Fig. 6.41).

Bilateral wedge resection was introduced in the 1970s as a nontraumatic method to reduce a prominent, narrow pyramid with a bony and cartilaginous hump (Huizing 1975). Bilateral resection of a wedge at the base of the pyramid, together with resection of a vertical and a

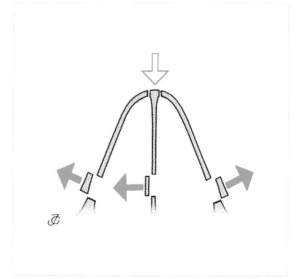

Fig. 6.42 Bilateral wedge resection and resection of septal strips to lower or let down the pyramid in cases with a bony and cartilaginous hump or a prominent, narrow pyramid.

horizontal strip from the septum and paramedian and transverse osteotomies allows let-down of the bony and cartilaginous dorsum (▶ Fig. 6.42, ▶ Fig. 6.43, and ▶ Fig. 6.44). This idea had already been put forward by Lothrop in 1914, but was rarely practiced. Today, the bilateral wedge resection technique is generally adopted as the method of choice to lower and broaden a prominent, narrow bony pyramid (▶ Fig. 6.45). Results in the long term are satisfying and complications are rare (Pirsig and Königs 1988).

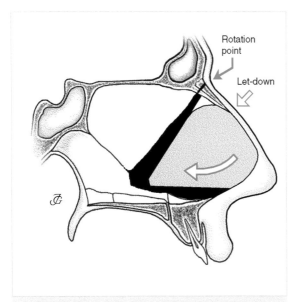

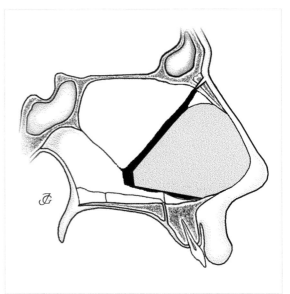

Fig. 6.43 A vertical and a basal horizontal strip are resected from the cartilaginous and bony septum to allow rotation of the pyramid in a dorsal direction around a pivot at the nasion.

Fig. 6.44 The pyramid is let down. The cartilaginous septum is rotated in a dorsal and caudal direction and positioned (fixed) on the premaxilla and maxillary crest. The dorsum is lowered and the hump is reduced.

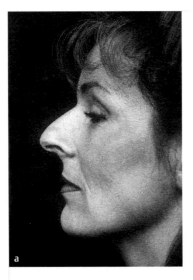

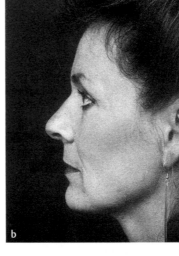

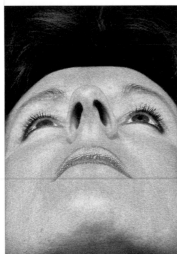

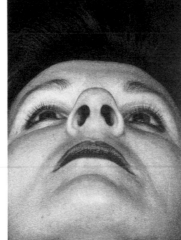

Fig. 6.45 Prominent, narrow pyramid ("tension nose") with a limited bony and cartilaginous hump and bilateral nasal obstruction due to a narrow valve area on both sides in combination with a moderate septal deformity. Before (**a, c**) and six months after (**b, d**) septal correction and let-down of the pyramid following bilateral wedge resection. Note the effect of the let-down on the bony and cartilaginous dorsum and the configuration of the lobule, nostrils, vestibules, and valve areas.
a, b Side view.
c, d Base view.

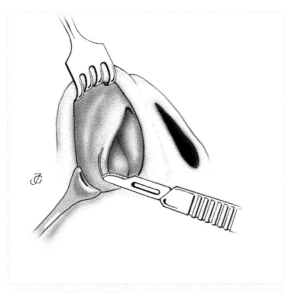

Fig. 6.46 A vestibular incision is made about 8 mm in length.

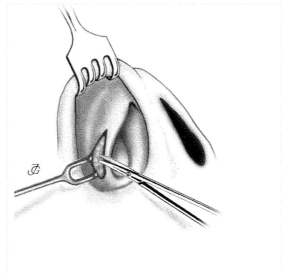

Fig. 6.47 The soft tissues are spread in a craniocaudal direction with blunt, slightly curved scissors.

Mobilization of the septum and resection of vertical and horizontal strips is an essential part of the technique of rotation and let-down of the pyramid by wedge resection. The septum must be fully mobilized. A vertical strip is taken from the anterior part of the perpendicular plate and a horizontal strip is resected from the base of the cartilaginous and bony septum to allow the necessary rotation and lowering of the dorsum (▶ Fig. 6.43 and ▶ Fig. 6.44).

6.2.2 Surgical Technique

The sequence of steps in unilateral and bilateral wedge resection is as follows:
1. Mobilization of the septum, resection of a vertical and a basal horizontal strip to allow the required rotation and/or let-down
2. Bilateral intraseptal paramedian osteotomies (may be omitted)
3. Unilateral or bilateral resection of a bony wedge at the base of the bony pyramid through vestibular incisions
4. Bilateral transverse osteotomies
5. Repositioning (rotation/let-down) of the pyramid
6. Adjustment of the septum to the new anatomy

Steps
- The cartilaginous septum is mobilized in the usual way. A posterior chondrotomy is made, and the septal base is dissected from its pedestal (see Chapter 5, page 166).
- A (more or less triangular) vertical strip of cartilage and bone is removed at the chondroperpendicular junction using a biting forceps.

- A horizontal strip is resected from the base of the cartilaginous septum and the vomer using angulated scissors and bone scissors or chisel, respectively (▶ Fig. 6.43). Initially, these strips should not be too large as we want to avoid a gap resulting at the septal base. An extra strip can always be resected later if required (see following text).
- The points and lines of reference (nasion, K area, tip, and NBL) and the lower margin of the bony pyramid are marked on the skin with surgical ink. The wedges to be resected are outlined. They are symmetrical when a let-down is planned, and may be asymmetrical when a let-down with some rotation is to be performed.
- Paramedial osteotomies are performed intraseptally in the standard way (see page 220).
- A vestibular incision is made (see Chapter 4). It should be of sufficient length (about 8 mm) to allow introduction of a narrow speculum (▶ Fig. 6.46).
- The subcutaneous tissues are spread with blunt, slightly curved scissors in a craniocaudal direction in line with the incision to avoid bleeding from the angular artery and to prevent unnecessary soft-tissue trauma (▶ Fig. 6.47).
- The caudal margin of the bony pyramid (frontal process of the maxilla) is identified and exposed with the sharp end of a Cottle elevator or with a McKenty elevator (▶ Fig. 6.48).
- The periosteum is incised with the elevator or a No. 64 Beaver knife. Subperiosteal tunnels are created both on the outside and the inside of the bony pyramid (▶ Fig. 6.49, ▶ Fig. 6.50, and ▶ Fig. 6.51).

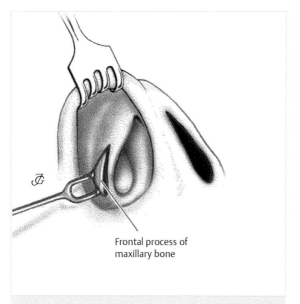

Fig. 6.48 The caudal margin of the bony pyramid (frontal process of maxilla) is exposed.

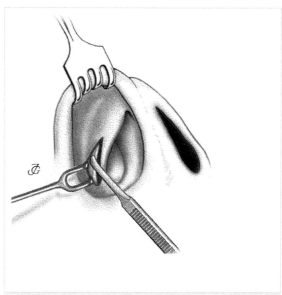

Fig. 6.49 An external subperiosteal tunnel is elevated using a McKenty elevator (or the sharp end of a Cottle elevator).

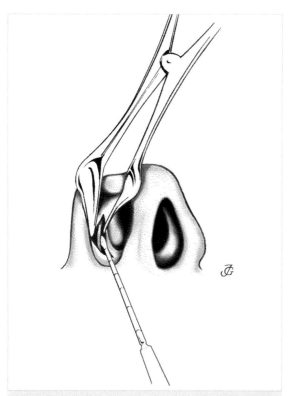

Fig. 6.50 An internal subperiosteal tunnel is elevated using the sharp end of a Cottle elevator.

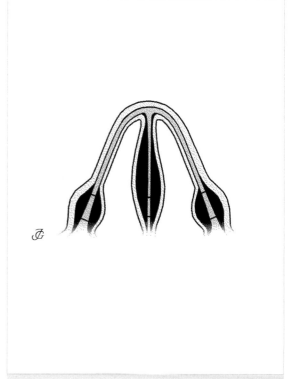

Fig. 6.51 External and internal subperiosteal tunnels are elevated to allow resection of wedges at the base of the pyramid bone under direct view.

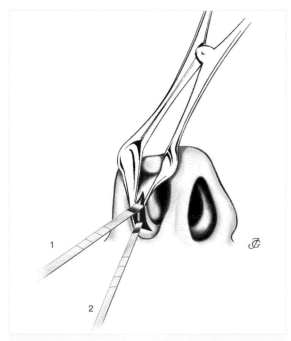

Fig. 6.52 Resection of the wedge. The upper (ventral) osteotomy (1) is made first, followed by the lower (dorsal) osteotomy (2).

- A narrow speculum of medium length is introduced. Any connective tissue fibers that are still in the way are pushed aside.
- The speculum is positioned with one blade on each side of the frontal process of the maxilla (▶ Fig. 6.52).
- The desired wedge is resected under direct view using a 7-mm or 4-mm chisel. The upper (most ventral) osteotomy is made first, the dorsal osteotomy second (▶ Fig. 6.52). In special cases, a parallel strip may be removed.
- To avoid fracturing of the wedge, it may be helpful to first make a small furrow in the external surface of the bone with a small saw. Another method to prevent accidental fracturing of the wedge is to make small perforations with the sharp edge of a narrow chisel.
- The wedges are taken out with a hemostat or a small forceps. They are inspected and compared. When desired, some extra bone can be removed with a narrow rasp.
- The defect is inspected. Care is taken that no loose bone fragments are left.
- Transverse osteotomies are carried out bilaterally.
- The bony pyramid can now be mobilized and repositioned:
  - *Rotation* is achieved by pushing the long, shallow side (where the wedge is resected) inward with the thumb, and intranasally lifting the short, steep side outward with the flat back end of a chisel.

- *Let-down* is accomplished by pushing down the bony cartilaginous pyramid and septum (in a dorsal direction) with a long angulated retractor (Aufricht type) introduced through the IC incision. If much pressure is required, an additional strip usually needs to be resected from the septal base (see following text).
  - The let-down may, if desired, be combined with some outfracture to broaden the bony pyramid and to widen the valve area.
- The septum is inspected again and adjusted to the new pyramidal height by additional resection of a basal and/or vertical strip, if necessary.
- After lowering of the bony and cartilaginous pyramid, the lobule may become too wide and the alae may be too convex. It may then be necessary to adjust the lobule to the new pyramid by bilateral resection of soft-tissue wedges from the alar base; it may also appear that the nose should be shortened (see following text).
- The pyramid and septum are fixed in their new position by internal and external dressings. The internal dressings support the bony and cartilaginous dorsum and fix the septum in the midline.

Adjusting the Lobule to the New Pyramid by Bilateral Resection of Soft-Tissue Wedges at the Alar Base

Lowering the bony and cartilaginous pyramid changes the configuration of the lobule. Its projection becomes less and its width increases. The nostrils widen and the alae become more convex. If these effects are too pronounced, we may have to bilaterally resect soft-tissue wedges from the alar base.

Steps

- The wedges to be resected are outlined on the skin.
- The lower incision is made first. Skin and subcutaneous tissues are incised with a No. 15 blade at the nasofacial and nasolabial groove, from superior to inferior. The incision is continued in the lateral wall of the vestibule. The outside and inside part of the incision are combined by cutting through the alar base. This will cause considerable bleeding, as a branch of the angular artery is severed. The bleeding is controlled by bipolar coagulation (▶ Fig. 6.53).
- The upper incision is made in a similar way: from superior to inferior and from outside to inside. The wedge is then removed (▶ Fig. 6.54**a**).
- Bleeding is controlled and the defect is closed by suturing the skin and subcutaneous tissue at the same time with a 5–0 monofilament nonresorbable suture (▶ Fig. 6.54**b**).
- Special attention is paid to the left–right symmetry of the procedure and its effect on the position of the alae.

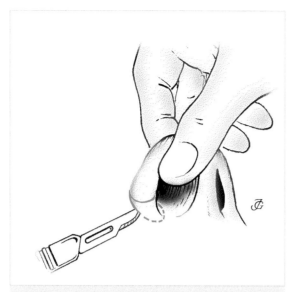

Fig. 6.53 A soft-tissue wedge is resected at the alar base to adjust the lobule to the new pyramid.

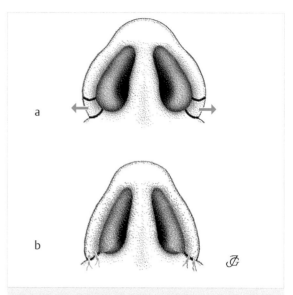

Fig. 6.54 The alar wedges are removed (a), and the defects are closed by suturing the skin and subcutaneous tissue at the same time with 5–0 monofilament nonresorbable sutures (b).

Shortening Nasal Length to Adjust the Lobule to the New Pyramid

Let-down of the pyramid reduces the prominence of both the bony and the cartilaginous pyramid; consequently, the nose will look longer. This may be a reason to shorten the nose, thereby re-establishing the original proportions. The nose may be shortened in the following ways:

1. Shortening of the septum by resection of a strip from its caudal end
2. Upward rotation of the tip by resection of small triangular strips from the upper margins of the lateral crura of the lobular cartilages by the inversion (retrograde) technique
3. Resection of small triangles of cartilage from the caudal margin of the triangular cartilages

For surgical techniques see Chapter 5, page 177 and Chapter 7, page 279.

6.2.3 Complications

Complications and adverse effects of wedge resections are relatively rare.

Asymmetries of the bony pyramid may occur if the resected wedges are unequal in size or shape. A deviating pyramid may then result.

Abnormal mobility of the pyramid may result when healing of the bony defect becomes fibrous instead of bony. To avoid this complication, special care is taken to bring the margins of the bony defect in good contact with each other during the let-down maneuver. It is also advisable to protect the let-down pyramid with a stent for a somewhat longer period of time than usual.

6.3 Hump Removal

Removal or reduction of a nasal hump is a common procedure in corrective aesthetic nasal surgery. Most patients who request hump reduction do so for aesthetic reasons. They dislike the prominence of their external nose and would prefer a straight nasal dorsum. Especially when the request comes from a young girl, some reserve on the part of the surgeon may be wise. It is well known that young people's taste often changes with age and experience.

Functional reasons for hump removal are relatively rare. Indications include posttraumatic and postsurgical irregularities when visible or palpable and when they cause discomfort (e.g., when using eyeglasses).

6.3.1 Types of Hump

Although the term *hump* could apply for any nasal convexity, it is most commonly used to indicate a convexity or prominence of the dorsum. A dorsal hump might be of genetic or traumatic origin, or both. It is important to distinguish various types, since humps of different origin may require a different surgical approach.

Humps may be classified as follows: bony; bony and cartilaginous; cartilaginous; part of the prominent-narrow pyramid syndrome; relative; and a localized irregularity. See also discussion on page 82 in Chapter 2.

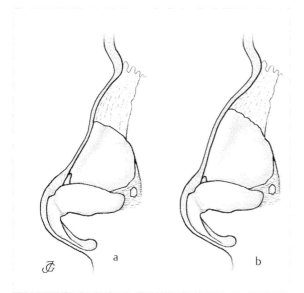

Fig. 6.55 Types of hump. (a) Bony hump. (b) Bony and cartilaginous hump.

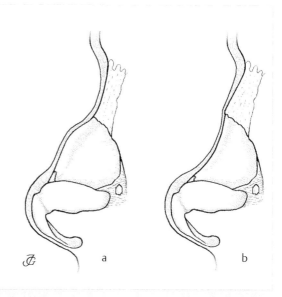

Fig. 6.56 Types of hump. (a) Cartilaginous hump. (b) Relative bony hump due to saddling of the cartilaginous pyramid.

Bony Hump

The bony dorsum is convex. Often this is of genetic origin. It is also frequently seen as a late effect of periosteal trauma due to previous trauma or surgery (▶ Fig. 6.55a; see also ▶ Fig. 2.48). A bony hump is either reduced with a rasp and file, or resected.

Bony and Cartilaginous Hump

Both the bony and cartilaginous dorsum are convex (▶ Fig. 6.55b; see also ▶ Fig. 2.47). This type of hump is the most common. Pronounced bony and cartilaginous humps are usually resected.

Cartilaginous Hump

The convexity is limited to the cartilaginous dorsum. This is more rare but may be seen after trauma and previous surgery (▶ Fig. 6.56a; see also ▶ Fig. 2.49). Resection is the only way to correct pronounced cartilaginous humps. In some cases with a limited convexity, they can be corrected by lowering the cartilaginous septum while keeping the dorsum intact.

Hump As Part of a Prominent-Narrow Pyramid Syndrome

A convexity of both the bony and cartilaginous dorsum is a common feature in patients with prominent-narrow pyramid syndrome (see ▶ Fig. 2.10, ▶ Fig. 2.11, and ▶ Fig. 2.12). This condition is described in detail in Chapter 2, page 69. Usually, this type of hump can be corrected by a let-down procedure, keeping the dorsum intact.

Relative Hump (Pseudohump)

The bony dorsum is prominent but its protrusion is relative. The hump is caused by sagging of the cartilaginous pyramid. Although the patient complains of a bony hump, nasal analysis reveals a relative or pseudohump. In most cases, it is the result of a defective septum due to trauma, septal abscess, or surgery without adequate septal reconstruction (▶ Fig. 6.56b; see also ▶ Fig. 2.50). The relative hump is corrected in the first place by reconstructing the septum. The dorsum is additionally augmented as required. The humped bony dorsum remains either untouched or is only slightly reduced with a rasp.

Localized Irregularity

Irregularities of the bony and cartilaginous dorsum may occur after trauma or previous surgery. They may be due to a periosteal reaction after trauma with spontaneous growth of bone, asymmetry of the nasal bones due to trauma, or inadequate surgical repositioning. Localized irregularities may also be due to a bony or cartilaginous sequester. Irregularities are corrected with a rasp or by resection.

6.3.2 Surgical Techniques

Humps may be removed or reduced in different ways. The most commonly used techniques are:
1. Reduction by rasp and file
2. Resection
3. Push-down with infracture of the pyramid
4. Let-down of the pyramid following bilateral wedge resection (see page 227).

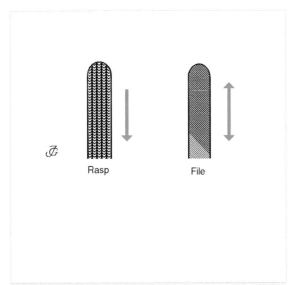

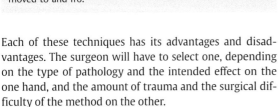

Fig. 6.57 Rasp to reduce a bony hump and file to smooth a raw bony surface. A rasp is only effective when pulled; a file can be moved to and fro.

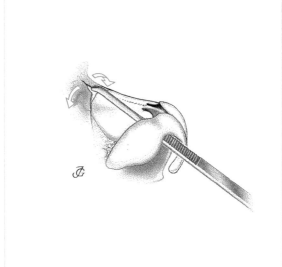

Fig. 6.58 The periosteum overlying the bony hump is incised in the midline, then scraped aside using a semi-sharp (McKenty or Cottle) elevator.

Each of these techniques has its advantages and disadvantages. The surgeon will have to select one, depending on the type of pathology and the intended effect on the one hand, and the amount of trauma and the surgical difficulty of the method on the other.

Instruments

Over the past century, a large number of instruments has been designed for hump resection. Various kinds of chisel, and osteotomes of different sizes and widths, protected and unprotected, have been proposed. Also saws, heavy scissors, strong biting forceps and special knives were developed enough to fill a small museum. The variety of instruments illustrates how the technique of hump resection has been a matter of great diversity among nasal surgeons.

Correcting a Bony Hump with Rasp and File

A bony hump may be reduced with a rasp and/or a file. This is performed through an intercartilaginous incision (or in special cases a caudal septal incision) with undermining of the dorsal skin. Only bony humps can be corrected with a rasp and a file as these instruments are not effective on cartilage. When using a rasp, one should realize that it will only take off bone when it is pulled; a file is effective in two directions (▶ Fig. 6.57). The technique of removing a bony hump with a rasp and file is relatively easy but rather traumatic. Rasping and filing will cause considerable damage to the periosteum over the bony dorsum. This may leave various minor and major undesired effects. Adhesions between the rough surface of the bone and the overlying thin skin, accompanied by atrophy and telangiectasias, are relatively frequent sequelae. Small irregularities are also rather common. They may lead to tenderness upon touching as well as to spontaneous pain sensations. Spontaneous growth of bone is another late complication. These adverse effects can be avoided to some extent by scraping the periosteum laterally before rasping, carefully smoothing and cleansing the rasped area, and reinforcing the skin with an underlay of connective tissue or well crushed autogeneic septal cartilage.

Because of the disadvantages mentioned above, it is better to restrict the use of the rasp and file as much as possible. We only use this technique for removing irregularities and for smoothing an (open) bony dorsum after hump resection or osteotomies.

Steps

- The hump to be reduced is outlined on the skin with surgical ink.
- The skin of the nasal dorsum is undermined through bilateral IC incisions (see ▶ Fig. 6.3). In cases with a medially localized small hump or irregularity, the caudal septal incision may be used.
- The skin is undermined with blunt, slightly curved scissors. The loose connective tissue plane is dissected as close to the perichondrium and periosteum as possible to preserve the overlying skin, which is usually thin.
- The periosteum over the hump is incised in a vertical direction and then scraped aside with a sharp elevator (sharp end of a Cottle elevator or a McKenty elevator) to prevent damage to the periosteum as much as possible (▶ Fig. 6.58).

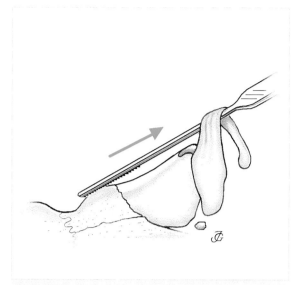

Fig. 6.59 The bony hump is reduced by pulling movements with a rasp.

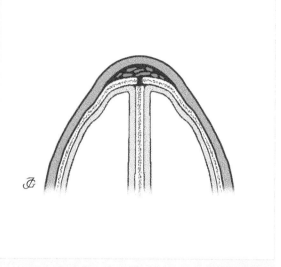

Fig. 6.60 Crushed cartilage or a sheet of connective tissue is inserted as an underlay. It is placed over the area where the hump has been removed to reinforce the dorsal skin and prevent adherence of the skin to the bony dorsum.

- The hump is reduced by pulling movements of the rasp (▶ Fig. 6.59).
- When sufficient lowering has been obtained, the raw surface is smoothed with a file.
- All bone dust is carefully removed by suction. The dorsum is carefully palpated to detect any irregularity that might also have to be removed.
- The lateralized periosteal flaps are swept back over the new dorsum by small movements from lateral to medial with the elevator.
- A limited underlay of crushed septal cartilage or a small sheet of compressed connective tissue may be inserted over the area to support the overlying skin and prevent adhesion (▶ Fig. 6.60).
- The dorsum is carefully taped.

Resecting a Bony and/or Cartilaginous Hump

Resection is the most common way to correct a bony and/or cartilaginous hump. The method was introduced by Joseph and others around 1900. In spite of the obvious disadvantages of the technique, it is still the most usual way of dealing with a bony and a cartilaginous hump. However, because of the drawbacks, several methods have been developed to diminish the unavoidable trauma to the bony and cartilaginous pyramid by hump resection. The first method is to close the open bony and cartilaginous roof after mobilizing the pyramid by performing osteotomies. Additionally, the dorsum is reinforced by inserting an underlay of connective tissue or crushed septal cartilage. Another option is to close the open roof with

a bony or cartilaginous transplant made from the removed hump. More recently, Jost has advocated elevating the mucoperiosteum of the inner surface of the nasal bones in a lateral direction. In this way, the mucosal lining is preserved when the hump is cut off.

Removal of the Hump in One Piece or in Parts?

We suggest resecting the bony part of the hump first and then the cartilaginous part. The bony part is resected with a chisel. This is followed by smoothing the defect with a rasp. The cartilaginous hump is then reduced step by step using small, straight or angulated scissors and/or a small knife (No. 64 Beaver knife or No. 15 blade). According to our experience, the proper sequence is to adapt the cartilaginous pyramid to the new bony pyramid and then to adjust the septum and reconstruct the dorsum.

Resecting a Bony Hump (or the Bony Part of a Combined Bony and Cartilaginous Hump)

Steps

- The hump to be resected is outlined on the skin (▶ Fig. 6.61).
- The dorsum is approached through bilateral (relatively wide) IC incisions. When the hump is large, the right IC incision is combined with the CSI. This allows wide access and a direct view of the dorsum (▶ Fig. 6.62). The access should always be wide to allow use of a broad chisel.

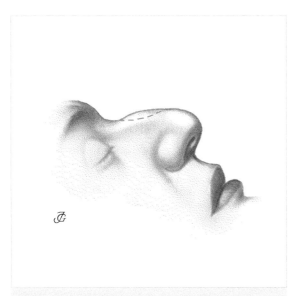

Fig. 6.61 The hump to be resected is outlined on the skin.

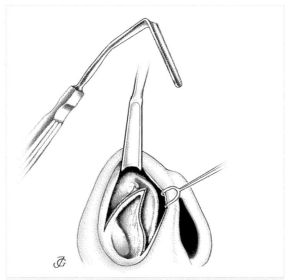

Fig. 6.62 The dorsum is approached by combining the right IC incision with the CSI. This is followed by wide undermining of the dorsal skin.

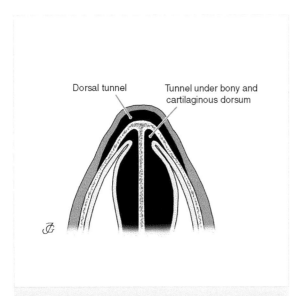

Dorsal tunnel | Tunnel under bony and cartilaginous dorsum

Fig. 6.63 The skin over the bony and cartilaginous dorsum is undermined supraperichondrially and supraperiosteally. The undermining is carried out widely enough to accommodate the instruments that are to be used. The mucosa lining the undersurface of the cartilaginous and bony pyramid is pushed aside to avoid damage when the hump is cut off.

- The skin is undermined with blunt, slightly curved scissors. The loose connective tissue layer is dissected as close to the perichondrium and periosteum as possible. The points of the scissors are therefore directed downward (see ▶ Fig. 6.3) The undermining is carried out widely enough to accommodate the instruments to be

used. Care is taken not to overstretch the usually thin skin overlying the bony part of the hump.
- The periosteum over the bony (part of the) hump is incised in a vertical direction and then scraped aside with a sharp elevator (sharp end of a Cottle elevator or a McKenty elevator) to prevent unnecessary damage to the periosteum (▶ Fig. 6.58).
- The mucosal lining of the undersurface of the cartilaginous and bony pyramid is pushed aside via the septal tunnels, using the blunt end of a Cottle elevator. This is done to avoid damage to the mucosal membranes when resecting the overlying bone (▶ Fig. 6.63).
- The hump is resected using a broad chisel (9-mm or 11-mm). It should be somewhat broader than the width of the hump to facilitate a symmetrical resection in one piece. We prefer a Cottle-type chisel as it can be used in two different ways, with the bevel up or down.
- The resection starts with the bevel up. The chisel then tends to go somewhat down while proceeding. Care is taken not to go too deep, however. Halfway, we retract the chisel and turn it 180°. With the bevel down, the instrument will slowly come up while proceeding (▶ Fig. 6.64a, b).
- The assistant uses the double-tap technique (see page 220). The surgeon lifts the skin with the thumb and index finger of the left hand to prevent damage to the skin by the edges of the chisel.
- The resected piece is mobilized by lifting it up with the chisel and/or a Cottle elevator. It is then grasped with a straight hemostat and removed (▶ Fig. 6.64c). Usually it is necessary to free it from adherent connective tissue and muscle fibers (procerus muscle) with scissors.

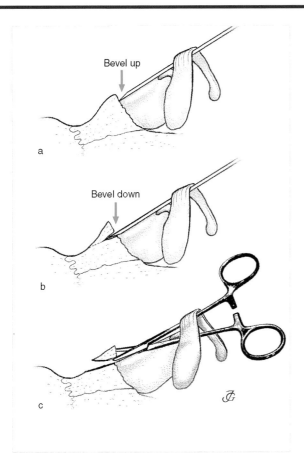

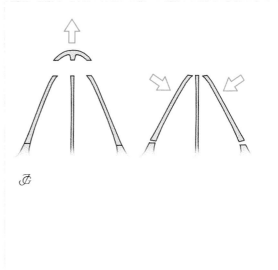

Fig. 6.65 The roof of the bony pyramid is closed. Paramedian, lateral, and transverse osteotomies are made. The bony pyramid is mobilized and modified as required, thereby closing the roof by pressing the ventral margins of the lateral bony walls together.

Fig. 6.64 Resection of a bony hump with a chisel. The chisel is introduced with the bevel up (**a**). The bevel is turned when the first part of the hump is cut; the bevel is down when the upper part is resected (**b**). The resected piece of bone is grasped with a straight hemostat and removed (**c**).

- The nasal roof is now open. Usually, the margins are somewhat unequal and irregular. They are equalized and smoothed with a rasp and a file.
- Medial, lateral, and transverse osteotomies are performed. The bony pyramid is mobilized and modified as required. The roof is closed by pressing the ventral margins of the lateral bony walls together (▶ Fig. 6.65).
- If no work on the cartilaginous dorsum has to be done, some crushed septal cartilage or fascia is inserted on top of the area. This helps smoothen the new contours and reinforce the skin.

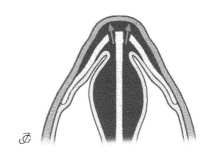

Fig. 6.66 The triangular cartilages are separated intraseptally from the septal cartilage using a No. 64 Beaver knife.

Resecting a Cartilaginous Hump (or the Cartilaginous Part of a Combined Bony and Cartilaginous Hump)

A cartilaginous hump is resected with sharp instruments. We recommend first separating the triangular cartilages from the septum, and then trimming the dorsum to the desired level under direct view.

Steps

- The dorsum is undermined as described in the previous text through bilateral IC incisions.
- The triangular cartilages are intraseptally separated from the septum with a No. 64 Beaver knife (▶ Fig. 6.66 and ▶ Fig. 6.67).

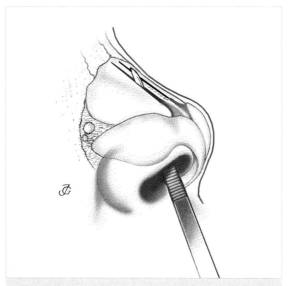

Fig. 6.67 The triangular cartilages are separated intraseptally from the septal cartilage using a No. 15 blade or a No. 64 Beaver knife.

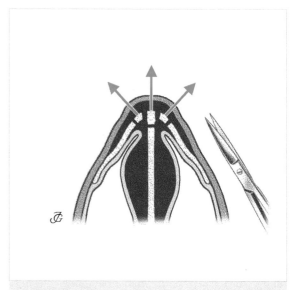

Fig. 6.68 The cartilaginous hump is resected stepwise. The height of the cartilaginous pyramid is adjusted to that of the modified bony pyramid.

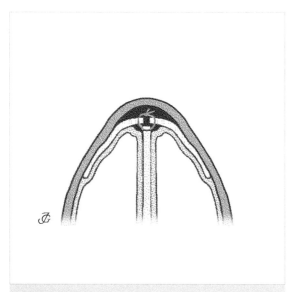

Fig. 6.69 The triangular cartilages are sutured to the septal cartilage to close the cartilaginous pyramid.

- The skin is lifted with an angulated retractor (Aufricht type). The anterior (ventral) margins of the septum and the two medial margins of the triangular cartilages are trimmed as required. This may be done with pointed, straight (or angulated) scissors or a knife (▶ Fig. 6.68).
- Care should be taken not to over-resect. After the resection, the retractor is removed. The height of the dorsum is then palpated and inspected. If required, some slices of cartilage may then be taken.

- The cartilaginous open roof is closed by readjusting the triangular cartilages. Generally, it is advisable to suture them to the septum with one or two 4–0 resorbable sutures (▶ Fig. 6.69).
- Some crushed cartilage is inserted on top to smooth the contours.
- A narrowing tape is applied to keep the triangular cartilages in position.

Push-Down and Let-Down

As previously discussed, hump reduction with a rasp and hump resection are rather traumatic techniques with a relatively high number of complications. Therefore, various surgeons have tried to develop less aggressive ways to reduce a dorsal hump. Two techniques that leave the bony pyramid intact have been suggested: the push-down technique, and let-down after resection of wedges at the base of the bony pyramid.

Push-Down

Cottle (1954) suggested reducing a hump by bringing the dorsum down. A vertical and a horizontal basal strip are resected from the septum, osteotomies are performed, and the nasal bones are infractured and pushed down. In this way the dorsum is kept intact; however, only small humps can be corrected. Besides, the effect of a push-down is often annihilated in the healing phase (Barelli 1975).

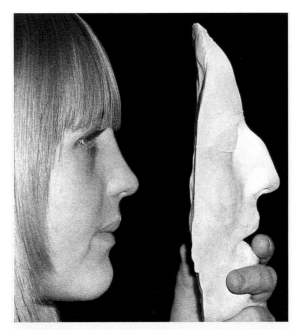

Fig. 6.70 Excessive reduction of a bony and cartilaginous hump has resulted in a ski-slope deformity.

Let-Down (After Resection of Wedges at the Base of the Bony Pyramid)

To overcome the shortcomings of the push-down technique, let-down after bilateral wedge resection was suggested (Huizing 1975). In our opinion, the let-down technique is the method of choice to reduce a limited or moderate hump, especially humps that are associated with a prominent, narrow pyramid. The method has been extensively discussed earlier in this chapter (page 227).

6.3.3 Complications

Hump removal is one of the procedures in nasal surgery with a relatively high risk of complications and adverse effects.

A *ski-slope deformity* is the most well-known complication. It is one of the most common "postsurgical looks" (▶ Fig. 6.70). Actually, it would be more correct to call it a technical failure instead of a complication. The bony and cartilaginous dorsa were lowered too much, especially in the region of the K area. Many surgeons do not take into account that the dorsal skin is thinner in this region, a fact stressed by Tardy (1990). At the same time, some sagging of the cartilaginous dorsum is a common occurrence due to inadequate fixation of the cartilaginous septum. A ski-slope deformity can be prevented by: (1) limiting the amount of reduction of the lower part of the bony dorsum; (2) fixating the cartilaginous septum to the premaxilla (or the anterior nasal spine) and the columella to prevent sagging of cartilaginous dorsum; and (3) transplanting some crushed septal cartilage under the skin in the K area.

An *open roof* is another well-known complication of a hump resection. This condition is often characterized by a special set of symptoms, the "open roof syndrome" (see Chapter 2, ▶ Fig. 2.19, ▶ Fig. 2.20 and Chapter 9, ▶ Fig. 9.76 ▶ Fig. 9.77). The bony dorsum is flattened, often irregular, and painful to the touch. Wearing eyeglasses and inhaling cold air may also produce pain. An open roof can be prevented by: (1) preserving the mucoperiosteum of the undersurface of the bony pyramid; (2) closing the bony dorsum by bringing the lateral walls together after osteotomies; and (3) inserting crushed septal cartilage under the skin in the area of the hump removal. Some surgeons prefer to reimplant part of the removed hump to cover the open roof. However, we find it difficult to avoid asymmetries and irregularities with this option.

A *local irregularity* is a third common complication of hump resection. This may be caused by: asymmetrical resection; asymmetrical repair of the cartilaginous dorsum; leaving behind a small particle of bone or cartilage; or transplantation of insufficiently crushed cartilage (see Chapter 9, ▶ Fig. 9.79).

Skin atrophy and telangiectasias: Removal of a hump with a rasp or by resection carries the risk of atrophy of the thin skin, adherence of the skin to the bone, and, in some patients, telangiectasias (see Chapter 9, ▶ Fig. 9.67). These complications can be avoided by: not overstretching the skin while undermining; closing an open roof; leaving a smooth dorsum; and inserting some crushed cartilage or connective tissue to reinforce the skin at the end of the operation.

6.4 Saddle Nose Correction

Saddling or sagging of the bony and/or cartilaginous dorsum is one of the most common and most difficult problems that we encounter in functional reconstructive nasal surgery.

Saddling and a *saddle nose* are generally accepted terms for a more or less severe depression of the bony and/or cartilaginous pyramid. It is seen after severe trauma and infection (septal abscess), but may also be a congenital anomaly or a sequela of a specific disease (e.g., Wegener granulomatosis and, in earlier times, syphilis).

Sagging is the common term for a limited depression of the cartilaginous pyramid, which may arise after trauma and septal surgery.

Saddling and sagging of the nasal pyramid usually cause both aesthetic and functional complaints. The disfigurement of the nose and the face is obvious, making the patient's cosmetic complaints easy to understand. The functional complaints that may be related to saddling and sagging vary considerably. Impaired inspiratory breathing is the most common symptom. Sometimes there are also signs of mucosal atrophy, crusting, and blood loss.

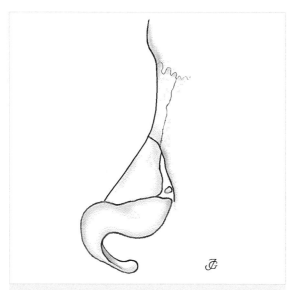

Fig. 6.71 Bony and cartilaginous saddle nose showing depressed and broadened bony and cartilaginous pyramid.

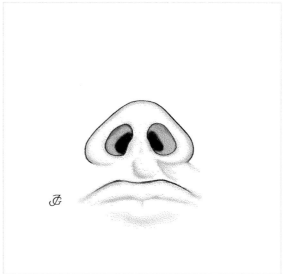

Fig. 6.72 Low, broad lobule; rounded nostrils; abnormally convex alae; short and often retracted columella.

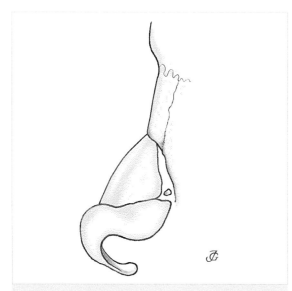

Fig. 6.73 Saddling of the bony pyramid due to frontal trauma.

6.4.1 Types of Saddling and Sagging

It is of paramount importance to analyze properly a saddle deformity and its pathogenesis. The surgical technique selected for correction will largely depend upon the type and cause of the saddling or sagging. The following types may be distinguished:
1. Bony and cartilaginous saddle nose
2. Low-wide pyramid syndrome
3. Bony saddle
4. Cartilaginous saddling or sagging

Bony and Cartilaginous Saddle Nose

Both the bony and the cartilaginous pyramid are more or less severely depressed (▶ Fig. 6.71; see also ▶ Fig. 2.51). These symptoms are usually accompanied by pathology of the septum, valve area, and lobule (▶ Fig. 6.72). If all nasal structures are involved, we prefer to speak of a low-wide pyramid syndrome. A bony and cartilaginous saddle nose is usually corrected by reconstruction of the septum, narrowing and push-up of the bony pyramid following osteotomies, and a dorsal transplant.

Low-Wide Pyramid Syndrome

Both the bony and the cartilaginous pyramid are severely depressed (see Chapter 2, page 69). The lobule is wide and low. The tip has lost its normal projection, the lobular base is broadened, the alae are more convex or ballooning, and the nostrils are rounded. The septal cartilage is defective or missing due to trauma, previous surgery, or infection. As a consequence, the valve area is lowered and widened, and the valve angle is increased, sometimes even to 90°. In many patients, depending on the cause of the deformity, the mucosa is atrophic, dry, and crusting. The main causes of this syndrome are septal abscess, severe trauma, congenital anomalies, and specific infections. The low-wide pyramid syndrome is corrected in the same way as described above. As part of the procedure, the lobule may be narrowed as well.

Bony Saddle

The dorsum of the bony pyramid is severely depressed and broadened, while the cartilaginous pyramid and the cartilaginous septum are normal (▶ Fig. 6.73; see also

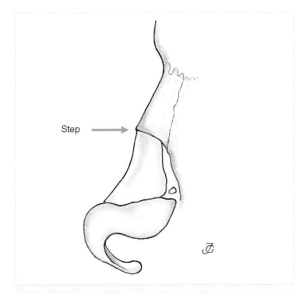

Fig. 6.74 Saddling of the cartilaginous pyramid. A "step" may be visible and palpable at the junction of the cartilaginous and bony septum.

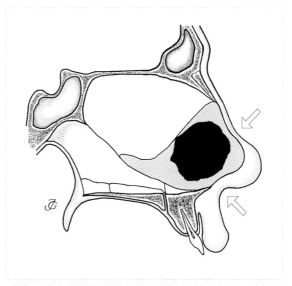

Fig. 6.75 Sagging of the cartilaginous dorsum and retraction of the columella due to submucous septal resection (Killian-Freer) without repair of the defect.

▶ Fig. 2.52). Deformities of the posterior septum may be present, however. A bony saddle is relatively rare compared with a bony and cartilaginous saddle and cartilaginous saddling. It is usually the result of severe frontal trauma with impression of the bony pyramid. Other possible causes are diseases of the nasal bones such as tertiary syphilis and congenital malformations. A bony saddle is corrected by narrowing and push-up of the bony pyramid following osteotomies and insertion of a dorsal transplant.

Cartilaginous Saddling and Sagging

The cartilaginous pyramid is severely (saddling) or moderately (sagging) depressed and broadened (▶ Fig. 6.74; see also ▶ Fig. 2.53 and ▶ Fig. 2.54). There may be atrophy or ballooning of the triangular cartilages. The continuity between the bony and cartilaginous pyramid may be disrupted. A "step" may then be visible in the region of the K area. There is loss of support and projection of the lobule (▶ Fig. 6.72). The cause of this deformity lies in the septum. It may result from frontal trauma, but the most common cause is septal surgery. In the heyday of the Killian-Freer submucous septal resection, postoperative sagging of the cartilaginous dorsum was a very common complication. The cause is loss of support and retraction of the mucoperichondrium at the septal defect during healing (▶ Fig. 6.75). Nowadays, the most frequent cause is backward rotation of the anterior septum after resection of (too large) vertical and horizontal strips and

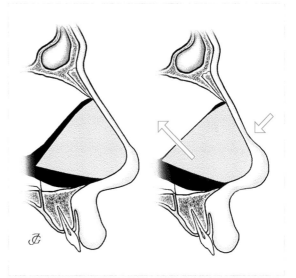

Fig. 6.76 Sagging of the cartilaginous dorsum due to backward rotation of the anterior septum after resection of excessively large vertical and horizontal strips without proper reconstruction and fixation.

inadequate fixation of the septal cartilage at the end of surgery (▶ Fig. 6.76). This type of pathology can be corrected by reopening the septum and anterior rotation of the septal cartilage (▶ Fig. 6.77).

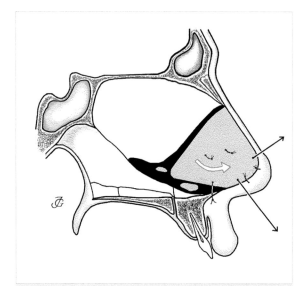

Fig. 6.77 The anterior septum is exorotated using guide sutures and fixed to the anterior nasal spine (chondrospinal suture) and the columella (septocolumellar sutures), and transseptally (transseptal sutures).

6.4.2 Surgical Techniques

Correcting saddling or sagging of the bony and/or cartilaginous dorsum is one of the most challenging tasks of the nasal surgeon, as in this type of pathology several nasal structures are usually involved.

- The septum is usually defective, in particular its anterior part, and the cartilaginous pyramid is low and wide, lacking normal septal support and projection. The triangular cartilages are often atrophic. The fibrous connections between the cartilaginous and bony pyramid may have been lost, making the lower margins of the nasal bones visible.
- The vestibule and the valve area are broad and low (see ▶ Fig. 2.17). The valve angle is depressed and considerably increased, sometimes even up to 90°.
- The bony pyramid is broad and lacks prominence. Its dorsum is flat and the nasal bones are usually thick.
- The lobule is underprojected and lacks support. The tip is broad and flat. The columella is short and retracted, especially at its base. The alae are more convex and thicker than normal. The nostrils are round and ballooning.

Because of the complexity of this pathology, it is advisable to consider a reconstruction of all essential anatomical elements: the cartilaginous septum, the cartilaginous pyramid, the bony pyramid, the lobular cartilages, and the columella.

The cartilaginous septum has to be reconstructed, positioned in the midline and fixed well to its bony base. This can very well be done endonasally. Many surgeons

(Rettinger) prefer the external approach, however, as it offers wider access and allows a complete reconstruction of the cartilaginous vault, the lobular cartilages, and the columella.

The cartilaginous pyramid may be reconstructed endonasally as well as via the external approach, depending on the pathology and personal preference. Reconstruction by an onlay of cartilage can very well be carried out endonasally; remodeling of the triangular cartilages and narrowing of the cartilaginous vault is best done by the external approach.

The bony pyramid may be mobilized by osteotomies, narrowed and pushed up as far as possible.

The lobular cartilages may be dissected and the domes may be sutured together to heighten the nasal tip.

The columella may be reconstructed by a cartilaginous batten.

In summary, patients with major pathology involving all nasal structures require surgery through an external approach. Surgery to correct limited pathology, such as cartilaginous sagging or columellar retraction, may be carried out endonasally.

We will here discuss the major elements that might be combined in reconstructing a saddle nose. Depending on the pathology, the surgeon has to decide which combination of the following procedures may be required and effective in the individual case:

1. Endonasal repositioning and/or reconstruction of the anterior septum
2. Reconstruction of the septum, cartilaginous dorsum, lobular cartilage, and columella using the external approach
3. Narrowing and push-up of the bony pyramid following osteotomies
4. Augmentation of the pyramid by a dorsal transplant
5. Increasing lobular projection and narrowing lobular width

Endonasal Repositioning and/or Reconstruction of the Septum

If the sagging of the cartilaginous dorsum is a complication of previous surgery, we attempt to correct this undesired side effect first of all by revision septal surgery. We mobilize the septum again, repair defects (especially those of its cartilaginous part), exorotate the anterior septum, and fix it in its new position. To this end, septopremaxillary sutures, septocolumellar sutures, and splints may be used (see page 174 and page 175).

Steps

- The septum is approached and mobilized in the usual way via a CSI. Generally, bilateral anterior–superior tunnels and one inferior tunnel are elevated (three-tunnel approach). The premaxilla and anterior nasal spine are fully exposed. The anterior septum is detached from its base and from the bony septum, apart from its attachment in the K area (see ▶ Fig. 5.26).

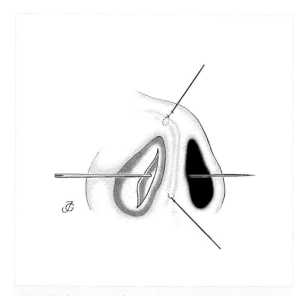

Fig. 6.78 The exorotated septum is temporarily fixed in its new position with a straight needle while septocolumellar mattress sutures are applied.

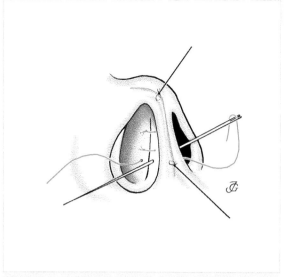

Fig. 6.79 Three septocolumellar mattress sutures are used to fix the caudal septal end to the columella and the medial crura.

- The skin over the nasal dorsum is undermined through bilateral IC incisions.
- The posterior septum is reconstructed (mosaic fashion) if required (see ▶ Fig. 5.34).
- Guide sutures are fixed to the caudal septal end at its ventrocaudal angle and its base (▶ Fig. 6.77).
- The assistant exorotates the anterior septum by pulling the guide sutures, while the surgeon fixes it in its new position with a straight needle (▶ Fig. 6.78).
- The septal base is fixed to the premaxilla or the anterior nasal spine (▶ Fig. 6.77). The caudal septal end is fixed to the columella by three slowly resorbable septocolumellar sutures (▶ Fig. 6.79).
- If desired, the septum can also be fixed by adding one or two transseptal sutures and/or septal splints.
- If the sagging is not completely abolished, some slightly crushed septal cartilage (or a small transplant of auricular cartilage) is introduced to augment the cartilaginous dorsum (▶ Fig. 6.80).

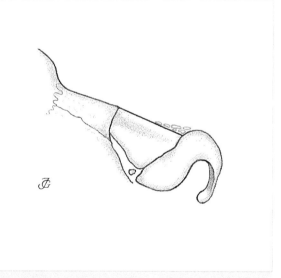

Fig. 6.80 The cartilaginous dorsum is augmented by inserting crushed septal cartilage through the IC incision.

Reconstruction of the Septum, Cartilaginous Dorsum, Lobular Cartilage, and Columella Using the External Approach

This is the preferred procedure in cases with severe pathology, as it allows correction of all anatomical structures.

Steps

- The pathology is approached by the external approach in the usual way (see page 264).
- The anterior part of the cartilaginous septum is dissected both from below (dissection starting at the caudal end) and from above. The triangular cartilages are exposed (extraperichondrially) and the valve angle is freed.
- The domes and the lateral crura of the lobular cartilages are dissected out extraperichondrially as much as required for redraping.
- The bony pyramid is mobilized and infractured, depending on the pathology.
- The septum is reconstructed applying the principles described in Chapter 5. Stabilization of the septum on the nasal spine and/or the premaxilla is of utmost importance, as the quality of the septal reconstruction greatly determines the functional and aesthetic outcome.
- The triangular cartilages are sutured to the ventral margin of the septum to obtain stability. Utmost care is taken to establish a valve angle of some 20°.
- The lobular cartilages are redraped to increase lobular prominence. The domes are sutured together to obtain a more prominent nasal tip.
- The medial crura may be fixed to the caudal end of the septum by two or three 5–0 sutures. This greatly adds to the stability and prominence, but may cause a certain stiffness of the lower third of the nasal pyramid.
- Depending on the result obtained by the previous procedures, a cartilaginous transplant may be required to obtain a straight dorsum (see below).

Narrowing and Push-Up of the Bony Pyramid

A bony saddle may be reduced by narrowing and push-up of the bony pyramid following mobilization of the pyramid by osteotomies. Although narrowing of the pyramid itself does not increase its projection, it gives the impression of a somewhat greater prominence. Push-up of the pyramid is difficult to accomplish but may be attempted. See page 218.

Augmentation by Dorsal Transplant

Crushed Septal Cartilage

A limited cartilaginous sagging may be corrected by inserting some crushed septal cartilage (without perichondrium) through the IC incisions or the CSI (▶ Fig. 6.80). Because crushed septal cartilage is easy to mold, it makes an almost ideal transplant material. Unfortunately, however, it is largely resorbed within 6 to 12 months. The amount of resorption is estimated at 30 to 60%, depending on the degree of crushing. Crushed septal cartilage is therefore only used to correct a limited

cartilaginous sagging, to fill minor lobular depressions, and to reinforce the dorsal skin following hump removal. If a more voluminous transplant is required, a sculpted transplant from septal, auricular, or rib cartilage is used.

Steps

- The septal cartilage to be (re)implanted is inspected. Care is taken that no perichondrium is left attached to avoid growth of the transplant.
- The cartilage is crushed to such an extent that a moldable substance is obtained. This is then cut into small pieces and inserted through the IC incision or the CSI using a narrow cup-forceps.
- We insert the crushed cartilage at the very end of surgery. The various incisions are closed first, leaving a small opening at the medial side of both IC incisions, or the upper end of the CSI.
- After insertion, the transplant is molded into place with the fingers and fixed by external taping.

Noncrushed Septal Cartilage or Auricular Cartilage

In patients with a moderate depression of the cartilaginous pyramid, a single or double transplant of noncrushed septal cartilage, or of auricular cartilage with perichondrium attached on one side, is a generally accepted method of augmentation. However, as stressed before, we will always first try to reconstruct and/or reposition the anterior septum. Augmentation of the dorsum by a transplant is performed as an additional procedure. The short-term results of auricular grafts in cases with moderate sagging are satisfactory. In the long term, however, a certain amount of resorption (rather variable in our experience) will take place. Therefore, additional surgery may be indicated after some years. Instead of auricular cartilage, one may use a graft sculpted from septal cartilage. Generally, septal grafts tend to become resorbed more readily, possibly because they are devoid of perichondrium.

Harvesting an Auricular Graft

Steps

- The transplant is taken from the auricle opposite the side on which the patient prefers to sleep.
- We like to resect the transplant by the anterior approach; others use the posterior one. The anterior approach has the advantage that the size and shape of the cartilage to be removed can be controlled more easily (▶ Fig. 6.81).
- The piece of cartilage to be removed is outlined with surgical ink. It is usually taken from the anterior cavity of the concha, but this depends on the size and the desired convexity of the transplant.
- The area around the piece of cartilage to be resected is infiltrated subcutaneously on both sides of the auricle with lidocaine–adrenaline 1:100,000.

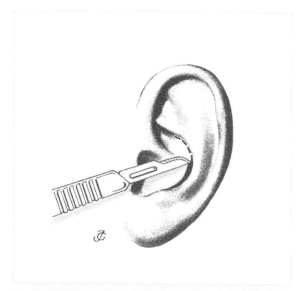

Fig. 6.81 Auricular cartilage is harvested by the anterior approach. An incision is made on the inside of the anthelix.

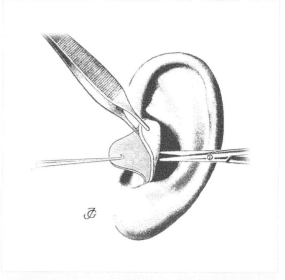

Fig. 6.82 The graft is dissected leaving the posterior perichondrium attached.

- The skin is incised on the inside of the anthelix to avoid a visible postoperative scar (▶ Fig. 6.81).
- Skin, subcutaneous tissue, and perichondrium are dissected in one layer from the anterior side of the cavity of the concha with pointed, slightly curved scissors.
- The graft to be taken is circumcised with a small knife and dissected out, leaving the posterior perichondrium attached (▶ Fig. 6.82). Skin and cartilage are handled with a delicate anatomical forceps (Adson-Brown type) and small, pointed, slightly curved scissors. Damage to the surface of the cartilage should be avoided as lesions to the cartilage may cause disfigurement of the graft and enhance resorption.
- The skin and subcutaneous layers are closed in one layer with a 5–0 monofilament nonresorbable suture.
- Care is taken to prevent blood from accumulating at the donor site. Therefore, the cavity of the concha is filled with gauze; in addition, a pressure dressing is applied to prevent a subcutaneous hematoma.

Sculpting, Inserting, and Fixing the Graft

Steps

- The graft is cut to the desired size and shape. Care is taken to not damage its surface. The margins are rounded off with a small knife, file, or sandpaper.
- In cases with more pronounced sagging, it may be advisable to construct a double or triple graft (▶ Fig. 6.83).
- A guide suture may be fixed at one or both ends of the transplant to maneuver and fix the graft in place.

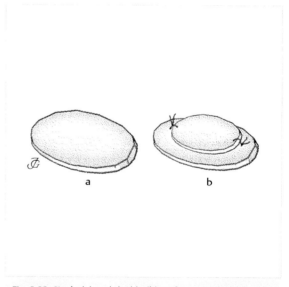

Fig. 6.83 Single (a) and double (b) grafts are sculpted from auricular cartilage to augment the nasal dorsum.

Note

Histological studies have shown that damage to the surface of grafts will enhance resorption. The same may occur in suture canals.

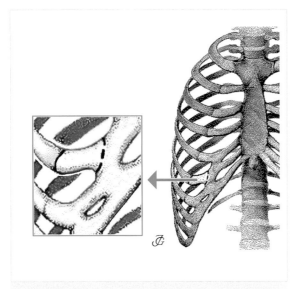

Fig. 6.84 Rib cartilage is harvested from the costochondral plate of the sixth or seventh rib.

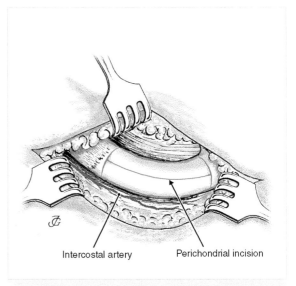

Intercostal artery   Perichondrial incision

Fig. 6.85 The perichondrium over the cartilaginous part of the rib is incised in an H-shaped manner.

Rib Cartilage

In patients with a more pronounced saddle, a large graft is required to restore a normal dorsal profile. Autogeneic rib cartilage is then the best choice. In the 20th century, a variety of nonbiological implants was introduced as alternatives to biological transplants (see following text and Chapter 9, page 354). However, they are not reliable. Generally, rib cartilage is considered the best material available for augmenting the nasal dorsum. Rib cartilage has several advantages: first, it is human tissue; second, it can easily be sculpted to the desired size and shape. However, it also has disadvantages: it tends to become resorbed, and its biomechanical properties make it difficult to cut it into a shape that remains unchanged.

Harvesting Rib Cartilage

Steps

- The cartilaginous part of the sixth or seventh rib is taken. Although the cartilaginous part of the eighth and ninth rib is larger, material from those ribs is not used because of the insertion of the rectus abdominis muscle.
- A slightly curved incision of about 8 cm is made over the sixth or seventh rib at the junction between its bony and cartilaginous part (▶ Fig. 6.84). The subcutaneous tissues are cut. The thin muscle fibers of the external oblique muscle are spread longitudinally and kept intact.
- The perichondrium is incised in an H-shaped manner (▶ Fig. 6.85). It is elevated from the cartilage in a cranial and caudal direction using a broad raspatory. Working subperichondrially, a pneumothorax and accidental injury of the intercostal vessels is avoided.

- A hook is introduced under the rib to elevate it while dissecting the inner side of the cartilage from its perichondrium.
- The cartilage is cut laterally from the bone and medially from the costochondral plate with a No. 20 or No. 21 knife. Generally, a piece about 5 cm in length can be removed.
- The donor site is examined for leakage of air by pouring saline into the wound and checking for air bubbles.
- The perichondrium is closed with slowly resorbable sutures. The muscle fibers of the external oblique muscle are sutured with resorbable suture material. The skin is closed in two layers.

Sculpting the Transplant

Steps

- The core of the rib is used to avoid bending and warping of the transplant (▶ Fig. 6.86). This is essential, as the outer layers of a rib contain asymmetrical amounts of elastic fibers to keep the rib in a curved shape.
- A biconvex transplant is cut (▶ Fig. 6.87). The graft should not only fit longitudinally but also in the transverse direction of the saddle (▶ Fig. 6.88).

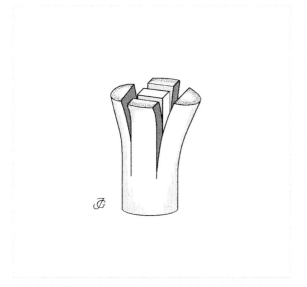

Fig. 6.86 The asymmetrically distributed elastic forces on the inner and outer curvature of a rib make rib cartilage liable to bending or warping. Therefore, the graft is cut from the center of the rib.

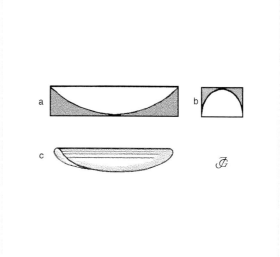

Fig. 6.87 a–c A biconvex transplant is sculpted to match the biconvex defect.

Inserting and Fixing the Transplant

Steps

- The transplant is usually inserted through the IC incision on the right.
- Care is taken that the graft can be positioned as required. Undermining of the dorsal skin should be sufficiently wide. Connective tissue and muscle fibers at the implant bed have to be cut. The skin should maintain its normal color after the transplant has been introduced. Ischemia greatly increases the risks of infection and extrusion.
- A small pocket is created between the two domes to accommodate the caudal end of the transplant. This will also help to keep it in the midline and prevent it slipping aside.
- Some crushed cartilage may be inserted on either side of the transplant to help keep the graft in position and to smooth the edges (▶ Fig. 6.89).
- The bony dorsum and K area may be "freshened up" with a rasp to enhance fibrous fixation of the cranial part of the transplant to the dorsum.
- The transplant is fixed with careful external taping and a stent. The benefit of sutures to keep a graft in place is debatable. It has been suggested that connective tissue may grow into the suture canals, thus enhancing resorption.

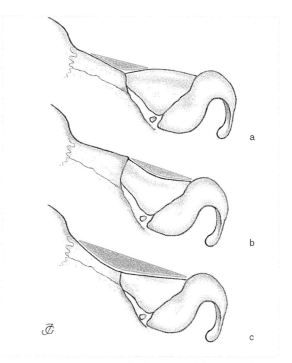

Fig. 6.88 a–c Most common shapes of dorsal transplants.

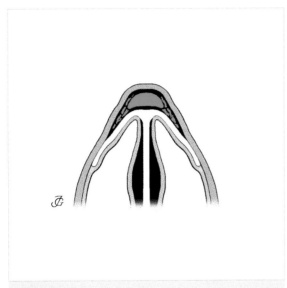

Fig. 6.89 The transplant is "dressed" with some crushed septal cartilage to help keep it in position and to smooth its edges.

Nonbiological Implants

Since the beginning of the 19th century, various nonbiological materials have been used to augment a saddling nasal dorsum. Unfortunately, none of them has withstood the test of time. Extrusion often occurred as an early or late complication. We therefore object to the use of foreign materials in the nasal dorsum and the septum. Nonbiological implants will never become incorporated in the surrounding tissues. Therefore, they may be extruded sooner or later. An overview of the nonbiological implants that have been applied over the last century is presented in Chapter 9 (page 354).

Engineered Cartilage Grafts

It will most likely be possible to produce biological materials in vitro in the near future. The availability of engineered cartilage grafts will undoubtedly have a great impact on the practice of reconstructive nasal surgery.

Increasing Lobular Projection and Narrowing Lobular Width

The contour and projection of the nose may be improved by increasing lobular projection and narrowing lobular width. Usually, these procedures are part of more extensive surgery, including septal reconstruction, osteotomies, and dorsal augmentation with a graft. For a discussion of the technique we refer to Chapter 7 (page 274).

Lengthening the Columella and Correcting Columellar Retraction

Lengthening the columella and correcting a columellar retraction may be performed as an additional procedure to improve nasal form and function in patients with a low, wide pyramid or a saddle nose. For a discussion of the techniques, the reader is referred to Chapter 7, page 294.

6.4.3 Complications

Infection is the most feared complication when a transplant is inserted. To reduce this risk, systemic antibiotic prophylaxis (e.g., amoxicillin) is started the day before surgery. The nasal vestibules are carefully trimmed to remove the vibrissae and thoroughly disinfected. Some surgeons put the transplant (or implant) in an antibiotic solution for some 30 minutes prior to insertion. If in spite of all precautions infection does occur, the IC incision is reopened and the dorsal pocket is drained. If a cartilage graft has been introduced, it may be left in place. By conducting daily check-up of drainage, administering systemic intravenous antibiotics (directed against penicillin-resistant staphylococci), and local application of antibiotics, a cartilaginous transplant can usually be saved. In contrast, bone transplants and nonbiological implants must be removed.

Resorption is the second most important problem. It occurs in all biological transplants, but its pace depends on the type of material. Crushed septal cartilage (without perichondrium) is usually resorbed within 1 year, though some connective tissue may remain. The degree of crushing is one of the factors that determines the speed of resorption. Grafts of auricular cartilage with perichondrium survive much longer and may become incorporated in the surrounding tissues. Transplants of rib cartilage remain intact for a long time. After 10 to 20 years, some resorption may become apparent, especially at the ends of the graft. Revision surgery may then be indicated.

Dislocation of the graft is another well-known complication. Symmetrical and sufficient undermining of the skin over the dorsum, careful positioning, and, above all, proper fixation by tapes and a stent, are the most important preventive measures.

Extrusion of transplants and implants is a feared complication. If a transplant or implant is extruded within days or weeks after surgery, infection is usually the cause. Another factor may be ischemia of the overlying skin as a result of insufficient undermining of the skin. Extrusion after months or years is rare with biological grafts. If it does occur, the most likely cause is trauma. Nonbiological implants, on the contrary, will never become part of the body. Consequently, they could be extruded years or even decades later (see Chapter 9, ► Fig. 9.91, ► Fig. 9.92, ► Fig. 9.93, ► Fig. 9.94, ► Fig. 9.95, ► Fig. 9.96, ► Fig. 9.97, ► Fig. 9.98, ► Fig. 9.99, ► Fig. 9.100, and ► Fig. 9.101).

Bending or warping of a rib transplant is avoided by using the central part of the rib, as previously described. This complication is seen more frequently in autogeneic than in allogeneic preserved transplants.

6.5 Valve Surgery

Surgery of the nasal valve is dictated by the structural and functional pathology of the valve area. Careful analysis of the anatomical and physiological abnormalities is of utmost importance. Both the anatomy of the valve area and its function during inspiration and expiration should therefore be carefully examined and measured.

6.5.1 Pathology of the Valve Area

Normal function of the valve area may be impaired by various anatomical abnormalities. The most common causes are:

- Septal pathology in area 2, such as a deviation, convexity, thickening, or a defect (see ▶ Fig. 2.112)
- Triangular cartilage pathology, in particular an irregular, twisted, or abnormally protruding caudal margin, or atrophied or missing cartilage (see ▶ Fig. 2.102)
- A narrow, high valve as part of a prominent, narrow pyramid (see ▶ Fig. 2.102)
- A wide, depressed valve as part of a saddle nose or a low-wide pyramid syndrome (see ▶ Fig. 2.103)
- Hypertrophy of the head of the inferior turbinate (see ▶ Fig. 2.117 and ▶ Fig. 2.118)
- Stenosis of the valve angle (see ▶ Fig. 6.106)
- Stenosis of the floor of the valve area (see ▶ Fig. 7.81)

These pathologies may occur in isolation, but they are often found in combination. For instance, a septal convexity in area 2 may be combined with hypertrophy of the head of the lower turbinate. A narrow, prominent pyramid may coincide with atrophy of the triangular cartilage. An excellent overview of the various types of pathology of the valve area was presented by Kern (1978).

6.5.2 Surgical Techniques

Various techniques have been described to correct disorders of the valve area. Some methods are said to be effective in almost all cases, for example a spreader graft or a valve plasty. We dispute this suggestion. In fact, we object to the propagation of a standard method to correct valve area pathology. Instead, we suggest addressing the specific cause(s) of the obstruction. If the valve area is narrowed by a septal deviation or convexity, we will correct the septum. If the obstruction is due to a narrow, high valve area, we may let down the pyramid. If the obstruction is caused by irreversible hypertrophy of the head of the inferior turbinate, we will perform anterior turbinoplasty; in other

words, we perform the procedure necessary to reconstruct a normal valve, including a normal valve angle.

Depending on the pathology, the following surgical modalities may be used, either as a single procedure or in combination:
1. Septal surgery
2. Inferior turbinate surgery
3. Triangular cartilage surgery

Septal Surgery

When obstruction at the valve area is caused by a deviation, convexity, or thickening of the cartilaginous septum, we will try to restore normal function by septal surgery. Dealing with a septal deviation or a convexity in area 2 is described and illustrated in detail in Chapter 5, page 187.

Inferior Turbinate Surgery

When hypertrophy of the head of the inferior turbinate is the cause of obstruction of the valve area, the logical treatment is submucous reduction of the turbinate head (anterior turbinoplasty). For techniques, see Chapter 8 (page 301). Whether or not the head of the turbinate is disturbing nasal breathing can be demonstrated by acoustic rhinometry before and after decongestion (see Chapter 2, page 119; ▶ Fig. 2.154 and ▶ Fig. 2.155). Generally, we would first investigate the effect of topical corticosteroids before definitely deciding to perform turbinate reduction by submucosal surgery.

Triangular Cartilage Surgery

Modifying the inferior margin of the triangular cartilage to improve valvular function is a delicate and risky type of surgery. First of all, the structural basis for the functional disturbance of the valve must be correctly diagnosed. Subsequently, the abnormality must be both anatomically and physiologically corrected in a technically flawless way. Otherwise, the result will be disappointing and the situation may even be worsened.

Steps

- An IC incision is made just above and parallel to the lower border of the cartilage from lateral to medial with a No. 11 (or No. 15) blade. The incision is continued beyond the valve angle (▶ Fig. 6.90).
- The caudal part of the triangular cartilage is exposed by careful subcutaneous dissection (on the lateral side of the valve) and submucoperichondrial dissection (on the medial side of the valve). This is best performed with delicate anatomical forceps (Adson-Brown) and pointed, slightly curved scissors. A No. 64 Beaver knife may be helpful as well. By dissecting subperichondrially, we preserve the connecting fibers between the lateral crus and the triangular cartilage as well as the vasculature, nerve supply, and musculature.

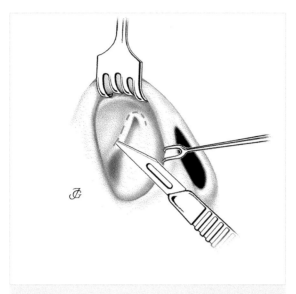

Fig. 6.90 An IC incision with extension around the valve angle is made to approach the caudal margin of the triangular cartilage and the valve angle.

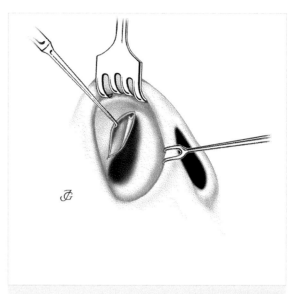

Fig. 6.91 The caudal margin of the triangular cartilage and the reflection of its most medial part are exposed.

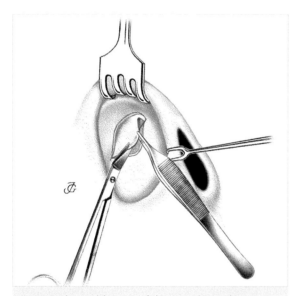

Fig. 6.92 The caudal margin of the triangular cartilage is trimmed.

- The extent of the dissection depends upon the type of the deformity. To free the valve angle completely, the mucoperichondrium of the septum may be elevated a few millimeters in a caudal direction.
- The structural basis of the functional disturbance is now identified (▶ Fig. 6.91).

Depending on the findings, one of the following corrective procedures is applied:
1. Trimming of the caudal margin
2. Resection of (excessive) reflection
3. Reinforcement or reconstruction of the triangular cartilage

Trimming the Caudal Margin of the Triangular Cartilage

If the caudal margin is protruding or irregular, it may be trimmed with small angulated scissors. Usually, only a small strip of cartilage is resected.

When shortening of the nose is desired, a small strip of the mucocutaneous covering of the caudal margin may also be removed. All resections should be bilateral and symmetrical to avoid postoperative asymmetry (▶ Fig. 6.92).

Resection of (Excessive) Reflection of the Triangular Cartilage

A certain amount of returning of the medial part of the lower margin of the triangular cartilage is normal. It helps to prevent inspiratory collapse of the lateral valvular wall. Resection of a reflection may weaken the lateral valvular wall too much, causing inspiratory breathing problems. On the other hand, the amount of reflection may be such that the valve may be too rigid. In this condition, resection of the reflecting part may be considered (▶ Fig. 6.93).

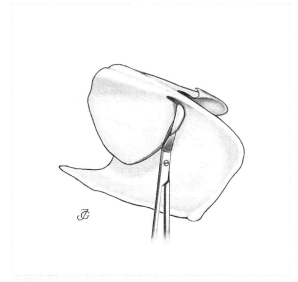

Fig. 6.93 The (excessive) reflection is resected.

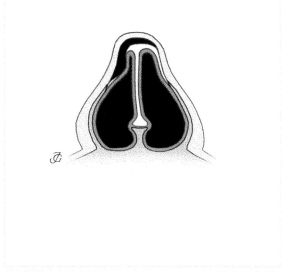

Fig. 6.94 A severely atrophied or missing triangular cartilage.

Reinforcing or Reconstructing the Triangular Cartilage

If the triangular cartilage is severely atrophied or missing, it may be reinforced or reconstructed by a thin plate of cartilage sculpted from septal or auricular cartilage.

Steps

- Generally, the external approach will be used.
- The defect to be restored or reinforced is carefully measured.
- A flat piece of autogeneic septal or auricular cartilage is cut to the desired dimensions.
- The transplant is fixed to the margin of the intact part of the cartilage or septum (▶ Fig. 6.94 and ▶ Fig. 6.95). The transplant should not be too bulky or convex, otherwise it may cause a hump.

Note

This procedure can also be performed endonasally through an IC incision. The transplant is then fixed transcutaneously.

Widening the Valve Area

A narrow valve area is a common type of pathology. Usually, it is part of a prominent-narrow pyramid syndrome. It is also observed following rhinoplasty. A well-known cause is scarring of the valve angle or the floor of the valve area (see ▶ Fig. 6.106). Another cause is too much infracture of the nasal bones. The following methods may be considered to widen the valve area:

1. Let-down of the bony and cartilaginous pyramid
2. Resection of a triangle from the lower margin of the triangular cartilage and its mucocutaneous covering

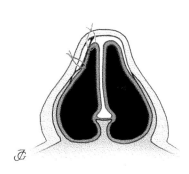

Fig. 6.95 The defect is reinforced or reconstructed by a septal or auricular transplant that is fixed to the intact part of the septolateral cartilage.

3. A spreader graft
4. Correction of a scarred valve angle by resecting the scar tissue and reconstructing the area with a free skin or a composite graft
5. Correction of stenosis of the floor of the valve area by resecting the scar tissue and reconstructing the area with a composite graft
6. Enlarging the piriform aperture

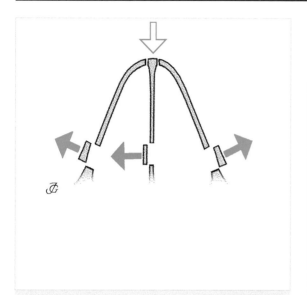

Fig. 6.96 In patients with a narrow valve area as part of a prominent-narrow pyramid syndrome, the pyramid is let down following bilateral wedge resection and resection of a horizontal and a vertical strip from the septum.

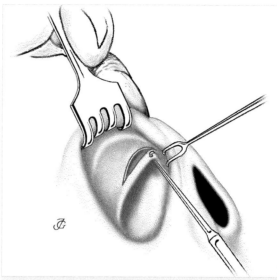

Fig. 6.97 A triangle is resected from the lower margin of the triangular cartilage. The cartilage with its overlying skin is hooked and pulled caudally.

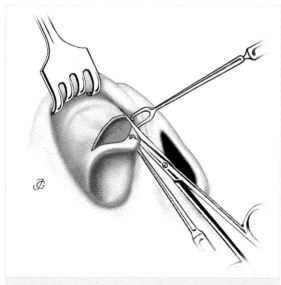

Fig. 6.98 The cartilage (and overlying skin) is separated from the septum over a distance of 2 to 3 mm.

The type of pathology will determine which method to use. In a patient with a narrow valve area due to a narrow pyramid, widening of the bony and cartilaginous pyramid is usually the best option. In a case with a narrow valve because of a protruding and twisted caudal margin of the triangular cartilage, "opening up" of the valve by resection of a triangle from its lower margin will be the best approach. In patients with scarring of the valve angle, resection of the obstructing scar tissue and reconstruction of the valve angle with a graft is the method of choice.

Let-Down of the Pyramid

In patients with a narrow valve area due to a prominent, narrow pyramid, a let-down of the bony and cartilaginous pyramid is the method of choice as it addresses the cause of the problem (▶ Fig. 6.96). The pyramid is let down following bilateral wedge resections and resection of a vertical and horizontal strip from the septum, as described and illustrated on page 227.

Resecting a Triangle of Cartilage from the Lower Margin of the Triangular Cartilage and Its Mucocutaneous Covering

A narrow valve angle may be effectively widened by resecting a triangle of cartilage from the caudal margin of the triangular cartilage with or without a strip of its cutaneous (lateral side) and mucosal (medial side) covering.

Steps

- The lateral and medial surface of the caudal margin of the triangular cartilage, including the valve angle, are dissected out (▶ Fig. 6.97).
- A triangle of cartilage is resected from its lower margin. To this end, the triangular cartilage is first separated from the septum over a distance of 2 to 3 mm with pointed straight scissors (▶ Fig. 6.98). Then a triangle of cartilage is cut off from lateral to medial using small angulated scissors (▶ Fig. 6.99).
- A somewhat smaller triangle of skin and mucosa may additionally be resected.

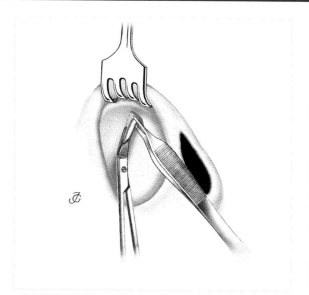

Fig. 6.99 A triangle of cartilage is resected along with some of the overlying skin and underlying mucosa.

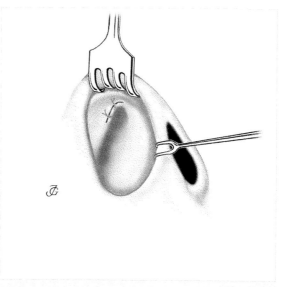

Fig. 6.100 The incision is carefully closed with two to three 4–0 resorbable sutures. The valve angle is thereby widened.

- The larger the triangle of cartilage and strips of soft tissue resected, the more the valve angle will be widened or "opened up."
- At the same time, the nose will be shortened and the nasal tip rotated upward when the incision is closed (▶ Fig. 6.100). This effect should be taken into account when using this technique.
- An internal dressing soaked in ointment, and external tapes, are applied to support the structures in their new position.

Spreader Graft

The spreader graft technique, introduced by Sheen (1985), is another method to widen a narrow nasal angle. The triangular cartilage is separated from the septum. A small rectangular strip of septal cartilage is inserted between the anterior margin of the septum and the medial margin of the triangular cartilage to widen the valve angle. This method is less physiological than the three previously described, but it is both easier to carry out and relatively atraumatic. A disadvantage is that the transplant may become resorbed so that an initial good effect may be lost. A small ball of cotton wool may be temporarily placed at the valve angle to determine whether widening of the valve will alleviate the breathing obstruction (see ▶ Fig. 6.115). If effective, it may convince both the patient and the doctor that a spreader graft can be helpful.

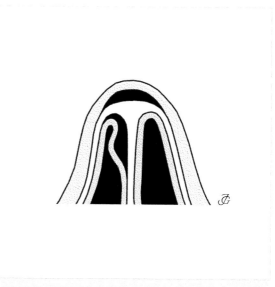

Fig. 6.101 A dorsal tunnel and a submucoperichondrial tunnel under the cartilaginous pyramid are elevated.

Steps

- The anterosuperior septal tunnel is extended up to the undersurface of the cartilaginous pyramid. The overlying dorsal skin is undermined via either the IC incision or the CSI (▶ Fig. 6.101).
- The triangular cartilage is intraseptally separated from the cartilaginous septum with a No. 64 Beaver knife (▶ Fig. 6.102).

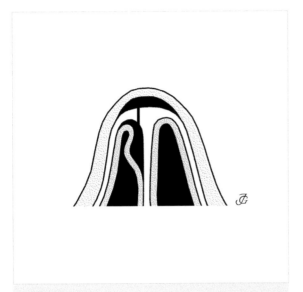

Fig. 6.102 The triangular cartilage and septal cartilage are separated intraseptally.

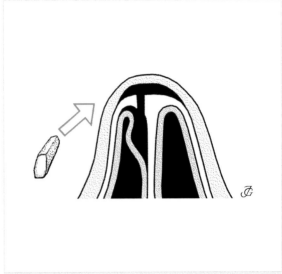

Fig. 6.103 A rectangular or wedge-shaped graft is made from septal or auricular cartilage.

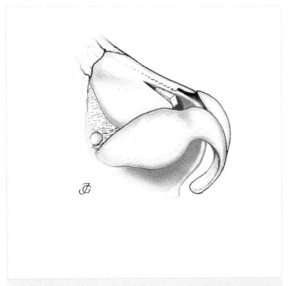

Fig. 6.104 A spreader graft is inserted as a spacer between the triangular cartilage and the septum.

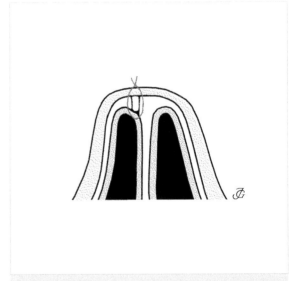

Fig. 6.105 The graft is fixed in place.

- A rectangular (or wedge-shaped) strip of autogeneic septal cartilage about 5 mm in length, 4 mm in height, and 2 to 3 mm in width is prepared (▶ Fig. 6.103).
- This strip is inserted intraseptally between the cartilaginous septum and the medial margin of the triangular cartilage (▶ Fig. 6.104). It is fixed in place with a small transdorsal suture (▶ Fig. 6.105). Care is taken to position the graft so that it will not interfere with the mobility of the cleft.

Correcting a Stenosis of the Valve Angle

If the valve angle is distorted by scar formation, it may be repaired by resecting the scar tissue and reconstructing the area with a free skin or a composite graft (▶ Fig. 6.106 and ▶ Fig. 6.107). A spreader graft may be inserted at the same time to widen the valve angle.

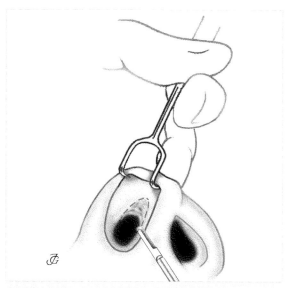

Fig. 6.106 The scar tissue obstructing the valve angle is resected.

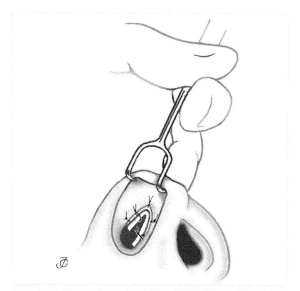

Fig. 6.107 The valve angle is reconstructed with a free full-thickness skin graft and fixed with a temporary stent.

Steps

- The stenosing scar tissue is resected with a No.15 blade or a No. 64 Beaver knife.
- A full-thickness skin graft is harvested from the post-auricular area and cut to the size of the defect that has been created at the valve angle.
- In cases where the triangular cartilage and the anterior margin of the cartilaginous septum are missing, a composite graft consisting of skin and cartilage from the auricle may be considered. It should be taken into account that a composite graft is rather bulky and may therefore not yield the desired widening. Besides, it may disturb the dorsal contour.
- The graft is placed in position by a transdorsal guide suture and fixed with two or three sutures (4–0 or 5–0).
- A Silastic stent is cut to support the skin graft and keep the valve angle open. It is fixed with a transdorsal guide suture as well as transseptal and transcartilaginous fixation sutures. The stent is left in place for about 2 weeks.

Correcting a Stenosis of the Floor of the Valve Area

Correcting a stenosis at the floor of the valve area is one of the most difficult procedures in nasal surgery. In our hands, resection of the scar and reconstruction of the floor of the valve area with a *composite graft* from the auricle has proven to be the most successful technique.

A *Z-plasty* is an alternative technique. In this region, however, the results of a Z-plasty are often disappointing. The method may be applied in patients with a localized and very limited stenosis.

Composite Graft

Steps

- The stenosis is incised from medial to lateral with an angulated Beaver knife. The scar tissue obstructing the floor of the valve area is resected. The adjacent skin and mucosa is undermined. In special cases, some bone may be removed from the piriform crest to widen the area.
- The defect is reconstructed with a composite graft (skin and cartilage) from the auricle (▶ Fig. 6.108). We prefer a composite graft over a full-thickness skin graft, as the cartilage inhibits retraction of the skin. See also Chapter 7 (▶ Fig. 7.83).
- The graft is fixed in place with tissue glue, and two or three sutures.
- The area is kept open for several weeks by a dressing with ointment.
- A custom-made vestibular prosthesis is worn until healing is complete.

Z-plasty

Steps

- The stenosis (at the floor of the valve area) is incised from medial to lateral with an angulated Beaver knife. Two small incisions are then made at a 45° angle to the first incision in opposite directions (▶ Fig. 6.109 and ▶ Fig. 6.110).
- The skin (and mucosa) is undermined in all directions. Subcutaneous scar tissue is resected where required.
- The two skin flaps are transposed and sutured as illustrated in ▶ Fig. 6.111. This should be possible without any tension. Otherwise, a free skin graft or a composite graft should be sutured in place (see following text).

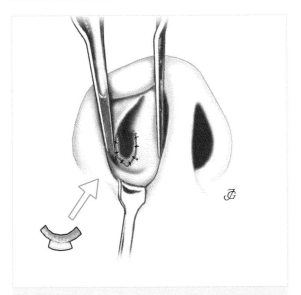

Fig. 6.108 The floor of the nasal valve is reconstructed with a composite graft taken from the auricle.

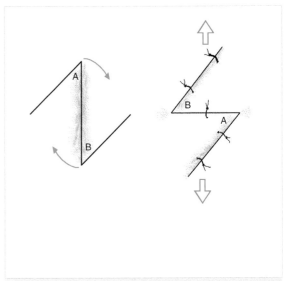

Fig. 6.109 Principle of a Z-plasty. A Z-shaped incision is made at the stenosis. Two triangular flaps are undermined and mobilized; they are rotated and sutured in their new position.

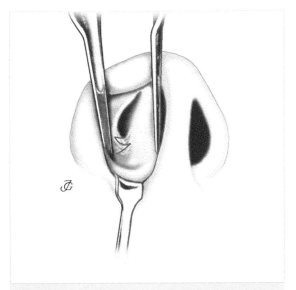

Fig. 6.110 A Z-shaped incision is made at the stenotic area.

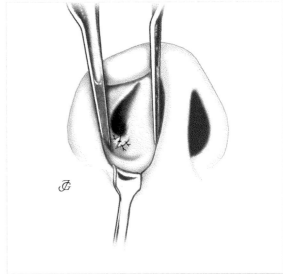

Fig. 6.111 The flaps are rotated and fixed in their new position.

- In some cases, it may be helpful to combine this procedure with enlargement of the bony piriform aperture, as described in the following text.
- A dressing with ointment is applied to help keep the transposed skin flaps in place.

Widening the Piriform Aperture

In special cases, the bony piriform aperture may be enlarged to widen the valve area. It is the method of choice in patients with a congenitally narrow bony aperture. It may also be the best option in cases with a deformity of the piriform aperture due to fracturing and dislocation of the maxilla. Generally, resection of some bone from the lateral wall of the aperture is carried out with a drill and cutting burr or biting forceps. In selected cases (maxilla fracture or stenosis of the nasal floor), resection of some bone from the piriform crest may be considered. Enlarging the piriform aperture may be performed as an isolated procedure or in combination with other types of surgery, such as resection of a stenosis (see previous text).

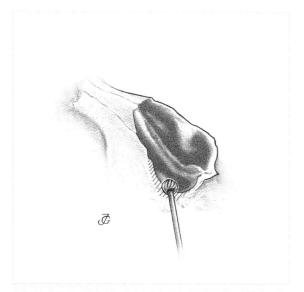

Fig. 6.112 The piriform aperture is enlarged by resecting bone from its lateral (or caudal) margin with a burr or a biting forceps.

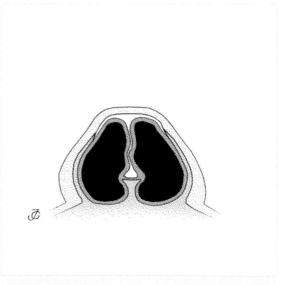

Fig. 6.113 Wide, depressed valve area in a patient with a saddle nose due to destruction of the anterior septum.

Steps

- The piriform aperture is approached either by a labio-gingival incision or by a modified vestibular incision. A labiogingival incision provides the widest access. It also avoids the need for an (extra) incision of the vestibular skin, which is quite often compromised in these cases.
- Depending upon the pathology, the lateral and/or the caudal margin of the piriform aperture will be exposed using a McKenty elevator.
- A small strip of bone (usually 2 to 3 mm) is resected with a burr or biting forceps (▶ Fig. 6.112).
- In some cases (e.g., stenosis due to scarring), it may be helpful to make two small holes in the newly created piriform margin and fix the skin of the valve area to the bone with slowly resorbable sutures.
- A dressing with ointment is applied to the valve area to keep the soft tissues in place.

Narrowing the Valve Area

A wide, depressed valve in patients with a saddle nose deformity is addressed by reconstructing the anterior septum (see Chapter 5, page 180). In this way, the valve angle is brought upward and narrowed (▶ Fig. 6.113 and ▶ Fig. 6.114). In patients with a long-standing low, wide pyramid, it may be impossible to restore a normal valve area because of retraction of the soft tissues. Surgery of the valve angle may then be considered as a secondary procedure after reconstructing the septum. It is important to realize that a dorsal transplant, although it may improve the nasal contour, does not improve valvular function. Because of the weight of the transplant, the valve angle may even become further depressed.

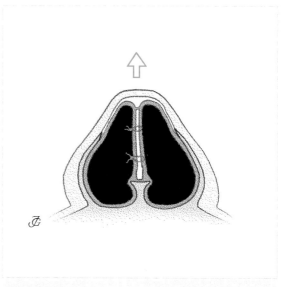

Fig. 6.114 The valve area is reconstructed by rebuilding the anterior septum.

6.5.3 Prosthesis

In some patients, none of the surgical procedures discussed above will lead to sufficient anatomical and physiological improvement. In these cases, use of a prosthesis should be attempted.

Cotton wool ball. In patients with a mobile but too narrow valve angle, a small cotton wool ball may be placed in the valve angle as a temporary measure (▶ Fig. 6.115).

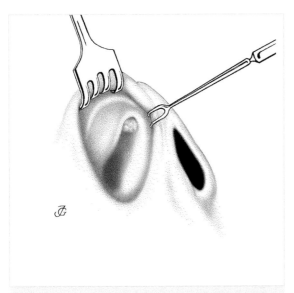

Fig. 6.115 A cotton wool ball is positioned at the valve angle to widen the valve area for diagnostic and therapeutic purposes.

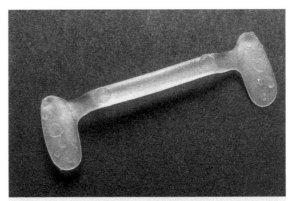

Fig. 6.116 Nozovent prosthesis (after Petruson).

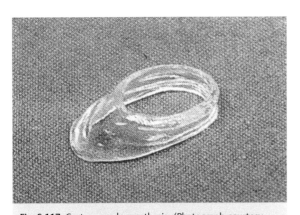

Fig. 6.117 Custom-made prosthesis. (Photograph courtesy Prof. Nolst Trenité.)

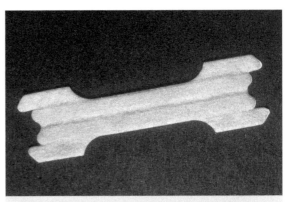

Fig. 6.118 Breathe-Right nasal strip (3 M, St Paul, Minnesota, United States).

Nozovent. Another option is to use a rubber Silastic vestibular dilatator as developed by Petruson (▶ Fig. 6.116). Many patients can be helped by this type of prosthesis during the night.

Custom-made prosthesis. Another option that might be tried is a custom-made prosthesis (▶ Fig. 6.117). Many patients do not tolerate such a device, however.

Breathe-Right nasal strips. A Breathe-Right nasal strip is often effective in cases where the stenosis is limited to the valve area (▶ Fig. 6.118). Care should be taken that the tape is glued at the correct place so that it opens on the valve area.

6.5.4 Complications

Obviously, the complications that may occur following surgery of the valve area are related to the type of surgery performed. The most frequent complication of surgery of the valve proper is stenosis of the valve angle. This serious complication can be avoided by careful suturing of the incisions used to approach the pathology.

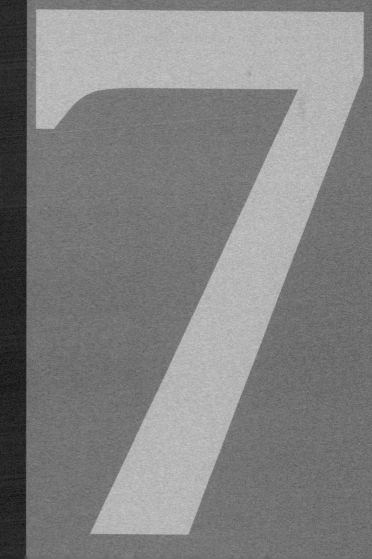

7 Lobular Surgery

7.1 Approaches to the Lobule

7.1.1 The Five Main Approaches: Advantages, Disadvantages, and Indications

The lobule and its cartilages can be approached in different ways. There are five generally accepted techniques:
1. Retrograde (or inversion) technique
2. Luxation (or delivery) technique
3. Infracartilaginous technique
4. External (or open) approach
5. Transcartilaginous (cartilage-splitting) technique

The retrograde and the cartilage-splitting technique are so-called nondelivery methods; whereas the infracartilaginous technique, the luxation technique, and the external approach are delivery methods.

None of these approaches is by definition the best. The choice of method to be used in a given case is based on the type and the degree of the pathology on the one hand, and the surgeon's skill and experience on the other (▶ Table 7.1).

The incisions that are used in these techniques are the intercartilaginous (IC) incision (see ▶ Fig. 7.3), the transcartilaginous incision (see ▶ Fig. 7.19), the infracartilaginous incision (see ▶ Fig. 7.12), and the midcolumellar transverse inverted-V incision (see ▶ Fig. 7.14). Their location and interrelationship is shown in ▶ Fig. 7.1. Outlining the cartilages and marking the two domes will provide helpful landmarks, in particular when the retrograde, the luxation or the infracartilaginous approach is used (▶ Fig. 7.2).

Retrograde (or Inversion) Technique

The retrograde (or inversion) technique is a relatively atraumatic and safe method to address minor deformities and asymmetries of the lobule and the tip. The cranial margin of the lateral crus and dome is inverted through an IC incision and exposed into the vestibule. This is always performed bilaterally to avoid postoperative asymmetry. A triangle or strip of cartilage may then be resected from the cranial margin of the lateral crus and dome. The method only allows limited corrections. It is used to refine a broad tip and supratip, to correct minor asymmetries, and to upwardly rotate the tip, although other techniques of tip rotation are more predictable (▶ Fig. 7.3, ▶ Fig. 7.4, ▶ Fig. 7.5, ▶ Fig. 7.6, and ▶ Fig. 7.7).

Luxation (or Delivery) Technique

The luxation (or delivery) technique is a more traumatic method that allows extensive modification of the lateral crus, dome, and upper part of the medial crus under direct view. The ventral (anterior) side of the lobular cartilage is mobilized supraperichondrially using an IC and an infracartilaginous incision. The medial two-thirds of the lateral crus, the dome, and the upper third of the medial crus are then delivered (luxated) outside the nostril. This is always performed on both sides to avoid postoperative asymmetry. In special cases, the lateral crus is completely dissected out and modified (redraped, rotated upward, or resected and reconstructed (▶ Fig. 7.8, ▶ Fig. 7.9, ▶ Fig. 7.10, and ▶ Fig. 7.11).

The luxation method is much more traumatic than the retrograde technique, and requires meticulous care in dissecting, modifying, and repositioning the cartilages as well as in closing the incisions.

Specific risks are loss of tip support, a drooping tip, and a "polly beak" nose. The technique is the classic way to address more pronounced abnormalities and asymmetries of the lobule. In the last decades, it has been partially replaced by the external approach.

Undermining the lobular skin and exposing the lobular cartilages is done supraperichondrially as close to the perichondrium as possible to avoid damage to the dermis, musculature, and the vascular and nervous supply.

Table 7.1 Advantages, disadvantages, and indications of the five main approaches to the lobule

Technique	Advantages	Disadvantages	Indications
Retrograde	Minimal trauma, relatively safe	Limited effect	Voluminous supratip, minor asymmetries
Luxation	Direct view, both cartilages simultaneously exposed	More trauma, requires special fixation measures	Pronounced tip deformities, modification of lateral crus
Infracartilaginous	Direct view	Limited exposure	Modification of lateral crus
External Approach	Wide overview of lobular cartilages, access to septum	More traumatic, skin complications, external scar	Severe deformities (e.g., cleft lip), revision surgery
Transcartilaginous (Cartilage-splitting)	Limited trauma, relatively safe	Limited possibilities, risk of weakness of lateral nasal wall	Bulbous supratip area

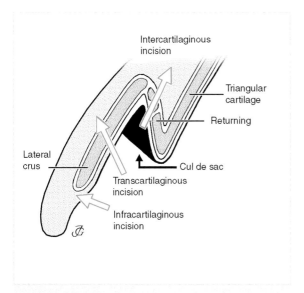

Fig. 7.1 Intercartilaginous (IC), transcartilaginous, and infracartilaginous incision.

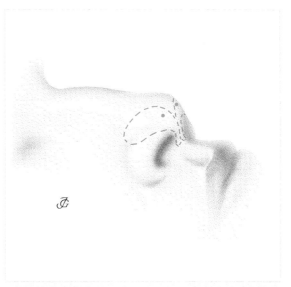

Fig. 7.2 The lobular cartilages are outlined on the skin. The domes are marked.

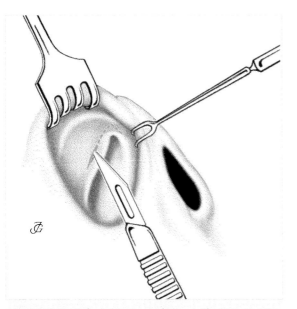

Fig. 7.3 Retrograde or inversion technique I. The IC incision is continued around the valve angle. The sharp angle helps to restore the valve angle in its original position when suturing the incision.

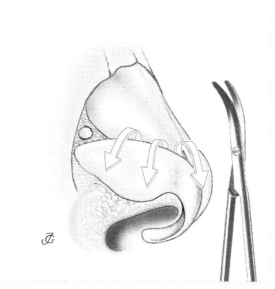

Fig. 7.4 Retrograde or inversion technique II. The skin over the lateral crura, domes, and interdomal area is undermined in a retrograde direction with fully curved, blunt scissors.

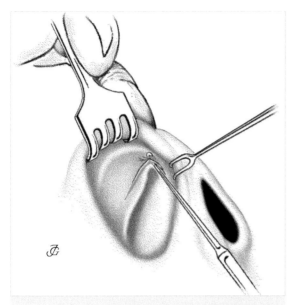

Fig. 7.5 Retrograde or inversion technique III. The dome and lateral crus are pulled caudally and inverted with a round hook that is poked through the cartilage and skin at the cranial margin of the dome.

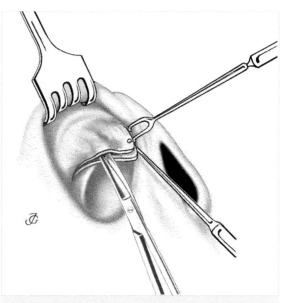

Fig. 7.6 Retrograde or inversion technique IV. The vestibular skin and the perichondrium are dissected from the vestibular side of the inverted cartilage. A cranial strip is then resected from the inverted lateral crus.

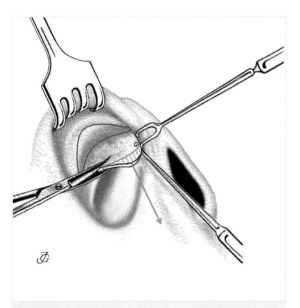

Fig. 7.7 Retrograde or inversion technique V. A cranial strip is resected from the inverted lateral crus to refine upwardly rotate the tip.

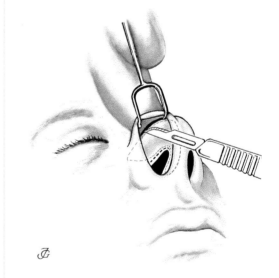

Fig. 7.8 Luxation technique I. IC and infracartilaginous incisions are made to allow dissection and delivery of the lateral crus, dome, and upper part of the medial crus of the lobular cartilage.

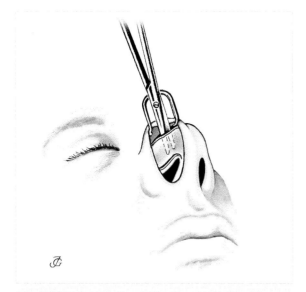

Fig. 7.9 Luxation technique II. The skin over the lateral crura, domes, and upper part of the medial crura is undermined through the infracartilaginous incision.

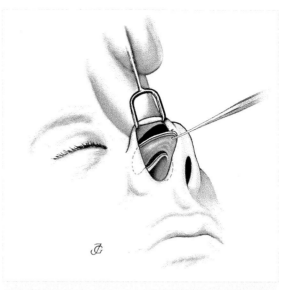

Fig. 7.10 Luxation technique III. The lateral crus and dome are pulled out with a hook poked through the cartilage and skin at the inferior margin of the dome.

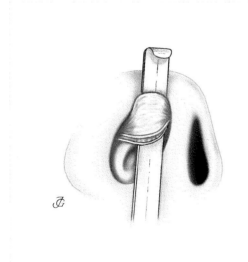

Fig. 7.11 Luxation technique IV. The lateral crus and dome are exposed with the vestibular skin over a Neivert retractor or the flat, back end of a chisel. They can now be modified under direct view.

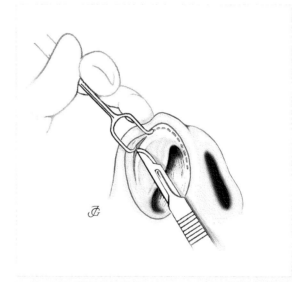

Fig. 7.12 Infracartilaginous technique I. An infracartilaginous incision is made to access the lateral crus and dome.

Infracartilaginous Technique

In this technique, the lateral crura and domes are exposed through an infracartilaginous incision. The infracartilaginous technique gives access to the ala, the lateral crus, and dome, and allows resection, modification, and reinforcement of the cartilage. The incision used in this method is much shorter than in the luxation technique and the external approach. The surgeon may then decide whether this approach is sufficient for the planned lobular surgery or if additional exposure is required, either by a luxation technique or an external approach (▶ Fig. 7.12 and ▶ Fig. 7.13).

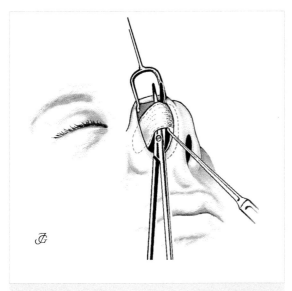

Fig. 7.13 Infracartilaginous technique II. The lateral crus and dome are dissected free using blunt scissors, and delivered by means of a round hook to allow modification under direct view.

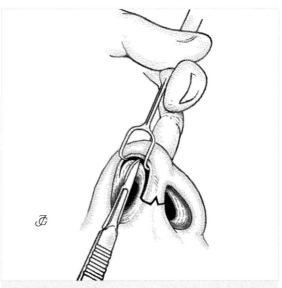

Fig. 7.14 External approach I. A transcolumellar inverted-V incision and bilateral infracartilaginous incisions are made using a No. 15 blade.

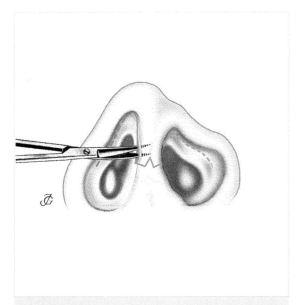

Fig. 7.15 External approach II. The columellar skin is carefully dissected from the caudal margin of the medial crura using pointed, slightly curved scissors.

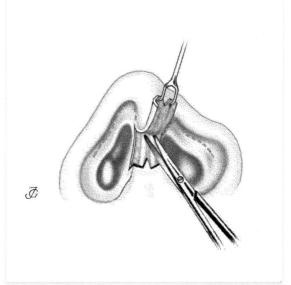

Fig. 7.16 External approach III. Upward dissection of the columellar skin from the medial crura using small, slightly curved scissors or angulated scissors and a delicate, sharp, two-pronged retractor.

External (or Open) Approach

The external (or open) approach implies complete exposure of the lobular cartilages, cartilaginous vault, bony dorsum, and overlying soft tissues. It offers superior exposure of the lobular cartilages, the triangular cartilages, the anterior nasal spine, and the anterior part of the septum. This is particularly important when correcting major deformities. The skin overlying the lobule and the nasal dorsum is elevated via a transcolumellar and two infracartilaginous incisions. The nasal structures are thus more or less "decorticated" or "degloved" (▶ Fig. 7.14, ▶ Fig. 7.15, ▶ Fig. 7.16, ▶ Fig. 7.17, and ▶ Fig. 7.18).

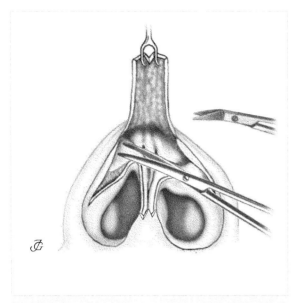

Fig. 7.17 External approach IV. The lobular cartilages and the cartilaginous dorsum are exposed supraperichondrially with pointed, slightly curved scissors or angulated scissors.

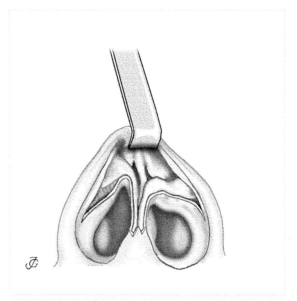

Fig. 7.18 External approach V. The columellar flap is inverted and retracted with a blunt hook.

The external approach gives a much wider access to most nasal structures than the two aforementioned endonasal approaches. At the same time, however, it is also the most traumatic of the five methods. Specific risks are a drooping tip, and necrosis and scarring of the lower end of the columellar flap. Although the external columellar incision remains visible, it is usually not seen unless looked for. Nowadays, the external approach is the method of choice in patients with more severe deformities and asymmetries of the lobule (e.g., cleft lip patients, bifid noses), as well as certain revision surgery. It may also be used to reconstruct the anterior septum in patients with a cartilaginous saddle nose.

Transcartilaginous (Cartilage-Splitting) Technique

The cartilage-splitting (or transcartilaginous) technique is an endonasal nondelivery method that allows resections from the cranial part of the lateral crus and dome (▶ Fig. 7.19). This method primarily aims at volume reduction of the cranial half of the nasal tip. It does not lead to significant rotation of the tip. A minimum of 6 mm of cartilage is left behind.

Too much resection may cause weakness of the lateral nasal wall, and inspiratory collapse. The resections should be carried out symmetrically, especially of the domes, as different heights of the remaining cartilages may lead to asymmetric buckling, "bossae," and tip asymmetry. These are the main drawbacks of the method.

First the vestibular skin is incised parallel to the lower margin of the lateral crus at a distance of about 6 mm,

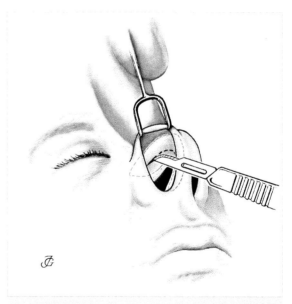

Fig. 7.19 Cartilage-splitting technique. A transcartilaginous incision is made 6 mm cranial to the caudal margin of the lateral crus using a No. 15 blade.

and dissected off the vestibular surface of the cartilage. Bilateral placement of fine needles from the outside into the vestibule at the level of the planned incisions may help obtain a symmetrical approach.

A strip of cartilage from the cranial part of the lateral crura (and domes) is then removed, leaving cartilage of sufficient width (minimum 6 mm) behind.

7.1.2 Surgical Techniques

Retrograde (or Inversion) Technique

The retrograde or inversion technique allows narrowing and upward rotation of the nasal tip. Bilateral resection of a cranial triangle of cartilage rotates the nasal tip somewhat upwards. In practice, this effect may be disappointing, however. Generally speaking, refinement and upward rotation of the nasal tip may be achieved in a more predictable way by other techniques.

The method requires a bilateral IC incision and undermining of the cartilaginous dorsum and the lobule. The modifications that can be achieved by this approach are limited. However, the procedure is relatively atraumatic and safe. The main risk is postoperative asymmetry.

Steps

- The domes and the margins of the lateral and medial crura are marked on the skin (▶ Fig. 7.2).
- IC incisions are made bilaterally and continued around the valve angle, preferably in an angled fashion. This helps to restore the valve angle in its original position when suturing the incision (▶ Fig. 7.3).
- The skin over the cartilaginous and the lower half of the bony dorsum is undermined with slightly curved, blunt scissors.
- The skin of the lobule over the lateral crura and domes is undermined in a retrograde direction with fully curved, blunt scissors (▶ Fig. 7.4). We do not undermine far laterally to avoid cutting the fibers of the dilator muscle that insert at the lateral end of the lateral crus. Cutting these fibers would increase the inspiratory collapsibility of the ala as the dilator muscle contracts during inspiration.
- The connective tissue between the domes and the upper part of the medial crura is slightly loosened. This should be done in a conservative way to avoid postoperative drooping of the tip.
- The ala is lifted with a blunt four-pronged retractor and inverted by pressure of the middle finger. The cranial margin of the dome is then grabbed with a sharp, round hook using the marks on the skin as points of reference. The hook is poked through the cartilage and the vestibular skin (▶ Fig. 7.5). The dome can then be pulled downward and inverted.
- The vestibular skin is subperichondrially dissected from the cranial margin of the cartilage with pointed scissors (▶ Fig. 7.6).
- The cranial margin of the lateral crus and the dome is now exposed and may be modified by resecting a cranial strip as required to narrow and/or upwardly rotate the tip (▶ Fig. 7.7).

Luxation (or Delivery) Technique

The luxation or delivery technique is a classic way to deal with abnormalities of the lobule, in particular of the tip and alae. The technique was developed in the 1940s and further refined in the 1950s. The lateral crura, domes, and the upper part of the medial crura are dissected on both sides and delivered outside the nostril. To this end, IC and infracartilaginous incisions are made bilaterally. The cartilages are exposed on a flat instrument (back end of a chisel or a Neivert retractor). The vestibular skin remains attached to cartilage. The lateral crura, domes, and the upper part of the medial crura can now be modified under direct view, as required. One risk specific to the luxation technique is loss of tip support. When wide exposure is required, a columellar strut may be inserted at the end of the operation to preserve support.

Steps

- The lobular cartilages are outlined on the skin; the domes are marked (see ▶ Fig. 7.2).
- IC incisions are made bilaterally and continued around the valve angle, preferably in an angled fashion (see ▶ Fig. 7.3).
- If wide exposure is required, the two IC incisions are continued downward in front of the caudal septum about halfway across the membranous septum (so-called transfixion; see ▶ Fig. 4.23).
- The skin over the cartilaginous and lower part of the bony dorsum is undermined. The skin over the lateral crura, domes, and medial crura is elevated in a retrograde direction with fully curved, blunt scissors (see ▶ Fig. 7.4).
- Infracartilaginous incisions are made on both sides with a No. 15 blade. The ala is inverted, for example with a two-pronged, sharp–dull (right side) or dull–sharp (left side) hook, while counterpressure is given by the middle finger of the left hand (▶ Fig. 7.8).
- The lower margin of the lateral crus is identified. The incision is started laterally and follows precisely the caudal margin of the cartilage (for details see Chapter 4, page 144).
- The incision is opened with slightly curved, pointed scissors. The skin over the lateral crus and dome is then supraperichondrially undermined with slightly curved, blunt scissors (▶ Fig. 7.9).
- A curved hook is poked through the skin and cartilage at the caudal margin of the dome. The cartilage is pulled downward and luxated out of the nostril (▶ Fig. 7.10).
- A flat instrument (the back end of a chisel or a Neivert retractor) is introduced through the IC incision to expose the cartilage (▶ Fig. 7.11). Care is taken to avoid overstretching or tearing the cartilage and the vestibular skin.
- The procedure is carried out again on the other side.
- Both cartilages can now be inspected and compared. They are modified as required by the pathology and the desired changes (for techniques see page 272).

Infracartilaginous Technique

The infracartilaginous technique may be used to address and correct deformities of the ala, the lateral crus, and the dome. As exposure is limited to the lateral crus, the method offers fewer possibilities but is at the same time less traumatic than the luxation technique or the external approach.

Steps

- The domes and the margins of the lateral and medial crura are marked on the skin (▶ Fig. 7.2).
- An infracartilaginous incision is made from lateral to medial using a No. 15 blade. The lower part of the ala is inverted with a sharp–dull two-pronged hook in combination with counterpressure of the middle finger of the left hand (▶ Fig. 7.12).
- The caudal margin of the lateral crus is identified and the skin is incised from lateral to medial. Care is taken to not incise the cartilage. After the first millimeters of the incision have been made, the hook is replaced more medially and the incision is continued (▶ Fig. 7.12).
- When the dome is reached, some extra pressure by the middle finger is needed to expose the ventricle of the vestibule.
- The incision is then continued for a few millimeters along the margin of the medial crus.
- The lateral crus and dome are now supraperichondrially dissected free from the overlying lobular skin with slightly curved, blunt scissors. The vestibular skin remains attached to the cartilage (▶ Fig. 7.13).
- The lateral crus and dome are now delivered by pulling the cartilage in a caudal direction by means of a round hook that is poked through the skin and the cartilage at the inferior margin of the dome.
- The cartilage is now exposed and resection, modification, and reinforcement may be carried out.

External Approach

The external or open approach is a recently redeveloped method to expose the lobular cartilages, cartilaginous vault, and anterior septum. The method originally dates from the 1920s, but was revived and refined in the 1980s.

Although more traumatic than the previously discussed approaches, the external approach is definitely the method of choice to address more pronounced deformities of the lobule. The technique has also proven its value in reconstructing the anterior septum, as demonstrated by Rettinger (1993).

Steps

- The incision is outlined.
- A transverse inverted-V incision is made in the columella one-third of the distance from its base using a No. 15 blade (▶ Fig. 7.14). Care is taken to avoid cutting into the medial crura.
- The medial leg of the infracartilaginous incision is made bilaterally. This part of the incision is made over the middle of the cartilage instead of at its caudal margin, to avoid postoperative retraction of the columella (▶ Fig. 7.14) (see Chapter 4, page 146).
- The columellar skin is gently dissected from the medial crura by pointed, slightly curved scissors through the lower end of the infracartilaginous incision (▶ Fig. 7.15).
- The columellar skin is separated from the medial crura in an upward direction, while the skin is gently lifted up with a delicate nontraumatic forceps or a small, sharp, two-pronged retractor (▶ Fig. 7.16). Damage to the skin and the soft tissues is avoided as much as possible to prevent postoperative scarring and retraction. Bleeding vessels (the columellar artery and its branches) are, for that reason, cauterized with utmost precision using bipolar coagulation.
- The skin over the domes is elevated supraperichondrially, while the infracartilaginous incision is continued in a lateral direction, following the caudal margin of the dome and lateral crus (▶ Fig. 7.17).
- The columellar flap is inverted and retracted with a blunt, angulated retractor (▶ Fig. 7.18).
- The lateral crura are exposed by continuing the dissection in a lateral direction, using slightly curved, blunt scissors or angulated scissors.
- The lobular cartilages are almost completely exposed. They may be modified while in position. They can also be dissected from the underlying vestibular skin and then either modified and fixed into another position, or resected and reconstructed.
- The incisions are carefully closed with a monofilament 5–0 or 6–0 suture, avoiding traction and ischemia. The transverse columellar incision is closed first.
- An internal dressing with ointment is applied in the vestibule. The lobule is externally taped to support the tissues in their new position and to prevent swelling and hematoma.

1920s: Sir Harold Gillies (London) introduces the "elephant trunk" pedicled flap that he developed to correct facial war injuries in British soldiers.

1929, 1933: Aurel Réthi (Budapest) introduces a high horizontal columellar incision for surgery of the lobular cartilages, the cartilaginous and bony dorsum, and for inserting a dorsal implant.

1938: EC Padget, very likely unaware of the publications in German by Réthi, describes "cross-cutting the columella and undermining the skin covering the tip and dorsum," and speaks of an "external exposure."

1951: H May publishes on "Réthi's incision."

1958, 1962: Ante Šerçer (Zagreb) uses a midcolumellar horizontal incision in combination with bilateral endonasal incisions, and elevates the skin up to the nasion to correct the nasal pyramid and lobule. He speaks of "decortication of the nose."

1960, 1966, 1972: Ivo Padovan (pupil and successor of Šerçer at Zagreb) and his pupil Jugo (New York) continue using this technique and introduce a V-shaped incision at the columellar base. In 1970, Padovan reports on this approach at the American Academy of Facial Plastic and Reconstructive Surgery (AAFPRS) in New York.

1970s: North American surgeons, especially Anderson (New Orleans), Goodman (Toronto) and Adamson (Toronto), further explore the potentials of the method.

1980s: Although controversial in the beginning, the "external approach" soon gained worldwide recognition as one of the standard approaches in nasal surgery. Some rhinosurgeons like to call the technique the "open (structure) rhinoplasty."

Transcartilaginous (Cartilage-Splitting) Technique

In the cartilage-splitting or transcartilaginous technique, the lobule is approached through a bilateral incision of the vestibular skin and the lateral crus (▶ Fig. 7.1 and ▶ Fig. 7.19). The incision is usually made at a distance of 6 mm from the caudal margin of the lateral crus. A so-called continuous strip of (lateral) cartilage is kept intact. This approach allows resection of a strip from the cranial margin of the lateral crus and dome to narrow a bulbous lobule and tip. At the same time, the tip may be rotated upward. The technique is relatively atraumatic. The level of the incision is of utmost importance. If it is too low, too much of the lateral crus will be resected, leaving a weak and depressed area which might cause inspiratory obstruction and a pinched-nose appearance.

Steps

- The lobular cartilages are outlined on the lobular skin (▶ Fig. 7.2).
- The endonasal incisions to be made in the vestibular skin are marked. They are usually made at a distance of about 6 mm from the lower margin of the lateral crus.
- The lateral wall of the vestibulum is subcutaneously injected with lidocaine–adrenaline to facilitate the next steps.
- The incisions are made in the vestibular skin only (▶ Fig. 7.19).
- The skin is dissected from the inside of the lateral crus in a cranial direction.
- The lateral crus and dome are incised endonasally under direct view and simultaneous outside control.
- The vertical dimension of the lateral crura and the domes is shortened under direct view as required. Care is taken to leave a strip of cartilage at least 6 mm in width.
- Resection of a small wedge at the domes has been advocated to (further) narrow the tip. This does not always lead to the desired degree of tip narrowing, however, and carries a relatively high risk of tip notching and asymmetry. Tip narrowing and tip rotation can be achieved more safely through one of the other techniques in combination with domal sutures.
- The incision is closed with resorbable sutures. A vestibular dressing is usually not needed. The lobule is taped in the usual way.

7.2 Tip Surgery

Surgery of the nasal tip is an important aspect of rhinoplasty. Most textbooks and instructional courses devote more attention to the surgical modification of this part of the nose than to any other nasal structure. Changing shape, volume, projection, and rotation of the tip is indeed of great importance for a pleasing outcome. Tip surgery should, however, never compromise nasal function. The nasal surgeon will first of all try to correct the septal pyramid and lobular pathology in order to restore normal anatomy and thereby physiology. Tip surgery for aesthetic purposes is secondary, but can go hand in hand with functional aspects.

7.2.1 Characteristics of the Tip

The nasal tip may be defined as the most prominent point or area of the external nasal pyramid. The tip has been defined (Sheen and others) by four landmarks: the *supratip breakpoint*, the left and the right *dome*, and the *tip–columellar breakpoint*. More recently, two important angles have also been added: the *angle of divergence* (the separation between the two intermediate crura), and *the angle of rotation* (the angle between the tip and the ventral end of the columella).

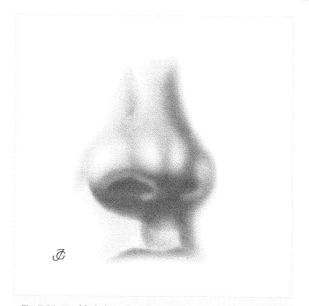

Fig. 7.20 Double light reflex of the tip.

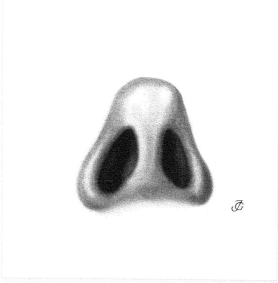

Fig. 7.21 Double light reflex of the tip.

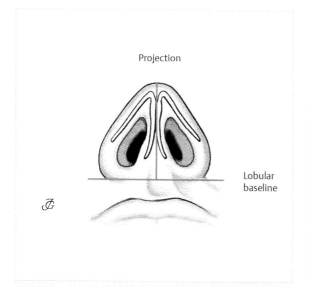

Fig. 7.22 Projection (prominence, salience) of the tip in relation to the lobular base line.

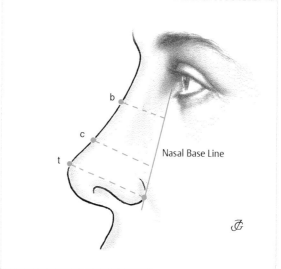

Fig. 7.23 Projection of the tip (t), and prominence of the cartilaginous (c) and bony (b) pyramid in relation to the NBL.

Definition

The nasal tip is defined by the two domes. Ideally, the two domes should not be visible as separate structures. On palpation they are usually easily distinguishable and they produce a double light reflex (▶ Fig. 7.20 and ▶ Fig. 7.21).

Projection

Tip projection, also called *tip prominence* (or salience), is determined by several factors, in particular, genetic influences (ethnicity, gender), age, trauma, infection, and previous surgery. Tip prominence is high in the prominent-narrow pyramid syndrome and low in the low-wide pyramid syndrome or saddle nose.

Tip projection may be related to:
- The lobular base line (▶ Fig. 7.22)
- The nasal base line (NBL) (▶ Fig. 7.23)
- The prominence of the bony and cartilaginous pyramid (▶ Fig. 7.23)
- Nasal length (nasion–tip distance) (see ▶ Fig. 1.12)

According to today's "beauty standard" for the Caucasian population, tip projection should be less than 0.6 of nasal length.

Position

The position of the tip in the vertical and horizontal axes of the face is determined by the aforementioned factors. If the tip is more cranial than normal, we speak of an upwardly rotated tip. If it is more caudal than average, we speak of a low, pendant, or drooping tip. In cases with an upwardly rotated tip, the nasolabial angle is large. If the tip is pendant, this angle is smaller than average.

Nasolabial Angle and Tip Rotation

The nasolabial angle has traditionally been accepted as the parameter for tip rotation. It is defined by the line from the subnasale to the upper lip vermilion border, and the tangent from the subnasale along the inferior border of the columella, or the line between the subnasale and the most ventral (anterior) point on the columella (Papel 2009). Yet, both the precise location of the subnasale (the point where the columella merges with the upper lip) and the most anterior point of the columella may be difficult to define, especially in patients with a curved transition between the upper lip and columella and a curved columella. The tip rotation angle has been suggested as an alternative parameter and more accurate measure. It is defined by the line between the long axis of the nostril and the Frankfurt horizontal plane.

Desirable Tip Rotation

It is generally accepted that a nasolabial angle in the range of 90 to 95° in men and 95 to 105° in women is perceived as attractive. These measures only offer a rule of thumb, however, as the desirable degree of tip rotation depends on ethnicity, gender, facial proportions, body height, culture, and personal preference. Many agree that in the past, nasal surgeons have often excessively increased tip rotation, answering to locally preferent aesthetic percepts. In a recent study based on modified profile photographs, 171 volunteers representing the general public in California ranked nasolabial angles of 104° and 108° as most attractive in women. Angles of 116° and 96° were rated least attractive (Biller and Kim 2009). Still, depending on facial proportions, more or less rotation of the tip may be preferred by individual patients. An earlier study also using computer-modified photographs indicated that over-rotation of the tip was preferred to tip droop (Mendelsohn and Farrel 1995). In both studies, the ratings were found to be poorly reproducible and inconsistent, however. Therefore, the surgeon should respect the patient's preference rather than aiming for a "standard ideal nose" (Tasman et al 2012).

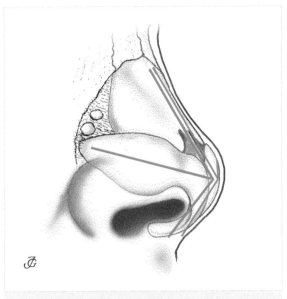

Fig. 7.24 Tripod configuration of tip support.

Desirable Nasolabial Angle

In a recent study, a nasolabial angle of 96° in men and 98° in women was considered the most attractive (Mendelsohn and Farrel 1995). In this study, the difference between men and women was smaller than in earlier reports.

7.2.2 Mechanics of the Tip

The nasal tip is often compared with a tripod. The concept of the single tripod was introduced by Anderson in 1969 and adopted and propagated by others as it helps understand the effect of certain modifications of the lobule on the position of the tip. In this idea, the two medial crura form the medial leg of the tripod, while the lateral crura form the second and third legs (▶ Fig. 7.24).

The medial crura and their neighboring soft tissues are essential in keeping up the tip. The main factors determining the supporting capacity are the rigidity and length of the paracrural connective tissue fibers, the connective tissue fibers of the septocrural area, the membranous septum, and the depressor septi muscle.

The support provided by the second leg is dependent upon the length and rigidity of the lateral crura and on the connection between the lateral crus and the triangular cartilage. The rigidity and elasticity of the caudal part of the cartilaginous septum is the third factor determining the strength of the tip-supporting tripod.

In the past, several authors have assumed the presence of transverse interdomal (sometimes called Pitanguy ligament), intercrural, and septocrural fibers. Histological studies have shown, however, that there are no interdomal and intercrural or septocrural fibers or ligaments, as could be expected if one takes the embryological development of the nose into account (Zhai et al 1995, 1996) (see ▸ Fig. 1.98, ▸ Fig. 1.99, ▸ Fig. 1.100, ▸ Fig. 1.101, ▸ Fig. 1.102, and ▸ Fig. 1.108, ▸ Fig. 1.109, and ▸ Fig. 1.110).

7.2.3 Deformities, Abnormalities, and Variations of the Tip and Their Surgical Correction

The human nasal tip is subject to a wide array of deformities, abnormalities, and anatomical variations. Whether we are dealing with a deformity is rarely a matter of discussion. Congenital malformations like those in a patient with a cleft lip, nasal hypoplasia, and bifidity are deformities. The same applies to pronounced lesions due to car accidents, bite injuries, or tumor removal. Whether a less pronounced anomaly is to be considered an "abnormality" or a "variation" may be more difficult to decide. This is often a matter of taste. We should keep in mind that several of the variations described here are, to a certain extent, race-dependent and therefore have to be considered as normal ethnic variations of the human nose.

It is sometimes said that it is the patient who decides whether the nasal tip is abnormal or not. Although understandable, this way of thinking may also be dangerous. It is necessary to warn against surgery that intends to make a "normal" nasal tip look "more beautiful."

The most common variations and deformities of the nasal tip have already been described and illustrated in Chapter 2 (page 88). In this section we briefly discuss the most common deformities and abnormalities in relation to the most important tip-modifying procedures.

Many of the deformities, abnormalities, and variations occur in combination. An amorphous tip is often underprojected at the same time, while an upwardly rotated tip is frequently overprojected.

Broad, Bulbous (Amorphous), Square, and Ball Tip

The tip is not well defined. This group includes the broad (wide) tip, the bulbous (amorphous) tip, the square tip, and the ball tip. In the broad tip, the domes are far apart. In the bulbous or amorphous tip, they are wide and massive. In the square tip, they are not arch-shaped but rectangular. In the ball tip, the domes are rounded. It should be stressed that these variations and abnormalities are not solely due to the form and thickness of the cartilage. The thickness of the lobular skin and the subcutaneous soft-tissue layers is another important factor (see ▸ Fig. 2.69, ▸ Fig. 2.70, and ▸ Fig. 2.71).

In all these cases, the tip might be given more definition by a narrowing procedure, as required. Function

should not be compromised. The continuity of the domes is therefore either respected or reconstructed.

Bifid Tip

The tip is duplicated due to an abnormally large distance between the two domes with an excessive amount of interdomal connective tissue. There is mostly a vertical groove or depression between the domes and in the columella (see ▸ Fig. 2.72). This abnormality is usually congenital and is the result of incomplete fusion of the two nasal primordia, although it may also be due to previous surgery. The congenital bifid tip illustrates the inaccuracy of the concept expressed by some surgeons that there is a transverse interdomal and intercrural ligament. This deformity requires dissection and repositioning of the lobular cartilages through an external or an endonasal approach.

Asymmetrical Tip

The domes are asymmetrical. This may occur as an isolated variation or deformity, in combination with bifidity, or as part of an asymmetrical lobule (see ▸ Fig. 2.73).

Underprojected Tip

The projection of the tip is abnormally low compared with that of the cartilaginous and bony pyramid. The tip is not the most prominent part of the external nasal pyramid; it is depressed and usually more flat. Tip support is mostly diminished (see ▸ Fig. 2.75). This abnormality usually requires a complete septorhinoplasty. Depending on the pathology, the anterior septum has to be exorotated or reconstructed. The projection of the domes may be increased by redraping the lobular cartilages or inserting a columellar strut, or by applying a tip or shield graft.

Overprojected Tip

The tip is abnormally prominent compared with the projection of the cartilaginous and bony dorsum. The nasolabial angle is mostly decreased (see ▸ Fig. 2.74). This condition usually requires a complete septorhinoplasty. The projection of the anterior septum may be reduced, while the projection of the domes may be diminished by redraping the lobular cartilages or by minor resections.

Upwardly Rotated Tip

The tip is more cranial than normal. An upwardly rotated tip is usually also overprojected. The nasolabial angle is abnormally large (see ▸ Fig. 2.76).

Hanging (Pendant, Drooping) Tip

The tip is more caudal than normal and underprojected at the same time. The nasolabial angle is abnormally small (see ▶ Fig. 2.77). A pendant tip is often seen in elderly individuals, combined with a long nose. A pendant, low tip is also a standard feature of the long, slightly humped Arabic nose.

7.2.4 Surgical Techniques

The number of tip-modifying techniques is almost endless. Many of them have proven their value. Some of them bear rather high risks. It is difficult for the beginner to find the right path in the vast literature.

First of all, it is important to realize that there is no such thing as the best technique. The type and severity of the deformity, on the one hand, and the skill and experience of the surgeon, on the other, should determine which technique is the most appropriate and safe in a given patient.

> "It is not so much what you resect but what you leave behind." (Eugene B. Kern)

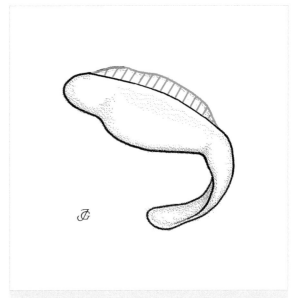

Fig. 7.25 Narrowing (and slightly upwardly rotating) the lobule and tip by resecting a cranial strip from the lateral crus. This may be achieved by the retrograde, the infracartilaginous and the luxation technique, as well as by the transcartilaginous technique and the external approach.

Narrowing the Tip and Supratip Area

The nasal tip and the lobule may be narrowed by:
1. Resecting a strip of cartilage from the cranial margin of the lateral crus
2. Suturing the domes together
3. Redraping the lobular cartilage

The method chosen depends upon the type of pathology, the surgical goals, and the personal preference of the surgeon.

Resecting a Strip of Cartilage from the Cranial Margin of the Lateral Crus

A strip of cartilage (▶ Fig. 7.25) can be resected from the cranial margin of the lateral crus and dome either by a nondelivery approach (retrograde technique or cartilage-splitting technique) or by a delivery approach (infracartilaginous technique, luxation technique or external approach).

The retrograde (or inversion) technique may be chosen when only a small degree of narrowing is required. The cartilage-splitting technique may be used when a larger resection is planned. The infracartilaginous and the luxation techniques have the advantage of working under direct view, albeit with the alar cartilages not in their anatomical position. The external approach has the advantage of combining direct view with an unaltered position of the alar cartilages.

Steps

- IC incisions are made in the usual way (see ▶ Fig. 7.3). The skin over the dorsum and lobule is undermined (see ▶ Fig. 7.4).
- The dome and lateral crus are pulled caudally and inverted with a round hook that is poked through the cartilage and the skin at the cranial margin of the dome (see ▶ Fig. 7.5).
- The cranial margin of the lateral crus and dome is now exposed (see ▶ Fig. 7.6).
- A cranial strip of cartilage is now resected (▶ Fig. 7.25).
- The hook is removed and the cartilage is repositioned. The effect of the resection is judged by gentle palpation with the index finger, or with the thumb and index finger (▶ Fig. 7.26).
- The other side is corrected in the same (usually symmetrical) way.
- If more narrowing is indicated, an extra sliver of cartilage may be resected. Apart from a strip of cartilage, a tiny triangular strip of skin may be removed to shorten the nose or upwardly rotate the tip. The amount of skin resected must always be less than the amount of cartilage removed to avoid uncontrolled retraction.
- One should always remove a small amount of cartilage (and skin) at one time. The effect of the previous resection must first be assessed and bilaterally compared before any further tissue is removed.

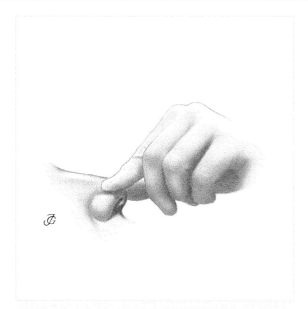

Fig. 7.26 The effect is assessed by inspection and palpation.

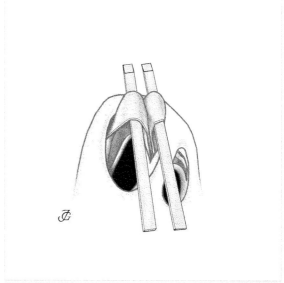

Fig. 7.27 Delivery of both domes through the right nostril and presentation over the back side of two 4-mm chisels to allow modification under direct view.

- The IC incisions are closed by two 4–0 resorbable sutures. The modified lobule is supported by an internal dressing and secured in its new form and position by a "tip-narrowing tape" and by "pressure tapes" (see ▶ Fig. 10.4, ▶ Fig. 10.6).

Note

- Take great care to resect in a symmetrical way (unless an asymmetry was present preoperatively).
- Do not resect too much medially, as this will give the tip a "pinched" appearance.
- Do not resect too much laterally, as this may weaken the lateral nasal wall, which may lead to depression of the lateral membranous area and inspiratory collapse.

Suturing the Domes Together

The tip may also be narrowed by bringing the domes together. This may be done either by the luxation technique, by the infracartilaginous technique, or by an external approach. We describe and illustrate this procedure using the luxation technique.

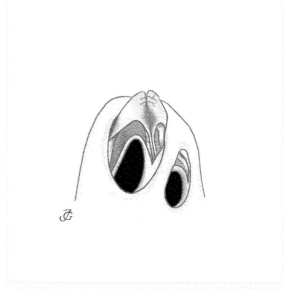

Fig. 7.28 The two domes are sutured together by two interdomal sutures and an intercrural suture.

Steps

- The lateral crura and domes are delivered end exposed.
- The right and the left dome are both delivered through the right nostril (▶ Fig. 7.27).
- The size and shape of the lateral crus and dome are adjusted, if required.
- Excessive interdomal connective tissue is resected, if necessary.

- Both domes are brought together by a preliminary suture. They are then replaced, and the result is assessed visually and by palpation.
- Both domes are delivered again and further adjusted if necessary. A second (and third) 5–0 non-resorbable (or slowly resorbable) suture and a high intercrural suture are applied for final fixation (▶ Fig. 7.28).

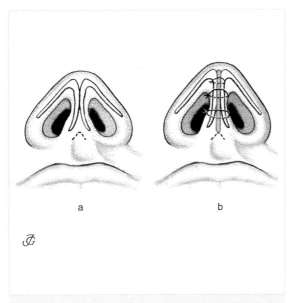

Fig. 7.29 a, b Increasing tip projection with a columellar strut using the endonasal approach.

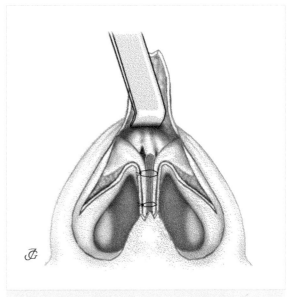

Fig. 7.30 Increasing tip projection with a columellar strut using the external approach.

Redraping the Lobular Cartilage

The domes may also be brought closer together by redraping the lobular cartilages using the so-called lateral crural steal technique. The lateral crura and domes are dissected free, modified where necessary, and repositioned. The domes are thereby brought together and fixed in a more prominent position. The surgical steps are described below under the heading *Increasing Tip Projection* (see ▶ Fig. 7.34, ▶ Fig. 7.35, ▶ Fig. 7.36, and ▶ Fig. 7.37).

Increasing Tip Projection

The projection of the nasal tip may be increased by:
1. A columellar strut (in combination with anterior septal reconstruction)
2. A tip graft (and a shield graft)
3. Redraping of the lateral crura and domes with lateral crural steal

The choice of method should depend primarily upon the underlying pathology. A broad lobule with a depressed tip may be addressed by reconstruction of the septum, reinforcement of the retracted columella, and an additional transplant in the tip and supratip area. A congenitally low, broad lobule with a flat, broad tip will be dealt with by the external approach with dissection, modification, and repositioning of the lobular cartilage.

Columellar Strut (Combined with Anterior Septal Reconstruction)

This technique is the method of choice in patients with a depressed tip due to retraction of the columella as a result of a missing anterior septum or (mostly surgical) trauma to the medial crura. In cases with severe pathology, the external approach is the best way to address the problem. However, in patients with moderate abnormalities, the endonasal approach through a caudal septal incision (CSI) usually provides sufficient access.

Steps

- The anterior septum is dissected and exposed. The medial crura are freed. When the endonasal approach is used, an intercrural (columellar) pocket is created by retrograde dissection with strongly curved scissors (see ▶ Fig. 7.68). The anterior nasal spine is exposed.
- The anterior septum is reconstructed.
- A batten (also called "strut") of septal cartilage about 3 mm in width and 20 to 25 mm in length is positioned on the anterior nasal spine between the medial crura. The strut is fixed to the crura by two or three transverse, slowly resorbable sutures. The two domes are hereby brought in a somewhat more prominent position (▶ Fig. 7.29 and ▶ Fig. 7.30).
- When the surgery is performed through a CSI, transcolumellar mattress sutures are applied for fixation.
- The upper end of the strut is lowered (if necessary) just below the level of the domes with small scissors. This prevents its end from becoming visible and palpable.

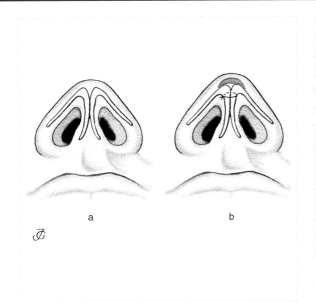

Fig. 7.31 **a, b** Increasing tip projection by a tip graft.

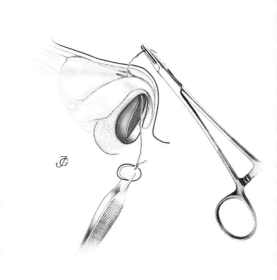

Fig. 7.32 Increasing tip projection by a tip graft. When the endonasal approach is used, the tip graft is brought into position through the CSI using an interdomal guide suture.

Tip Graft and Shield Graft

A relatively simple means to increase tip projection is with a tip graft. A single or double graft of auricular or septal cartilage is inserted and fixed in place on top of the two domes (▶ Fig. 7.31 and ▶ Fig. 7.32). This may be combined with a shield graft (▶ Fig. 7.33). The early effects of this technique are better than the long-term results, as an unpredictable amount of resorption of the cartilage will eventually take place. Besides, these transplants may become visible in patients with a thin skin.

External Approach

Steps

- Tip and shield grafts can be best positioned and fixed under direct view using the external approach (▶ Fig. 7.33). Tip grafts can also be applied through a CSI, however (▶ Fig. 7.32). See the following text.
- The grafts are sculpted according to requirements.
- They are sutured to the domes with two 5–0 or 6–0 slowly resorbable sutures. A one-layer, two-layer, or even three-layer transplant may be applied, as required. Care is taken to ensure that all edges of the graft are smooth.

Endonasal Approach

Steps

- A tip graft can also be applied through a CSI.
- A small subcutaneous pocket is created over the domes with blunt scissors, which are introduced through the upper part of the CSI, to accommodate the graft (see ▶ Fig. 5.4).
- The graft is brought into position with an interdomal guide suture (▶ Fig. 7.32) and fixed by external taping.

Fig. 7.33 Increasing tip projection by a tip and a shield graft fixed in position with two or three 5–0 slowly resorbable sutures (external approach).

Note

Some surgeons prefer to use nonresorbable sutures to fix a tip and a shield graft. Others, ourselves included, favor slowly resorbable materials to avoid late extrusion of nonresorbable sutures through the skin.

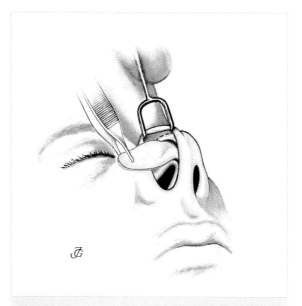

Fig. 7.34 Increasing tip projection by redraping the lateral crus and the dome I. The lateral crus and dome are exposed using the infracartilaginous or the luxation technique.

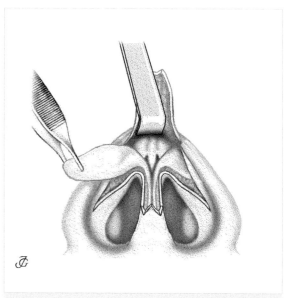

Fig. 7.35 Increasing tip projection by redraping the lateral crus and the dome II. The lateral crus and the dome are dissected from the underlying vestibular skin. The medial crura remain attached to the skin and soft-tissues (external approach).

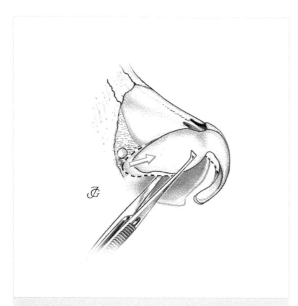

Fig. 7.36 Increasing tip projection by redraping the lateral crus and the dome III. The lateral crus and the dome are redraped and fixed in a medial direction to increase tip projection.

Redraping the Lateral Crus and Dome with Lateral Crural Steal

Redraping the lateral crus and dome with lateral crural steal is an elegant way to narrow the tip and increase its projection. The technique is performed by either the external approach or the luxation technique. This method is more sophisticated but also more risky than the previously described methods.

Steps

- The lobular cartilages are exposed in the usual way with the luxation technique (▶ Fig. 7.34) or the external approach (▶ Fig. 7.35).
- The lateral crus and the dome are dissected from the underlying vestibular skin with small scissors. The medial crura remain attached to the soft-tissue structures.
- The cartilage is modified as required.
- It is then repositioned or "redraped" into the desired position (▶ Fig. 7.36 and ▶ Fig. 7.37a). The lateral crura are moved in a ventral direction. New, more projecting domes are created by "stealing" cartilage from the lateral crura.
- The cartilages are sutured together in their new position with a transcrural and a transdomal 5–0 nonresorbable suture (▶ Fig. 7.37b).
- A tip and/or a shield graft may be added as required.

Note

The redraping technique also allows repositioning of the lateral crura more cranially. This may be done to reestablish contact between the cranial margin of the lateral crus and the triangular cartilage in cases where this relationship has been lost. In this way, the lateral nasal wall is made more resistant to inspiratory collapse (see ▶ Fig. 7.46, ▶ Fig. 7.47, and ▶ Fig. 7.48).

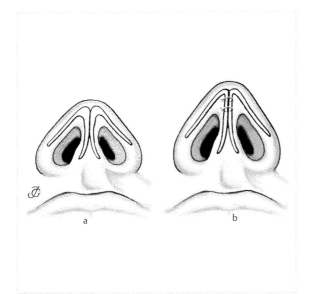

Fig. 7.37 **a, b** Tip projection is increased by redraping the lateral crura with lateral crural steal, and bringing the domes together.

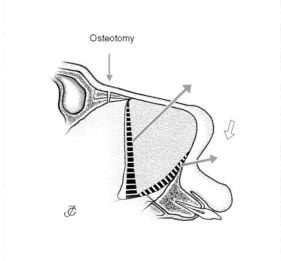

Osteotomy

Fig. 7.38 Decreasing tip projection by let-down (or push-down) of the whole nasal pyramid. This is accomplished by resecting a horizontal basal strip and a triangular vertical strip from the cartilaginous septum, and performing osteotomies with bilateral wedge resections.

Reducing Tip Projection

Nasal tip projection may be reduced in various ways:
1. Let-down of the pyramid and lobule
2. Lowering the domes by the dome resection–reconstruction technique
3. Resecting strips from the medial crura

The method chosen will, as always, depend upon the pathology. If the overprojected tip is part of a prominent, narrow pyramid, a let-down of the whole pyramid is the best technique. If an overprojected tip is combined with asymmetry of the domes, partial resection and reconstruction of the domes is a logical choice. If the domes are symmetrical, we prefer to preserve them. Shortening the medial crura may then be the better choice.

Let-Down of the Pyramid and Lobule

When an overprojected tip is part of a prominent-narrow pyramid syndrome, the bony and cartilaginous vault and the lobule are lowered by removing a horizontal basal and a vertical triangular strip from the septum and performing bilateral resection of bony wedges at the base of the bony pyramid (► Fig. 7.38). Let-down of the bony and the cartilaginous pyramid will broaden the lobule and reduce tip projection. For a discussion of this technique, see Chapter 6, page 227.

Lowering the Domes by the Dome Resection–Reconstruction Technique

Nasal tip projection can also be reduced by resecting small strips of cartilage just beneath the domes. Since the domes are critical to tip definition and tip position, immediate restitution of their integrity is mandatory. Otherwise, the result will be a cosmetic and functional disaster. The main risk of this technique is a pinched nose due to the loss of spring of the domal vault (see ► Fig. 9.82 and ► Fig. 9.83).

Steps

- A delivery approach is required, either the luxation technique or the external approach.
- The domes and upper parts of the crura are dissected.
- The upper part of the domes is resected (► Fig. 7.39**a**).
- Small strips (1 to 2 mm) are resected from the lateral and the medial crura (► Fig. 7.39**b**).
- The domes are modified as far as required, replaced, and fixed again to the crura (► Fig. 7.40**a**).
- A tip graft may be applied to reinforce the new construction (► Fig. 7.40**b**).

Note

Because of the risk of postoperative deformities, only an experienced nasal surgeon should carry out the dome resection–reconstruction technique.

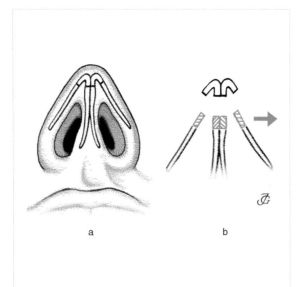

Fig. 7.39 a, b Decreasing tip projection by resecting small strips from the lateral and medial crus just lateral and medial to the domes. The domes are separated from the lateral and medial crura, the strips are removed, and the domes are reconstructed.

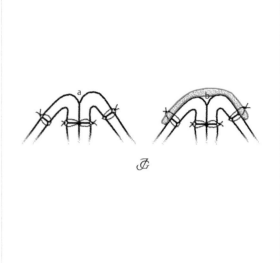

Fig. 7.40 The domes are sutured to the medial and lateral crura **(a)**. A tip graft from the auricle may be applied to reinforce the new construction **(b)**.

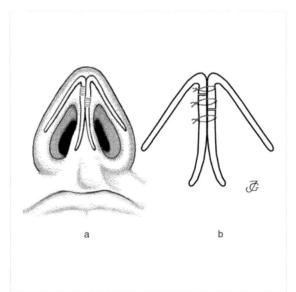

Fig. 7.41 a, b Decreasing tip projection by resecting non-opposing strips from the medial crura. The lateral ends of the lateral crura are somewhat shortened to allow reduction of the lateral leg of the tripod.

Resecting Strips of the Medial Crura

This method is an alternative to the dome resection–reconstruction technique. The procedure is just as delicate but somewhat less dangerous, as the domal superstructures determining the tip remain intact (▶ Fig. 7.41).

Steps

- An external approach is mandatory.
- The medial and lateral crura are exposed.
- The lateral crura and domes are dissected from the underlying skin.
- A small strip is resected from the upper part of both medial crura. It is advisable to do this at different levels.
- The end of the lateral crura may be slightly shortened. This is not essential, however.
- The domes are lowered and sutured to the medial crura (6–0 slowly resorbable sutures).

Upward Positioning (Rotation) of the Tip

Rotation of the nasal tip may be accomplished in various ways. It is advisable to rotate the tip at two or three different levels, especially if shortening of nasal length is desired at the same time. The following methods may be used (▶ Fig. 7.42):

1. Resecting a triangle of cartilage from the caudal septal end, with or without resecting a triangle of skin from the membranous septum
2. Trimming the cranial margin of the lateral crus with resection of a triangle of vestibular skin
3. Resecting a triangle of cartilage, skin, and mucosa from the lower margin of the triangular cartilage

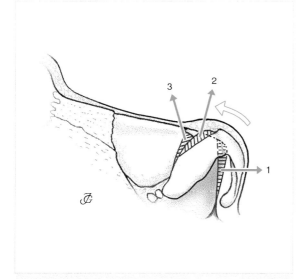

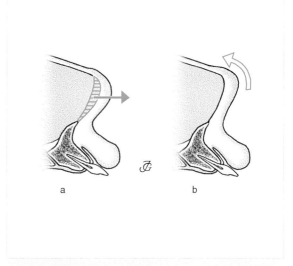

Fig. 7.42 Upward rotation and shortening of nasal length by limited resections from: the caudal end of the septum (1); the cranial margin of the lateral crura (2); and the caudal margin of the triangular cartilages (3).

Fig. 7.43 a, b Upward rotation of the tip and shortening of nasal length by resecting a ventrally based triangle of cartilage from the caudal septal end.

Resecting a Triangle of Cartilage from the Caudal Septal End with or without Resecting a Triangle of Skin from the Membranous Septum

The tip can be rotated upward by resecting a triangular piece of cartilage from the caudal end of the septum as shown in ▶ Fig. 7.43. This is done in combination with creating a columellar pocket. (See also Chapter 5, ▶ Fig. 5.48.) The method may be combined with resecting a similar triangle of skin from the membranous septum (▶ Fig. 7.44).

Trimming the Cranial Margin of the Lateral Crus with Resection of a Small Triangle of Vestibular Skin

A second effective way of upwardly rotating the tip and shortening the nasal length is to resect a strip from the medial part of the cranial margin of the lateral crus together with a small triangle of vestibular skin. The cranial margin of the cartilage can be trimmed by various methods: the retrograde technique, luxation technique, or external approach. Resection of a triangular piece of vestibular skin can only be performed endonasally through an IC incision (▶ Fig. 7.45). See also page 272 and ▶ Fig. 7.25.

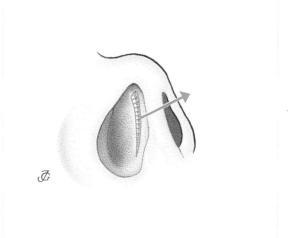

Fig. 7.44 Upward rotation of the tip and shortening of nasal length by resecting a triangle of skin from the membranous septum.

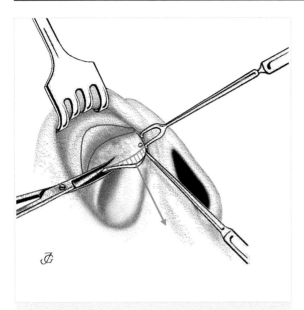

Fig. 7.45 The medial part of the cranial margin of the lateral crus is resected together with a triangle of vestibular skin, using the retrograde technique.

Resecting a Triangle of Cartilage, Skin, and Mucosa from the Lower Margin of the Triangular Cartilage

A third way to upwardly rotate the tip and shorten the nose is to resect a triangle of cartilage with skin (cul de sac) and mucosa from the free caudal margin of the triangular cartilage. This requires meticulous surgery and reconstruction of the valve to avoid functional damage (▶ Fig. 7.45). This method is extensively discussed in Chapter 6 (page 249) and illustrated in ▶ Fig. 6.97, ▶ Fig. 6.98, ▶ Fig. 6.99, and ▶ Fig. 6.100.

Downward Positioning of the Tip

In certain lobular pathology, it may be desirable to bring the tip somewhat downward (i.e., in a caudal direction). This results in an increase of nasal length. In general, downward positioning of the tip is difficult to accomplish. It is mostly accompanied by reduction of tip projection. The following techniques may be attempted, depending upon the pathology:

- Let-down of the pyramid. If the prominence of the pyramid is diminished, tip projection will be less. At the same time, the tip will become more caudal (see Chapter 6, page 227).
- Resection of a dorsally based triangle of cartilage from the caudal end of the septum, as described in Chapter 5 (page 176). This shifts the columellar base in a cranial direction. It diminishes the nasolabial angle, bringing the tip somewhat more caudal.

- Redraping of the lateral crura and fixating the domes more caudally. The effect of this method is limited.
- Inserting spreader grafts between the triangular cartilages and the septum to bring the medial crura somewhat more caudal (see Chapter 6, page 253).

Shortening Nasal Length and Lifting the Tip by Resecting an Ovaloid Piece of Skin and Subcutaneous Tissue from the Nasal Dorsum (Rhinopexia or "Tip Lift")

In patients with extreme lengthening of the nose and severe drooping of the tip, one may consider shortening nasal length by resecting an ovaloid piece of skin and subcutaneous tissue from the nasal dorsum. This may be indicated in elderly patients where drooping of the tip causes breathing impairment. The nasal tip is lifted upward by resecting a double wedge of skin over the bony dorsum just above the K area.

The method is described and illustrated in detail on page 336.

7.3 Alar Surgery

7.3.1 Deformities, Abnormalities, and Variations of the Ala and Their Surgical Correction

The nasal alae may show numerous anatomical variations, abnormalities, and deformities. Whereas some of them produce functional symptoms, others may prompt aesthetic complaints.

Thin, Flaccid Ala

The ala is thin and flaccid. It is drawn inward and may collapse at inspiration (see ▶ Fig. 2.78). Thin, "overstretched" alae are common in the prominent-narrow pyramid syndrome. Atrophy due to old age is another frequent cause of alar weakness. It may also occur after lobular surgery if the cranial margin of the lateral crus has been trimmed too much. The overlap and fibrous connections between the lateral crus and the triangular cartilage may then be lost. The lateral crus loses its cranial support, the supra-alar groove becomes deeper and wider, and the ala easily collapses (see ▶ Fig. 9.80, ▶ Fig. 9.81). Alar flaccidity in patients with a prominent pyramid and lobule is corrected by deprojection of the nose, with or without reinforcement of the ala. The most logical and elegant method is the let-down procedure (see Chapter 6). Nowadays only a limited number of nasal surgeons master this technique. Collapsibility of the ala following surgery or trauma is treated by reconstructing or reinforcing the lateral crus.

Thick Ala

Abnormal thickness of the ala is usually caused by a thick skin, excessive connective tissue, and an abundance of sebaceous glands. The lobular cartilage may also be more massive than normal (see ▶ Fig. 2.79). Surgical treatment usually includes narrowing of the tip and thinning of the lateral crura. In rare cases, it may involve slight thinning of the subcutaneous soft-tissue layers as well.

Abnormal Convexity or "Ballooning" of the Ala

An abnormal convexity of the ala (which some authors call "lateral convexity") is seen in Caucasians with a wide lobule and a broad, bulbous, square, or bifid tip (see ▶ Fig. 2.80). In black people and some Asians, a strong alar convexity is a common feature. In functionally or aesthetically relevant cases, segments of the lateral crus may be inverted, or the excessive curvature may be corrected with sutured alar strut grafts. Complete dissection of the lateral crus followed by redraping is another option. In cases with an abnormally thick skin, some of the deep subcutaneous and fatty tissue layers may be resected. This is a risky type of surgery, however.

Abnormal Concavity of the Ala

An abnormal concavity of the ala is generally of genetic origin. It may lead to aesthetic as well as functional complaints (see ▶ Fig. 2.81). The lateral crus is usually thin, and the ala may collapse at the level of the vestibule. Surgical treatment requires complete subperichondral dissection of the lateral crus and dome. The cartilage may be modified and repositioned, or may be reinforced by a graft. In patients with a limited degree of concavity, it may be sufficient to insert an appropriately sized alar batten or strut onlay graft.

Congenital Anomalies of the Ala

There are many kinds of congenital anomalies of the alae. They are part of a malformation of the whole lobule. The most well known examples are the lobular deformities found in cleft lip patients and in cases with nasal hypoplasia (see ▶ Fig. 2.82).

7.3.2 Surgical Techniques

This section presents the most important methods used to reconstruct or modify the alae. Techniques addressing the lateral crus of the lobular cartilage as part of tip surgery are reviewed in the section on tip surgery (see page 272).

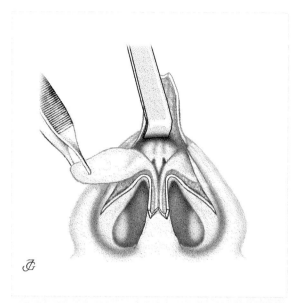

Fig. 7.46 The lateral crus is dissected from the underlying vestibular skin (external approach).

Reinforcing the Ala

Thin and atrophic alae may have to be reinforced to diminish their collapsibility. This can be done in many ways. The choice of method depends on the pathology of the lateral crus and the cause of the defect. Most surgeons prefer the external approach as the means of access. In some cases, and in some hands, an endonasal technique may suffice, however.

Reinforcement may be carried out by repositioning, reinforcement with a graft, or reconstruction of the lateral crus using a transplant. In the majority of cases, a combination of these principles is used, as required by the findings.

- *Repositioning* is chosen when the quality of the cartilage is satisfactory but its relationship with other supporting structures, in particular the triangular cartilage, is disturbed.
- *Reinforcement* by a graft is preferred when the cartilage can be left in place but has to be strengthened because of weakness. Such a graft is preferably cut from septal cartilage or, as second choice, from auricular cartilage.
- *Reconstruction* using a graft is carried out when the lateral crus is defective, abnormally twisted, or concave. Both autogeneic auricular cartilage with perichondrium as well as septal cartilage may be used.

Repositioning

In cases where the relationship between the lateral crus and the lower margin of the triangular cartilage has been lost (due to previous surgery in which too much of the cranial margin of the lateral crus has been resected, or as a result of trauma), it may be mobilized and shifted (rotated) upward. Its cranial margin is then sutured to the caudal margin of the triangular cartilage (▶ Fig. 7.46 and

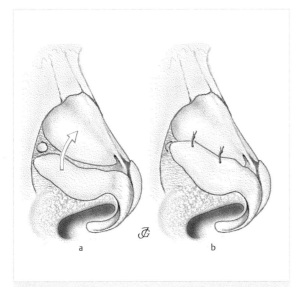

Fig. 7.47 The lateral crus is upwardly rotated **(a)** and fixed to the caudal margin of the triangular cartilage **(b)** (external approach or luxation technique).

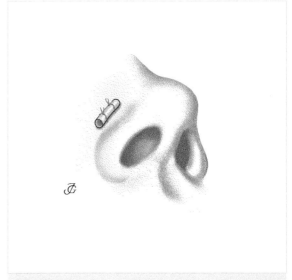

Fig. 7.48 The upwardly rotated lateral crus may be temporarily fixed transcutaneously (luxation technique).

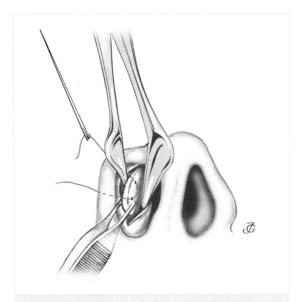

Fig. 7.49 An atrophied lateral crus is reinforced with a cartilaginous graft inserted through an infracartilaginous incision.

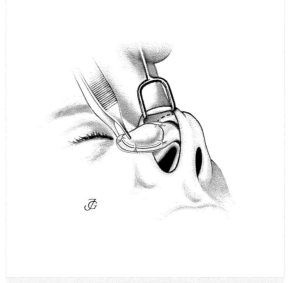

Fig. 7.50 An atrophied lateral crus is reinforced with a graft sutured on the lateral crus (luxation technique).

▶ Fig. 7.47). This procedure was first described by Rettinger and Masing (1981) using the luxation technique. We too have used it successfully. The disadvantage of the rotation is that it produces torsion between the lateral crus and the dome. We therefore prefer to sever the lateral crus from the dome and then reposition and fixate it as illustrated in ▶ Fig. 7.53. The cartilage may be temporarily fixed into its new position by transcutaneous fixation (▶ Fig. 7.48).

Reinforcement

The lateral crus is reinforced by a cartilage transplant from septal, auricular, or rib cartilage. In uncomplicated cases, the graft may be inserted through an infracartilaginous incision and fixed as shown in ▶ Fig. 7.49. In more difficult cases, the lateral crus is delivered using the luxation technique, and the graft is sutured on top (▶ Fig. 7.50). In complicated cases, the external approach

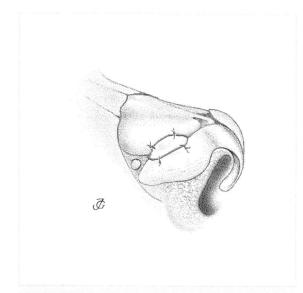

Fig. 7.51 The ala is reinforced with a cartilaginous patch sutured to the lateral crus and the triangular cartilage (external approach).

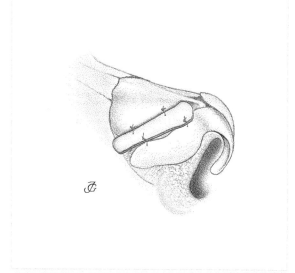

Fig. 7.52 The ala is reinforced with a cartilaginous batten between the anterior septum and the piriform aperture (external approach).

is preferred. Depending on the pathology, reinforcement may be accomplished by bridging the gap between the cartilages with a thin shield of auricular cartilage. The transplant is fixed with its perichondrial side lateral to the caudal margin of the triangular cartilage and the remnant of the lateral crus (▶ Fig. 7.51). Another way to reinforce the ala is to use a batten sculpted from rib cartilage. Toriumi (1997) has suggested positioning the batten in such a way that its lateral end rests on the edge of the piriform aperture, while its medial end lies against the anterior rim of the septum (▶ Fig. 7.52).

Reconstruction

If the lateral crus is severely defective or atrophic, it may be resected and replaced by a transplant from auricular, septal, or rib cartilage with perichondrium. The graft is medially fixed to the lateral side of the dome (preferably by two sutures) and laterocranial to the caudal margin of the triangular cartilage (by two sutures). This technique should only be used in cases where the lateral crus is severely defective (▶ Fig. 7.53).

Resecting a Protruding End of the Lateral Crus

The vestibule may be obstructed by a protrusion of the end of the lateral crus (▶ Fig. 7.54). This may occur as a result of "tip-refining" surgery, when the connections between the upper margin of the lateral crus and the lower margin of the triangular cartilage have

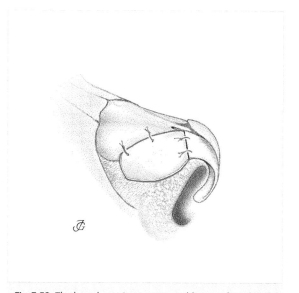

Fig. 7.53 The lateral crus is reconstructed by a graft sculpted from auricular cartilage (external approach).

inadvertently been destroyed. It is also seen in elderly patients because of laxity of the soft tissues of the lobule. The end of the lateral crus may then become inverted and protrude into the vestibule, resulting in inspiratory breathing obstruction. Resection of the protruding end of the lateral crus and/or reinforcement of the ala may then be an effective treatment.

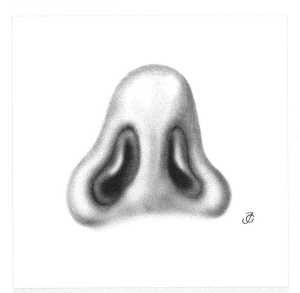

Fig. 7.54 The vestibule is obstructed due to abnormally protruding ends of the lateral crura.

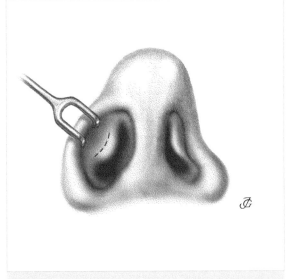

Fig. 7.55 Incision of the vestibular skin overlying the protruding end of the lateral crus.

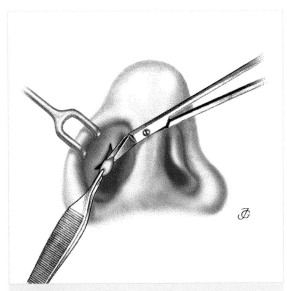

Fig. 7.56 The protruding part of the lateral crus is resected.

Steps

- A small incision into the vestibular skin overlying the protruding end of the lateral crus is made with No. 15 blade or a No. 64 Beaver knife (▶ Fig. 7.55).
- The lateral protruding part of the lateral crus is dissected subperichondrially using a delicate anatomical forceps and small, slightly curved scissors.
- The protruding part of the lateral crus is resected (▶ Fig. 7.56).

- The incision is carefully closed with 5–0 sutures.
- Supporting internal dressings and outside pressure tapes are applied.

Reducing Alar Convexity

Abnormal convexity or ballooning of the ala is addressed by decreasing the spring of the overly convex cartilage. This has formerly been attempted by superficial gridding, cross-hatching, or resecting two or three minute wedges (▶ Fig. 7.57). These techniques may weaken the cartilage too much, however, and they have therefore largely been replaced by suture techniques respecting or reconstructing the structural integrity of the alar cartilages. All three methods require a delivery approach, either the luxation technique or the external approach. In cases with an extreme degree of convexity, it may be necessary to resect, modify, and reposition the crus or replace it or splint it by a graft, as illustrated in ▶ Fig. 7.53.

Gridding

A few superficial vertical incisions are made using a No. 64 Beaver blade (▶ Fig. 7.57a). Utmost care is taken to not weaken the cartilage too much. It must remain sufficiently rigid to withstand the negative pressure in the vestibule during inspiration.

Cross-hatching or Morcellation (Crushing)

The cartilage is slightly cross-hatched (▶ Fig. 7.57b). This method bears an even greater risk of weakening the alae too much, however.

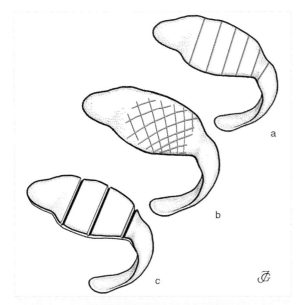

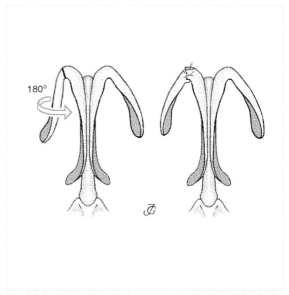

Fig. 7.57 Superficial gridding (**a**), cross-hatching (**b**), or resecting of minute wedges (**c**) may be performed to reduce an abnormal convexity, but is a risky method as the cartilage may easily become too flaccid.

Fig. 7.58 An abnormal concavity may be corrected by resecting and turning the lateral crus 180°.

Resecting Small Wedges

In cases with extreme ballooning of the lateral crus, two or three tiny wedges may be resected from the cartilage with a No.64 Beaver knife (▶ Fig. 7.57c). Care is taken to not damage the vestibular skin. These minute resections must be performed with utmost precision, as this procedure carries a great risk of causing too much loss of alar rigidity.

Reducing Alar Concavity

In cases where the lateral crus is concave, surgical correction may be indicated for functional (alar collapse at the level of the vestibule) as well as aesthetic reasons. Surgical treatment can best be achieved using the external approach. The lateral crus (and dome) is subperichondrially dissected and modified. In patients with a limited degree of concavity, it may be sufficient to splint it with a batten or strut onlay graft. In other cases, the lateral crus is resected, repositioned by turning it 180°, and sutured in a new position.

Steps

- The external approach (or the luxation technique) is used.
- The lateral crus is exposed and dissected *sub*perichondrially on both sides (see page 260).

- Sometimes, the cartilage straightens out when it is liberated from its perichondrial envelope and freed from surrounding scar tissue.
- If the concavity still remains, the lateral crus will have to be resected, modified, and repositioned, or splinted with a batten or strut that is sutured on the cartilage as illustrated by ▶ Fig. 7.52.
- Another option is to resect the lateral crus, turn it 180°, and fix it again to the dome (▶ Fig. 7.58). The most stable fixation of the repositioned lateral crus is achieved if both edges overlap.

Shortening the Ala by Wedge Resection at Its Base

When reducing a prominent lobule and tip, it may be wise to shorten the ala as part of the procedure. A well-known example is let-down of the bony and cartilaginous pyramid. When the bony and cartilaginous pyramid are lowered, the lobule will become lower and wider. The nostrils will become rounder and the alae more convex. To restore the normal configuration of the lobule, it may then be necessary to bilaterally resect a soft-tissue wedge at the alar base.

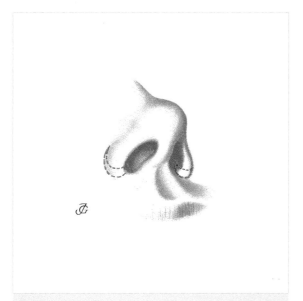

Fig. 7.59 The wedges to be resected from the alar base are outlined on the skin.

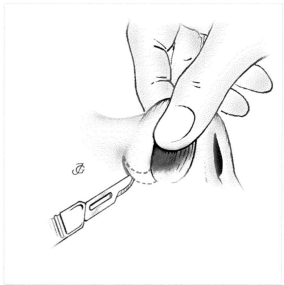

Fig. 7.60 The lower part of the incision is made first. The ala is cut from its base.

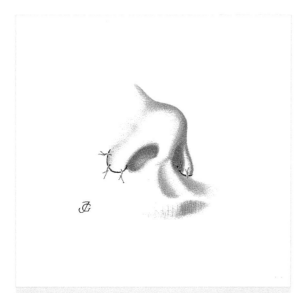

Fig. 7.61 The ala is sutured at its base with 5–0 nonresorbable sutures.

Steps

- The wedges to be resected are outlined on the skin (▶ Fig. 7.59).
- The ala is taken between the thumb and index finger. The skin of the alar base is then incised at the nasofacial fold with a No. 15 or a No. 11 blade. The incision should be made precisely in the nasofacial and nasolabial fold. The ala is cut from its base (▶ Fig. 7.60).

- A second incision is made at the upper margin of the wedge that has been outlined. The wedge is now resected. Bipolar coagulation is applied to control bleeding from small branches of the angular artery.
- The ala is sutured at its base with multiple nonresorbable sutures (▶ Fig. 7.61). This is done both externally and in the vestibule. Care is taken to avoid any left–right asymmetry.

Displacing the Alar Base

A wide lobular base with a wide floor of the nostril and vestibule may be corrected by medial displacement of the alar base. In extreme cases, a Z-plasty is an excellent solution. In the majority of cases, it usually suffices to excise a wedge on the vestibular side of the vestibular sil.

Steps

- The ala is disconnected from its base as described above.
- A Z-plasty is carried out. A triangular flap of vestibular skin is cut and elevated (▶ Fig. 7.62).
- The skin of the alar base and the vestibule is undermined.
- The skin flap is sutured to the lateral part of the incision at the nasofacial fold. The ala is sutured into the vestibular defect (▶ Fig. 7.63).

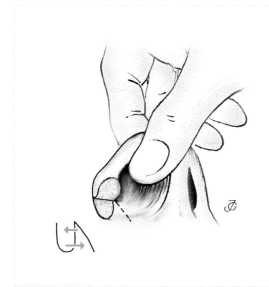

Fig. 7.62 The ala is cut from its base. A triangular skin flap is mobilized from the nasal floor.

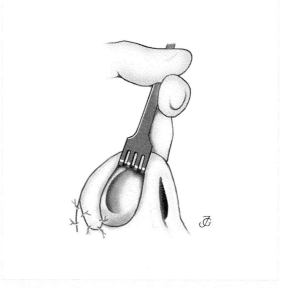

Fig. 7.63 The ala is displaced and sutured medially.

Thinning the Ala

In patients with abnormal thickness of the lobular skin, it may be advisable to resect some of the abundant subcutaneous tissues. This should be performed with utmost care in a symmetrical way. Resecting too much soft tissue, or asymmetrical resection leads to ugly retractions that are almost irreparable. In this case, the external approach is advised as it allows the surgeon to work under direct view.

Narrowing the Lobular Base

The lobular base can be narrowed by making one or sometimes two so-called bunching sutures. These narrowing sutures will only be effective if the soft tissues have been widely undermined.

Steps

- The lobular base is undermined using blunt, slightly curved scissors through the CSI (see ▶ Fig. 5.16).
- A slowly resorbable 4–0 (or 3–0) suture is introduced through the CSI with a straight needle, and directed towards the left alar-labial fold. Then the needle is stabbed back and comes out of the CSI again (▶ Fig. 7.64**a**).
- The needle is once more introduced into the CSI but now towards the right alar-labial fold. Again, the needle is stabbed back into the alar-labial fold towards the CSI (▶ Fig. 7.64**b**).
- Small stab incisions are made in the alar-labial folds to bury the suture.
- The suture is pulled and knotted in the septal space.
- The CSI is closed over the knot (▶ Fig. 7.64**c**).

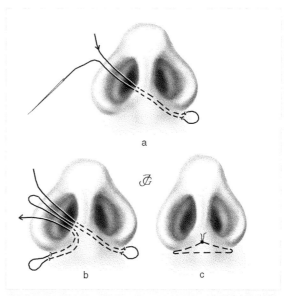

Fig. 7.64 a–c The alar base is narrowed using a bunching suture.

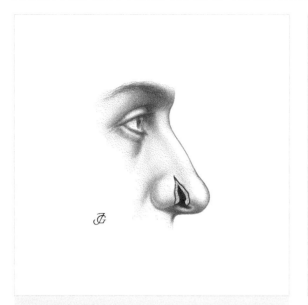

Fig. 7.65 Alar defect after trauma. The edges of the wound are cleaned and freshened up.

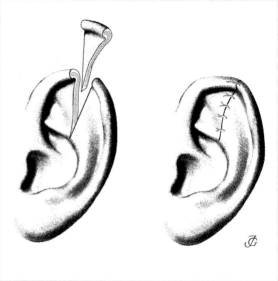

Fig. 7.66 A composite graft is taken from the auricle.

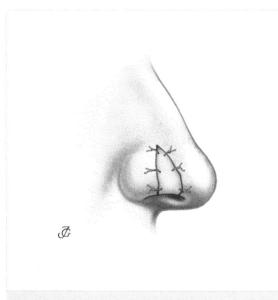

Fig. 7.67 The graft is sutured into the defect.

Reconstructing the Ala

Alar defects are common deformities after tumor resection or trauma. Car accidents and dog bites are well known causes. In some cases, primary closure of the wound may be attempted. In most patients, however, there will be a certain tissue defect. To avoid an ugly upward and dorsal retraction of the ala, it is necessary to repair the defect. If it is small (5 to 6 mm), this may be accomplished with a composite graft from the auricular helix. The best results are obtained when the reconstruction is carried out within a few days. Larger defects are repaired in three layers: an internal lining (e.g., septal mucoperichondrial flap), a structural support (septal or auricular cartilage), and an outer cutaneous layer (nasolabial flap or forehead flap).

It goes beyond the scope of this book to deal with all types of nasal and paranasal skin defects and their surgical correction. However, to give an example, we discuss the alar defect.

Steps

- The wounded surfaces are cleaned and freshened up (▶ Fig. 7.65).
- A triangular wedge (skin–cartilage–skin) is resected from the auricle. The resection is carried out up to the cavum conchae as the defect can then be closed without causing malformation of the auricle (▶ Fig. 7.66).
- From the resected piece, a graft is carefully shaped to fit into the defect. It should be slightly oversized, as some tissue retraction will take place in the healing process.
- It is sutured in place with interrupted skin sutures, both externally and in the vestibule. Ischemia is avoided as much as possible by approximating the wound edges without compression, and placing single stitches further apart than usual when closing a facial incision (▶ Fig. 7.67).

7.4 Columellar Surgery

Modification of the dimensions and the position of the columella is an essential part of functional reconstructive nasal surgery. Columellar surgery may serve aesthetic as well as functional purposes.

Inspiratory breathing is often impaired in patients with a broad, retracted, or oblique columella. Aesthetic complaints may be expressed by patients with a narrow, short, retracted, hanging, or asymmetrical columella.

7.4.1 Deformities, Abnormalities, and Variations of the Columella and Their Surgical Correction

The columella shows a great variety of deformities, abnormalities, and variations. They may result from genetic factors, trauma, disturbed growth, previous surgery, or infection. Analysis of the deformity and its pathogenesis is of utmost importance. The outcome of that analysis determines which surgical method will be used.

Long Columella

The columella is displeasingly long and narrow (see ▶ Fig. 2.85). This is seen, for example, in the prominent-narrow pyramid syndrome. This may be corrected by letdown of the pyramid, by deprojection through a transfixion incision, or by a medial crural overlay procedure (Lipsett procedure).

Short Columella

The columella is both short and broad (see ▶ Fig. 2.86). This is normal in the black and Asian nose. It also occurs in Caucasians as part of several congenital anomalies (see also broad columella). A short columella may be lengthened by a columellar strut with or without a V–Y-plasty.

Broad Columella

The columella is broad and usually short (see ▶ Fig. 2.87). This is seen in congenital anomalies such as the bifid nose, the cleft lip nose, and nasal hypoplasia. It is also a common feature in the black and Asian nose. The most common causes are excessive intercrural connective tissue, abnormal thickness of the medial crura, or an abnormal protrusion of the lower ends of the medial crura. Narrowing may be achieved by resecting some (excessive) intercrural connective tissue, trimming the protruding lower ends of the medial crura, and applying a narrowing suture.

Protruding Ends of the Medial Crura

The lower ends of the medial crura are abnormally bent in a lateral direction. They protrude into the nostril and vestibule where they may cause (or contribute to) inspiratory obstruction. The columellar base is usually abnormally broad (see ▶ Fig. 2.88). Correction is carried out by trimming the protruding ends or approximating the footplates with a suture.

Narrow Columella

The columella is narrow and usually long (see ▶ Fig. 2.89). A narrow (and long) columella may be part of a congenitally prominent, narrow pyramid. It may also result from scarring due to previous surgery (or infection), for example after transfixion of the membranous septum or surgery of the caudal septal end. The columella is usually retracted as well. A narrow columella may be broadened by an intercrural cartilaginous transplant (columellar strut), or by reconstruction of the caudal septum and a tongue-in-groove technique.

Oblique Columella

The columella runs obliquely. This is a common symptom in cases with deviation of the anterior septum and the cartilaginous pyramid (see ▶ Fig. 2.90). It is also observed in congenital anomalies, in particular in patients with a cleft lip nose. The method used to correct this abnormality depends upon its cause.

Retracted ("Hidden") Columella

The columella, especially its base and lower part, is retracted in a cranial direction. Viewed from the side, the columellar base is not visible as it is hidden behind the ala (see ▶ Fig. 2.91). This is almost always caused by a missing caudal septum due to infection, trauma, or surgery. Too much resection of the anterior nasal spine is another well known cause. A retracted columella is frequently observed in combination with saddling of the cartilaginous dorsum. It may be corrected by reconstructing the anterior septum and reinforcing the columella by transplanting a cartilaginous strut between the medial crura.

Hanging ("Showing") Columella

The caudal margin of the columella is lower and more convex than normal. Viewed from the side, too much (more than 4 mm) columella is visible. Sometimes, even part of the membranous septum is in view (see ▶ Fig. 2.92). This often leads to cosmetic complaints. A hanging columella may be corrected by resecting an ovaloid area of skin from the membranous septum in combination with removal of cartilage, or better, by suturing the medial crura over the caudal septum (tongue-in-groove technique). The hanging columella must be differentiated from a retracted ala, which may also cause a columellar show of more than 4 mm.

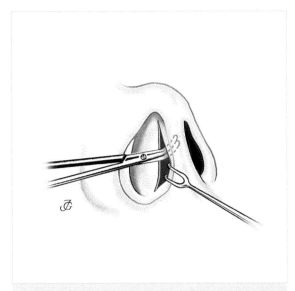

Fig. 7.68 The intercrural area is loosened up, and a columellar pocket is created through a CSI.

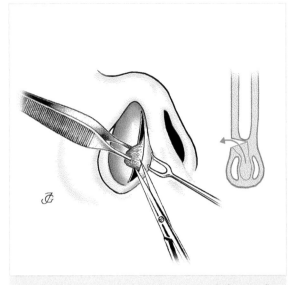

Fig. 7.69 Excessive connective tissue is resected (if required) from the intercrural area through the CSI.

Asymmetrical Columella

Asymmetry may be due to (unequal) scarring after nasal trauma or surgery (see ▶ Fig. 2.93). It may also be caused by pathology of the caudal end of the septum or the medial crura. The surgical technique to be used depends upon the cause of the condition.

7.4.2 Surgical Techniques

Narrowing the Columella

The columella may be narrowed in different ways. The method selected will depend first of all on the type of pathology. The following techniques have proven effective:
1. Resecting intercrural connective tissue
2. Trimming protruding ends of the medial crura
3. Applying narrowing ("bunching") sutures

In many cases, a combination of these three techniques will be used.

Resecting Excessive Intercrural Connective Tissue

Steps
- If surgery is performed endonasally, this is done through a CSI.
- The caudal septal end is exposed and freed. The membranous septum and the intercrural area are then loosened up along the midline with fully curved scissors. A columellar pocket is created (▶ Fig. 7.68).

- Excessive connective tissue is resected as required using pointed, slightly curved scissors and a small (Adson–Brown–type) forceps (▶ Fig. 7.69). To avoid postoperative asymmetry, this is performed very carefully and symmetrically.
- If no further narrowing is required (see following text), two or three vertical (or horizontal) mattress sutures are applied to narrow the columella and close the CSI.

Trimming Abnormally Protruding Ends of the Medial Crura

Steps
- An incision 3 to 4 mm in length is made in the skin over the lower ends of the medial crura (▶ Fig. 7.70)
- The abnormally protruding parts are dissected and exposed using delicate anatomical forceps and pointed, slightly curved scissors.
- The lower part of the protruding ends are trimmed as required by the pathology and the surgical goals (▶ Fig. 7.71).
- When no other columellar surgery is carried out, the columella may narrowed by two horizontal transcolumellar mattress sutures.
- When a CSI has been made, a special bunching suture may be applied (see below).

Applying Narrowing Sutures

Depending on the pathology and the surgical goals, vertical or horizontal mattress sutures may be applied to narrow the columella (▶ Fig. 7.72 and ▶ Fig. 7.73). A small, straight needle is used with a 4–0 slowly resorbable suture. These sutures will only be effective if a wide intercrural pocket has been made.

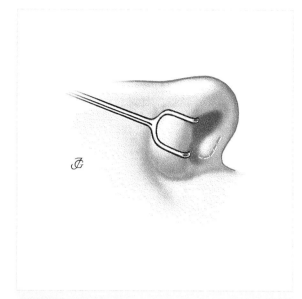

Fig. 7.70 An incision of 3 to 4 mm is made over the medial crura to expose abnormally protruding lower ends.

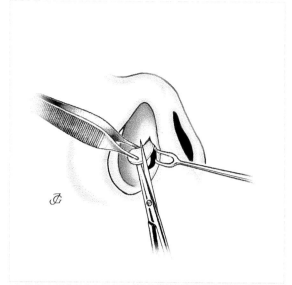

Fig. 7.71 An abnormally protruding lower end of the medial crus is trimmed.

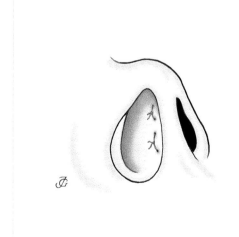

Fig. 7.72 The columella is narrowed by two vertical mattress sutures.

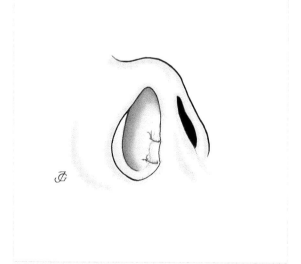

Fig. 7.73 Horizontal transcolumellar mattress sutures are used to narrow the columella after wide intercrural undermining, and resecting connective tissue and/or the protruding ends of the medial crura.

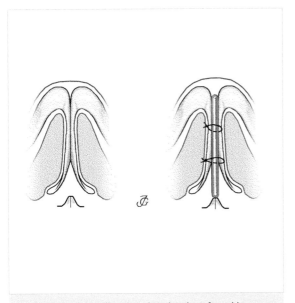

Fig. 7.74 The columella is broadened and reinforced by transplanting and fixing a cartilaginous strut between the medial crura.

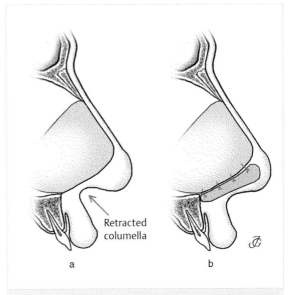

Fig. 7.75 A retracted columella (a) is corrected by a septal extension graft (b).

Note

Excising a double vertical triangle of columellar skin from an abnormally broad columella has been suggested in some older textbooks. We do not advise this technique, as it may lead to an ugly retracted vertical scar.

Reinforcing the Columella

A narrow (retracted) columella may be reinforced and broadened by fixing a strut of cartilage between the two medial crura (▶ Fig. 7.74).

Steps

- An intercrural pocket is created with blunt, fully curved scissors. This is done either through the CSI (▶ Fig. 7.68) or through the external approach.
- A strut is sculpted from septal cartilage. Auricular cartilage is another option, though it is difficult to cut a straight batten with sufficient rigidity from this type of cartilage.
- If projection is to be increased, the columellar strut should ideally rest on the anterior nasal spine, and when possible, be fixed to it; if only straightening of the columella is planned, the strut may be "floating" and sutured to both medial crura.
- The strut is fixed to the medial crura (▶ Fig. 7.74).

Note

Care should be taken to ensure that a columellar strut is not visible or palpable between the domes.

Correcting a Retracted Columella

To correct a retracted columella, the following surgical options should be considered:
- Reconstructing the caudal end of the septum and/or extending it by a so-called caudal septal extension graft (see also Chapter 5, page 177).
- In selected cases, reconstructing the anterior nasal spine by a bony transplant
- Reinforcing the columella by an intercrural cartilaginous strut

The technique chosen depends (as always) on the pathology found. In many cases, these methods will be combined.

Reconstructing the Caudal End of the Septum by a Septal Extension Graft

If the columellar retraction is caused by a defective caudal septal end following trauma or previous surgery, the missing part is reconstructed by a triangular graft of septal cartilage (▶ Fig. 7.75). The procedure is extensively discussed and illustrated in Chapter 5 (see page 177).

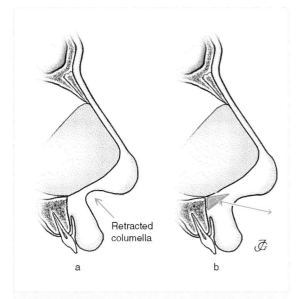

Fig. 7.76 A defective anterior nasal spine **(a)** is repaired by a triangular piece of bone usually taken from the bony septum (e.g., vomeral spur) and fixed by columellar base guide suture and a bunching mattress suture **(b)**.

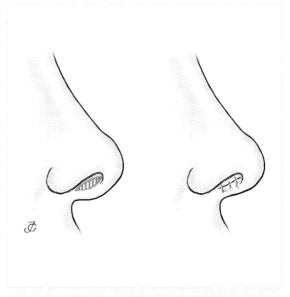

Fig. 7.77 An ovaloid piece of skin is resected from the membranous septum to correct a hanging columella.

Reconstructing the Anterior Nasal Spine by a Bony Transplant

If the columellar base is retracted because of a missing anterior nasal spine, a bony transplant is fixed at the defective area. This will shift the columellar base more caudally and increase the nasolabial angle. If only the protruding part of the spine is missing, a more or less triangular transplant will suffice. We then speak of "spine repair." In patients who have a defective anterior nasal spine with retrusion of the maxilla, a broader transplant is inserted, often referred to as a premaxillary transplant or "plumping graft."

Steps

- The anterior nasal spine is exposed. In endonasal surgery, this is done through the CSI.
- A piece of bone of the required size is resected from the bony septum. Part of a vomeral spur is usually a good choice.
- Depending on the pathology, either a small pyramid or a broader premaxillary transplant is cut using heavy bone scissors.
- A guide suture is usually brought through the middle of the columellar base (▶ Fig. 7.76). Another option is the labiogingival fold.
- The transplant may be secured in place by a bunching mattress suture (see ▶ Fig. 7.64). Some surgeons prefer to use tissue glue.

Reinforcing the Columella by an Intercrural Cartilaginous Strut

The columella may be reinforced and somewhat lengthened by inserting an intercrural batten made from septal or auricular cartilage. To shift the columellar base in a more caudal direction, the lower end of the strut is made wider than its upper end (▶ Fig. 7.74). The method may be combined with reconstruction of the anterior nasal spine, as previously described (▶ Fig. 7.76).

Correcting a Hanging Columella

A hanging columella may be corrected by resecting an ovaloid strip of skin from the membranous septum in combination with a tongue-in-groove technique if the caudal septum is intact.

Steps

- This technique may be carried out as an isolated procedure or as part of an endonasal or external septorhinoplasty.
- When an endonasal rhinoplasty is performed, the CSI is made somewhat more cranial than normal.
- The ovaloid area of skin to be resected is bilaterally outlined. If the columella is symmetrical, care is taken to resect the same amount on both sides. If the columella is asymmetrical, somewhat more tissue may be resected from one side.
- The defect is closed bilaterally with three or four monofilament 5–0 sutures (▶ Fig. 7.77).
- The columella is stabilized in its new position by a vestibular dressing and upward-pulling tapes (▶ Fig. 7.78).

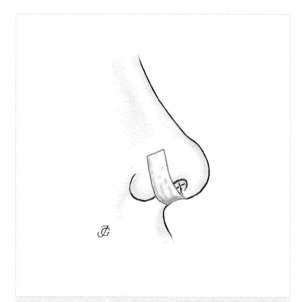

Fig. 7.78 Upward-pulling tapes are applied to fix the columella in its new position.

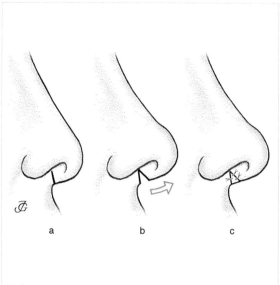

Fig. 7.79 a–c The columella is lengthened with a composite graft.

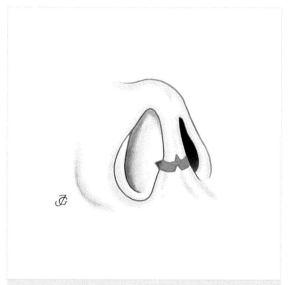

Fig. 7.80 The columella is shortened by resecting a double inverted-V-shaped piece of soft tissue.

Lengthening the Columella

In cases where the columella is short, we may try to lengthen it by inserting an intercrural strut of sufficient length. If the subnasale is retracted and the nasolabial angle acute, a strut can increase both rotation and projection while bringing the subnasale forward, which can be pleasing, especially in women. Many older textbooks have suggested a V–Y-plasty at the columellar base in patients with a congenitally short columella. In our experience, this method accentuates the nasolabial angle and may be indicated in men with a short columella and a displeasingly obtuse nasolabial angle, or in patients with a bilateral cleft (see ▶ Fig. 4.21). In selected cases, an abnormally short columella may be lengthened by transplanting a composite graft taken from the auricle (▶ Fig. 7.79).

Shortening the Columella

Shortening of the columella is rarely indicated. An exception may be a pronounced prominent, narrow nasal pyramid. The let-down technique may then be combined with wedge resections at the lobular base (see ▶ Fig. 6.54) and shortening of the columella. This is done by resecting a small triangle of soft tissue from the lower third of the columella using a double-V incision, as illustrated in ▶ Fig. 7.80.

Correcting an Oblique Columella

An oblique position of the columella is usually due to deviation of the anterior septum and the cartilaginous vault. Correct analysis of the causative factors of this type of pathology is of utmost importance. We should not try to correct an oblique columella without first correcting the septum and pyramid. Only in exceptional cases would additional correction of the columella itself be required. If so, this may be best performed in a secondary intervention 6 to 12 months later. For correction of an oblique columella in cleft lip patients, see Chapter 9 (page 331).

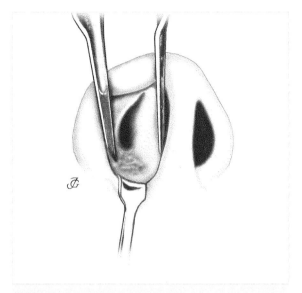

Fig. 7.81 Stenosis of the vestibular floor.

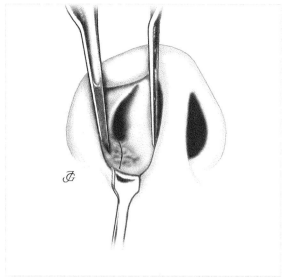

Fig. 7.82 The stenotic area is incised from dorsal to ventral.

7.5 Vestibular Surgery

Surgery of the vestibule is one of the most difficult types of nasal surgery. In most cases, vestibular surgery serves both functional and aesthetic purposes. The most common reason to operate is congenital or posttraumatic deformity and stenosis of the vestibule with impairment of breathing.

Deformity and stenosis of the vestibule may be caused by various types of pathology:

- Deformities of its medial wall (dislocated caudal end of the septum, protruding end of the medial crus, retracted columella, broad columella)
- Deformities of its lateral wall (cleft lip deformity, abnormal alar concavity, alar flaccidity, protruding end of the lateral crus)
- Pathology of its floor and attic (cleft lip deformity, scarring)

Surgical correction of the deformities of the medial and lateral vestibular wall is covered in the sections on surgery of the dislocated caudal end of the septum (Chapter 5, page 176), columella (Chapter 7, page 289), and ala (Chapter 7, page 280). In this chapter, we discuss the surgical techniques dealing with correction of a stenosis of the vestibular floor and attic.

7.5.1 Deformities

The main causes of a stenosis of the floor of the vestibule are:

- Congenital malformations, in particular cleft lip syndrome
- Trauma, especially avulsion of the ala or the lobule
- Previous surgery with stenotic scarring as a result of inadequate repositioning of tissues and/or closure of incisions

For patients with a vestibular stenosis, we have two therapeutic options: surgical correction or a prosthetic device. Generally, we first consider the surgical options. For patients in whom surgery has failed or is expected to fail, we have to resort to a custom-made vestibular prosthesis to keep the stenotic vestibule open.

7.5.2 Surgical Techniques

Widening the Vestibule

In the past decades, the literature has described an overwhelming variety of techniques to widen a stenotic vestibule (▶ Fig. 7.81). Their sheer number is indicative of the difficulty of this type of surgery. In this chapter, we describe the method that has proven effective in our hands: resection of the stenotic area and repair by a composite graft.

Steps

- The stenosis is incised from dorsal to ventral (▶ Fig. 7.82). The skin is widely undermined in all directions.
- Scar tissue is resected where necessary (▶ Fig. 7.83**a**).
- A composite graft consisting of cartilage and overlying skin is harvested from the auricle (see ▶ Fig. 6.81 and ▶ Fig. 6.62).
- The graft is cut to fit and sutured into the defect with monofilament 5–0 nonresorbable sutures (▶ Fig. 7.83**b**). The use of tissue glue may be helpful to position the transplant.
- An internal dressing is carefully applied for a relatively long period of time. It may be renewed every 5 to 7 days. The stitches are removed no earlier than 7 to 10 days after surgery.
- A custom-made prosthesis (see following text) is worn in the vestibule and nostril at night for 6 months until healing and scar retraction is complete.

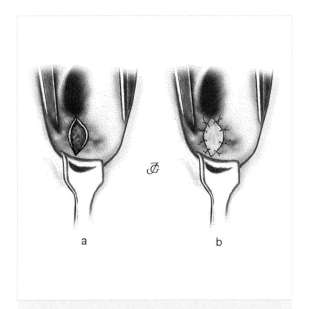

Fig. 7.83 Scar tissue is excised **(a)**. A composite graft (cartilage with overlying skin) taken from the auricle is glued and sutured into the defect **(b)**.

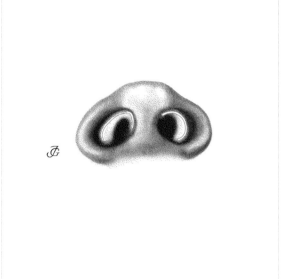

Fig. 7.84 Custom-made vestibular prosthesis for patients with an irreparable vestibular stenosis.

7.5.3 Prosthesis

For patients in whom surgical repair of a stenosis is impossible or has been unsuccessful, a vestibular prosthesis should be considered. Such a device must be custom-made to meet the specific requirements of the individual patient. It is advisable to make the prosthesis in collaboration with a technician experienced in making ear molds.

Steps

- All vibrissae are carefully clipped and removed.
- The vestibulum is covered with a thin layer of Vaseline.
- The technician prepares the impression compound as used for making ear molds. The material is injected into the vestibule and allowed to settle for a few minutes.
- Care is taken to not inject too much of the impression compound. If the vestibule is expanded too much, the prosthesis will become too large. The device will then not be tolerated.
- The impression is removed and a "nose shoe" is made by a technical laboratory (▶ Fig. 7.84).
- In most cases, the prosthesis needs some additional adjustment and polishing to obtain a perfect and thus painless fit.

Chapter 8

Surgery of the Nasal Cavity

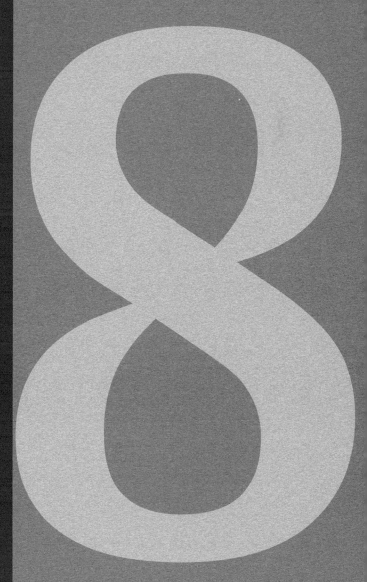

8 Surgery of the Nasal Cavity

8.1 Turbinate Surgery

8.1.1 General

Pathology of the turbinates is one of the most frequent causes of nasal complaints. Obstructed breathing, hypersecretion, sneezing, itching, hyposmia, and pressure sensations are the most common symptoms. Remarkably, most textbooks and courses on nasal surgery pay little or no attention to turbinate pathology and its treatment. Instead, they concentrate on the septum, pyramid, and lobule. Nonetheless, disorders of the turbinates are extremely common in daily rhinological practice.

Types of Turbinate Pathology

Therapy of turbinate disorders should take account of the character and the cause of the pathology. Remarkably, however, specific types of turbinate pathology are rarely distinguished. Most textbooks and articles refer to "hyperplastic," "hypertrophic," "engorged," or "congested" turbinates. In an attempt to provide grounds for choice of treatment, this chapter differentiates between various types of turbinate pathology.

Function-Preserving Treatment

The choice of a therapy for turbinate disorders has been a matter of dispute for over a century. What all authors do agree on is that conservative treatment—with topical steroids, antihistamines, or systemic antibiotics, depending on the cause of the pathology—should be the first choice. Medications are permanently effective only in a limited number of cases, however. Surgical treatment—usually some kind of turbinate reduction—may then be considered. When choosing a method of turbinate reduction, we must keep in mind that the turbinates are the most important functional structures that enable the nose to perform its tasks by:

1. Regulating the course of the airstream
2. Humidifying, warming, and cleansing inspired air
3. Being the main organs of defense for the upper respiratory tract

Preservation of these functions is therefore obligatory. We must also realize that the head of the inferior turbinate is part of the nasal valve, and thus of inspiratory breathing resistance. In all surgery of the inferior turbinate, it is therefore essential to preserve the turbinate head and leave it in its proper position in the valve area.

8.1.2 Inferior Turbinate

Pathology

As previously noted, we need a workable classification of turbinate pathology. In our experience, the following types may be distinguished:

1. Compensatory hypertrophy
2. Protrusion (i.e., abnormal medial position of the turbinate)
3. Hyperplasia of the turbinate head
4. Hyperplasia of the entire turbinate
5. (Degenerative) hyperplasia of the turbinate tail

Compensatory hyperplasia is a very well-known pathological entity. In patients with septal deviation, it develops on the wide side of the nose (see ► Fig. 2.117). It is a physiological reaction that serves to diminish the size and normalize the configuration of the breathing space in the pathologically wide nasal half. Therefore, it is questionable whether septal surgery has to be combined with turbinate reduction in these cases. There are compelling reasons to wait and see if a physiological correction takes place. In a prospective study, Grymer et al (1993) found that septal surgery combined with turbinate surgery did not yield a better functional outcome than septoplasty alone.

Protrusion is identified less frequently. The experienced rhinologist will recognize it at rhinoscopy, but it may show up more clearly on a CT scan. The angle between the turbinate bone and the lateral nasal wall is larger than average, sometimes even up to 90° (► Fig. 8.1). See also ► Fig. 2.118. As a consequence, the turbinate protrudes further into the nasal cavity than usual. Lateralization by fracturing the turbinate bone in combination with a limited submucosal resection of the anteroinferior part of the bone is usually an effective treatment.

Hyperplasia of the turbinate head is a very common type of pathology. It is observed in most patients suffering from allergic and hyperreactive rhinitis. The congested head of the turbinate protrudes in a medial and anterior direction and obstructs the valve area. It is important to distinguish this condition from hypertrophy of the whole turbinate and of the tail. Topical or systemic use of corticosteroids and/or antihistamines is the preferred therapy. If ineffective, an anterior turbinoplasty is usually the best solution, as this type of surgery reduces turbinate volume at a critical area without loss of function.

Hyperplasia of the whole turbinate is an even more common symptom of allergic and hyperreactive rhinitis (see ▶ Fig. 2.121). Our therapeutic approach is the same: first treat with medications; if ineffective, resort to surgical reduction of the whole turbinate by intraturbinal resection of bone and parenchyma, or by crushing and trimming (see following text).

Hyperplasia of the turbinate tail is frequently seen in patients with chronic sinusitis and postnasal discharge. The mucosa and submucosa have become hyperplastic due to continuous infection, and they degenerate irreversibly with the formation of polypoid, papillomatous, or fibrous new growth (see ▶ Fig. 2.122). Resection of the pathology with some trimming of the turbinate is usually the best remedy.

Treatment

Conservative Treatment

As previously noted, we will first consider conservative treatment, as we would in the majority of cases of turbinate pathology. The effect of a corticosteroid spray and/or systemic or topical antihistamines should be tested in allergic or hyperreactive patients for at least 3 months. Where infection plays a role, a course of antibiotics (sometimes in combination with antihistamines or corticosteroids) should be given first. In patients who do not respond within 3 to 6 months, surgery must be considered.

Surgical Treatment

Methods

Over the past 130 years, some 14 different methods have been used to treat hypertrophy of the inferior turbinate. These are, in chronological order: thermal coagulation (electrocautery), chemocoagulation (chemocautery), (partial) turbinectomy, lateralization, submucosal resection of the turbinate bone, crushing and/or trimming, injection of corticosteroids, injection of sclerosing agents, vidian neurectomy, cryosurgery, turbinoplasty, laser surgery, reduction using powered instruments like shavers, and high-radiofrequency coablation. While several of these procedures have been abandoned, quite a few are still in use. An overview is given in ▶ Table 8.1. In our opinion, the majority of techniques that are still in use are to be condemned, as they are unnecessarily destructive to nasal function. An extensive review of the literature and a discussion on the various techniques was presented by Hol and Huizing (2000).

Criteria for Evaluating Methods of Reducing Turbinate Volume

Procedures to reduce a turbinate should be judged by two basic criteria. The first is the efficacy of the technique in alleviating breathing obstruction, hypersecretion, recurrent infection, sneezing, and headaches. The second is an

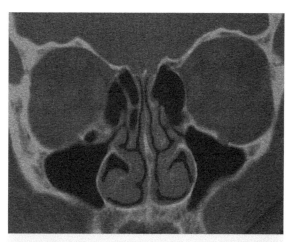

Fig. 8.1 Protrusion and hyperplasia of the inferior turbinates. The angle between the turbinate bone and the lateral nasal wall is wide.

Table 8.1 Different modalities of treatment for inferior turbinate hypertrophy (data from Hol and Huizing 2000)

Method	Time of introduction	(Still) in use	Abandoned
Thermal coagulation (electrocautery)	1845–1880	+	
Chemocoagulation	1869–1890	+	
Turbinectomy	1882	+	
Lateralization	1904	+	
Submucosal resection of turbinate bone	1906–1911	+	
Crushing and trimming	1930–1953	+	
Injection of corticosteroids	1952		+
Injection of sclerosing agents	1953		+
Vidian neurectomy	1961		+
Cryosurgery	1970		+
Turbinoplasty	1982	+	
Laser surgery	1977	+	
Powered instruments (shavers)	1994	+	
High-radiofrequency radiation	1998	+	

assessment of the procedure's side effects, both in the short term and the long term. It would be a mistake to focus solely on the degree of widening of the nasal passages in terms of endoscopic findings, rhinomanometry, and acoustic rhinometry. A wider nasal cavity does not necessarily mean the nose functions better. The aim of turbinate surgery must be to *reduce volume (pathology) while preserving function.*

Surgical Techniques

A Critical Evaluation

Thermal coagulation or electrocautery was initially introduced in the period 1845 to 1860. The method gradually gained in popularity, eventually coming into widespread use when cocaine became available as a topical anesthetic in the 1880s. Even today, electrocautery is still carried out. Historically, in surface electrocautery two parallel furrows are usually cut into the turbinate. As a result of coagulation of the tissues, the turbinate is diminished in size. During the healing process, further reduction takes place by retraction of the scar tissue. However, irreversible damage has been done to the mucosa, with its cilia, glands, and defense systems. The epithelium becomes metaplastic, and mucociliary transport is abolished. Crusting may occur, and patients often complain of nasal dryness and irritation. Synechiae are another common side effect. In terms of function, surface electrocautery is a destructive procedure and does not meet the requirement of "diminishing volume (pathology) while preserving function." Modern variations, such as submucosal bipolar diathermy and the recently propagated high-frequency diathermy coablation, may cause less superficial damage.

Chemocoagulation or chemocautery with chromic acid or trichloric acid was introduced as an alternative to electrocautery in the last decades of the 19th century. In our opinion, chemocautery of the turbinate mucosa is the worst treatment imaginable. It does not reduce the turbinate volume but causes damage to all functional elements of the mucosa.

Turbinectomy also dates from the last decades of the 19th century. Resection of the inferior turbinate became one of the most frequently practiced rhinological surgical procedures in the first quarter of the 20th century. Special instruments were designed, such as Struycken's scissors. Soon after its introduction, however, reports about postoperative atrophic rhinitis and "secondary" ozena appeared. This led many surgeons to use more conservative techniques such as lateralization, partial resection, and submucous resection of the turbinate bone. In the 1970s and 1980s, turbinectomy was again recommended by several authors. Many of them disputed claims that it might lead to atrophic rhinitis or a "wide nasal cavity syndrome." Noting the numerous complications, others disagreed. Stenquist and Kern coined the term "empty nose syndrome." In our opinion, turbinectomy is a nasal crime.

Total turbinectomy must be considered a nasal crime.

Lateralization by outfracturing the turbinate was introduced as early as 1904 by Killian, among others. This conservative function-preserving method is still widely used, particularly as a flanking procedure along with septoplasty. Its effect is rather limited.

Submucosal resection of the turbinate bone was presented by several authors in the years 1906 to 1911, as an alternative to the more aggressive techniques previously discussed. Despite its attraction, this procedure gained only limited popularity. In 1951, Howard House revived the method. The anterior part of the bony lamella, together with some of the parenchyma, is resected through an incision at the head of the turbinate (Freer 1911). Mabry (1982, 1984) refined the technique and introduced the term "turbinoplasty." As the mucosa and submucosa are preserved, the method meets our requirement of "volume reduction with preservation of function." In a comparative study by Passali et al (1999), this technique came out as the best method.

Crushing and/or trimming have been recommended as a less destructive alternative to turbinectomy since early 1930s. The turbinate is first crushed in an effort to damage and thus reduce the amount of the parenchyma and, at the same time, to leave the mucosal surface intact. It is then trimmed to size. From the viewpoint of preserving function, the technique appears to be acceptable, provided it is performed in a conservative way.

Injection of a long-acting corticosteroid solution was introduced in 1952. The method was soon discouraged because of its temporary results and reports of acute homolateral blindness.

Injection of sclerosing agents was suggested for the first time in 1953. The method did not come into general use because of its unpredictable results and complications.

Vidian neurectomy was introduced by Golding Wood in 1961 as a completely different approach to the problem of turbinate hypertrophy and hypersecretion. Parasympathetic innervation was severed by cutting the nerve fibers in the Vidian canal through a transantral approach or endonasal coagulation of the sphenopalatine ganglion. Usually, some decrease of hypersecretion was obtained. The effect on blockage was poor. Since the effects appeared to be temporary, the method was abandoned in the 1970s.

Cryosurgery was the next step in the long history of the treatment of inferior turbinate hypertrophy. It was widely used in the 1970s, but its popularity soon declined. The amount of reduction appeared to be rather unpredictable.

Laser surgery is a more recent approach to turbinate reduction. It was introduced in 1977 by Lenz and others, and has become increasingly popular. A huge number of enthusiastic reports have appeared over the past 15 years. Some describe the results achieved with a CO_2

laser, others report on the results of using a KTP or an Nd: YAG laser. It is unlikely that the type of laser has much influence on the outcome. More important is the way the laser is applied. Is it used superficially on the mucosa to make a large number of small craters ("surface laser treatment")? Or is it applied as a means to resect a part of the turbinate? The latter seems to be the more acceptable method, since it uses the laser as scissors or a knife. The part of the turbinate that is left behind then has a normal structure and function. Surface laser treatment, on the contrary, evaporates a large part of the mucosa and submucosa, as shown by histological studies. There will be considerable loss of function, while the reduction of turbinate volume is limited. In our opinion, laser treatment of the turbinate surface should therefore not be performed.

> "As soon as we have got a new instrument, you will see that it is immediately tried out on the turbinates." (Wolfgang Pirsig).

Powered instruments like "shavers" have recently come into use in turbinate surgery. These instruments are used on the turbinate surface as well as intraturbinally, often in combination with an endoscope. Use of a powered instrument appears to be a matter of personal preference. The results depend less on the instrument that is used than on the surgical concept.

High-frequency coablation is another more recent technique for reducing turbinate hypertrophy. Again it makes a difference whether it is used superficially or endoturbinally.

In Conclusion

When accepting that the aim of turbinate surgery must be to diminish complaints while preserving function, we have to come to the conclusion that only four of the methods discussed above are acceptable:
1. Submucosal turbinoplasty
2. Lateralization
3. (Crushing and) trimming
4. Local resection of irreversibly degenerated mucosa (polyps, granulations)

The choice of technique in an individual case will depend on the type of pathology. All procedures may be carried out under general or local anesthesia (for techniques see Chapter 3, page 132). If local anesthesia has been chosen, care is taken to thoroughly block the branches of the pterygopalatine and nasopalatine nerves, as they innervate the posterior part of the inferior turbinate (see ▶ Fig. 1.57).

> In reducing a turbinate, it depends not so much on the instrument that is used. Rather, it is the surgical concept that counts.

Submucosal Turbinoplasty

In our opinion, submucosal turbinoplasty is the method of choice in cases of turbinate hypertrophy. It is the most function-preserving technique of reducing a turbinate. The method is based on the principle of submucosal resection of a part of the turbinate bone and parenchyma. It was developed into an elegant plastic procedure by Mabry, Lindsay Gray, Pirsig, and others. If the hyperplasia is limited to the head of the turbinate, only an anterior turbinoplasty is carried out. Acoustic rhinometry before and after decongestion may provide definite proof of this diagnosis (see ▶ Fig. 2.154 ▶ Fig. 2.155). If the posterior part of the turbinate and/or its tail is involved, the crushing and trimming technique may be used.

Steps

- The (anterior part of the) turbinate is medialized (see previous text).
- An L-shaped incision is made at the head and the inferior margin of the turbinate with a No. 15 blade or a No. 64 Beaver knife (▶ Fig. 8.2).
- The soft tissues are elevated from both sides of the anterior half of the bony lamella. If only an anterior turbinoplasty is planned, elevating over an area of 1 to 2 cm will suffice.
- A medial mucosal flap is mobilized to obtain sufficient access (▶ Fig. 8.3).
- The anterior part of the bone is resected with a biting forceps. A certain amount of parenchyma is resected using small scissors (▶ Fig. 8.4). In an anterior turbinoplasty, a resection of 1 to 2 cm of the turbinate bone is usually sufficient.
- The mucosal flaps are trimmed until they can be adjusted properly. The newly created anterior part of the turbinate is hereby not only reduced but also somewhat displaced in a posterior direction, thus unblocking the valve area (▶ Fig. 8.5).
- The redressed mucosa is fixed in place with one or two resorbable sutures or plates of compressed gelfoam or Merocel, and strips of Adaptic or gauze with ointment (▶ Fig. 8.6).

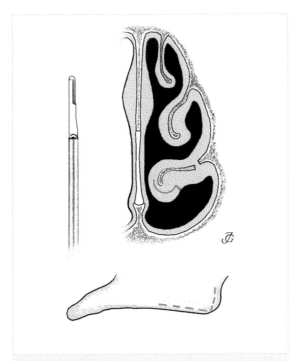

Fig. 8.2 Submucosal (anterior) turbinoplasty. An L-shaped incision is made in the mucosa of the anterior and inferior margin with a No. 64 Beaver knife.

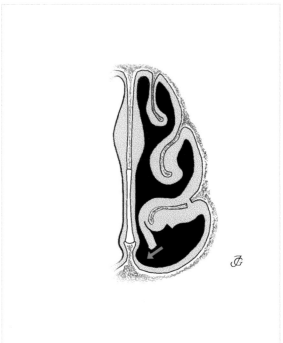

Fig. 8.3 A medially based mucosal flap is dissected.

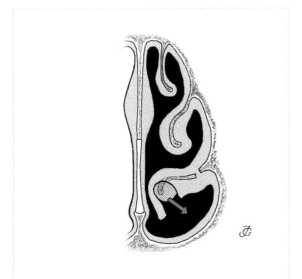

Fig. 8.4 The anterior or the anteroinferior part of the turbinate bone is resected, usually by 1 to 2 cm, together with some of the parenchyma as required.

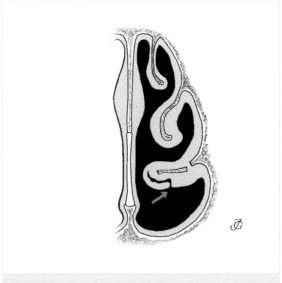

Fig. 8.5 The mucosal flap is repositioned.

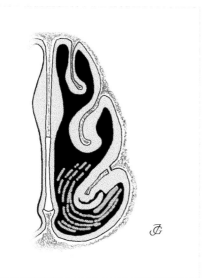

Fig. 8.6 The reduced turbinate is repositioned and fixed in its new position with gelfoam and an (anointed) internal dressing.

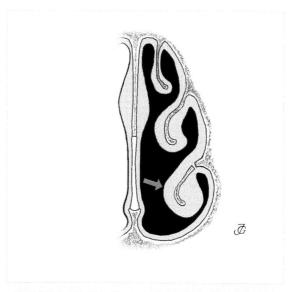

Fig. 8.7 Lateralization of a protruding or hyperplastic inferior turbinate is performed using the flat, blunt end of a Cottle chisel.

Lateralization

Lateralization (lateral displacement) of the inferior turbinate by outfracturing the turbinate bone is the most conservative method to address turbinate obstruction. It is mostly used in combination with another procedure, as lateralization alone is rarely effective enough. It is often combined with septal surgery or one of the volume-reducing techniques described in the following text.

Steps

- The turbinate is outfractured with a flat and blunt instrument, such as the handle of a Cottle chisel. The use of a speculum is not advisable, as the pressure exerted by the blades of the speculum will damage both the septal and the turbinate mucosa. This may result in a synechia.
- The turbinate is lateralized into the desired position (▸ Fig. 8.7). An internal dressing may be used to keep it in place.

(Crushing and) Trimming

When the inferior turbinate is hypertrophic both anteriorly and posteriorly, crushing and trimming would be the best compromise between reduction and preservation of function. The whole turbinate is first compressed using a special forceps, and then reduced by resecting a parallel or slightly diagonal strip from its inferior margin. The technique respects the functional capacity of the remaining part of the turbinate.

Steps

- The turbinate is fractured medially with a flat and blunt instrument, such as the handle of a Cottle chisel.
- The turbinate is squeezed with a modified Kressner forceps (▸ Fig. 8.8). This is done at two different levels, both posteriorly and anteriorly.
- The now somewhat flabby inferior part of the turbinate is trimmed with long, angulated Heymann scissors (▸ Fig. 8.9). When indicated, an inferior strip of the turbinate bone is resected. The cut is made parallel or slightly oblique to the nasal floor. Resecting too much from the turbinate tail is avoided. Besides, care is taken not to resect too much at one time. It is better to later remove an extra slice of tissue than to remove too much at once.
- The reduced turbinate is moved into the desired position (▸ Fig. 8.10).
- A dressing with ointment is applied to prevent bleeding. It is usually removed after 1 to 3 days.

Resection of Degenerated Tissue

When part of the turbinate mucosa (e.g., the tail), is irreversibly degenerated, the diseased tissue is resected using long angulated scissors or, in special cases, a snare.

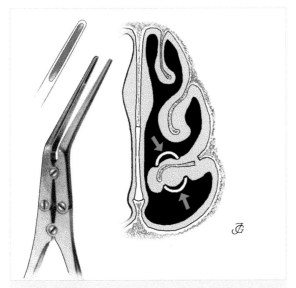

Fig. 8.8 The inferior turbinate is crushed and trimmed in cases with hypertrophy of the whole turbinate, including the tail. The soft tissues are squeezed using a modified Kressner forceps.

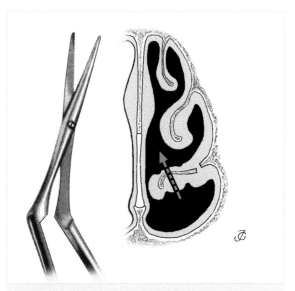

Fig. 8.9 The turbinate is trimmed to size by resecting a strip from its inferior margin with Heymann-type scissors.

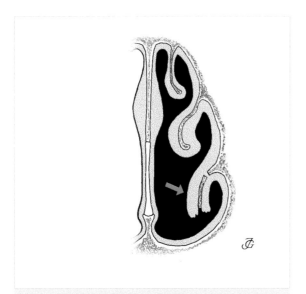

Fig. 8.10 The reduced turbinate is repositioned laterally.

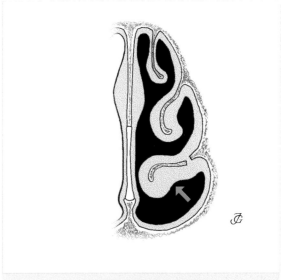

Fig. 8.11 Medialization of the inferior turbinate.

Steps

- The turbinate is fractured medially with a flat and blunt instrument, such as the handle of a Cottle chisel (▶ Fig. 8.11).
- The pathological tissue is resected using sharp scissors (Heymann type, ▶ Fig. 8.12) or, in patients with a polypous type of degeneration, with a snare (▶ Fig. 8.13).
- The turbinate is lateralized again. An internal dressing is applied.

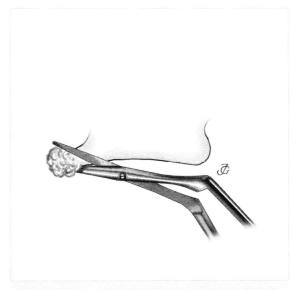

Fig. 8.12 Resection of irreversibly degenerated tissue from the turbinate tail with Heymann scissors.

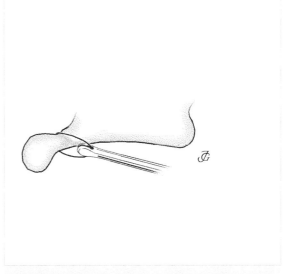

Fig. 8.13 Resection of a degenerative tissue mass from the turbinate tail using a snare.

8.1.3 Middle Turbinate

Pathology

Abnormalities of the middle turbinate may be divided into two types: anatomical variations and pathological conditions. The most common anatomic variations are:
1. Concha bullosa
2. Concha spongiosa
3. Paradoxically curved turbinate
4. Double turbinate
5. Concha polyposa

The most common type of pathology is concha polyposa. Usually, these abnormalities can be easily recognized by nasal endoscopy. Decongestion and palpation may help in making the correct diagnosis. Concha bullosa and a spongiotic turbinate bone can be also be confirmed by coronal and axial CT scanning (▸ Fig. 8.14).

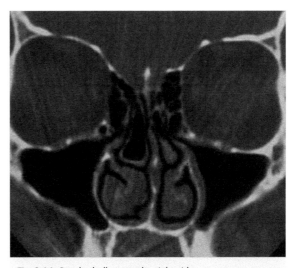

Fig. 8.14 Concha bullosa on the right side.

Concha Bullosa

Concha bullosa is an anatomical variation found in about 25% of the population. The skeleton of the turbinate consists of a bony cell (in rare cases multiple cells) instead of a more or less curved lamella. This cell or bulla, which is in fact an ethmoidal cell, may be of considerable size, obstructing the middle nasal passage and the infundibulum. The general opinion is that individuals with a concha bullosa are more inclined to develop sinusitis and polyposis. Unequivocal confirmation of this hypothesis is lacking, however. See also ▸ Fig. 1.46 and ▸ Fig. 2.120.

Concha Spongiosa

The bony skeleton of the turbinate consists of a massive bone with a cortex and spongiotic bone in its center instead of a lamella. This condition may be suspected at rhinoscopy and palpation, but can only be definitively diagnosed by a CT scan or during surgery. It is a normal variation that may have consequences similar to those of a bullous turbinate.

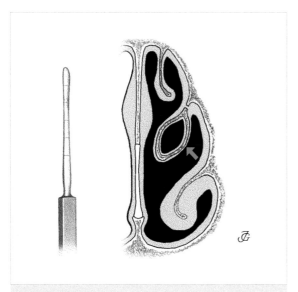

Fig. 8.15 The middle turbinate is medialized with the blunt end of a Cottle elevator

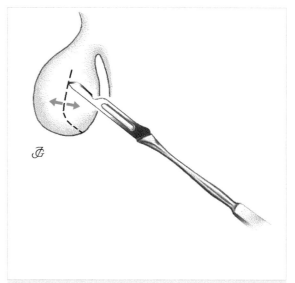

Fig. 8.16 An L-shaped incision is made in the mucosa of the turbinate head and inferior margin with a No. 15 blade or a No. 64 Beaver knife.

Paradoxically Curved Turbinate

Paradoxically curved turbinate is a relatively rare anatomical variation (see ▶ Fig. 2.119). When present, it may compromise the middle nasal passage and the infundibulum. Surgical correction is then advisable.

Double Middle Turbinate

Double middle turbinate is another rare anatomical variation that may have consequences similar to those of the abnormally curved turbinate.

Concha Polyposa

Concha polyposa is a very common type of pathology usually related to chronic purulent rhinosinusitis. It may be part of a vicious circle: infection–swelling–polypoid degeneration–obstruction–infection.

Surgical Techniques

When indicated, the pathology and abnormalities of the middle turbinate may be corrected by resecting parts of the skeleton and trimming the mucosa. The surgical goal is to create a turbinate that fits anatomically and physiologically. Middle turbinate reduction may be carried out as a single procedure. More frequently, it is performed as a flanking procedure in combination with septal or sinus surgery. Using the endoscope is of great help.

Steps

- The middle turbinate is medialized with a slender blunt instrument, such as the handle of a Cottle chisel, a Freer elevator, or the blunt end of a Cottle elevator. Medializing a middle turbinate with a speculum may lead to opposing mucosal lesions and synechia (▶ Fig. 8.15).
- An L-shaped incision is made in the mucosa with a No. 15 blade or a No. 64 Beaver knife (▶ Fig. 8.16).
- The mucoperiosteum is elevated with the semi-sharp end of a Cottle elevator. The bulla (or the spongiotic bone) is exposed (▶ Fig. 8.17).
- The bulla is opened and inspected. Mucus, pus, and the complete mucosal lining of the inside are removed (▶ Fig. 8.18).
- Half of the bulla is then resected in a piecemeal manner with a slender Blakesley forceps (▶ Fig. 8.19). (Spongiotic bone is usually partially removed.)
- The soft tissues and remaining skeleton are then compressed using a forceps (▶ Fig. 8.20). The mucosa is trimmed with special angulated scissors. A new and smaller turbinate is created (▶ Fig. 8.21).
- The new and smaller turbinate is positioned and fixed between the septum and the lateral wall of the infundibulum with Merocel or gauzes with ointment, which are left in place for several (5 to 7) days to avoid synechiae.

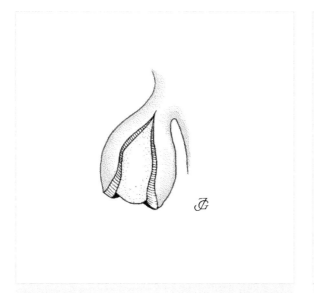

Fig. 8.17 The mucoperiosteum is bilaterally elevated; the bulla is exposed.

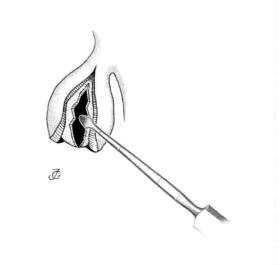

Fig. 8.18 The bulla is opened using the sharp end of a Cottle elevator.

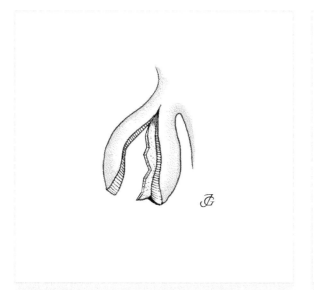

Fig. 8.19 The mucosal lining of the inside of the bulla is removed together with the medial half of the bulla.

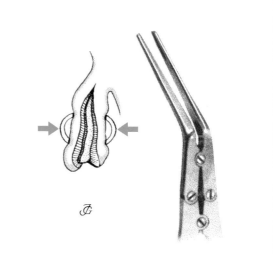

Fig. 8.20 The remaining bone and the soft tissues are compressed.

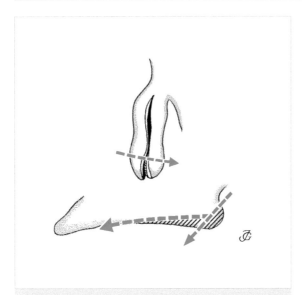

Fig. 8.21 The head and the inferior margin of the turbinate are trimmed to the desired size with Heymann scissors and angulated scissors.

Preservation or Resection of the Middle Turbinate in Infundibulotomy and Ethmoidectomy

Whether or not the middle turbinate should be preserved or resected in ethmoid surgery for chronic sinusitis with polyposis is an old debate. It dates from the 1920s and has led to several vehement discussions. There have been middle turbinate "preservers" and "removers." Among the well-known surgeons who routinely resected the middle turbinate in the old days were Mosher, Yankauer, Lederer, and more recently, Friedman. Their ideas were opposed by Pratt, Williams and Eichel, and others, who advocated preservation of the turbinate when possible. This discussion has recently been revived with respect to endoscopic sinus surgery. Some surgeons remove the middle turbinate, claiming a lower incidence of synechiae and more patency of the maxillary ostium. Others stress that the middle turbinate should be respected as much as possible, as it plays an important role in nasal physiology. In our opinion, routine resection is unnecessarily aggressive in many cases, and thus difficult to defend as a standard. Here too, pathology must dictate the extent of surgery. Irreversibly degenerated tissues have to be removed, while drainage and ventilation should be restored. On the other hand, reversibly diseased mucosa and important anatomical–physiological structures must be preserved as much as possible.

8.2 Surgery of the Wide Nasal Cavity

8.2.1 Pathology

The wide nasal cavity is a well-known pathological entity. Because of its specific set of symptoms, one might speak of the "wide nasal cavity syndrome," or in severe cases of the "empty nose syndrome." The most frequent causes are atrophic rhinitis, ozena, and postoperative widening of the nasal cavity following turbinate resection or surgery for polyposis and tumors. The symptomatology of the wide nasal cavity syndrome is highly variable. Several factors play a role, in particular the quality of the mucosa and submucosa, and the anatomical configuration of the widened nasal cavity.

Atrophic Rhinitis

This condition is characterized by a dry, atrophic and metaplastic mucosa and an atrophic submucosa with signs of chronic infection. There is loss of cilia, goblet cells, and seromucous glands. As a consequence, mucociliary transport (MCT) is abolished. Usually, the mucosal membrane has a pale color and small crusts may appear. The nasal cavity is usually wide. Atrophic rhinitis is generally secondary. The most common causes are:

- Iatrogenic damage to the nasal mucosa due to (repeated) electrocoagulation, chemocautery, or surface laser surgery
- Radiation therapy
- Repeated and/or excessive turbinate surgery in youngsters suffering from cystic fibrosis
- Systemic diseases such as sicca syndrome, relapsing polychondritis, and Wegener granulomatosis

Patients usually complain of dryness of the nose, irritation, crusting, bleeding, and a feeling of nasal obstruction.

Ozena

Ozena is a primary disease characterized by severe atrophy of the nasal mucosa and submucosa with formation of foul-smelling crusts. *Klebsiella ozaenae* can be cultured in most of the cases. The pathogenesis of ozena has not yet been fully elucidated. It may occur as a separate disease entity or as part of a syndrome such as ectodermal dysplasia. The disease has been known for ages. It has been described in almost all ancient cultures, very likely because of the foul odor that affected individuals produced, making them social outcasts.

Epidemiology

The disease usually starts at a young age and becomes fully developed after puberty. It is more frequently observed in girls than in boys. In Western Europe, ozena was once a common disease. After World War II, its incidence gradually decreased. By 1969, we were still able to report on the surgical results of 102 operations performed in 50 patients in the years 1962 to 1967 (van Bolhuis 1967). Nowadays, only a few cases are treated each year in our department. The generally accepted explanation for this sharp decline is the great improvement in the general physical condition of young people. Their good health is mainly due to better nutrition and the decreased incidence of chronic rhinosinusitis and other chronic infections in childhood.

Etiology

The known causative factors of ozena are genetic predisposition, poor nutrition, and chronic infection.

Pathology

The disease is characterized by severe atrophy of the whole nasal mucosa, submucosa, cavernous parenchyma of the turbinates, cartilage, and bone of all nasal structures. Sometimes the maxilla is involved too. As a result of the atrophy, an abnormal widening of the whole nasal cavity occurs, especially in its posterior and inferior regions. Chronic inflammation of the mucosa and submucosa with formation of large, foul-smelling crusts is seen on inspection. *Klebsiella ozaenae* and other pathogenic and nonpathogenic micro-organisms can be cultured. These bacteria are considered to be opportunistic parasites.

Symptoms

The main symptoms of the disease are fetor, formation of greenish–brown crusts, anosmia, and headache. A feeling of nasal obstruction, in spite of the widening of the nasal cavity, is often reported. This symptom is very likely due to abnormal breathing patterns and involvement of the sensory innervation of the mucosa. If the external nasal pyramid is involved, saddling of the bony and cartilaginous dorsum will gradually develop, sometimes in combination with hypoplasia of the midface and maxillary sinuses (▶ Fig. 8.22).

Postoperative Widening of the Nasal Cavity

Pathological enlargement of the nasal cavity is a common rhinological entity. Its most frequent cause is resection of the inferior and/or middle turbinate. It is also seen following surgery for polyposis and sinusitis, or tumor resection.

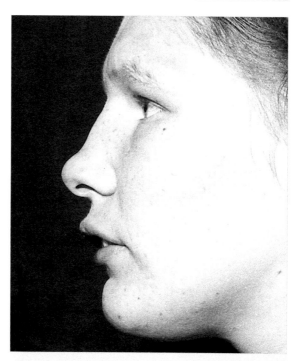

Fig. 8.22 Characteristic sagging of the cartilaginous nasal dorsum and maxillary hypoplasia in a patient with ozena.

Turbinate Reduction and Resection

Unfortunately, a wide nasal cavity syndrome due to reduction or resection of the inferior turbinate (and/or middle turbinate) is still frequently seen. When caused by (subtotal) turbinectomy, it can hardly be considered a complication. In our opinion, it is a "nasal crime." This iatrogenic condition can easily be avoided by reducing a hypertrophic turbinate using one of the intraturbinal function-preserving techniques (see page 301).

Ethmoidosphenoidectomy

Surgery for polyposis and/or chronic sinusitis is another well known cause of wide nasal cavity syndrome. Symptoms may occur particularly when the middle turbinate is resected. Whether or not symptoms occur depends upon the extent and the location of the widening and the quality of the mucosa.

Tumor Removal

Tumor removal may also result in pathological widening of the nasal cavity. Fortunately, symptoms occur only in a limited number of cases. Why some patients develop crusting while others do not is not easy to explain. Various factors play a role, for instance the geometry of the cavity and the quality of the mucosa.

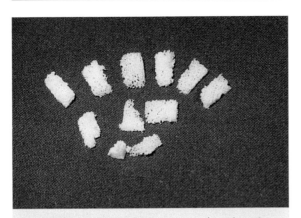

Fig. 8.23 Processed heterogeneic spongiotic bone (e.g., Osteovit) is cut into small pieces and soaked in isotonic saline with antibiotics.

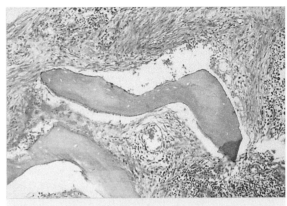

Fig. 8.24 Processed heterogeneic spongiotic bone is invaded by connective tissue and not resorbed. Histological section of biopsy obtained 5 years postoperatively at revision surgery.

8.2.2 Treatment

Conservative Treatment

Treatment of ozena has an extremely long history. For many centuries, conservative treatment was the only option. Various methods have been used to clean the nasal cavity and improve the quality of the mucosa. Today, cleansing of the nose by irrigation, ointments (e.g., lanolin, Vaseline, glycerin), or oils (sesame oil) is still one of the basic modes of therapy. Insufflation of glucose powder may also be of great help in reducing crusting and fetor.

Attempts to improve the quality of the mucosa have also been numerous (e.g., topical application of estrogens and oral supplementation of iron). To treat concomitant infection, several antibiotics have been advocated. Long courses of systemic broad-spectrum antibiotics and topical antibiotic drops and ointments have both been tried, but the results have been only temporary.

Surgical Treatment

Historical Development

The insight that surgical narrowing of the wide nose might be effective dates from the early 1900s, when submucous injection with paraffin was introduced. Lautenschläger (1926) developed a surgical technique to narrow the nasal cavity by detaching and inwardly displacing the lateral nasal walls and the inferior turbinates. In the 1920s, various authors tried to narrow the nasal cavity by submucosal implantation of autogeneic bone (tibia, iliac crest) or processed ox bone (Eckert-Moebius 1923). This method remained popular until the end of the 1950s. From the 1930s on, all types of nonbiological materials have been tried (acrylic, tantalum gauze, dolomite, Proplast, and hydroxyapatite). These attempts were not very successful, however. Nonbiological materials are poorly accepted between the thin mucosa and the

atrophic cartilage and bone. Unterberger (1929) was the first to implant bone submucosally in all three nasal walls. This technique was further improved by Cottle (1958) and ourselves (Huizing 1969, 1974, 1976). In the 1980s, Jones working in India, (re)introduced a method of surgical closure of the nasal entrance at the level of the valve area. As this procedure makes nasal breathing and olfaction impossible, we do not consider this method a realistic therapeutic option.

8.2.3 Surgical Techniques

Narrowing the nasal cavity by submucous implantation of processed heterogeneic spongiotic bone is the best treatment available. In patients suffering from ozena, the fetor is mostly abolished, while crusting either disappears or is considerably diminished.

Choice of Implant Material

As discussed above, a great variety of nonbiological and biological materials has been used to narrow a wide nasal cavity. Experience has shown that only biological materials yield satisfactory results. Nonbiological materials are mostly extruded (see ▶ Fig. 9.92 and ▶ Fig. 9.95). Of the available biological materials, we have tried autogeneic bone (spongiotic bone from the iliac crest), cartilage (rib), and fascia. All these transplants were well accepted but showed a very high rate of resorption. Processed xenogeneic spongiotic bone, on the contrary, is well accepted and only resorbed to a limited degree (▶ Fig. 8.23 and ▶ Fig. 8.24). Others prefer using auricular cartilage.

Unilateral Surgery

It is advisable to narrow one side at a time. Bilateral implantation on the septum deprives the usually thin and atrophic cartilage of its nutrition over a large area. This can easily lead to a perforation.

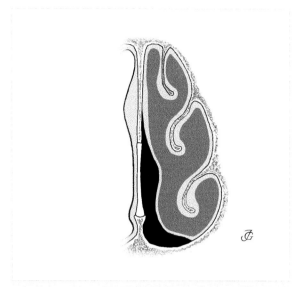

Fig. 8.25 The septal mucosa and the mucosa of the nasal floor is elevated using a right CSI and the MP approach. Both tunnels are joined.

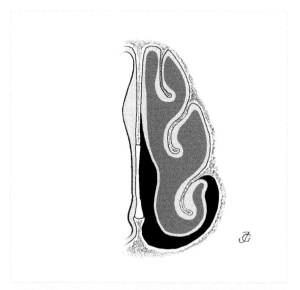

Fig. 8.26 The mucoperiosteum of the lateral nasal wall caudal to the attachment of the inferior turbinate is elevated through a vestibular incision. This tunnel is joined with the other tunnels.

Local or General Anesthesia

We prefer to perform this type of surgery under local anesthesia. If general anesthesia is chosen, a bloodless surgical field is an absolute condition for a good result (for techniques see Chapter 3, page 135).

Area of Implantation

In primary ozena, widening generally takes place in the posterior and inferior parts of the nasal cavity. It is therefore advisable to implant most of the material in area 5. Care is taken not to narrow the region of the valve area.

Importance of Keeping the Mucosa Intact

Keeping the mucoperichondrium/mucoperiosteum fully intact while elevating the tunnels is a necessary condition for successful narrowing. If a perforation is inadvertently made in the mucosa, implantation must not be conducted. A damaged mucosa will not heal over a nonvital bony or cartilaginous implant. Infection will occur, and the material will be extruded. The surgeon then has no other choice but to seal the defect with an underlay of fascia or dura, and reoperate after some months. Only if the perforation is made anteriorly could some material be implanted in the posterior part of the nasal cavity.

Revision Surgery and Additional Implantation

If resorption takes place and symptoms of crusting reappear over the course of time, additional implantation may be considered. Contrary to expectation, such a reoperation is usually less difficult than the primary one. Elevating the mucosa for a second time is usually easier and less risky since some of the implanted material is still present.

Technique of Narrowing the Nasal Cavity

Steps

- A caudal septal incision (CSI) is made in the usual way.
- The caudal end of the septum is dissected, and the anterior nasal spine is exposed.
- An anterosuperior tunnel is elevated on the side that is to be narrowed.
- An inferior tunnel is created on the same side. Both tunnels are joined (▶ Fig. 8.25).
- The inferior tunnel is extended in a lateral direction over the nasal floor.
- A vestibular incision is made, and the lateral wall of the piriform aperture is exposed.
- The mucoperiosteum of the lateral nasal wall caudal to the attachment of the inferior turbinate is elevated (lateral nasal tunnel). The orifice of the nasolacrimal duct is thereby preserved. The lateral tunnel is joined with the inferior tunnel (▶ Fig. 8.26).

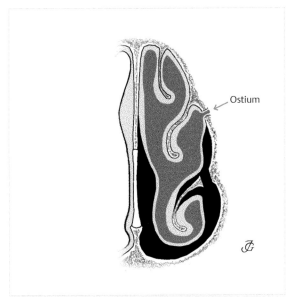

Fig. 8.27 The bone of the inferior turbinate is detached submucosally using a narrow, straight chisel. The turbinate is medialized, and the lateral nasal tunnel is extended in a cranial direction towards the middle meatus. Care is taken not to damage the maxillary ostium.

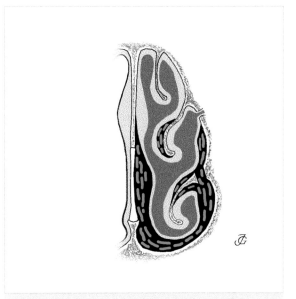

Fig. 8.28 Pieces of processed heterogeneic, spongiotic bone are implanted in all tunnels to narrow the nasal cavity in all its dimensions. When indicated, some material may also be implanted on the medial side of the middle turbinate.

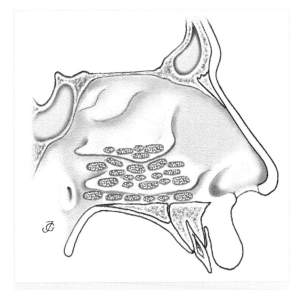

Fig. 8.29 The nasal cavity is narrowed, in particular posteriorly and inferiorly.

- All three tunnels are extended in a posterior direction up to the choana. The septal tunnel is extended to the sphenoid bone and choana; the lateral tunnel is extended up to the tubal orifice; the tunnel on the nasal floor is extended up to the soft palate. Utmost care is taken to avoid perforating the mucoperiosteum (see previous text).

- The inferior turbinate bone is submucosally detached from the lateral wall with a 7-mm chisel or osteotome. The turbinate is subsequently medialized (▶ Fig. 8.27).
- The lateral tunnel is extended in a cranial direction towards the middle meatus. Care is taken not to damage the maxillary ostium.
- The processed spongiotic bone that is to be implanted is soaked in isotonic saline (with antibiotics, if desired) to make it soft enough to be cut and compressed. Rectangular pieces of varying size are prepared.
- The pieces are inserted one by one with a long (16-cm) bayonet forceps. This is performed simultaneously in all three tunnels, proceeding from posterior to anterior (▶ Fig. 8.28). Utmost care is taken to obtain regular narrowing. In general, the greatest narrowing is effected posteriorly and inferiorly (▶ Fig. 8.29). Narrowing of the valve area is to be avoided.
- The pieces of cancellous bone are lightly pressed together to avoid gaps and accumulation of blood. Some overcorrection is advisable to compensate for resorption.
- In patients with an abnormally wide middle nasal passage, some material may be implanted submucosally on the medial side of the middle turbinate. To that end, a vertical incision is made at the head of the turbinate with a No. 64 Beaver knife. The mucoperiosteum on the medial side of the turbinate is then elevated.
- The incisions are closed, and an internal dressing with antibiotic ointment (Terracortril) is applied for 2 or 3 days. A systemic broad-spectrum antibiotic is prescribed for at least a week.

8.3 Endonasal Surgery of the Infundibulum, Ethmoid Bone, and Maxillary Sinus

Disorders of nasal function and form are frequently associated with pathology of the osteomeatal complex, ethmoid bone, maxillary sinus, sphenoid bone, and frontal sinus. Although this book is not intended to deal with sinus problems, a discussion on endonasal sinus surgery should not be left out.

In many patients with impaired nasal function, septal pyramid or turbinate surgery has to be combined with some type of endonasal sinus operation. Likewise, in cases of infection and polyposis, sinus surgery is often flanked by septoplasty and/or turbinoplasty. For more information on the diseases and pathology of the paranasal sinuses, we refer the reader to one of the many recent books on endoscopic sinus surgery. Here, we restrict ourselves to a brief discussion of the pathology of the infundibulum and the middle meatus, and the most common endonasal surgical techniques.

8.3.1 Pathology of the Infundibulum and Middle Meatus

Obstruction of the infundibulum and the middle nasal meatus is a common type of pathology. It may lead to a common set of symptoms, in particular postnasal discharge, breathing impairment, hyposmia, and pressure headache (see also Chapter 2, page 73). Due to impairment of the drainage and aeration of the maxillary sinus, anterior ethmoidal cells, and frontal sinus, sinusitis may result. In most cases, obstruction of the middle meatus and infundibulum is caused by a combination of three factors: anatomical abnormalities and variations; infection; and polypoid degeneration of the mucosa.

A septal deformation in the cranial part of area 4 is one of the common causes of obstruction of the middle nasal passage. Permanent contact between a deviated septum and the middle turbinate may be one of the underlying factors of a middle meatus obstructive syndrome.

Abnormalities and variations of middle turbinate anatomy, such as concha bullosa or spongiosa, may act in a similar way. An abnormally massive middle turbinate may permanently impact on the septum and/or the lateral wall of the infundibulum, thereby impairing sinus drainage and aeration.

Rhinosinusitis is another major cause of infundibular pathology. Chronic production of mucopurulent secretions leads to polypous degeneration of the mucosa, and ultimately to polyp formation in the infundibulum and ethmoidal cells. Swelling and polyposis impairs aeration and drainage of the sinuses involved. This enhances the chronicity of the infection, creating a vicious circle.

Polypoid degeneration of the nasal and sinus mucosa is one of the most common rhinological diseases of our time. Evidently, several factors play a role in the origin of this pathology. First of all, hereditary and infectious factors are involved. Previously, allergy was considered a causative factor as well. It has been amply demonstrated, however, that an immediate-type IgE-mediated allergy is not involved. Recently, Ponikau and Kern have suggested that an immunological reaction to a chronic fungal infection might play a role in the pathogenesis of polyposis.

8.3.2 Surgical Techniques

Surgical treatment of nasal obstruction by polyposis and sinusitis has a very long history. The first attempts date back to the ancient Egyptian, Greek, and Roman cultures. By the end of the 19th century, major new therapeutic modalities were introduced to treat sinus infections and polyposis. The main modalities were: antral irrigation through the inferior meatus; surgery of the antrum by the canine approach; nasoantrostomy; and ethmoid and frontal sinus surgery by the external and the endonasal approach. In the years 1910 to 1970, these methods were further developed by various authors in several countries.

In the 1950s, fiber optics were introduced by Harold Hopkins. In the 1960s, he designed the rod lance system. Soon afterwards, Karl Storz made this instrument available for general practice. Messerklinger (1970, 1972), Buiter (1976), and Wigand (1977, 1981) introduced the endoscope for diagnosis and therapy. In the 1980s, endonasal sinus surgery was propagated further by Stammberger (1985) in Europe and Kennedy (1985) in the United States. Some authors prefer the use of the microscope or magnifying glass to the endoscope.

Infundibulotomy and Middle Meatal Antrostomy

Infundibulotomy is a surgical procedure combining widening of the region between the middle turbinate, anterior ethmoid bone, and lateral nasal wall by resecting the uncinate process and the ethmoidal bulla and enlarging the natural ostium of the antrum.

The objective of infundibulotomy and middle meatal antrostomy (MMA) is to abolish infundibular obstruction. At the same time, it is meant to establish better drainage and ventilation of the maxillary sinus, the anterior ethmoidal cells, and the frontal sinus. In patients with concomitant pathology of the middle turbinate and/or a septal deformity, the procedure may be combined with reduction of the middle turbinate and/or surgery of the septum. In cases with more extensive pathology, anterior ethmoidectomy, (sub)total ethmoidectomy, or enlargement of the frontal sinus orifice may be mandatory (see following text).

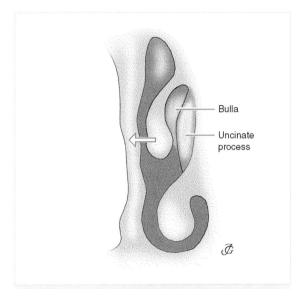

Fig. 8.30 The uncinate process and ethmoidal bulla are exposed after medialization of the middle turbinate.

Bulla

Uncinate process

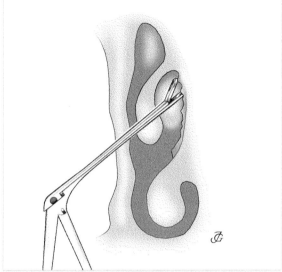

Fig. 8.31 The uncinate process is resected with a Blakesley forceps.

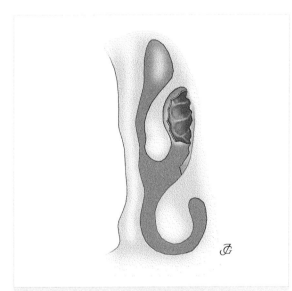

Fig. 8.32 The ethmoidal bulla is opened and resected.

Infundibulotomy can be performed under local anesthesia as an outpatient treatment. If more extensive surgery is required, general anesthesia is preferable.

Steps

- Local anesthesia and mucosal decongestion is obtained by applying small gauzes soaked in a solution of cocaine 7% with adrenaline 1:20,000. The gauzes are applied in particular medial and lateral to the middle turbinate (see also Chapter 3, page 133). It is advisable to do this in two steps. The first step serves to anesthetize the nasal mucosa in general; the second step (new gauzes may be used) is to anesthetize and decongest the surgical field proper. Care is taken to bring the gauzes into direct contact with the mucosa. The anesthesia may be reinforced if anterior ethmoidectomy seems advisable after the infundibulotomy. Although submucosal injection of an anesthetic solution is sometimes advised, we avoid this as there have been reports of blindness following injection in the lateral nasal wall.

- The middle turbinate is medialized with the blunt end of an elevator. Damage to the mucosa should be avoided to prevent synechiae (▶ Fig. 8.30).

- A middle-sized speculum with broad blades is introduced, and the infundibulum is inspected. The uncinate process, ethmoidal bulla, and maxillary ostium are identified using a 30° endoscope.

- The mucosa over the uncinate process is incised with a No. 15 blade on a long handle. The uncinate process is resected using a slender Blakesley-type forceps. Access to the infundibulum is thereby widened (▶ Fig. 8.31).

- The ethmoidal bulla is opened and resected using a small forceps (▶ Fig. 8.32). If the bulla is filled with polypous mucosa, the anterior ethmoidal cells are resected as well until normal aerated cells are reached. If required, the surgery may be extended by resecting all diseased ethmoidal cells (see following text).

- The ostium is visualized and probed with a curved Ritter probe (▶ Fig. 8.33). If no ostium can be found, the probe is used to penetrate the membranous part (fontanel) of the lateral nasal (antral) wall.

- The ostium is enlarged by punching away some of the tissue anterior and/or inferior to the (newly created) ostium, using a Blakesley forceps and a backward-biting forceps (▶ Fig. 8.34 and ▶ Fig. 8.35).

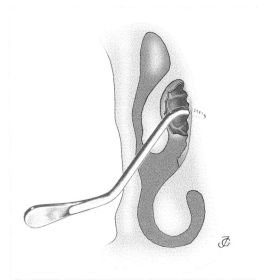

Fig. 8.33 The ostium of the maxillary sinus is identified and probed with a Ritter probe.

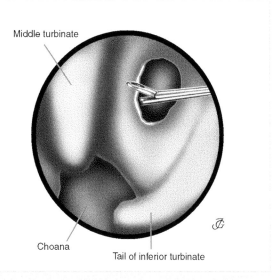

Fig. 8.34 The ostium is enlarged posteriorly with a Blakesley forceps.

- The middle turbinate is adjusted, depending on its size and pathology (for techniques, see page 306).
- Merocel or small gauzes with ointment are applied in the infundibulum between the middle turbinate and the septum. Usually, the gauzes are left in place for several days. We feel that synechiae (the most common complication of infundibulotomy) can be prevented in this way.

Endonasal Anterior and (Sub)Total Ethmoidectomy

If the preoperative CT scan and the findings at infundibulotomy demonstrate pathology of the anterior ethmoidal cells, the operation will be extended by resecting all anterior ethmoidal cells.

If the posterior cells appear to be diseased as well, these cells are also resected. A (subtotal) ethmoidectomy is then performed. To this end, the basal lamella of the middle turbinate has to be removed. There is some controversy as to how extensive the resections should be. The present debate concerns the following issues: (1) To what extent should the mucosa be resected? (2) Should the walls of all cells be completely removed to create a smooth cavity? (3) Should the middle turbinate be routinely resected, left in place, or trimmed?

Should All Mucosa Be Removed?

As a rule, irreversibly diseased mucosa or polypous tissue should be resected, whereas healthy mucosa should be left in place. However, much depends on the individual

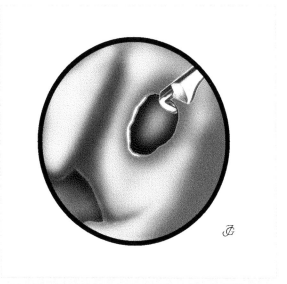

Fig. 8.35 The ostium is enlarged in an anterior direction with a backward-biting forceps.

case. In patients with extensive disease and those with recurrences requiring revision surgery, resection of mucosa will be more aggressive than in cases with limited pathology.

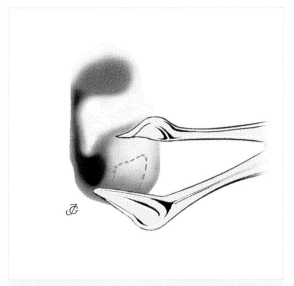

Fig. 8.36 A rectangular, caudally based mucoperichondrial flap about 2 × 1 cm is cut off.

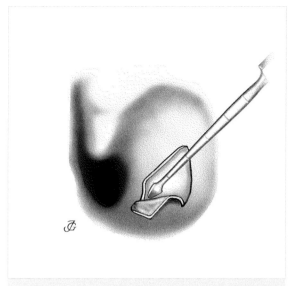

Fig. 8.37 The mucoperiosteal flap is elevated in a caudal direction exposing the lateral bony nasal wall.

Should All Cell Walls Be Resected?

The general rule presented under point 1 also applies to the controversy about whether or not the cell walls are to be resected completely. In cases with limited pathology, drainage of the diseased cells usually suffices. In revision surgery, one may have to decide to resect all cell walls as well as all diseased mucosa, thus creating a smooth cavity. Such a cavity will not become lined with functional ciliated epithelium, however. Crusting and other symptoms of an irreversible wide nasal cavity syndrome may occur.

Should the Middle Turbinate Be Routinely Resected, Left in Place, or Trimmed?

In our opinion, the middle turbinate should be treated conservatively. It is either trimmed or left untouched. There is no justification for routinely resecting a functional nasal organ, except in special circumstances. This issue has been discussed more extensively on page 308.

Inferior Meatal Antrostomy

We consider inferior meatal antrostomy (IMA) to be a beneficial surgical procedure, even though some recent publications may suggest otherwise. The procedure should be carried out with a modern tissue-conserving technique, as described, for example, by Buiter (1988). Lund (1985) has demonstrated that the window should measure at least 1 × 1.5 cm to guarantee that the opening will be permanently draining and ventilating.

Steps

- Local anesthesia and mucosal decongestion are achieved in the usual way.
- The inferior turbinate is fractured upward to an almost horizontal position to allow a sufficient view of the inferior lateral nasal wall. A self-retaining speculum may be used to allow the surgeon to work with two hands.
- An incision is made in the mucoperiosteum, as illustrated in ▶ Fig. 8.36.
- A rectangular mucoperiosteal flap, which has its base in the nasal floor, is cut and elevated in a craniocaudal direction. The flap is about 2 cm long (anteroposterior) and 1 cm high (craniocaudal) (▶ Fig. 8.37).
- A window of about 2 × 1 cm is resected from the lateral bony nasal wall with a 4-mm chisel and removed with a Blakesley forceps (▶ Fig. 8.38). A small chisel or burr is used to lower the base of the window to the level of the nasal floor (▶ Fig. 8.39).
- Polypous tissue present on the floor of the antrum is removed.
- The mucosal flap is rotated into the antrum to cover the floor of the window and prevent early closure (▶ Fig. 8.40).
- The inferior turbinate is trimmed or reduced by an anterior plasty and then repositioned (for techniques, see page 301).
- A dressing with ointment is applied, which may be removed after 1 or 2 days.

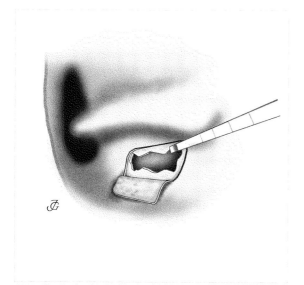

Fig. 8.38 A window is chiseled in the bony wall with a straight 6-mm chisel. The pieces are removed with a slender forceps.

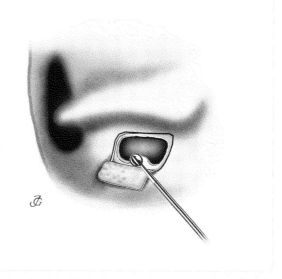

Fig. 8.39 The margins of the bony window are smoothed with a burr.

8.3.3 Complications

Infundibulotomy and endonasal ethmoidectomy are surgical procedures with a relatively high risk of complications. As early as the 1920s, Mosher warned of serious consequences. Some of his warnings are still cited ("intranasal ethmoidectomy is one of the most dangerous and blindest of all surgical operations," and "ethmoidectomy is the easiest way to kill a person"). The recent literature usually distinguishes between major and minor complications. Major complications are, among others, orbital hematoma, cerebrospinal fluid (CSF) leakage, cerebral damage, eye muscle lesion, blindness, and severe hemorrhage. Minor complications are permanent crusting, synechiae, and closure of the ostia. According to the literature, the incidence of the major complications is between 0.3 and 3%. However, we should keep in mind that complications are generally under-reported.

High-Risk Areas

The *roof and medial wall of the anterior ethmoid bone* are the most important high-risk areas. A minor injury of these thin bony walls may tear the dura mater and result in CSF leakage. Meningitis, pneumoencephaly, cerebral damage, and intracranial hemorrhage may occur as well.

The *medial wall of the orbit or lamina papyracea* is another well-known, high-risk area. It is a thin bony lamella that bulges towards the ethmoid bone and can therefore be easily penetrated with a forceps. If the surgeon is not aware of the error, there is a risk of permanently damaging the medial rectus, inferior rectus, or inferior oblique muscle.

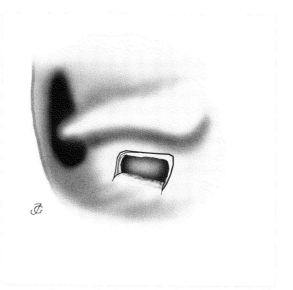

Fig. 8.40 The mucoperiosteal flap is rotated into the antrum and covers the inferior margin of the window.

The *roof of the posterior ethmoid bone*, where it continues in the anterior wall of the sphenoid bone, is a third vulnerable region. Perforation may lead to CSF leak and serious intracranial complications.

Posterior ethmoidal cells (Onodi cells): In some cases, a posterior cell that compromises the optic nerve may be present. Resection of the posterior cells may cause blindness.

The *lateral wall of the sphenoid bone* shows a slight bulging because of the internal carotid artery (ICA). The bone should be kept intact. If it is dehiscent, the artery may bulge into the sinus.

Major Complications

As mentioned previously, the list of major complications that may occur in ethmoidal surgery is long and impressive. It includes: severe bleeding, orbital hematoma, CSF leakage, ocular muscle lesions, meningitis, pneumoencephaly, cerebral damage, intracranial hemorrhage, blindness, and carotid artery damage.

Prevention

To avoid these very serious complications as much as possible, the following measures are taken:

1. A *coronal and axial CT scan* is made preoperatively. The CT scan is systematically studied before surgery is started. The following aspects are examined in detail: the ethmoidal roof and its relation to the cribriform plate; the lamina papyracea; and the lateral wall of the sphenoid bone.
2. A *good view* of the surgical field is an essential condition for endonasal ethmoidal surgery. This is established by providing good illumination, a bloodless surgical field, and proper magnification.
3. The *proper use of instruments* means using them parallel to the cranial and lateral wall of the ethmoid bone as much as possible. This applies in particular when a cutting forceps is used.
4. *Surgery is terminated if the surgeon is disorientated.* If the surgeon is losing control of the procedure due to difficulty in orientation, the operation must be stopped.

Treatment

Discussing all the treatment options for all major complications would go beyond the scope of this book. The reader is referred to other textbooks. Here, some general remarks may suffice:

- If a complication occurs, the surgeon should immediately consult an ENT colleague. Depending on the type of complication, a neurosurgeon and/or an ophthalmologist may also have to be consulted.
- Permanent damage can often be prevented by taking immediate action. An orbital hematoma requires immediate orbital decompression. A dural defect is closed with a fascia and mucosal graft as soon as possible. As to the handling of complications in general and the legal issues involved, we refer to Chapter 9, page 355 and page 370.

Minor Complications

The most frequent minor complications of ethmoidal surgery are permanent crusting, synechiae, closure of the sinus ostia, and neuralgia.

Whether or not *permanent crusting* will result depends on the anatomy of the resulting cavity and the quality of the remaining mucosa. See previous text under the heading "Endonasal Anterior and (Sub)Total Ethmoidectomy."

In our experience, *synechiae* between the middle turbinate and the lateral nasal wall (or the middle turbinate and the septum) can be avoided by introducing a dressing with ointment or Merocel and leaving it in place for 5 to 7 days.

Closure of the sinus ostia is a more difficult complication to prevent. Creating a wider window certainly helps, but this may interfere with restoring nasal and sinus physiology. Leaving a small slip of dressing in the opening for several days is another option.

Neuralgia may be related to the anatomy of the created cavity, a diseased cell, or damage to the anterior or posterior ethmoidal nerve endings. Generally, one should wait at least 6 to 12 months before deciding to perform revision surgery, as neuralgic complaints often subside gradually.

Chapter 9

Special Subjects

9 Special Subjects

9.1 Acute Nasal Trauma

On the subject of nasal trauma, Hippocrates (460–377 BC) wrote in his book "Joints" that its treatment does not require any particular skill on the part of the doctor. Although his writings on how to treat fresh nasal injuries contain several recommendations that are still valid, he was certainly mistaken on this point. On the contrary, taking good care of a fresh nasal injury is a difficult art. Both correct diagnosis and adequate treatment require great skill.

We know that most nasal deformities that we see in daily practice would not have occurred if the underlying trauma had been addressed correctly in the acute phase. Nasal injuries in childhood, if not properly treated, may have a great impact on later nasal form and function. A minor dislocation of the cartilaginous septum may lead to a septal deviation, crest, and spur during later nasal growth (see ▶ Fig. 9.7 and ▶ Fig. 9.8). A hematoma that has not been recognized and treated will cause scarring and retraction of the nasal dorsum, cartilaginous vault, and columella. A septal abscess in childhood, if not treated in its acute stage by reconstruction of the septal defect, will have grave consequences on growth of the midface and the nose (see ▶ Fig. 5.89). We have the best chance to prevent these deformities if we see the patient when the injury is still fresh. Treatment at that time may prevent many of the functional and aesthetic problems that could arise in later life.

Hippocrates on Treating Nasal Fractures

"For a simple fracture what is recommended is simple bandaging, so as to avoid the possible deformation caused by complicated bandages used to draw attention. When in addition to the fracture, the ridge of the nose is depressed or the nose is laterally dislocated, the recommended course of action includes reduction (which must take place in the first few days), the placement of wads into the nostrils, and very careful bandaging. This applies for complicated fractures as well, since the injury is not considered an obstacle in performing the above."

Hippocrates ("Joints")

9.1.1 Nasal Trauma in the Newborn

Deviation of the nose and compression of the lobule are frequently observed in the newborn. About 30% of all newborns exhibit some flattening of the lobule immediately after birth. This flattening disappears quickly in most cases, although in some a deformity remains. Although individual cases of nasal deformity at birth were described long ago,

the study of its incidence, causes, and treatment only started in the 1970s (e.g., Lindsay Gray, Jazbi, Jeppesen, Pirsig). In describing neonatal nasal deformities, we should distinguish between nasal deformities due to birth trauma and those occurring in utero.

Nasal Deformity due to Birth Trauma

Nasal deformity in the newborn following vaginal birth is rather common. The incidence reported varies from 1 to 23%. This variation is very likely due to differences in definition, time lapse between examination and birth, and ethnic factors. The majority of these deformities correct themselves in a few days. The tissues are apparently flattened or pushed during birth, later returning to their original position due to their elasticity. In a minority of cases, however, the deviation remains and nasal breathing may be impaired (Jeppesen 1977, 3.2%; Jazbi 1977, 1.9%; Collo 1978, 1.6%; Podoshin et al 1991, 0.93%; Hughes et al 1999, 0.6%). Concern about disturbed nasal growth is then justified.

Nasal trauma due to vaginal birth is characterized by a deviation of the cartilaginous pyramid and lobule to one side and dislocation of the cartilaginous septum from its base to the opposite side. The columella is deviated, while the shape of the nostrils and alae is distorted and asymmetrical. Sometimes, bulging instead of a luxation of the anterior septum is found. Jeppesen and Windfield (1976) postulated that presentation of a child in the left occipitoanterior position would lead to luxation of the septal base to the right, whereas presentation in the right occipitoposterior position would cause luxation to the left. Other authors (e.g., Kent et al 1998) have not been able to confirm this hypothesis, however.

Diagnosis

A proper diagnosis of these fresh birth trauma deformities is of paramount importance. The most important questions are:
- Is the septum dislocated?
- Is the nose obstructed?
- Are there other congenital anomalies (e.g., choanal atresia and piriform aperture stenosis)?

Steps
- The nasal mucosa is decongested and slightly anesthetized by putting a few drops of xylometazoline 0.025% and xylocaine 1% in the nasal cavity.
- The pyramid and lobule are inspected and palpated. The following aspects are investigated: Is the nose deviating? Is the lobule compressible? Are the nostrils equal in size and shape? Is the columella symmetrical? Is there loss of support of the cartilaginous dorsum and tip, indicating a septal dislocation?

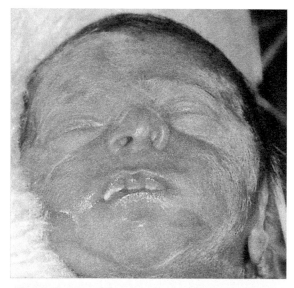

Fig. 9.1 Deviation of the pyramid and septum in a neonate delivered by cesarean section; the septum appeared to be immobile.

- The vestibule, valve, and nasal cavity are inspected using a straight, small diameter endoscope or electric otoscope. The septum is palpated with a cotton wool applicator. The following questions are answered: (1) Is the caudal septum in the midline? (2) Has the septal base slipped off the premaxilla? (3) Is there a septal hematoma? (4) Are the choanae open?
- When a septal dislocation is found, the cartilaginous septum is gently grasped and examined for abnormal mobility using a straight anatomical forceps with protected legs (e.g., with a piece of silicone tube cut from a narrow suction tube).

Treatment

A septal dislocation is corrected as soon as possible.

Steps

- If the septum is found to be displaced and mobile, it is gently lifted up with the anatomical forceps (see preceding text) and replaced in the midline.
- If it is immobile, no further action is taken. A watchful waiting policy is adopted, and the child is followed up.
- In babies with breathing obstruction, isotonic saline or decongestive nose drops are put into the nose before feeding.

Deformities Occurring in Utero

In rare cases, a neonatal nasal deformity is observed that cannot be attributed to birth trauma, as the delivery is by cesarean section. The incidence is estimated at 0.5 to 1.0% or lower. Whether the condition is due to intrauterine trauma or hereditary factors is unclear. On examination,

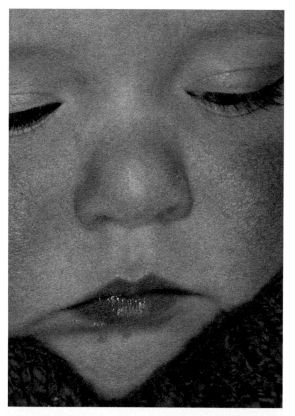

Fig. 9.2 Spontaneous correction of the deformity after 18 months.

the external pyramid and septum are found to be deviating and immobile. Repositioning of the septum is impossible. Long-term follow-up has shown that the deformity disappears spontaneously in about two-thirds of cases (► Fig. 9.1 and ► Fig. 9.2), whereas it remains in about one-third of the children, as found by Pentz, Pirsig and Lenders, 1999 (► Fig. 9.3 and ► Fig. 9.4)

9.1.2 Acute Nasal Trauma in Childhood

Nasal trauma is one of the most common injuries during childhood. No child reaches puberty without having suffered several minor and major falls and bumps on the nose. The majority of these accidents do not need special attention. However, some eventually lead to a nasal deformity.

Pathology

Septal and pyramid deformities may gradually develop in later life when the septum becomes dislocated from its base by an accident with a frontolateral or basolateral impact. Even minor trauma may have this effect. A frontal injury may cause disruption of the cartilaginous pyramid from the bony pyramid. In these cases, sagging of the cartilaginous dorsum occurs. It is generally assumed that

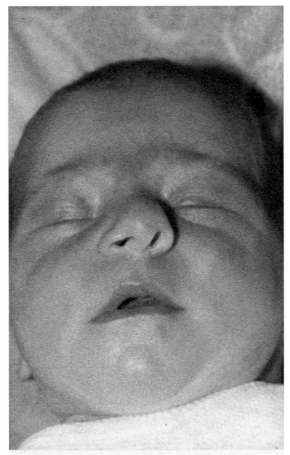

Fig. 9.3 Severe nasal deviation to the left after birth that was irreparable and therefore left untreated. (Photograph courtesy Prof. Pirsig.)

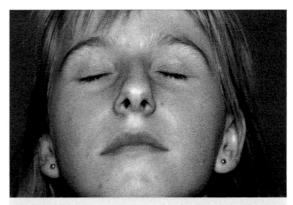

Fig. 9.4 At age 12 years, the girl presented with an inverted C-shaped deviation of the pyramid and a shortening and compression of the left maxilla. Septorhinoplasty was performed at the age of 15 years. (Photograph courtesy Prof. Pirsig.)

a high percentage of nasal deformities in adults are due to incomplete fractures of the cartilages as a result of minor injuries during childhood.

Hematomas, especially septal and dorsal, should not be overlooked. In infants and children, septal hematomas occur rather frequently. They pose a major threat, as they usually lead to a septal abscess and destruction of the septum.

Soft-tissue lesions, such as avulsion of the alae, columella, or the head of the inferior turbinate, have to be treated as soon as possible. This also applies to dog and monkey bites and to lesions of the columella caused by intubation.

Diagnosis

The external nose, septum, and nasal cavity are inspected and palpated after mucosal decongestion under general or local anesthesia. Special attention is paid to the septum. A septal hematoma is excluded by palpating the septum with a cotton wool applicator.

Examining the nose in a child with a fresh injury puts quite a strain on the child, its parents, the doctor, and the hospital staff. Therefore, appropriate intranasal inspection is often omitted. This may be acceptable in some cases, but in other cases such negligence may have grave consequences. Navigating the gray area between doing too much and too little requires experience. Plain radiographs have almost no value in diagnosing fresh nasal injuries in children. CT scans may provide important information but cannot be performed routinely.

Treatment

Depending on the findings, we have to decide whether it is best to wait and see what happens, or arrange for surgery. The parents or caregivers must be told that an accurate prediction of the final outcome after growth is completed is impossible, and that a second intervention may be indicated after puberty.

Wait-and-See Policy

When we decide to follow a wait-and-see policy, the parents are asked to watch out for the following developments over the next days:
- Is nasal breathing possible, or does the nose remain obstructed?
- Is the swelling of the external nose decreasing?
- Is there improvement in the child's general condition (no fever)? The signs and symptoms of a septal abscess are briefly described.

Closed Correction ("Reduction")

In some cases, an immediate correction, or so-called closed reduction may be attempted.

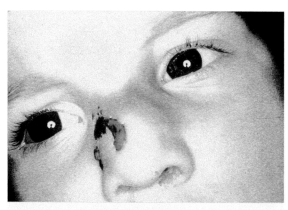

Fig. 9.5 Pronounced dorsal hematoma in a young child, which was evacuated through an IC incision.

Steps

- The nasal mucosa is anesthetized in the usual way, and depending on the case, a brief general anesthesia may be needed as well.
- To prevent damage of the nasal mucosa, a strip of cotton wool or gauze is positioned underneath the nasal bones before they are lifted up by an instrument (e.g., the blunt end of an elevator).
- With the help of a middle speculum and a blunt elevator, the nasal bones are lifted up and repositioned as much as possible, using three fingers of the other hand as an external guide.
- Repositioning of a fresh septal deviation or fractures may also be attempted but is usually less successful. While the bony and cartilaginous pyramid is lifted up by an instrument in the left hand, the septum is repositioned using a blunt or flat instrument in the right hand.
- Internal and external dressings with a stent are then applied.

Surgical Treatment

Surgical treatment is indicated under the following circumstances:

- *Septal hematoma*
  A septal hematoma should be opened and evacuated through a caudal septal incision (CSI). This is necessary to avoid necrosis of the septal cartilage and to prevent a septal abscess.
- *Dorsal hematoma*
  A limited dorsal hematoma may be left alone. However, in children with a pronounced localized hematoma, the accumulated blood might be evacuated through a small intercartilaginous (IC) incision (▶ Fig. 9.5). Internal dressings and external tapes are applied to prevent recurrence. If left untreated, large hematomas may lead to atrophy of the triangular cartilage and scarring of the soft tissues (▶ Fig. 9.6). If the septum is dislocated, it is repositioned and fixed as required. Internal dressings are applied, and antibiotics are prescribed.

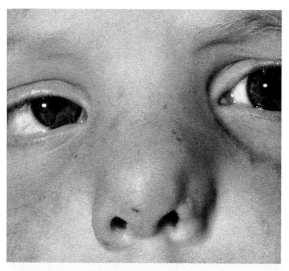

Fig. 9.6 Scarring of the ala and atrophy of the triangular cartilage on the left due to an untreated dorsal hematoma.

- *Septal fracture with dislocation*
  If the septum is dislocated, it is reconstructed in the usual way through a CSI. The dislocated parts are mobilized and repositioned. Resections and cross-hatchings are avoided (see Chapter 5, page 190).
- *Fracture and dislocation of the bony pyramid*
  A minor dislocation of the bony pyramid may be left untouched. We know, however, that a slight deviation or impression may become more pronounced in later years, especially during pubertal growth (▶ Fig. 9.7 and ▶ Fig. 9.8). Nevertheless, a wait-and-see policy is adopted in many cases, as septal pyramid surgery can be performed later with less risk, if required. In children with more severe fractures of the nasal bones, one should not hesitate to operate in the acute stage (immediately or within 3 to 5 days). Usually, osteotomies are required to complete the fractures and allow repositioning of the dislocated parts. We know from follow-up studies that the results of surgery in the acute stage are often the best.
- *Soft-tissue lesions*
  Soft-tissue lesions are treated immediately with 6–0 sutures under magnification by a loupe or a microscope (see following text).

9.1.3 Acute Nasal Trauma in Adults

Nasal trauma is one of the most common injuries in adults. It is usually caused by sports, traffic accidents, and fights. Males are most frequently affected, especially young males between 15 and 25 years of age. A nasal trauma may be an isolated injury or part of a major maxillofacial and/or skull trauma. If it is part of a larger trauma, a completely different approach to diagnosis and treatment is required.

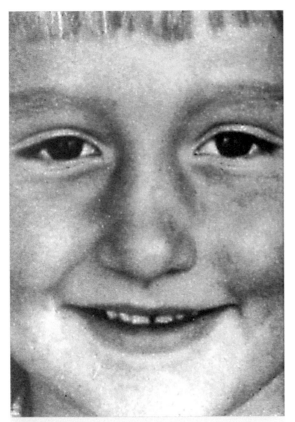

Fig. 9.7 Untreated nasal injury with a slight deviation of the bony pyramid to the right in a 6-year-old girl. (Photograph courtesy Prof. Pirsig 1992.)

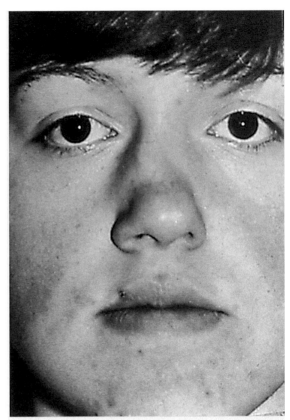

Fig. 9.8 At age 17 years, a severe deformity had occurred. The external pyramid is underdeveloped ("child's nose"); the maxilla shows retrusion; the bony pyramid deviates markedly to the right, while the cartilaginous pyramid deviates to the left (C-shaped deformity). There is severe saddling of the cartilaginous dorsum with a step at the junction between the cartilaginous and the bony pyramid. (Photograph courtesy Prof. Pirsig 1992.)

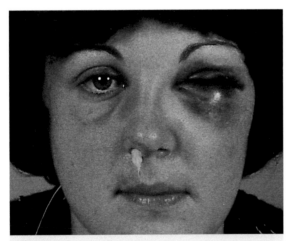

Fig. 9.9 Classic example of a fresh nasal fracture with a C-shaped deformity of the nasal pyramid and septum to the right, caused by trauma with frontolateral impact.

Pathology

Nasal injuries may involve the bony–cartilaginous skeleton, the soft tissues, or both.

Fractures and Dislocation of the Bony and Cartilaginous Skeleton

Depending on the impact of the trauma and the resulting fractures and dislocations, we may distinguish five types of trauma: those with a lateral, frontal, frontolateral, basal, or basolateral impact. In special circumstances, a combination of these main types may occur.

Lateral Impact Trauma

This is one of the most common types of trauma. It may be inflicted by a fist during a fight, or by an elbow or knee in sports. The bony and/or cartilaginous pyramid and the septum are fractured. The bony and/or cartilaginous pyramid will deviate to the opposite side. The nasal bone on the side of the impact is impressed. The septum is usually fractured vertically or diagonally in its anterior part. Depending on the injury, the result may be a deviated bony and cartilaginous pyramid, a C-shaped or reversed C-shaped pyramid, or a deviated cartilaginous pyramid (▶ Fig. 9.9). See also Chapter 2, page 66.

Frontal Impact Trauma

This is another very frequent type of trauma. It is usually caused by a traffic accident, fall, or sports injury. The bony and/or cartilaginous pyramid will be impressed. The dorsal skin may be lacerated. In patients who received a severe impact on the bony bridge, the result may be a bony saddle nose with multiple fracturing of the nasal bones, skin lesions, and a septal fracture. In cases where the force has hit the cartilaginous pyramid, the triangular cartilages may be disconnected from the bony pyramid, resulting in a saddling nose and a vertical septal fracture. Lobular soft-tissue injuries may also occur (e.g., of the ala and the head of the inferior turbinate).

Frontolateral Impact Trauma

Some injuries are caused by both lateral and frontal forces. Usually, one of the deformities previously described will result.

Basal and Basolateral Impact Trauma

This is another common type of trauma. It is caused by a fist blow, traffic accident, sports injury, or fall. The most common sequelae are horizontal fractures of the cartilaginous septum, and soft-tissue lesions such as avulsion of the columella, alae, and the head of the inferior turbinate. This type of trauma may be combined with dental damage. Therefore, an examination of the bite is mandatory. In adults, dental lesions are usually evident. In children, the damage may be more difficult to recognize. When in doubt, a dental expert should be consulted.

Diagnosis

It is not as simple to make a correct diagnosis of fresh nasal injuries as is usually thought. Edema, hematoma, bleeding, pain, and anxiety of the patient make it difficult to determine precisely what has been fractured, dislocated, or bruised.

History

For a correct diagnosis of the nasal injury, we first need to obtain a full history of the cause and the angle of impact. Furthermore, information is needed about preexisting nasal complaints and deformities, previous surgery, and earlier injuries.

Examination

The bony and cartilaginous pyramid, the lobule, and the internal nasal cavity are carefully inspected, palpated, and examined for any abnormal mobility. This is done after decongestion and anesthesia of the mucosal membranes. In patients with a fracture of the bony pyramid, local anesthesia of the bony pyramid by paranasal infiltration of lidocaine–adrenaline may be added (for

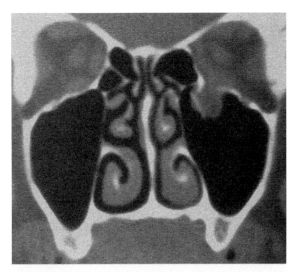

Fig. 9.10 The CT scan showed a blowout fracture of the left orbital floor.

techniques, see Chapter 3, page 132). In some cases, sedation prior to examination (and subsequent treatment) may be of great help.

Plain Radiographs and CT Scans

The diagnostic value of plain radiographs is limited. A negative outcome does not exclude a fracture, especially at young age when cartilaginous fractures are mostly invisible. They may be helpful, however, when swelling interferes with reliable palpation. They may also help diagnose an orbital blowout fracture, as well as fractures of the maxilla and frontal sinus. In addition, they may be important for legal reasons.

CT scans are performed in patients with maxillofacial and skull trauma (▸ Fig. 9.10). In special cases, scans are performed to examine in detail the relationships between the cartilaginous and the bony pyramids.

Color Photographs

Color photographs of the nose and face are required for documentation. They are particularly important in legal cases when another party is involved.

Consultation

Depending on the type and severity of the trauma and the general condition of the patient, it may be necessary to arrange for an ophthalmologic, maxillofacial, and neurological examination.

Treatment

First of all, treatment depends on whether we are dealing with an isolated nasal injury or with an injury as part of a major maxillofacial and/or skull trauma.

Primary general care to secure the airways, bleeding, and circulation is provided first. The airway is secured by intubation or tracheotomy; bleeding is controlled as much as possible by anterior nasal tamponade or anterior and posterior nasal tamponade (Bellocq type); and circulation is ensured.

If the nasal injury is part of a major accident, reconstruction of the nasal septum and external pyramid is usually the last phase of surgical treatment. Surgery of the anterior skull base, repositioning and fixation of maxillofacial fractures, and orbital surgery should always precede nasal reconstruction.

Closed Reduction or Surgical Reconstruction?

There is no doubt that the best way to treat a fresh septal and pyramid fracture is by surgical repositioning and reconstruction. Nevertheless, "closed reduction" is more commonly practiced. It is less invasive and takes less time to perform. Those who defend closed reduction also argue that the results are not too bad and that most patients are satisfied with the outcome. Finally, if complaints remain or recur, functional and/or aesthetic surgery can always be performed later. All these arguments are certainly valid. However, they do not dispel the evidence that surgical reconstruction in the acute or semi-acute phase produces the best results. Thus the question is when to choose closed reduction and when to prefer surgical correction? As many factors are involved, this decision has to be made for each patient individually. Some of the factors to take into account are the extent and type of the injury, the cause of the trauma, the wishes of the patient, the skill of the surgeon, and the hospital facilities.

Injuries that may be treated by a so-called closed reduction are uncomplicated septum–pyramid fractures.

Immediate Surgical Reconstruction

The following injuries require immediate surgical reconstruction:
- Open skin lesions, avulsions, bites
- Septal hematomas and pronounced paranasal or dorsal hematomas
- Nasal bleeding that does not stop in spite of repeated intranasal tamponade
- Bony fractures with severe dislocation, open fractures, and multiple fractures
- Severe depression of the bony and/or cartilaginous pyramid
- Septal fractures obstructing nasal breathing

Conservative Treatment

Injuries that may be treated conservatively by internal dressings, taping, and stents are limited hematomas and ecchymoses.

Optimal Time for Surgery

The best timing for surgical treatment of nasal injuries is within hours after the injury. Skin lesions and avulsions are taken care of as soon as possible. A septal hematoma is evacuated the same day. Repositioning of septal and pyramid fractures is also performed the same day. When indicated, this may be postponed, however. It has often been stated that injuries to the septum and pyramid should be addressed either within hours or after 3 to 5 days when the posttraumatic edema has subsided. Although it is certainly true that surgery in swollen and hyperemic tissues is more difficult, there are, in our opinion, no strong arguments against performing surgery during the first days after the trauma.

> The majority of septal and pyramidal deformities could be prevented by adequate treatment of the primary injury.

Technique of Closed Reduction

For many surgeons, closed reduction is the preferred treatment in the majority of cases. The reason is that if the attempt proves unsuccessful, surgical correction can always follow at a later stage. In many cases, however, the effect of a closed reduction is limited for two main reasons: First, it is difficult and sometimes impossible to reposition the dislocated bones, as the traumatic fracture is usually incomplete. Second, it is impossible to redress the bony pyramid without repositioning the deviated or fractured septum.

Steps
- Local anesthesia is applied to the mucosa and paranasally as required.
- Bimanual repositioning with the thumb and the forefinger may be attempted first. It sometimes works when the pyramid is deviated without impression of one of the lateral walls.
- In cases with impression of the lateral bony wall, a blunt elevator or a Walsham or Asch forceps is used. To protect the nasal mucosa, a strip of cotton wool or gauze is introduced under the bony and cartilaginous pyramid before the elevator (or one leg of the forceps) is introduced and positioned under the impressed bone. The dislocated bone is then outfractured while the pyramid is simultaneously rotated towards the midline. The fingers of the other hand are used as an external guide.
- The repositioned pyramid is supported by internal dressings and protected by external tapes and a stent for several days.

Technique of Repositioning and Reconstruction

Septal fractures and septal hematomas are addressed as described and illustrated in Chapter 5, page 196. The septum is mobilized through a CSI using a two-tunnel approach. A hematoma is aspirated. Fractured parts are mobilized and repositioned (if necessary after minimal resections), and then fixated.

Fractures of the bony pyramid are repositioned after complete mobilization of the fractured parts. Traumatic fractures are almost always incomplete. The lateral wall of the bony pyramid may be impressed, but the bony vault is usually still attached to the frontal bone and the frontal nasal spine. Therefore, closed reduction usually has a limited effect. To allow repositioning of the fractured fragments, the incomplete fractures have to be completed by osteotomies. It should be kept in mind that repositioning the external pyramid also requires mobilization of the septum.

Disruption of the cartilaginous vault is corrected by taking the following steps: (1) mobilizing and exorotating the septum; (2) performing osteotomies; and (3) repositioning and fixating the septolateral cartilage in its original position with guide sutures, fixating sutures, and splints.

Skin lesions are meticulously closed in two layers without delay. The wound is carefully cleaned. Irregular wound edges are not resected. They usually heal better than expected. In contrast, defects in the nasal domain often leave unsightly scars and lead to retractions.

Avulsions of the columella or alae are closed in four layers: (1) vestibular skin; (2) connective tissue layer; (3) subcutis; and (4) external skin. Lesions of the head of the inferior turbinate may be closed by one or two resorbable sutures. In most cases, adjusting the tissues with Merocel, gelfoam, or a dressing with ointment usually suffices.

Technique of Rebuilding a Severely Damaged Nose

In some cases with severe nasofacial trauma, the nose may have to be completely rebuilt.

Steps

- The septum is rebuilt first. The anterior septum is reconstructed by one or two plates. The posterior septum is repaired by several smaller plates mosaic-style.
- An internal dressing with ointment is applied to fix the septum and provide support for the pyramid and lobule.
- The bony pyramid is reconstructed. Dislocated parts are repositioned. Loose fragments may be used. Miniplates may have to be applied.
- The triangular cartilages are reconstructed and fixed to the bony pyramid and the septum. The cartilaginous pyramid is rebuilt working from the inside to the outside in four layers: (1) mucosa (resorbable sutures);

(2) cartilage (slowly resorbable sutures); (3) subcutaneous layers (continuous resorbable suture); and (4) skin (nonresorbable monofilament sutures). Special care is taken to recreate a functioning valve area.
- The lobule is reconstructed working from inside to outside. Usually, internal dressings are applied first. The lobule is then reconstructed over it in the following sequence: (1) vestibular skin (resorbable sutures); (2) lobular cartilages (slowly resorbable sutures); (3) connective tissue layer (continuous resorbable sutures); and (4) external skin (5–0 or 6–0 nonresorbable monofilament sutures).

9.2 Nasal Surgery in Children

9.2.1 General

Nasal surgery in children differs from that in adults. Neither the indications nor the surgical techniques are the same. The reason is that surgery in children influences further growth of the nose and the midface. The effects of surgery may be similar to those of other injuries. This applies in particular to surgery of the septum and the triangular cartilages (in other words, the septolateral cartilage), and to a lesser extent to surgery of the bony pyramid.

The influence of surgery on nasal growth has become evident in many ways. It was first reported in follow-up studies in children following submucous septal resection by Ombrédanne in 1942. In later years, it was convincingly shown by various studies on identical twins (Huizing 1966, Pirsig 1992, Grymer 1997). Finally, it was systematically investigated in a large number of animal studies (Sarnat and Wechsler, 1966, 1967; Verwoerd et al 1979, 1980, 1990, 1991).

9.2.2 Clinical and Experimental Evidence

The conclusions drawn from the information gathered so far may be summarized as follows:

1. The septolateral cartilage (septum and triangular cartilages) is the main determining factor controlling outgrowth of the nose and the maxilla. Injury or surgery to the septum and/or cartilaginous pyramid is likely to impair development of the nose and midface.
2. The earlier in childhood the injury or surgery takes place, the more influence it will have on nasal and facial development. When possible, nasal surgery should be postponed until after puberty: in girls earlier than in boys. This waiting period is recommended in spite of the great progress that has been made in conservative and reconstructive surgical techniques.

3. A traumatic deviation of the septum and external pyramid increases during nasal growth mainly due to incomplete healing of the growing nasal cartilages. This process can only partly be prevented by early repositioning of the septum and the pyramid. The long-term outcome of nasal surgery in cases of lateral nasal trauma is better than in cases of frontal nasal injuries.

4. Elevation of the septal mucoperichondrium and mucoperiosteum, either unilaterally or bilaterally, does not cause any substantial impairment of nasal growth.

5. Resection of parts of the septal cartilage interferes with nasal growth. Resections of the thicker and supporting central zones extending from the sphenoid bone to the anterior nasal spine and the nasal dorsum cause more damage than resections of the thin anterocentral areas.

6. Transection of the cartilaginous septum (chondrotomy), especially in a vertical direction, immediately leads to overlap of the resulting free cartilage margins. Consequently, anterior nasal growth may be negatively influenced, resulting in shortening of the nose. When possible, a posterior chondrotomy is to be avoided, as the zone of progressive ossification of the septal cartilage will be interrupted.

7. Reconstruction of septal defects by reimplantation of plates of autogeneic cartilage or bone does not restore normal nasal growth.

8. Mobilization or partial resection of the caudal part of the vomer (as recommended in cases of bilateral choanal atresia) does not lead to specific deformities. However, defects do not become closed by new bone formation; instead they remain fibrous.

9. Injuries to the triangular cartilage may cause a progressive deviation of the cartilaginous pyramid and the septal cartilage.

10. Damage to the thick caudal part of the septum and disconnection of the septal base from the nasal spine also cause growth inhibition of the maxilla.

9.2.3 When Should Nasal Surgery in Children Be Performed?

Fresh Injuries

- *Fractures with dislocation of the nasal bones*
  Closed reduction is performed as early as possible, but at least within the first 3 to 5 days, as nasal fractures in children are relatively easily reduced.
- *Septal hematoma and septal abscess*
  Immediate action is required. The hematoma (abscess) is drained through a CSI (hemitransfixion). The septum is explored; a defect is immediately reconstructed by transplantation of auricular cartilage to avoid dorsal saddling and columellar retraction. Internal dressings

are applied, and antibiotics are administered systemically (see Chapter 5, page 196).
- *Septal fractures with (severe) dislocation*
  This type of fracture is corrected within a few days. The dislocated parts are dissected, repositioned, and fixed in the midline. Resections, cross-hatching, and cartilage crushing are avoided as much as possible (see page 192).
- *Dorsal hematomas*
  When large, these are immediately drained via an IC incision. A supporting internal dressing and external taping is applied (see page 129 and page 130).
- *Disruption of triangular cartilage*
  The cartilage is readjusted in its position and fixed to the septum and the bony pyramid.

Long-Standing Deformities

- *Septal deformity*
  Whether and when surgery is performed is extensively discussed in the section on septal surgery in children (see Chapter 5, page 192).
- *Deviation of the bony pyramid*
  Minor deviations are not corrected before puberty. Major deformities and asymmetries may be corrected by osteotomies after mobilizing and repositioning the septum.
- *Humps*
  Humps are left untouched unless they are very pronounced and cause severe psychological problems.
- *Saddling*
  Saddling is preferably corrected after puberty. However, in some patients with a pronounced congenital nasal and septal hypoplasia or a severe traumatic saddle nose, the septum may be reconstructed and the dorsum augmented at an earlier age. Usually, this is done for psychological and aesthetic reasons. The patient and his or her parents or caregivers should be informed that a second and sometimes a third surgical intervention may be needed later.
- *Lobular deformities*
  The best results are obtained after puberty. Lobular surgery should therefore be postponed when possible. In children with a pronounced congenital or acquired deformity (e.g., cleft lip nose, bifid nose, defect due to a bite or injury), the first stage of a multistage operation may be carried out earlier.

9.2.4 Conclusions

The present status of nasal surgery in childhood can be summarized as follows:

1. Despite our increased knowledge, the late effects of nasal surgery in childhood are still unpredictable in an individual case. The amount of damage to the septolateral cartilage dictates future growth of the nose and midface.

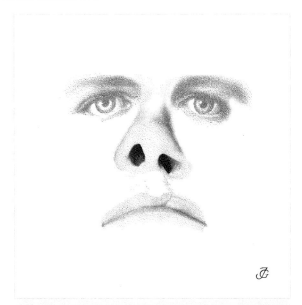

Fig. 9.11 Cleft-lip and palate on the left side. The bony and cartilaginous pyramid leans slightly to the NCS. The lobule is severely deformed: the dome and ala on the CS are depressed; the nostril is more horizontal.

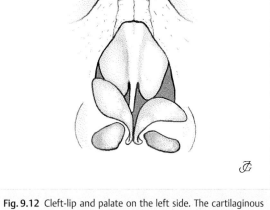

Fig. 9.12 Cleft-lip and palate on the left side. The cartilaginous pyramid and lobule deviate to the NCS. The lobule is severely asymmetrical. The lobular cartilage is depressed and the lateral crus is flattened, less convex, and located more caudally.

2. The later in life surgery is carried out, the less negative the effects will be on further development of the nose and midface. This applies in particular to surgery of the cartilaginous septum and triangular cartilages.
3. The old notion that nasal surgery should be postponed until after puberty is basically still valid.
4. Obstructing deviations of the septum and pyramid are the exception to this rule. Early repositioning of the septum and cartilaginous pyramid, whereby resections are avoided as much as possible, may prevent development of a severely deviated and obstructed nose during further growth.
5. It is the task of the nasal surgeon to weigh, in each individual case, the likely advantages of surgery against the disadvantages.

9.3 Nasal Surgery in the Unilateral Cleft-Lip Nose

9.3.1 Pathology

In cleft-lip patients, all nasal elements and adjacent structures are more or less affected.
- *The bony and cartilaginous pyramid* is asymmetrical and leans slightly to the noncleft side (NCS) (▶ Fig. 9.11 and ▶ Fig. 9.12; see also ▶ Fig. 9.15**a**).
- *The piriform aperture* is asymmetrical, the aperture on the cleft side (CS) being lower and narrower. The anterior nasal spine deviates to the CS or may be hypoplastic. The premaxilla is severely deviated to the CS with its median axis up to 40° (▶ Fig. 9.13).

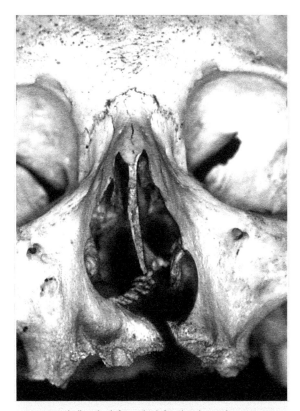

Fig. 9.13 Skull with cleft on the left side. The piriform aperture on the CS is lower and narrower. The anterior nasal spine and the premaxilla are strongly deviating to the CS. A pronounced crest and spur are present on the CS. The bone of the inferior turbinate on the CS is lower and more lateral than on the NCS. (Photograph courtesy Prof. Pirsig.)

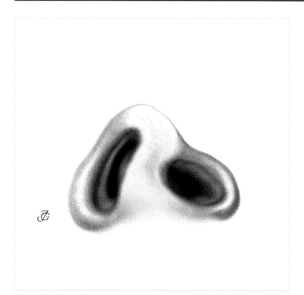

Fig. 9.14 Characteristic deformity of the lobule in a cleft lip nose with the cleft on the left. The lobule is severely asymmetrical: the dome and lateral crus on the CS are depressed and rotated in an anterior direction. The nostril is ovaloid and has an almost transverse axis. The vestibule is narrow. The columella is short and its ventral part is deviating to the CS. The caudal septum is deviating to the NCS.

- *The lobule* is deviated to the CS and strongly asymmetrical. The tip is bifid and flat and deviates to the CS. The dome and lateral crus on the CS are severely depressed, less convex, and more caudally located; the ala is elongated, flat, and displaced in a lateral and caudal direction; the vestibule is narrow and has a more horizontal axis. The columella is short, broad, and oblique. Its upper end leans to the CS, its base is retracted. The medial crus on the CS is somewhat displaced in a caudal direction and looks shorter than the opposite medial crus (▶ Fig. 9.14 and ▶ Fig. 9.15).

The septum is severely deformed. Its caudal end is dislocated to the NCS and may thereby narrow the vestibule on this side (▶ Fig. 9.15**b**). More posteriorly, the cartilaginous septum, vomer, and perpendicular plate are strongly deviated to the CS, obstructing the valve area and the nasal cavity (▶ Fig. 9.16). At the chondropremaxillary and perpendicular–vomeral junction, a pronounced cartilaginous and bony crest and spur are present. Due to these skeletal distortions, the inferior part of the vomer is part of the nasal floor on the NCS (▶ Fig. 9.16 and ▶ Fig. 9.17).

The depressed ala usually contributes to the stenosis of the valve area. The inferior turbinate on the CS is lower and compressed in a lateral direction. Its bony lamella is lower than normal. On the NCS, the inferior turbinate usually undergoes compensatory hypertrophy. The middle turbinate on the CS is generally somewhat more slender than on the NCS (▶ Fig. 9.16 and ▶ Fig. 9.17).

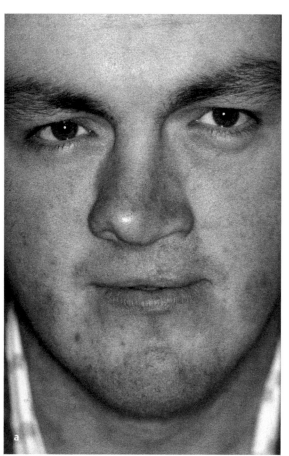

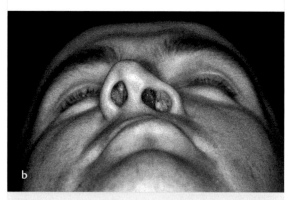

Fig. 9.15 a, b Characteristic nasal pathology in a 16-year-old male with a repaired cleft lip on the left side. Note the asymmetry of the bony and cartilaginous pyramid that deviates to the NCS, the depressed oval nostril with its almost horizontal axis, the severely depressed and elongated ala and lateral crus on the CS, and the obstructive septal deformity.

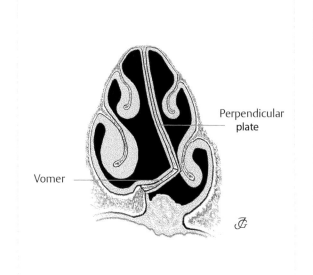

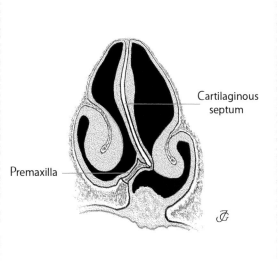

Fig. 9.16 Deformity of the septum and turbinates at the level of the vomer. The perpendicular plate and vomer deviate to the CS. A pronounced crest and spur are usually present at the chondrovomeral and the perpendicular–vomeral junction. The inferior turbinate on the CS is compressed and positioned lower. The inferior turbinate on the NCS usually shows compensatory hypertrophy.

Fig. 9.17 Septal deformity at the level of the premaxilla. The premaxilla deviates to the CS at a 45° angle. A huge crest is present at the chondropremaxillary junction. The inferior turbinate on the CS is located lower and is somewhat compressed; the inferior turbinate on the NCS shows compensatory hyperplasia.

9.3.2 Treatment

Rehabilitation of cleft lip patients requires close cooperation between various specialists. Nowadays, all large medical centers have a so-called Cleft Team. In such a team, specialists of the following disciplines work together: plastic surgery, maxillofacial surgery, otorhinolaryngology, orthodontics, and speech therapy. Usually, a general pediatrician completes the team.

Rehabilitation Schedule

Most teams treat a cleft lip patient according to a locally accepted schedule. An internationally accepted schedule is still in preparation. Such a schedule usually consists of three major phases of rehabilitation: a *primary* phase which is carried out within the first year of life, a *secondary* phase which is performed between 4 and 10 years of age, and a *final* phase which is completed after puberty (▶ Table 9.1).

Nowadays, there is a tendency to correct the skeletal deformities of the hard palate and the septum at a younger age than before. Closure of the periosteum of the bony palate and the nasal floor at an early age may inhibit the further increase of some of the anomalies, for instance those of the maxillary and premaxillary bones.

Despite the importance of adopting a general treatment schedule in cleft lip rehabilitation, treatment of cleft lip deformities must be tailored to the patient's needs and particular deformities.

9.3.3 Surgical Techniques

In this chapter, we only deal with the rhinological aspects of rehabilitation of cleft lip patients. Here, we discuss only the specific surgery of the septum, pyramid, and lobule in these cases. For surgery of the lip, maxilla, and palate, as well as the various orthodontic options, we refer the reader to other textbooks.

Table 9.1 Schedule of rehabilitation of cleft lip patients, to be adapted according to the patient's individual circumstances

Phase 1	
2–4 m	• Closure of lip, alveolus, maxilla, and hard palate
12 m	• Closure of posterior velum
Phase 2	
4–5 y	• Speech therapy, velopharyngoplasty
5–6 y	• Correction of lip/elongation of lip in bilateral clefts • Vestibulum oris–plasty
8–10 y	• Septal surgery, first phase • Orthodontic treatment
Phase 3	
16–18 y	• Septorhinoplasty, first septal pyramid surgery • 12 m later lobular surgery • Orthodontic surgery/prosthesis

Septal Surgery

Until recently, it was general policy to delay septal surgery until after puberty. However, the development of more conservative techniques has allowed intervention at an earlier age, if indicated. Repositioning of the septum in childhood may first of all have a beneficial effect on nasal breathing. Whether or not a first phase of septal surgery is performed before puberty depends on several factors, in particular the quality of nasal breathing. A typical case for early septal correction is the patient with a cleft lip nose deformity and marked additional nasal obstruction due to trauma. For the techniques of septal surgery, we refer to Chapter 5 (page 159).

Pyramid Surgery

Surgery of the bony and cartilaginous pyramid is postponed until after puberty almost without exception. Deformity of the bony pyramid does not need early correction. Pyramid surgery is usually performed in combination with secondary septal surgery (and anterior turbinoplasty) as required in the final phase of rehabilitation (▶ Table 9.1). In patients with a limited septal and pyramid deformity, it may be performed in one stage as part of the correction of the lobule. In other cases, however, septal and pyramid surgery is carried out first, whereas lobular surgery is done as one of the final steps some 12 months later. For techniques, we refer to Chapter 6.

Lobular Surgery

Lobular surgery is performed in the final phase of rehabilitation. This means that it can be performed in the same stage as septal and pyramid correction, or in a separate procedure 1 year after correction of the septum and the bony pyramid. Reconstructing the nasal lobule in cleft lip patients is one of the most difficult surgical procedures in nasal surgery, requiring great skill and experience.

Over the past decades, several techniques have been developed worldwide. Here, we limit ourselves to a description of the method that is applied by a great majority of nasal surgeons.

In the past two decades, primary closure of the unilateral cleft lip and palate in infancy has not—or only minimally—involved nasal structures. This means that the septum, and especially the lobular cartilage, on the CS are not inhibited during nasal growth, but only deformed and distorted. Therefore, septorhinoplasty postpuberty in these patients principally means readjustment of the congenitally deformed and distorted nasal structures, either endonasally or, mostly, via an external transcolumellar approach.

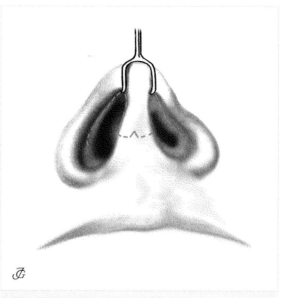

Fig. 9.18 A transcolumellar incision and bilateral infracartilaginous incisions are made according to the same principles as in the external approach technique.

Steps

- A transcolumellar inverted-V incision is made in combination with bilateral infracartilaginous incisions as usual in the external approach. The incision is made while lifting the lobule on the CS into its desired position to define the exact position of the incision (▶ Fig. 9.18). Making the infracartilaginous incision on the CS may be more difficult than usual, as the caudal margin of the lateral crus is often indefinite because of an underdeveloped or lacking soft triangle. The transcolumellar incision is made as usual at about one-third of the distance from the columellar base.
- The medial crura, domes, and lateral crura of both lobular cartilages and the anterior part of the cartilaginous septum and the cartilaginous dorsum are exposed (▶ Fig. 9.19).
- Septoplasty is performed first and carried out according to the principles and techniques described in Chapter 5. Sometimes, removal of the whole septum may be advisable. A new, straight, septal plate is then extracorporally sculpted and reimplanted, a so-called extracorporal septoplasty (Gubisch 1995).
- Correction of the asymmetric lobule is started by dissecting the lateral crus on the CS from the vestibular skin, whereas the vestibular skin on the NCS remains attached to the lateral crus. If the lateral crus on the CS is severely depressed, its very lateral end is cut and left attached to the vestibular skin so that the lateral part of the ala does not lose its stability.

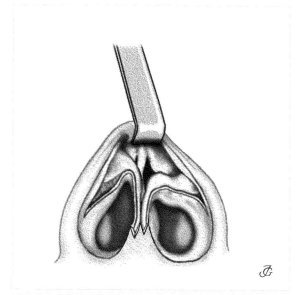

Fig. 9.19 The lobular cartilages, anterior septum, and cartilaginous dorsum are exposed. On the CS the vestibular skin is dissected from the lateral crus. On the NCS it remains attached to the cartilage.

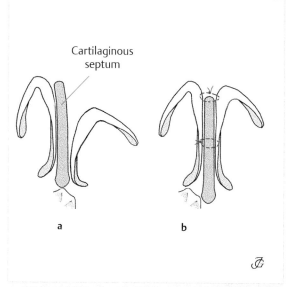

Cartilaginous septum

Fig. 9.20 (a) The cartilaginous septum with its base on the CS is fixed laterally to the premaxillary spine using a 4–0 or 5–0 nonresorbable suture. **(b)** The foot of the medial crus of the lobular cartilage on the CS is freed, and its dome and lateral crus are redraped in a medial and upward direction and fixed to the septum. The domes are brought together by interdomal sutures to achieve a more narrow, projecting and symmetrical tip.

- Both lateral crura are now sculpted. The cephalic margins of the lateral crus on the CS, and sometimes on the NCS as well, are trimmed to make the craniocaudal width of the crura as symmetrical as possible. The resected strip(s) of cartilage may later be used as an onlay or shield graft to augment the dome at the CS when repositioning of the alar cartilage alone does not lead to a good result.
- To straighten and lengthen the columella, the base of the medial crus on the CS is almost completely freed. This helps to create symmetry of the domes.
  - The freed lateral crus on the CS is now rotated in a cranial and medial direction until both domes are of symmetrical height. It is fixed to the triangular cartilage and the septum by a nonresorbable suture and to the lobular cartilage of the NCS by one or two interdomal nonresorbable sutures (▶ Fig. 9.20).
- Special care is taken to leave a distance of about 1 to 2 mm between the two domes. On the CS, an intradomal suture may be used to give the wide and flat dome on this side normal curvature.
- The next step is fixation of the mobilized septum laterally to the premaxilla on the CS. This is done by suturing its base to the premaxillary fibers by a 4–0 nonresorbable suture. In this way, the bent caudal septal end can mostly be straightened (▶ Fig. 9.20).

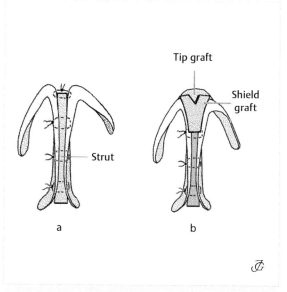

Tip graft / Shield graft / Strut

Fig. 9.21 (a) The medial crura are reinforced by a strut of cartilage taken from the posterior part of the cartilaginous septum and fixed by 2 or 3 sutures. **(b)** A shield and/or tip graft may be applied to give the tip more projection.

- To straighten and reinforce the columella and at the same time increase lobular projection, a rectangular strut taken from the posterior part of the cartilaginous septum is fixed between the medial crura using 5–0 nonresorbable suture material (▶ Fig. 9.21**a**).
- In case of remaining asymmetry between the two domes, a cartilaginous "onlay graft" is fixed on top of the less prominent dome.
- A shield and/or tip graft may be added to give the tip more projection and definition (▶ Fig. 9.21**b**).
- All incisions are closed by 5–0; onlay grafts by 6–0 sutures.
- If the nostril sill and floor of the vestibule on the CS is too low, this should be corrected in a second step in combination with recreation of the facet in the nostril, which is usually lacking on the CS.

9.4 The Nose and Sleep Disordered Breathing

According to International Classification of Sleep Disorders (ICSD-2), obstructive sleep apnea (OSA), also named *obstructive sleep apnea syndrome* (OSAS) or *obstructive sleep hypopnea–apnea* (OSHA), belongs to the group of sleep disordered breathing (SDB), a subgroup of 95 different sleep disorders which cause nonrestful sleep.

Primary snoring is not considered a disease because it does not cause symptoms of daytime sleepiness or hypersomnia.

OSA is a sleep disorder with a significant decrease in airflow due to obstruction of the upper airway. It is characterized by recurrent episodes of upper airway collapse with oxyhemoglobin desaturation and arousals from sleep. It is the most common type of sleep apnea. OSA is mostly associated with daytime sleepiness and may cause cardiovascular and neurological disorders due to chronic intermittent hypoxia and sleep fragmentation. The most serious adverse consequences associated with OSA are myocardial infarction, stroke, hypertension, and traffic accidents.

The medical profession has long ignored OSA, which, because of snoring, was considered more a social than a medical issue. In the late 1970s and the 1980s, however, greater interest arose in SDB and in the past 30 years, enormous progress has taken place in classifying and standardizing symptoms, diagnosis, and treatment. This is an important aspect of the broad field of the new specialty, "sleep medicine."

9.4.1 Pathology and Causative Factors

There is evidence that both neurologic disturbances and abnormal anatomy of the upper airway contribute to OSA to different extents in individual patients. Snoring noises are produced at the level of the pharynx. Hypopneas and apneas are caused by temporary collapse of one or more pharyngeal airway segments. A major causative role is abnormal dimensions of the upper airway and the oral cavity. Other important factors are alterations (condition) of the soft tissues, in particular the mucosa, the nerves and musculature of these areas, and the size of the adenoids and tonsils. Other causative factors are obesity, alcohol intake, use of certain medications, and sleeping position.

Impaired nasal breathing may play a role in OSA, but recent studies have demonstrated that this is less important than previously thought and only a very small group of patients with OSA will be cured by nasal surgery alone (Rappai et al 2003, Verse and Pirsig 2003, Rombaux et al 2005). From these reviews, it can be concluded that nasal obstruction may have a negative impact on sleep quality; however, it can only be considered as a cofactor in the pathophysiology of SDB.

The Role of the Nose in Sleep Disordered Breathing

In former decades, obstruction of nasal breathing was widely believed to be one of the main causes of SDB. Patients were sent to the ENT surgeon to have their septum straightened or their nasal polyps removed. However, restoration of nasal breathing turned out to have considerably less effect on snoring than expected. In some cases, complaints of snoring and apnea have even been found to increase after improving nasal breathing. Unfortunately, we do not yet have methods to predict the effects of nasal surgery on SDB in an individual case. Therefore, the unpredictable response of SDB to nasal surgery must be discussed with the patients preoperatively. They should be informed that nasal surgery is not a primary treatment of SDB and has proven to be effective only in about 10% of cases. Nonetheless, there are several indications to treat nasal obstruction in patients suffering from snoring, hypopneas, and apneas. In cases with allergic rhinitis, antiallergic treatment may be given. An intranasal dilator, an extranasal dilator, or the intranasal valve Provent (Ventus Medical, San Jose, California, United States) may reduce symptoms of SDB. In patients with polyposis or septal pyramid deformities, surgery is performed, especially if nasal continuous positive airway pressure (nCPAP) or oral appliances are not tolerated.

Surgery is performed primarily because most patients report a considerable improvement in quality of life after improvement of nasal breathing. This means that an ENT examination should always be included in the diagnostic work-up of each patient with SDB. Moreover, nasal surgery can reduce pressure in nCPAP ventilation treatment and thus increase the compliance to use nCPAP ventilation. On the contrary, nCPAP treatment is not tolerated by some patients with OSA because of the nasal side effects (see below). Finally, some patients with SDB have a high pathological nasal resistance and are treated with oral appliances (mandibular advancement splints). It has been shown that high nasal resistance negatively impacted on success of oral appliances for the treatment of OSA (Sugiura et al 2007; Zeng et al 2008).

9.4.2 Treatment

We restrict ourselves here to a discussion of the effects of nasal surgery, intranasal and extranasal dilators, and the benefits and adverse effects of nCPAP ventilation.

Nasal Surgery

In all patients with SDB and impaired nasal breathing, surgery (after failed conservative and instrumental treatment) must always be considered as discussed earlier. However, surgery has a beneficial effect on snoring and apneas in a limited number of patients. This applies in particular to OSA patients. For such patients, therefore, nasal surgery is not a primary treatment.

In general, snoring is estimated to decrease to a socially acceptable level in up to 40% of patients when normal breathing is restored, as shown by studies using questionnaires or analog scales. However, it is difficult to measure snoring objectively, and studies on primary snoring have not been standardized. In OSA patients, the success rate is much lower. In polysomnographic studies using data from two reviews, it was found to be less than 15% (▶ Table 9.2) (Rombaux et al 2005, Verse and Pirsig 2010).

Nasal surgery is usually followed by temporary obstruction of the nasal cavities by internal dressings. Even in healthy people, internal dressings may cause hypopneas or apneas and sleep disturbance. Therefore, the combination OSA and nasal tamponade is dangerous. In patients with OSA, one should seriously consider nasal surgery under local anesthesia that does not require internal dressings, such as radiofrequency reduction of the inferior turbinate. In patients treated with nCPAP after surgery and a temporary full-face mask, supervision in a medium or intensive care unit is necessary. If internal dressings are applied, oral CPAP may be helpful (Dorn et al 2001).

It has to be emphasized that in patients suffering from massive nasal polyposis or severely deformed nasal anatomy, OSA may deteriorate after successful nasal surgery despite improvement in nasal breathing and subjective sleep quality. Therefore, follow-up of these patients by polygraphy or polysomnography is recommended.

Internal and External Nasal Dilators

An internal nasal dilator (Nozovent) that serves to decrease inspiratory breathing resistance and to reduce snoring was introduced by Petruson in 1988. Positive results have been reported by some authors but not by others. At present, no controlled study has demonstrated long-term effectiveness of this device alone in patients

Table 9.2 Effect of nasal surgery on the severity of obstructive sleep apnea

Author	N	Follow-up (months)	Preoperative AHI	Postoperative AHI	p Value	EBM
Rubin et al 1983	9	1–6	37.8[a]	26.7[a]	<0.05	4
Dayal 1985	6	4–44	46.9	28.2	n.s.	4
Caldarelli et al 1985	23	No data	44.2[a]	41.5[a]	n.s.	4
Aubert-Tulkens et al 1989	2	2–3	47.5[a]	48.5[a]	–	4
Sériès et al 1992	20	2–3	39.8	36.8	n.s.	4
Sériès et al. 1993	14	2–3	17.8[a]	16[a]	n.s.	4
Utley et al 1997	4	No data	11.9	27	–	4
Verse et al 1998	2	3–4	14	57.7	–	4
Friedman et al 2000	22	>1.5	31.6	39.5	n.s.	4
Verse et al. 2002	26	3–50	31.6	28.9	n.s.	4
Kim et al 2004	21	1	39	29	<0.0001	4
Balcerzak et al 2004	22	2	48.1	48.8	n.s.	4
Nakata et al 2005	12	No data	55.9	47.8	n.s.	4
Virkkula et al 2006	41	2–6	13.6	14.9	n.s.	4
Koutsourelakis et al 2008	49	3–4	31	31	n.s.	4
All	**272**	**1–50**	**33.0**	**31.8**		4

Abbreviations: AHI, Apnea Hypopnea Index; EBM, level of evidence-based medicine; N, number of subjects; n.s., Not statistically significant
[a]Apnea Index
Source data: Verse T, Pirsig W. Nasal surgery. In: Hörmann K, Verse T. Surgery for Sleep Disordered Breathing (2nd edition). Heidelberg: Springer: 2010: 24–31

with OSA. The same applies to the external nasal dilator developed by the 3 M company under the name Breathe Right.

Nasal appliances may help identify some of the patients with OSA in whom nasal surgery is indicated. Improvements in subjective parameters, such as subjective sleep quality, daytime sleepiness, quality of life, and nonapneic snoring, have been reported after using nasal dilators. Reviews of subjective and objective data on the effect of nasal dilators have been published by Rappai et al 2003, Verse and Pirsig 2003, and Rombaux et al 2005.

Nasal Continuous Positive Pressure Ventilation

nCPAP ventilation is currently the first option to treat more serious types of SDB. There are only a few reports on the effect of nasal surgery on CPAP. In a prospective, randomized, double-blind, placebo-controlled clinical study in 22 patients, Powell et al (2001) compared the effect of intraturbinal radiofrequency reduction of the nasal turbinates with that of a sham operation. Both nasal breathing and self-reported CPAP adherence were statistically ($p = 0.03$) superior in the treatment group than in the control group 4 weeks after surgery. Several other studies (▶ Table 9.3) have also shown that corrective nasal surgery may be an effective method to enhance the compliance of nCPAP, as it may reduce the CPAP by 2 to 5 cm H_2O (Verse and Pirsig 2010). Therefore, when indicated, nasal surgery is commonly performed prior to nCPAP treatment. Unfortunately, nCPAP is only tolerated by some 60% of patients in the long term. A large number of side effects have been reported, such as nasal dryness,

crusting, rhinorrhea, and epistaxis. The high air pressure causes an inflammatory response of the nasal mucosa causing watery rhinorrhea or a dry nose. Sugiura et al (2007) demonstrated that increased nasal resistance is significantly correlated with inability to tolerate nCPAP and suggested that nasal resistance measured by active anterior rhinomanometry might be used as an indicator of initial CPAP acceptance. Topical steroids, anticholinergic medication, and saline irrigation may help control rhinorrhea, while a humidifier and a warming device in the CPAP equipment may help reduce the symptoms of a dry nose. Nevertheless, some patients still give up nCPAP ventilation because of noncurable nasal side effects. In case of noncompliance of nCPAP therapy, oral appliances or multilevel surgery from the nose to the larynx may help treat SDB. In special cases, maxillomandibular advancement surgery or, very rarely, a tracheotomy might be considered. For both types of surgery, a long-term success rate of about 90 to 99% is documented in the literature.

9.5 Rhinopexy in the Elderly

As patients age, the connections between the triangular cartilages and the lower lateral cartilages often become lax, resulting in a lobule that begins to droop downward. This may result in impaired inspiratory breathing due to narrowing of the valve area. Patients have frequently noted that elevating the nasal tip with a finger improves their breathing. They often sleep with tape fixed to the skin of the nose to elevate the tip, which improves breathing. In certain cases, it might be advantageous to correct the drooping of the tip and lobule by a surgical elevation called rhinopexy. Rhinopexy is a conservative operation designed to raise the lobule and can be performed under attended local anesthesia.

The principle of the method is to raise the nasal tip and ventral part of the lobule by undermining the skin over the nasal pyramid (dorsum) and resecting an elliptical piece of skin at the nasion, and then bring the mobilized dorsal skin and suture it upwards (▶ Fig. 9.22, ▶ Fig. 9.23, and ▶ Fig. 9.24). The method was introduced to us by Vernon Gray of Los Angeles.

Steps

- Local anesthesia is given as outlined in Chapter 3 (page 132).
- IC incisions are performed bilaterally.
- The skin is elevated over the nasal pyramid subcutaneously (at the level of the superficial musculoaponeurotic system [SMAS]) up to the nasion using long double-blunt dissecting scissors.
- The elliptical piece of skin and subcutaneous tissue to be resected is outlined on the skin. Its horizontal cranial base should measure 2 to 3 cm; the height of the ellipse is about 2 cm (▶ Fig. 9.25).

Table 9.3 Effect of corrective nasal surgery on continuous positive airway pressure (nCPAP) according to the literature

Author	N	Preoperative CPAP (cm H_2O)	Postoperative CPAP (cm H_2O)	p Value
Mayer-Brix et al 1989	3	9.7	6.0	No data
Friedman et al 2000	6	9.3	6.7	< 0.05
Dorn et al 2001	5	11.8	8.6	< 0.05
Masdon et al 2004	35	9.7	8.9	n.s.
Nakata et al 2005	5	16.8	12.0	< 0.05
Zonato et al 2006	17	12.4	10.2	< 0.001
All	70	11.0	9.1	

Abbreviation: n.s., not significant
Source data: Hörmann K, Verse T. Surgery for Sleep Disordered Breathing (2nd edition). Heidelberg: Springer; 2010

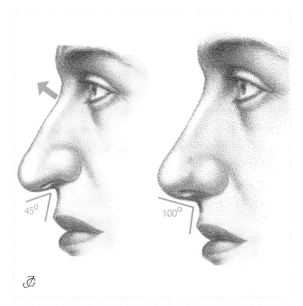

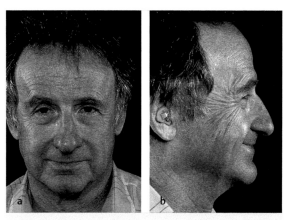

Fig. 9.23 a, b Elderly man with drooping lobule and impaired inspiratory breathing before rhinopexy. (Photographs courtesy Prof. Kern.)

Fig. 9.22 Principle of rhinopexy in the elderly patient with a drooping lobule due to increased laxity of the soft tissues resulting in impaired inspiratory breathing at night.

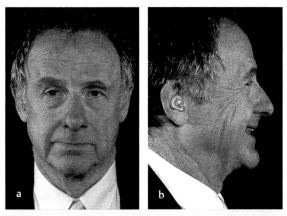

Fig. 9.24 a, b Elderly man with drooping lobule and impaired inspiratory breathing 1 year after rhinopexy. (Photographs courtesy Prof. Kern.)

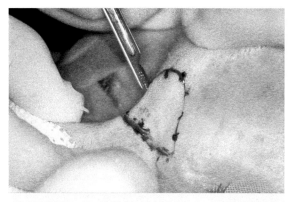

Fig. 9.25 The triangle of skin and subcutaneous tissue to be resected is outlined. (Photograph courtesy Prof. Kern.) (Photograph courtesy Prof. Kern.)

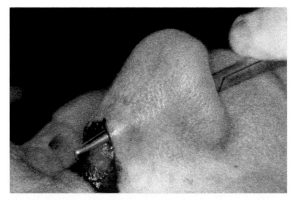

Fig. 9.26 The skin overlying the middle and lower part of the external pyramid is mobilized in the cranial direction. (Photograph courtesy Prof. Kern.)

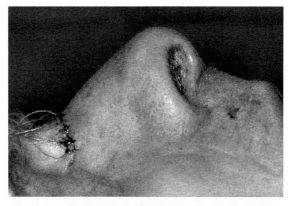

Fig. 9.27 The skin overlying the middle and lower part of the external pyramid is sutured. (Photographs courtesy Prof. Kern.)

- The horizontal incision through the skin and subcutaneous tissue layers overlying the upper margin of the bony pyramid is made first.
- Then the incisions at the sides of the piece of skin to be resected are made.
- The piece of skin is then dissected out.
- The skin overlying the middle and lower part of the external pyramid is now gently mobilized in the cranial direction and sutured in one layer with interrupted 4–0 absorbable sutures (▶ Fig. 9.26 and ▶ Fig. 9.27).
- Tapes are applied to fix the skin into its new position.
- The IC incisions are closed and gentle pressure dressings are applied both internally and externally.

9.6 Retrusion of the Mandible and Mentoplasty

Retrusion (retrognathia) and protrusion (prognathia) of the mandible and maxilla have a strong influence on our aesthetic appreciation of the nasal profile.

Retrusion of the chin is frequently seen in Caucasians, mainly in individuals with dolichocephaly and a prominent, narrow external nasal pyramid. In these individuals, retrognathia accentuates the prominence of the nose. These patients may benefit from a reduction of their nasal prominence by a let-down procedure with bilateral wedge resections in combination with an augmentation mentoplasty (▶ Fig. 9.28 and ▶ Fig. 9.29).

Protrusion of the mandible is relatively rare. Surgical retroposition of the mandible as part of surgery of the nasal profile is only performed exceptionally.

9.6.1 Diagnosis

With the patient's mouth closed, the position of the chin is examined in relation to the face and nose from a front, side, and oblique perspective. Apart from the standard photographs, preoperative evaluation should also include a submental photograph and a lateral cephalometric

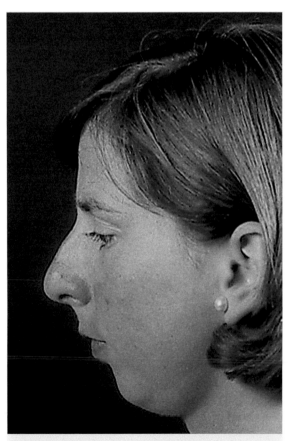

Fig. 9.28 Patient with retrusion of the mandible and a prominent, narrow nasal pyramid with impaired nasal breathing.

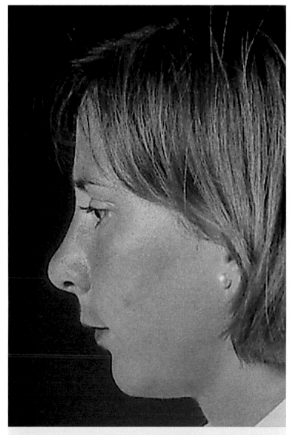

Fig. 9.29 Six months after septal surgery, the external nasal pyramid is let down and a Silastic chin implant is inserted through the intraoral route.

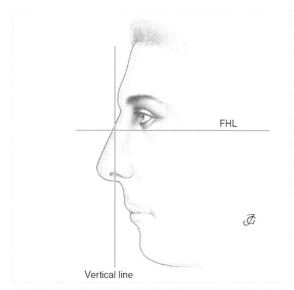

Fig. 9.30 Mandibular retrusion. The pogonion is situated dorsal to the vertical line.

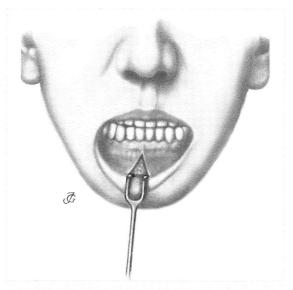

Fig. 9.31 Intraoral approach to insert a chin implant. A vertical labiogingival incision is made in the midline.

radiograph. The Frankfort horizontal line (FHL) and a vertical line at right angles to the FHL are drawn on the standard side-view photographs. Normally, the pogonion is situated some millimeters posterior to the border of the lips. If the chin is posterior to the vertical facial line, we speak of mandibular retrusion, retrognathia, or mandibular underprojection (▶ Fig. 9.30). If the pogonion is situated anterior to the vertical line, the chin is considered protruding.

9.6.2 Treatment Modalities

The following are the main surgical modalities from which the surgeon may choose to augment the chin:
• Implanting a nonbiological prosthesis
• Mandibular advancement by horizontal osteotomies with interposition of a bone graft or by a sliding genioplasty

Chin augmentation by implant is done in the same procedure as the rhinoplasty. It is a part of profile surgery and is usually performed by the rhinoplastic surgeon. Mandibular advancement is performed prior to a rhinoplasty. This surgery is carried out by a maxillofacial surgeon.

Materials

Over the past decades, a wide variety of materials has been used for chin augmentation. In the 1930s, Aufricht used a resected osteocartilaginous hump. After World War II, nonbiological implants (such as Proplast, Mersilene mesh, and polyamide mesh) became increasingly popular. Nowadays, Silastic implants are generally used. Solid Silastic (silicone rubber) is firm but flexible and can be autoclaved. The

material can easily be sculpted as required. When preparing the implant, the horizontal contours should be considered as well as the anteroposterior dimension. Silastic chin implants are available in various sizes and shapes.

Surgical Technique

Preparation

Steps

• The pogonion, midline, and caudal mandibular border are marked on the skin. The intended position of the implant is outlined.
• The implant is selected and its shape is adjusted as required.
• The implant is soaked in a broad-spectrum antibiotic solution for 0.5 to 1 hour prior to implantation.

Approach

Many surgeons prefer an extraoral approach, whereas others use an intraoral approach. Both have advantages and disadvantages.

Intraoral Approach

Steps

• A vertical gingivolabial incision is made in the midline in the frenulum (▶ Fig. 9.31).
• The loose submucosal tissue is opened up in a vertical direction.
• The periosteum of the mandible is incised in the midline and undermined in lateral directions. A subperiosteal pocket is created that just accommodates the implant.

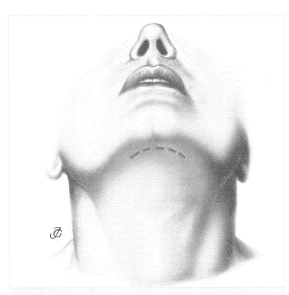

Fig. 9.32 Extraoral approach to insert a chin implant. A 2-cm incision is made in the skin at the inner margin of the chin.

- The implant is inserted and the effect is assessed.
- The incision is closed in two layers (periosteum and mucosa).
- The implant is carefully secured with external tapes that are left in place for several days.

Extraoral Approach

Steps

- A curved incision of about 2 cm is made at the inner margin of the mandible (▶ Fig. 9.32).
- The subcutaneous tissues are incised at a somewhat more anterior and cranial level to stagger the approach.
- The periosteum is incised at the lower margin of the mandible and elevated with a McKenty elevator in superior and lateral directions.
- Care is taken to make the pocket just wide enough to accommodate the implant.
- Bleeding is controlled by careful hemostasis.
- The implant is inserted and positioned. The result is assessed.
- The incision is closed in three layers: periosteum, subcutaneous tissue, and skin (intracutaneous running suture).
- The transplant is carefully fixed in place with outside taping.

Complications

Damage to the mental nerve is avoided by not extending the pocket too laterally and by remaining caudal to the mental foramen.

Hematoma is prevented by careful hemostasis and a pressure tape dressing.

Infection is prevented by careful asepsis, soaking the implant in antibiotic solution prior to insertion, and intravenous administration of a broad-spectrum penicillin before surgery.

Extrusion is the most feared complication of nonbiological implants. This may lead to visible scarring when the external approach is used. The implant has to be removed as soon as possible, preferably by the intraoral route.

Malalignment of the implant is prevented by outlining the intended position of the implant on the skin, taking care that the subperiosteal pocket will be symmetrical and not too wide.

Resorption of the underlying bone is a common long-term radiographic finding in follow-up studies. The clinical significance of this complication is usually limited.

9.7 Special Approaches

9.7.1 Endonasal and Transseptal–Transsphenoidal Approach to the Hypophysis

The idea of approaching the hypophysis transnasally dates back to the beginning of the 20th century. Harvey Cushing (1909, 1913, and later years) is usually credited as being the first to suggest the sublabial route to the pituitary gland. In 1910, Oskar Hirsch (Vienna, later Boston) was the first to describe the endonasal approach. This access was then used by several other authors (e.g., Spiess, Segura, and Dott). In 1912, von Chiari reported for the first time on the transethmoidal route.

Despite the advantages of these approaches to pituitary pathology, they were eventually forgotten. For decades, hypophysectomy and surgery for tumors of the pituitary gland were usually carried out via a transcranial–subfrontal approach. In the 1960s and 1970s, however, the transsphenoidal approach was revived. The transethmoidal–transsphenoidal approach was reintroduced by Angel James, Bateman (London), and Escher (Bern), whereas Hamberger (Stockholm) used transantral access. A major disadvantage of this technique is that the sella was approached obliquely. In the meantime, septal surgery techniques had been greatly refined and as a consequence, the transethmoidal and transantral approach were soon replaced by the transseptal–transsphenoidal approach (Guiot 1973, Kern 1978, and others). The surgery was usually performed using magnifying glasses or a microscope.

Since the late 1980s, the rigid endoscope has become more and more the instrument of choice. The endoscopic surgery may be carried out endonasally or transseptally. In the endonasal approach, the right-handed surgeon will use the endoscope in the left nasal cavity and the working instruments in the right one. The advantage of the endonasal approach is that no septal surgery is needed. However, some surgeons still prefer the transseptal approach.

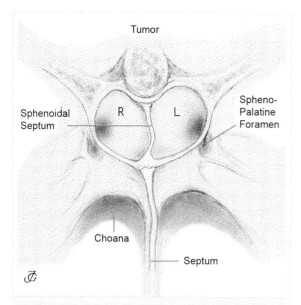

Fig. 9.33 Anatomy of the sphenoidal sinuses, the sella with a tumor, the choanae and the posterior part of the bony septum seen from above (cranial view).

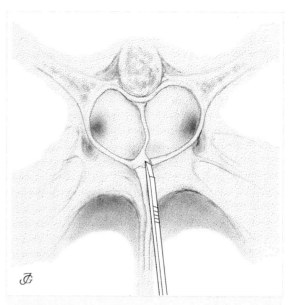

Fig. 9.34 The anterior wall and the ostium of the sphenoidal sinus are identified and opened using a narrow 4-mm chisel (or a burr).

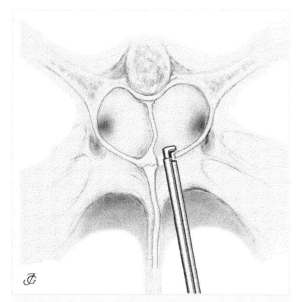

Fig. 9.35 The anterior wall of the sphenoidal sinuses is resected with a slender Hajek-type punch.

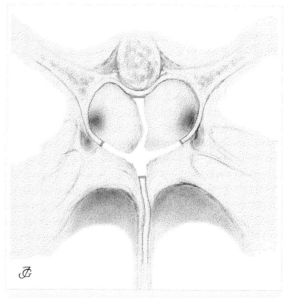

Fig. 9.36 The posterior part of the bony septum is resected to obtain a sufficiently wide overview. The intersphenoidal septum is then removed and the sella is identified.

Endonasal Approach

Steps

(▶ Fig. 9.33, ▶ Fig. 9.34, ▶ Fig. 9.35, and ▶ Fig. 9.36)

- The mucosa of the nasal cavity is decongested bilaterally in the usual way, in particular its dorsal and cranial area.

- The middle turbinates are lateralized to widen access to the sphenoid.
- A 0° endoscope is introduced and the superior turbinates and choanae are identified. The ostia of the sphenoidal sinuses are localized (superomedially of the turbinate tail and about 1.5 cm cranial to the choana).

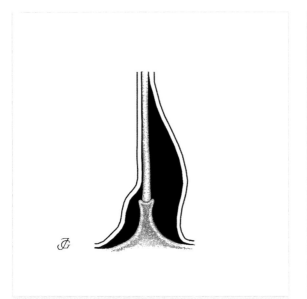

Fig. 9.37 An anterosuperior septal tunnel is made on the right side followed by limited bilateral inferior tunnels (three-tunnel approach). Both inferior tunnels are extended over the nasal floor. The mucoperichondrium on the right side remains attached to the septal cartilage.

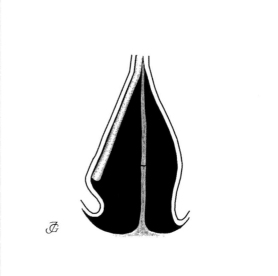

Fig. 9.38 The cartilaginous septum is mobilized and displaced to the right.

- The mucosa of the sphenoidal–ethmoidal recess and the anterior wall of the sphenoids are infiltrated with local anesthetic and adrenaline.
- The ostia of the sinuses are enlarged by resecting the anterior sphenoidal wall in a medial direction with a diamond burr and/or a small bone punch. Some surgeons prefer the use of the slender 4-mm chisel to penetrate the anterior wall of the sphenoid and continue the resection with a small punch (▶ Fig. 9.34 and ▶ Fig. 9.35).
- The rostrum sphenoidale and a part of the posterior bony septum are resected to obtain a sufficiently wide overview (▶ Fig. 9.36).
- The septum between the two sphenoidal sinuses is resected and the mucosal lining is removed. The posterior wall of both sphenoids as well as the sella are now widely exposed.
- The posterior wall is resected using a micro-punch and a small forceps, and the pituitary gland is exposed (see ▶ Fig. 9.42).

Transseptal Approach

Approach

Steps

- A CSI is made in the usual way.
- An anterosuperior septal tunnel is elevated on one side —for the right-handed surgeon, the right side. Then limited inferior tunnels are made bilaterally. The mucoperichondrium on the right side remains attached to the septal cartilage (so-called three-tunnel approach).

Both inferior tunnels are somewhat extended laterally on the nasal floor (▶ Fig. 9.37).
- A posterior chondrotomy is made at the junction between the cartilaginous septum and the perpendicular plate. The cartilaginous septum is dissected from its base and mobilized to the right (▶ Fig. 9.38).
- Bilateral posterior tunnels are elevated to expose the perpendicular plate and vomer.
- The lower part of the perpendicular plate and the upper part of the vomer are resected using Koffler scissors and a Craig forceps (▶ Fig. 9.39).
- The removed pieces of bone are preserved in isotonic saline so they can be used to repair the sphenoidal and septal defects at the end of the surgery.
- The endoscope is now introduced (▶ Fig. 9.40).
- The anterior wall of both sphenoidal sinuses is freed by elevating the mucoperiosteum in a lateral direction. Both sinuses are then opened at a thin area using a 4-mm chisel, and subsequently resected piecemeal with a small Hajek-type punch (▶ Fig. 9.41).
- The mucosal lining of both sphenoidal cavities is removed, and the posterior wall is resected using a micro-punch and small forceps. The pituitary gland is exposed (▶ Fig. 9.42).
- Surgeons who prefer to use the microscope instead of the endoscope in addressing pituitary pathology will now make a sublabial incision (▶ Fig. 9.43) and introduce a wide self-retaining speculum (▶ Fig. 9.44). To obtain a maximal overview, it may be necessary to resect the anterior nasal spine. The removed bone piece is replaced and fixed at the end of the surgery according to the principles described and illustrated on page 293 and in ▶ Fig. 7.76.

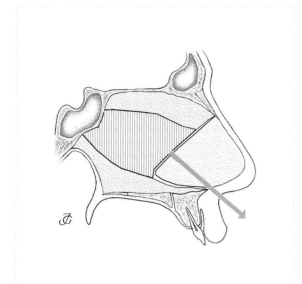

Fig. 9.39 The lower part of the perpendicular plate and the upper part of the vomer are resected. The anterior wall of the sphenoid bone is exposed. The removed bone is temporarily preserved in saline and later used to repair the sphenoidal and septal defects.

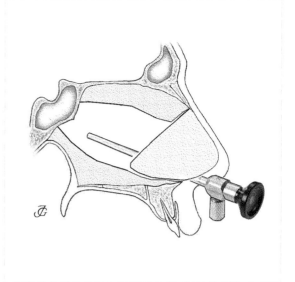

Fig. 9.40 The endoscope is introduced.

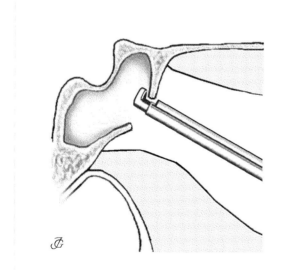

Fig. 9.41 The anterior wall of the sphenoidal sinuses is resected with a small Hajek-type punch.

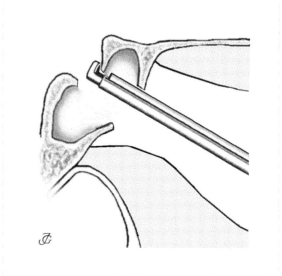

Fig. 9.42 The posterior wall is resected, exposing contents of the sella.

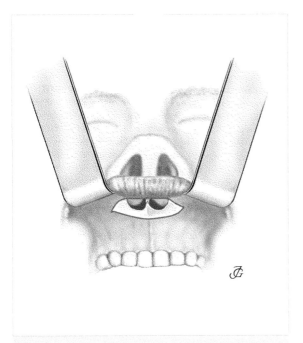

Fig. 9.43 A sublabial incision is made. The anterior nasal spine and the crest of the piriform apertures are exposed.

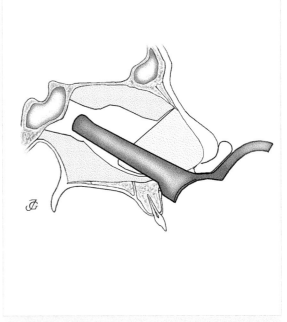

Fig. 9.44 A self-retaining speculum according to Cushing–Landolt is introduced.

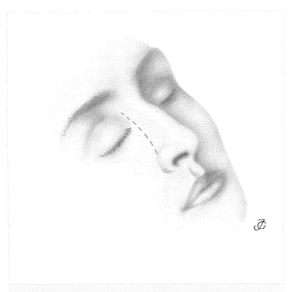

Fig. 9.45 A paranasal incision is made at the NBL.

Closure

Steps

- The posterior wall of the sphenoid is sealed by a layer of autogeneic fascia. Tissue glue may be used to safeguard the sealing.
- The sinus cavity is filled with fat tissue harvested from the abdomen.

- The nasal cavity is loosely packed.
- If the transseptal approach has been used, the defective part of the posterior septum is repaired by implanting the removed plates of bone, and the CSI is closed with 4–0 resorbable sutures as usual.

9.7.2 Lateral Rhinotomy

Lateral rhinotomy is the classic approach to the nasal cavity, paranasal sinuses, orbit, and anterior skull base. The method was introduced by Moure (Bordeaux) in 1902. He made use of a paranasal and an infraorbital incision. In later years, a number of other incisions have been advocated, the most common being the paranasal incision (▶ Fig. 9.45). Depending on the pathology, this incision may be extended in a caudal direction by an alatomy and a Z-shaped vertical incision at the midline of the upper lip. In a cranial direction, it may be continued in or just below the upper brow (▶ Fig. 9.46).

Approach

Steps

- The incision to be made is outlined on the skin.
- A paranasal incision is made at the nasal base line using a No. 15 and/or a No. 10 blade. Usually, the skin and periosteum are cut simultaneously.
- The periosteum is elevated in a ventral and a lateral direction.

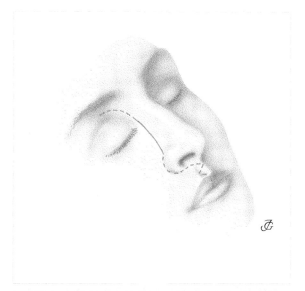

Fig. 9.46 The paranasal incision may be extended in a caudal direction by an alatomy and cleavage of the upper lip. It may also be extended cranially by an incision just below the eyebrow.

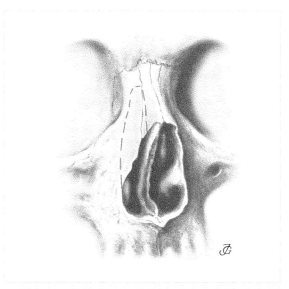

Fig. 9.47 Lateral, transverse, and intermedial osteotomies are performed.

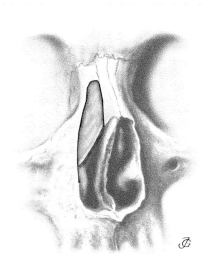

Fig. 9.48 The frontal process of the maxilla and part of the nasal bone is resected, leaving the inner nasal mucoperiosteum intact. The removed piece of bone is replaced at the end of the procedure.

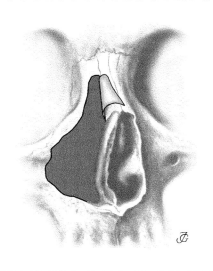

Fig. 9.49 The approach is enlarged using a Hajek-type punch. The mucoperiosteum of the inside of the bony pyramid is cut laterally and folded medially, where it is temporarily fixed.

- A lateral osteotomy is performed as dorsally as possible. Then a cranially situated transverse osteotomy and a ventral intermediate osteotomy are carried out (▶ Fig. 9.47).
- The frontal process of the maxilla, together with a part of the nasal bone, is resected from the underlying mucoperiosteum. The removed pieces of bone are placed in isotonic saline and may be used to repair the defect of the bony nasal vault (▶ Fig. 9.48).
- The mucoperiosteum of the inside of the nasal vault is mobilized and folded medially.
- The bony defect is enlarged by resecting parts of its margins with a heavy Hajek-type punch, as required (▶ Fig. 9.49).

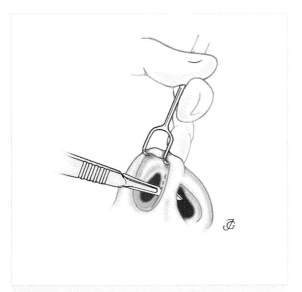

Fig. 9.50 Circumferential vestibular incision. The membranous septum is cut through just anterior to the caudal end of the septum (transfixion).

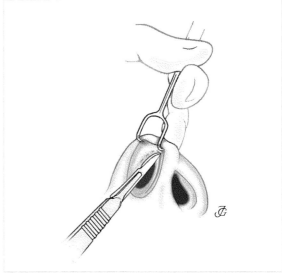

Fig. 9.51 The transfixion is continued into bilateral IC incisions.

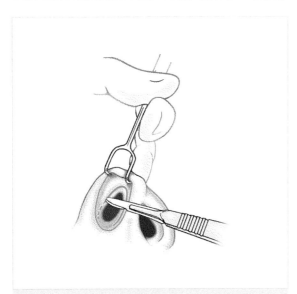

Fig. 9.52 The IC incisions are continued into vestibular incisions.

Closure

Steps

- Inner dressings are applied.
- The mucoperiosteum of the inside of the bony pyramid is repositioned and closed as far as possible.
- The bony defect is repaired by reimplantation and fixation of the removed bone segments. This is only feasible if the fragments have a reasonable chance of survival. Otherwise sequesters will occur. The bony defect may also be left open.

9.7.3 Sublabial Rhinotomy

In recent years, sublabial rhinotomy or the degloving technique has become one of the most favored approaches to the nasal cavity, paranasal sinuses, maxillary bones, orbit, anterior skull base, and hypophysis. This approach was initially suggested by Conley and Price (1979) and Allen and Siegel (1981). It has become increasingly popular as it offers wide access and leaves no visible scars. In this approach, a sublabial incision is combined with a bilateral circumferential vestibular incision. The upper lip and the nasal lobule are then dissected ("degloved") from the maxillary bones and the cartilaginous and bony pyramid. This provides wide access to the nasal cavities and adjacent structures.

Approach

Steps

- A circumferential vestibular incision is made bilaterally, thereby separating the lobule from the septum and the cartilaginous pyramid. This incision consists of a combination of a transfixion, an IC incision, a vestibular incision, and an incision at the vestibular floor (▶ Fig. 9.50, ▶ Fig. 9.51, ▶ Fig. 9.52, and ▶ Fig. 9.53). The incision at the vestibular floor is V-shaped to facilitate reconstruction but also to prevent skin retraction and stenosis (▶ Fig. 9.53).
- The connective tissue fibers between the lobule and the pyramid are cut with slightly curved scissors.
- The skin and subcutaneous tissue overlying the cartilaginous and bony pyramid are elevated through the IC and vestibular incisions.

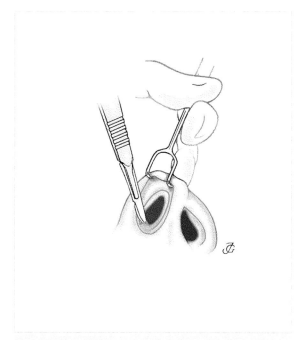

Fig. 9.53 The vestibular incisions are continued towards the floor of the vestibule. The incision is completed by making a V-shaped incision at the nasal floor that joins the transfixion.

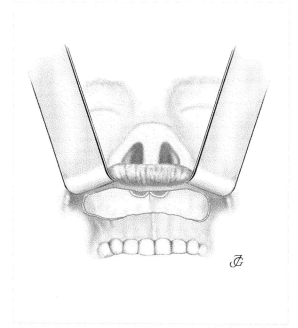

Fig. 9.54 A wide sublabial incision is made. The periosteum of the maxillary bones is elevated. The anterior nasal spine and the piriform aperture are exposed.

- A wide sublabial incision is made with a No. 15 or a No. 10 blade (▶ Fig. 9.54).
- The mucoperiosteum of the maxilla is elevated in a cranial direction. The anterior nasal spine and the crest of both piriform apertures are exposed (▶ Fig. 9.54).
- The upper lip is retracted upward. Elevation of the periosteum is continued bilaterally up to the infraorbital foramen, the inferior margin of the orbit, and the nasion.
- The nasal cavities, maxillary bones, and inferior rim of the orbits are now exposed (▶ Fig. 9.55).

Closure

Steps

- The circumferential vestibular incision is closed with 4–0 or 5–0 slowly resorbable sutures. This is done meticulously to avoid stenosis of the vestibule and valve area.
- The sublabial incision is also closed with 4–0 resorbable sutures.
- The valve areas and vestibules are carefully dressed, according to personal preference, with or without antibiotic ointment.
- The skin is closed in two layers.

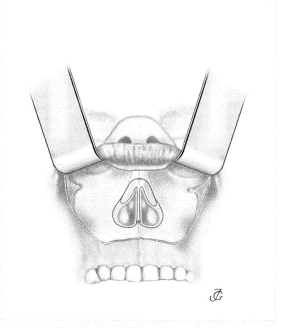

Fig. 9.55 The sublabial incision is connected with both circumferential vestibular incisions. The upper lip is lifted upward. The lobule is dissected ("degloved") subperichondrially/subperiosteally from the cartilaginous and bony pyramid. The infraorbital nerves are identified and secured.

9.8 Transplants and Implants

9.8.1 Terminology

Until recently, authors have used different terms when dealing with the various aspects of transplantation and implantation of tissues (organic) and other materials (inorganic). The words *transplant*, *implant*, and *graft*, for example, have been used in some publications as synonyms, whereas they have a different meaning in other articles and books.

Adapting an international standardized terminology is therefore of utmost importance. At present, the following definitions are generally accepted:

- *Transplant*: A tissue or an organ taken from the body for grafting into another area of the same body or into another individual
- *Implant*: Nonbiological (inorganic) material inserted into the body
- *Graft*: Any tissue or organ that is transplanted
- *Biological material*: Tissue from a living creature
- *Nonbiological material*: Inorganic material, present in nature or artificially produced
- *Autogeneic or autogenous (old: autologous) transplant*: Tissue originating from the same individual
- *Allogeneic (old: homologous) transplant*: Tissue originating from a different individual of the same species
- *Xenogeneic (old: heterologous) transplant*: Tissue originating from a living creature of a different genus or species
- *Orthotopic transplantation*: Tissue transplanted in the same area from which it was harvested; the recipient area is the same as the donor area
- *Heterotopic transplantation*: Tissue transplanted into an area different from the donor area

9.8.2 Requirements for the "Ideal" Transplant and Implant

The criteria for the "ideal" transplant and implant have been listed in numerous publications. It is easier to describe them than to comply with them, however. The ideal transplant or implant should:

- Be well tolerated by the recipient and the recipient area, also in the long run
- Not transmit diseases or cause diseases
- Show no resorption or disintegration
- Not become deformed while in the body

Finally, the material should be easily available. As far as reconstructive and aesthetic nasal surgery is concerned, it is evident that these criteria have not yet been met by any transplant or implant.

9.8.3 Materials

The list of materials that has been used in nasal and facial reconstruction over the past 150 years is almost endless.

Biological Transplants

Biological transplants were introduced in the middle of the 19th century by Dieffenbach (bone; 1845) and Bert (rib cartilage; 1869). Since then, various types of autogeneic tissue, as well as processed allogeneic and xenogeneic tissue, have been tried out. In chronological order, the main ones are tibial cortex, iliac crest, calf bone, rib cartilage, auricular cartilage, various types of processed spongiotic and cortical bone, connective tissue, bovine collagen, and fat (▶ Table 9.4).

Nonbiological (Nonorganic) Implants

The history of using nonbiological (inorganic) implants in nasal surgery dates back to the first half of the 19th century, when gold and silver were first used. Around the turn of the century, subcutaneous and submucosal injection of paraffin became highly popular for use in patients with a saddle nose and ozena, respectively. Because of severe adverse reactions, other materials were tried, for example (in chronological order), ivory, various metals, different kinds of natural materials, and an almost endless variety of synthetic materials. A survey is presented in ▶ Table 9.5 and ▶ Table 9.6. Most of these materials were enthusiastically adopted initially but later abandoned for various reasons. This has induced such cynical remarks as, "Each decade has its own nonbiological

Table 9.4 Biological transplant materials used in nasal surgery

Material	Publishing author(s) (year)
Bone	
Autogeneic	
Frontal bone	Dieffenbach (1845)
Tibial cortex	Israel, Joseph (1907)
Iliac crest	Unterberger (1929)
Processed xenogeneic	
Calf tibia	Eckert-Möbius (1923)
Boplant	
Kiel bone	University of Kiel (1966)
Osteovit	
Cartilage	
Autogeneic	
Rib	Von Mangold (1900)
Auricular	1980s
Allogeneic	
Rib	Bert (1869)
Connective tissue	
Autogeneic	1960s
Allogeneic	1960s
Xenogeneic	
Bovine collagen	1980s
Fat	
Autogeneic	1990s

Table 9.5 Most popular nonbiological implant materials used in nasal surgery before 1950

Material	Introduction	Use
Gold, silver	Fallopius (1600) Rousset (1828) Dieffenbach (1845)	Skull defect Saddle nose
Paraffin, petrolatum	Gersuny, Broeckaart (1900)	Saddle nose, ozena
Ivory	Joseph, Safian, and many others (1920s)	Saddle nose
Celluloid		
Acrylic	Eyries and many others (1930s)	Saddle nose, ozena
Marble	1940s	
Tantalum gauze	1930s	Saddle nose, ozena
Stainless steel	1930s	Saddle nose

Note: Less commonly used and not listed are Vaseline, glass pearls, Dolomite, and Paladon

Table 9.6 Most popular nonbiological implant materials used in nasal surgery since 1950

Material	Developed	Still in use?
Polyethylene	Early 1950s	No
Silicone • Solid silicone • Silicone rubber • Silicone gel	1950s–1960s	Yes
Teflon	1960s	Yes
Dacron velour	1970s	No
Polyamide/Supramid mesh	Mid 1970s	No
Proplast I, II	1970s–1980s	No
Mersilene mesh	Early 1980s	
Med-Pore	1980s	No
Gore-Tex	1980s	Yes

implant that was inserted by one surgeon and had later to be removed by another."

Choosing between Biological and Nonbiological Material

There has been considerable divergence of opinion concerning the materials chosen for reconstruction and augmentation in nasal surgery. Many nasal surgeons, like ourselves, use and have always used biological materials, preferably autogeneic tissues. They never insert nonbiological materials in the septum, and only very rarely subcutaneously.

Other surgeons have been in favor of using nonbiological materials to augment the dorsum, increase tip projection, or fill defects. This divergence was not only related to conceptual differences, but also to differences in the types of patient treated. Surgeons specialized in functional and reconstructive nasal surgery preferred biological materials. Among surgeons who were mainly involved in aesthetic surgery, nonbiological compounds were rather popular. Because of the complications (infection, extrusion) that have been observed following implantation of nonorganic materials, the use of nonbiological materials has considerably decreased.

Biological Materials—Transplants

Various biological materials have been successfully used for reconstruction and augmentation: cartilage, bone, connective tissue, fat, skin, and mucosa. In special cases, combinations are used, particularly composite grafts of auricular cartilage and skin for reconstruction of the ala or vestibule.

In general, we try to restore or replace tissues with the same type of tissue material. Cartilage is used to reconstruct the cartilaginous septum and the triangular and lobular cartilages, plates of bone to reconstruct the posterior septum. This is not always possible, however. For instance, to augment a bony saddle nose, we use cartilage instead of bone, and to repair a missing cartilaginous septum, we may use one or more plates of bone if no cartilage is available.

Cartilage

Types of Cartilage

On the basis of their function and histological structure, we can distinguish four types of cartilage: morphological cartilage, elastic cartilage, fibrocartilage, and articular cartilage (Caplan 1984).

• *Morphological cartilage* is supple and elastic and maintains its shape. It is genetically programmed in such a way that the chondrocytes make new cartilage in its original configuration. Two examples are lobular and auricular cartilage. Auricular cartilage is therefore our first choice material to repair or reinforce defective lobular cartilage.

• *Elastic cartilage* is less supple than morphological cartilage. Even though it is stiffer, it has a certain degree of elasticity. The main examples are septal cartilage and rib cartilage. Especially in its superficial layers, elastic fibers are arranged in such a way that the shape of the cartilage is maintained. The forces keeping elastic cartilage in form are called interlocked stresses (Gibson and Davis 1957). When these elastic fibers are cut unilaterally (or asymmetrically), the cartilage will bend to the other side (▶ Fig. 9.56). For this reason, we avoid damaging the surface of the septal cartilage when elevating the mucoperichondrium. This is also why we take the central part of a rib to sculpt a dorsal or septal transplant.

• *Fibrocartilage* is found in intervertebral disks. It is stiffer than elastic cartilage.

• *Articular* cartilage is found in joints.

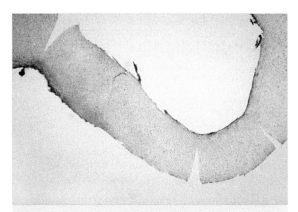

Fig. 9.56 Disfiguration of septal cartilage caused by making small superficial incisions. As the superficial elastic fibers are cut through, the cartilage bends to the side opposite the cuts. (Photograph courtesy Prof. Hellmich.)

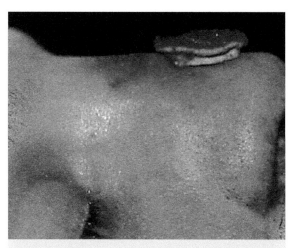

Fig. 9.57 Transplants sculpted from autogeneic auricular cartilage to correct a limited sagging of the cartilaginous dorsum.

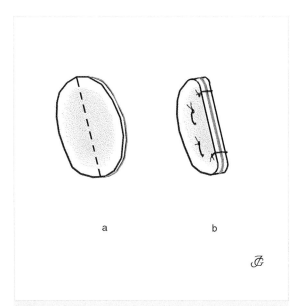

a   b

Fig. 9.58 Back-to-back transplant for reconstructing a missing caudal end of the septum. A graft is taken from the cavum conchae with its posterior perichondrium attached. It is cut into two halves leaving the attached perichondrium intact **(a)**, and then folded and sutured to make a semi-ovaloid transplant **(b)** to be used for reconstruction.

Use of Different Types of Cartilage

In reconstructive nasal surgery, septal, auricular, and rib cartilage may be used in many ways.

Plates or struts may be cut from septal cartilage to reconstruct the septum, to reinforce the columella, to correct a retracted columella, and to restore the triangular cartilage.

Single or double plates of septal or auricular cartilage are cut to measure to fill a sagging cartilaginous dorsum if still required after reconstruction of the anterior septum (▶ Fig. 9.57).

Battens of cartilage may be used to straighten and reinforce the septum, and wedges as spreader grafts. All kinds of small strips, battens and "shields" may be used to repair or reinforce the lobular and triangular cartilages.

Auricular cartilage is the best choice if septal cartilage is not available. A "back-to-back" transplant according to Pirsig, Kern and Verse (2004) has proven to be an excellent alternative to replace a missing caudal septal end (▶ Fig. 9.58). A graft is taken from the cavum conchae with its posterior perichondrium attached (see ▶ Fig. 6.82). It is cut into two halves, leaving the attached perichondrium intact **(a)**, and then folded and sutured to make a semi-ovaloid transplant **(b)** to be used for reconstruction.

Crushed cartilage is used subcutaneously to support a thin dorsal skin and to fill depressions and grooves.

Rib cartilage may be used to sculpt a transplant to correct a bony and cartilaginous saddle nose (▶ Fig. 9.59).

Resorption

The major disadvantage of using biological materials for reconstruction and augmentation is their tendency to be resorbed (▶ Fig. 9.60 and ▶ Fig. 9.61) or become deformed, warped or twisted (see ▶ Fig. 9.88 and ▶ Fig. 9.89) The rate and degree of resorption depends on many factors:

- Cartilage tends to survive better when the perichondrium is left attached (at least on one side).
- Orthotopic transplants are less rapidly resorbed than heterotopic transplants.
- The greater the surface of the transplant in relation to its volume, the quicker the resorption. Plates are resorbed more rapidly than blocks.
- Damage to the cartilage (e.g., lesions of its surface and puncture holes resulting from sutures) will enhance absorption. Between 30 and 60% of crushed cartilage is resorbed, depending on the degree of crushing.

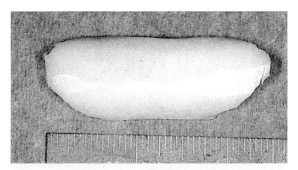

Fig. 9.59 Transplant sculpted from rib cartilage for dorsal augmentation.

- Transplants survive better in areas with low metabolic and immunological activity (e.g., in the connective tissue layers of the dorsum and the lobule) than in areas where such activity is high (e.g., underneath the septal mucosa).
- Microtrauma is often said to play a role in resorption. In our opinion, this rapid resorption is more likely related to immunological activity of the mucosa than to microtrauma.

Deformation

Disfiguration of the transplant (e.g., bending [or warping] and growth) is another common problem of using cartilage for transplant material. The most important factors are the following:

- Type of cartilage: Curved elastic cartilage such as rib cartilage, and morphological cartilage like auricular cartilage, have a relatively high tendency to deform after transplantation (see ▶ Fig. 9.88, and ▶ Fig. 9.89).
- Incisions into the cartilage: Any incision into septal cartilage will lead to bending to the other side (▶ Fig. 9.56).
- Technique of sculpting: When rib cartilage is taken to correct a saddle nose, the center of the rib is used. This will considerably decrease the chances of warping (▶ Fig. 9.59; see also ▶ Fig. 6.86, ▶ Fig. 6.87, and ▶ Fig. 6.88).
- Growth of a transplant: Although rare, this does occur. This phenomenon has been described for cartilage transplants in which the perichondrium remained attached (see ▶ Fig. 9.90).
- Preservation of cartilage: Freeze-drying, Cialit, and other methods of preserving cartilage denature its structure to certain extent and may therefore decrease the chance of disfiguration.

Incorporation

Histologic studies of rib grafts (removed because of dislocation or disfigurement) have demonstrated that these transplants may become incorporated to a certain extent. They are first surrounded by a capsule of dense connective tissue and then gradually invaded by connective

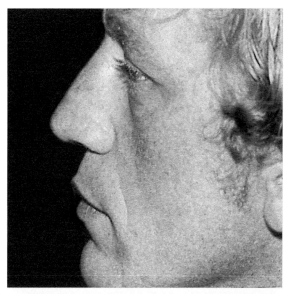

Fig. 9.60 Long-term follow-up of preserved allogeneic rib cartilage transplant in the nasal dorsum 3 months after septal reconstruction and augmentation of the cartilaginous dorsum with Cialit-preserved allogeneic rib cartilage in a patient with severe saddling of the cartilaginous vault due to septal trauma.

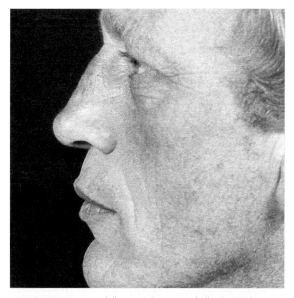

Fig. 9.61 Long-term follow-up of preserved allogeneic rib cartilage transplant in the nasal dorsum 9 years after surgery, demonstrating some resorption of the transplant.

tissue and some small blood vessels. The cartilage itself remains amorphous (▶ Fig. 9.62).

Calcification

Rib cartilage grafts in the nasal dorsum may also become partially calcified in the long run. An example is presented in ▶ Fig. 9.63.

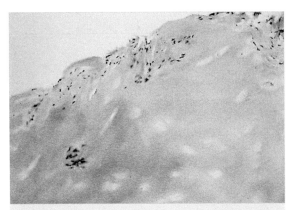

Fig. 9.62 Preserved allogeneic rib transplant removed because of dislocation 1 year after insertion in the nasal dorsum for augmentation purposes. The cartilage is amorphous; invasion of connective tissue can be observed in several areas.

Harvesting

The surgical techniques for harvesting rib cartilage and auricular cartilage are described in detail in Chapter 6 (see ▶ Fig. 6.84, ▶ Fig. 6.85, ▶ Fig. 6.81, and ▶ Fig. 6.82, respectively).

Bone

Bone (cortical calvarial bone, spongiotic bone from the iliac crest) can only be used to a limited extent in reconstructive nasal surgery because of its rigidity. A plate of bone, preferably septal perpendicular plate or vomer, may be taken to rebuild a missing anterior septum. A bone transplant sculpted to the demands may be used to reconstruct a severe bony saddle nose.

Types of Bone

The following types of bone may be used: cancellous bone (spongiosa), cortical bone, and septal bone. Cancellous bone is usually well accepted and incorporated, but it may become resorbed rather quickly. Cortical bone survives much better. It is usually not incorporated but encapsulated within a fibrous envelope.

Septal bone (lamina perpendicularis) has proven to be an excellent material for septal reconstruction (▶ Fig. 9.64).

Autogeneic versus Processed Allogeneic and Xenogeneic Bone

Generally, autogeneic bone is our first choice. Nonetheless, allogeneic bone may be a very good substitute, provided that essential precautions are taken to avoid transmitting disease. Over the years, processed bone of non-human origin (for instance calf bone) has proven to be a good alternative, unlike xenogeneic cartilage. Processed bovine spongiosa is successfully used to narrow the nasal

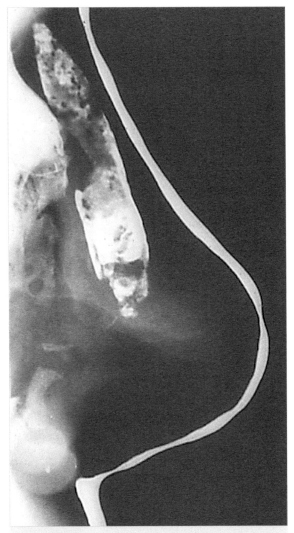

Fig. 9.63 Calcification of preserved allogeneic rib cartilage 7 years after transplantation. The dorsal skin has been painted with a radiopaque substance to show the position of the transplant. The graft is intact and the nasal profile is normal.

cavity (see ▶ Fig. 8.23 and ▶ Fig. 8.24) and repair the anterior nasal spine, for instance.

Use of Different Types of Bone

Autogeneic cancellous bone from the iliac crest has been used for many decades as a dorsal transplant in saddle noses. Its use has been limited for a number of reasons. First, bone is too rigid to repair a cartilaginous dorsum; second, it is rather rapidly disfigured by resorption; and third, a bone transplant might break after trauma.

Processed cancellous bone has been used to repair a missing anterior nasal spine, to correct a localized depression of the maxilla, and to narrow the nasal cavity.

Cortical bone is becoming increasingly popular for reconstructing the bony pyramid, maxilla, and mandible.

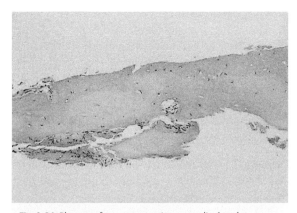

Fig. 9.64 Plate cut from autogeneic perpendicular plate to reconstruct a missing anterior septum, which had to be removed because of repeated trauma 16 months after surgery. The bone appears to be histologically normal.

Septal bone is an excellent material for reconstruction of the bony and cartilaginous septum and, for example, the nasal bones. Sherris and Kern (1998) described an autogeneic ninth rib bony transplant that was fixed by small screws to construct a missing bony pyramid.

Advantages and Disadvantages

The advantages of using a bone graft are its rigidity and limited resorption. It can therefore be used as supporting and augmentation material in certain areas. These advantages are also limitations. The rigidity of bone makes it unsuitable as a graft for the mobile and soft parts of the nose, such as the cartilaginous pyramid and lobule. A bony transplant in the nasal dorsum gives the nose an unnaturally rigid appearance. When used in these areas, bone grafts tend also to become dislocated more easily than cartilaginous transplants.

Connective Tissue and Collagen

Connective tissue may be used in nasal surgery subcutaneously as a skin underlay or a filler in the cartilaginous dorsum and lobule. Sometimes it is applied in closing septal perforations or a defect of the dura. Autogeneic fascia and allogeneic dura are the most commonly used materials.

- *Autogeneic connective tissue* is taken from the temporal fascia. This donor area is near our surgical field. In addition, the harvesting technique is well known to ENT surgeons. Another option is autogeneic deep fascia of the thigh, with or without muscle, which is often used to close the skull base defect after transsphenoidal hypophysectomy (see page 340). More recently, autogeneic fibroblasts generated in tissue culture for injection have become available.

- *Processed allogeneic material* is a well-known alternative. AlloDerm (LifeCell Corporation, Bridgewater, New Jersey, United States), originally developed (1994) for treating burns, is a freeze-dried de-epithelialized, acellular dermal graft processed from tissue-banked skin. It is available both in sheets and in an injectable form.

- *Xenogeneic (bovine) connective tissue* became available as injectable filler in the early 1980s. Zyderm (Inamed Corporation, Fremont, California, United States) consists of 95% type I and 5% type II collagen, thereby imitating human dermal collagen. Dermalogen is a mixture of allogeneic collagen, elastin and glycosaminoglycans.

Unfortunately, the effect of xenogeneic collagen injections is short-lived: generally, no more than 6 to 9 months. The procedure thus has to be repeated. Before bovine collagen is injected, a skin test must be performed, as about 3% of the population appears to be allergic to bovine collagen.

Fat

Fat is not a commonly used material for reconstructive nasal surgery. It may be used as a filler in subcutaneous defects, however. Generally, fat cells survive better than cartilage cells. Moreover, fat is easily harvested through a small paraumbilical incision. It may be inserted either in small pieces through a small intranasal incision, or injected as a suspension. Any leftover fat may be preserved by deep-freezing. It can then be injected or implanted after some months as an additional procedure.

Skin and Mucosa

Free grafts or pedicled grafts of skin or mucosa may be used to reconstruct cutaneous or mucosal defects.

A *split-skin graft* may be used to cover external skin defects after trauma or ablative surgery. In the past, split-skin grafts have often been used to replace irreversibly diseased nasal mucosa in patients with hereditary telangiectasias (Rendu–Osler–Weber disease). The results of this so-called Saunders operation were disappointing, however. Nasal irritation, dryness, and crusting were disturbing side effects. We therefore prefer to replace nasal mucosa with a full-thickness graft of buccal mucosa.

A *full-thickness skin graft* may be used to reconstruct the valve angle or the floor of the vestibule in patients with a posttraumatic or postsurgical stenosis. As an alternative, a composite graft may be used for this type of repair (Chapter 6, page 255 and Chapter 7, page 295). Free and pedicled skin grafts are used to repair larger and deeper external skin defects. Reconstructions of that kind are not discussed in this book, however.

Free mucosal grafts harvested from the buccal mucosa may be used to replace severely diseased nasal mucosa. They are also taken to cover the endonasal surface of a skull base defect, and to cover a surgically widened ostium of the frontal sinus.

Pedicled mucosal grafts are the preferred material for closing a septal perforation. The most well-known methods are the "rotation flap technique," the "bridge flap technique," and the "buccogingival flap technique." These are extensively dealt with in Chapter 5 (page 207 and page 208).

Composite grafts are a very important material to reconstruct multilayered defects. Alar and columellar defects may be repaired with a free composite skin–cartilage or a skin–cartilage–skin graft taken from the auricle. A congenital or posttraumatic stenosis of the valve area or vestibule is restored by reconstruction with a free skin–cartilage graft (see Chapter 6, page 255 and Chapter 7, page 295).

Nonbiological (Nonorganic) Materials—Implants

The 20th century has witnessed a continuous search for the "ideal" nonbiological implant for nasal and facial surgery. The North American literature in particular abounds in reports on the use (actually try-outs) of diverse natural substances and synthetic compounds (see ▶ Table 9.5 and ▶ Table 9.6).

Advantages and Disadvantages

There are clear advantages to using nonbiological implants: they are easily available, they do not require a second surgical field or a tissue bank, and their quantity is always sufficient. At the same time, they have major disadvantages. First of all, nonbiological materials—at least, those that have been developed so far—do not become integrated within the living tissues. Thus, there is a higher risk that they will cause infection and become extruded, both in the short and long term. A nonorganic implant may still be extruded after 10 or 20 years, usually after a minor infection or trauma. Some examples are presented in ▶ Fig. 9.91, ▶ Fig. 9.92, ▶ Fig. 9.93, ▶ Fig. 9.94, ▶ Fig. 9.95, ▶ Fig. 9.96, ▶ Fig. 9.97, ▶ Fig. 9.98, ▶ Fig. 9.99, ▶ Fig. 9.100, and ▶ Fig. 9.101. Other disadvantages are immunological reactions, carcinogenesis, degradability, and migration. In fact it may take years, even decades, to determine that a certain nonbiological material is biocompatible, noncarcinogenic, nonimmunogenic, and nondegradable. For this reason, we are reluctant to use nonbiological materials in functional nasal surgery.

Historical Overview of the Materials Used

Silicone is marketed as solid silicone, silicone rubber (Silastic), and silicone gel.
- *Silicone rubber* was introduced in the late 1950s and early 1960s. It is available in soft, medium, and firm consistencies, and can easily be contoured with a sharp blade.

- *Silicone gel or injectable silicone* was introduced in the 1960s. It enjoyed widespread application, particularly in the face where it was, and sometimes still is, used to fill furrows and creases. Various adverse reactions and complications have been described. Some of them are related to incorrect injection technique. It should be kept in mind that we are injecting a foreign material that may give rise to tissue reactions, both in the short and long term.

Polytetrafluoroethylene (PTFE) is a rather well-tolerated material that is available in various forms. It is marketed under the trade names Teflon, Proplast, and Gore-Tex.
- *Teflon* has been available since the late 1940s. Teflon paste was used for vocal cord augmentation. It may migrate and cause chronic inflammatory responses. It may also break down.
- *Proplast* is a porous material. In its primary form, it consisted of PTFE and elemental carbon (Proplast I, black). Later it was substituted by Proplast II, which consists of Teflon and aluminum (white). Finally, it was replaced by Proplast–Hydroxyapatite. It was eventually withdrawn from the market due to its association with various forms of morbidity.
- *Gore-Tex* is a fibrillated PTFE that was developed in the late 1960s. Initially, it was used in vascular surgery, later in hernia surgery. Since the 1980s, it has also been used for soft tissue augmentation. Gore-Tex has been used for facial surgery, including rhinoplasty, since 1993. The material has a relatively good safety record: it does not induce foreign body reactions, has a low infection rate, and is rarely rejected. It is available in sheets with a thickness of 0.4, 0.6, 1.0, and 2.0 mm, and can be sterilized using gas or steam. It could well be the best nonbiological implant material for nasal application that has been introduced thus far.

High-density polyethylene is on the market as Med-Pore. It is a wide-woven, high-density porous polyethylene. Although it is a hard substance, it can be contoured with a knife. It is supposed to allow osseous integration and to be nonresorbable. However, it is not appropriate for use in stress-bearing areas. The reason is that it may delaminate with particle formation, producing a chronic inflammatory response. It has been advocated for insertion into a subperiosteal pocket in chin augmentation.

Polyamide (Supramid mesh) is a polyamide with relatively high biocompatibility. Available as a mesh, it was introduced in the mid 1970s, among others for dorsal augmentation. It is not used much, since progressive resorption and extrusion has been reported.

Polyether (Mersilene) is similar to Supramid and part of the same family as Dacron. A wide-woven mesh, it can be folded and rolled and then sutured to retain the desired shape. It is considered relatively nonreactive, although some resorption seems to take place.

Hydroxyapatite: The most well-known form of hydroxyapatite is its ceramic form, calcium phosphate. This compound is synthesized at a very low pH and then heated (sintered) to create a hard, nonresorbable material. It is available in solid and porous forms, and has been in use for over 20 years. The material is too rigid to be used successfully in facial and rhinoplastic surgery, however. The porous type resembles marine coral. It is invaded by fibro-osseous tissue and becomes fixed to the bone.

Titanium: Because of its osseointegrative properties, titanium was introduced to fixate epitheses. The results have been remarkably good, and several applications have been developed.

9.9 Complications—Prevention and Treatment

9.9.1 Complications or Mistakes?

Do complications really exist or are they mostly the result of errors and negligence? This is an awkward question. When reviewing the "complications" that have occurred during or after nasal surgery, we have to admit that many of them could have been avoided. The majority of the complications that we see are either caused by mistakes, whether major or minor, or by lack of proper care. Terms such as "undesired side effect" and "adverse reaction" or "adverse event" are basically euphemisms. We should be aware of the fact that many complications could have been prevented by better preoperative analysis, a more extensive preoperative discussion with the patient, better anesthesia and vasoconstriction, more conservative surgery, more intensive aftercare, and so on.

We should therefore always ask ourselves the following two questions: "What did I do wrong?" and "What am I going to do differently next time to prevent a similar mishap?" If we do not know the answers to these questions, we will very likely not improve our skills or build on our experience. It has often been said that experience comes from making mistakes. This is only true if we take the time to analyze the results and complications of our work. The fewest complications are found among surgeons who are prepared to make this effort.

This does not mean that someone or something should be blamed whenever a complication arises. Sometimes, an unfortunate and unpredictable sequence of events may occur. There is no point in blaming the patient or the healing process. It is more productive to look for the real cause.

Remarkably, complications are still rarely discussed. Most surgeons seem reluctant to face up to them. Very few of the books on rhinoplasty devote a chapter to complications, and usually only the best results are shown in congress presentations.

> Do complications really exist, or are they mostly the result of major or minor errors, shortcomings or negligence?

9.9.2 General Recommendations on Prevention

Based on their long experience, some authors have formulated some general recommendations on how to keep complications to a minimum. The following guidelines may prove helpful:

Preoperatively

- Take a careful history.
- Analyze whether the findings of the physical and functional examination fit with the patient's complaints. If not, be cautious.
- Do not decide too quickly to go ahead with surgery. Discuss the options with your patient and give him or her ample information about the chances, risks, and alternatives (see Chapter 2, page 105).
- Ensure thorough documentation. Record the history, the findings, and any matters discussed with the patient.

During Surgery

- Ensure proper anesthesia and a bloodless field.
- Do not do too much at a time. It may be better to postpone part of the surgery to a secondary stage.
- Do not use techniques that you do not master.
- Limit your resections to those that are really necessary.
- Reconstruct all defects. Try to reconstitute normal anatomy instead of "creating" a new anatomy.
- Fixate the tissues in their new position and carefully close the incisions.

Postoperatively

- Do not leave all aftercare to your coworkers. Check your patient personally to avoid embarrassing "surprises."
- In case of complications, consult a colleague.

(See also the section on page 370.)

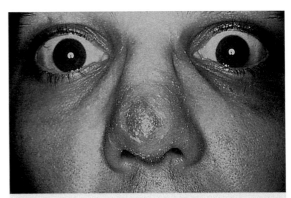

Fig. 9.66 Ischemia of the skin of the tip caused by incorrect taping, leaving the tip free. (Photograph courtesy Prof. Cottle.)

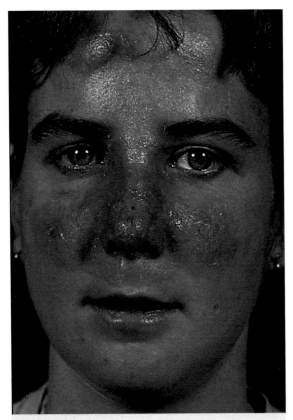

Fig. 9.65 Allergic reaction of the skin to tapes, prevented by carefully taking the patient's history.

9.9.3 Prevention and Treatment of Specific Complications

Skin Problems

Allergic Reactions to Tape

This is a common but avoidable complication (▶ Fig. 9.65). It has become less frequent since improvements have been made in the quality of the taping material.

Prevention: When taking the history, the patient is asked about known allergies, in particular to tape or antibiotics. In case of doubt, the patient is tested by placing a piece of the tape on the cheek or forehead for 24 to 48 hours. This test is not done on the arm, as a negative reaction there does not exclude a reaction of the facial skin.

Treatment: All tapes are removed. A corticosteroid cream is applied. The area is covered with a cotton wool or linen dressing fixed with paper tape. The stent may be replaced.

Ischemia of the Skin

Ischemia of the skin may occur at various sites: (1) at the dorsum after inadequate undermining of the skin and introduction of an oversized transplant or implant; (2) at

the tip after extensive undermining of the lobule and incorrect postoperative taping (▶ Fig. 9.66); or (3) at the columella after using the external approach (which implies severing the columellar artery) and suturing under tension (see ▶ Fig. 9.72).

Prevention: Ischemia of the skin is avoided by: (1) undermining the dorsal skin widely enough and checking the color of the skin for some time after inserting the transplant; (2) taping the lobule and cartilaginous pyramid completely after surgery. The tip is not left bare as this may lead to interference with venous blood flow.

Treatment: Very little can be done. The only guideline is to keep the ischemic skin dry and free of infection.

Reactions to Suture Material

Nowadays, suture materials very rarely cause adverse reactions. In earlier days, granulomas in reaction to chromic catgut were reported.

Telangiectasias

Telangiectasias may occur after undermining the skin over the bony dorsum, in particular after repeated surgery (▶ Fig. 9.67).

Prevention: Care is taken to undermine at the proper level (immediately above the periosteum) and to avoid stretching the skin when spreading the tissues. After resecting or rasping a bony hump, it may be helpful to insert a thin layer of connective tissue or crushed septal cartilage.

Treatment: Camouflage using a cosmetic ointment and powder is usually the best solution. Laser therapy may be discussed with an expert.

Discoloration of the Skin

After osteotomies and hump resection with wide undermining of the dorsal skin, a brownish-blue discoloration of the skin beneath the lower eyelids may persist for several weeks (▶ Fig. 9.68), which may alarm the patient. This minor side effect will gradually subside completely. It may be helpful to massage the skin.

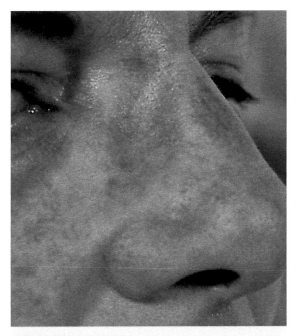

Fig. 9.67 Telangiectasias of the skin over the bony dorsum due to repeated undermining and overstretching of the thin skin.

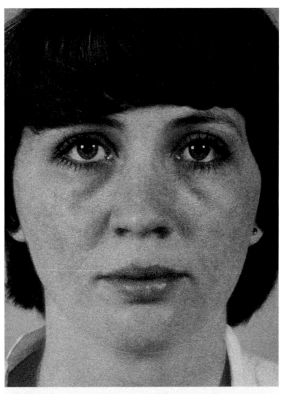

Fig. 9.68 Discoloration of the skin beneath the eyelids after extensive pyramid surgery. This side effect usually disappears spontaneously after some months.

Hematomas

Ecchymoses and hematomas are common after nasal surgery. Various factors play a role: the extent and duration of surgery; the quality of surgery (sequence of surgical steps; prevention of bleeding [decongestion, pressure during surgery, postoperative taping]); and the patient's characteristics.

Prevention: The most important measures that can be taken are to ensure a bloodless surgical field and to prevent bleeding and any accumulation of blood by applying pressure (manual pressure, temporary internal dressings, postoperative taping).

Treatment: Septal hematomas must be drained immediately, either by reopening the CSI or by making a horizontal basal incision. The blood clot is removed with a sterile suction tube. The septal mucosa is readjusted bilaterally using Merocel or gauzes with ointment, and antibiotics are given systemically to prevent infection (see also Chapter 5, page 196). A dorsal hematoma is removed by reopening one of the IC incisions. The blood remnants are removed by suction, and a gentle pressure dressing is applied. Paranasal hematomas should also be drained as they may become infected. Eyelid and lip hematomas do not require treatment. They occur within loose connective tissue, not in a surgically created pocket. As a consequence, they resolve.

Infections

Rhinosinusitis

Some degree of rhinitis and sinusitis will invariably occur following extensive septal pyramid surgery. Therefore, many surgeons prefer to administer systemic antibiotics, usually starting the day before surgery (see Chapter 3, page 136). The length of time the internal dressings are left in place is an important factor causing nasal and sinus infection.

Septal Abscess

A postoperative septal abscess must be treated immediately. Otherwise, necrosis of the septal cartilage will occur within hours, which leads to sagging of the dorsum and retraction of the columella (see Chapter 5, page 198).

Dorsal Abscess

A dorsal abscess is drained by reopening the IC incision (▶ Fig. 9.69). After cleansing the abscess by suction, the incision is left partially open. An antibiotic solution may be placed in the dorsal pocket. The skin is adjusted to the dorsum with tapes using slight pressure (see following text on complications of transplants and implants).

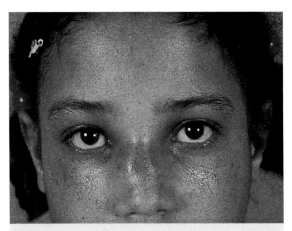
Fig. 9.69 Dorsal abscess after augmentation of the external pyramid by a cartilaginous transplant.

Infected Implant or Transplant

If a nonbiological implant has been introduced for augmentation, there is no choice than to remove it (see ► Fig. 9.91► Fig. 9.92, ► Fig. 9.93, ► Fig. 9.94, ► Fig. 9.95, ► Fig. 9.96, ► Fig. 9.97, ► Fig. 9.98, ► Fig. 9.99, ► Fig. 9.100, ► Fig. 9.101, ► Fig. 9.102, ► Fig. 9.103, ► Fig. 9.104, and ► Fig. 9.105). If a biological transplant has been inserted, one may try to preserve it. A paranasal abscess is treated according to the same principles. If a bony sequester has occurred, it should be removed (see following text).

Intranasal Synechiae

Intranasal synechiae are well-known complications of nasal and sinus surgery Although often asymptomatic, they should nevertheless be prevented as much as possible. Synechiae most frequently occur: (1) between the septum and the inferior turbinate (after septal and inferior turbinate surgery); (2) between the septum and the middle turbinate (after septal and middle turbinate surgery); (3) between the middle turbinate and the lateral nasal wall (after infundibulotomy); (4) under the nasal bony dorsum (after hump resection and/or osteotomies); and (5) at the valve angle (after valve and septal surgery).

Prevention: Synechiae are prevented by: (1) avoiding opposing mucosal lesions; (2) interposition of a dressing (or splints) between the septum and the turbinates, and between the middle turbinate and the lateral nasal wall; and (3) carefully adjusting and closing endonasal incisions.

Treatment: Most synechiae can be cut (or better resected) easily after applying some local anesthesia. In most cases, however, some special measures must be taken to prevent recurrence. An effective method is to slightly coagulate the opposing areas. This will produce two small crusts that prevent a new synechia while the

mucosa is healing underneath. Another measure is to suture a small Silastic sheet to the septum, which is left in place for 1 to 2 weeks.

Complications of Septal Surgery

Septal Perforation

Septal perforations are among the most feared complications of septal surgery. This topic is dealt with extensively in Chapter 5.

Sagging of the Cartilaginous Dorsum

Sagging of the cartilaginous dorsum was a common complication of the submucous septal resection (SMR) operation. This was due to the fact that a relatively large part of the cartilaginous septum was resected and the defect was not repaired. As a consequence, the dorsum lost support. At the same time, the nasal mucosa at the defective area retracted as it was devoid of its underlying cartilage. This led to a sagging of the cartilaginous pyramid and, in many cases, to retraction of the columella.

Since the introduction of more conservative and reconstructive methods of septal surgery (septoplasty) in the 1960s and 1970s, this complication has become less frequent. It is still seen, however (► Fig. 9.70). In most instances, it occurs when too large a strip is resected from the base of the anterior septum and when the posterior chondrotomy has been continued up to the cartilaginous dorsum. As a consequence, the anterior part of the septum exorotates unless it is repositioned and fixed properly (see ► Fig. 5.31).

Complications of Incisions

Some of the worst complications in nasal surgery are related to incisions. External scars may have serious aesthetic consequences, while scars in the vestibule and valve area may cause severe inspiratory breathing problems. Secondary correction of these scars and stenoses is very difficult, in some cases even impossible.

Two factors may play a causative role: the surgery itself, and subsequent infection. Surgical factors include the choice and number of incisions, the specific combination of incisions, inadequate closure of the incisions, and insufficient aftercare. All of these shortcomings are related either to a lack of knowledge or to carelessness on the part of the surgeon.

External Incisions

External incisions are generally more risky than internal ones. Columellar incisions and rim incisions cause the most problems. Vertical columellar incisions should be avoided (► Fig. 9.71). Transverse columellar incisions are to be made in a broken line, but even then they will probably remain visible. Two well-known complications are

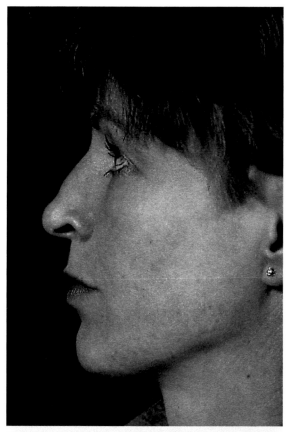

Fig. 9.70 Sagging of the cartilaginous dorsum after septal surgery due to endorotation of the cartilaginous septum. This is usually caused by excessively extensive disconnection of the cartilaginous from the bony septum and resection of too wide a strip from the septal base without proper repositioning and fixation of the cartilaginous septum.

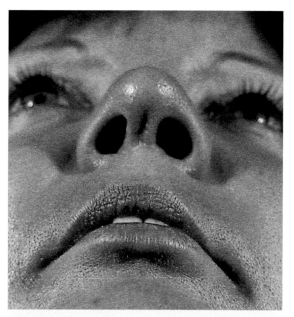

Fig. 9.71 Scarring and retraction of the columella following a vertical columellar incision. This incision is to be avoided.

asymmetrical healing, and necrosis of the lower end of the upper skin flap due to tension (▶ Fig. 9.72). Rim incisions have a risk of asymmetrical healing and upward retraction of the alar margin (see ▶ Fig. 9.84).

Endonasal Incisions

The CSI (hemitransfixion) is relatively safe. It very rarely leads to undesired scarring or retraction.

The IC incision should always be closed by one to three sutures, depending on the length of the incision and type of surgery. Utmost care is taken to avoid distortion of the valve and the valve area. Stenosis of the valve angle may lead to serious functional problems that are very difficult to repair (▶ Fig. 9.73).

The vestibular incision is usually closed by one or two sutures. This incision rarely leads to complications.

The infracartilaginous incision may cause cosmetic as well as functional complaints if not closed properly and symmetrically (see ▶ Fig. 9.83).

Complications of Osteotomies

Too Much Infracture of the Lateral Wall of the Bony Cartilage

In attempting to narrow the external nasal pyramid, the nasal bones may be infractured too much. This is a well-known problem which usually causes both aesthetic and functional complaints. Inspiratory breathing may be impaired as the valve area has become too narrow (▶ Fig. 9.74). Wearing eyeglasses too soon after surgery may also be a factor (▶ Fig. 9.75).

Prevention: The mobilized bony pyramid should be placed carefully in the desired position. The nasal bones are then fixed by supporting internal dressings. At the end of the operation, external tapes and a stent are applied for further stabilization and protection. Postoperative wearing of eyeglasses is discussed with the patient in advance. Temporary devices to prevent the eyeglasses from pushing the mobile bony walls inward may be made as required.

Treatment: Revision surgery is the only option.

Recurrence of Bony Deviation and Asymmetry

Achieving complete symmetry, midline position, and optimal width of the bony pyramid is one of the most difficult tasks in nasal surgery. Even very skilled surgeons may experience disappointments in this respect. The following factors may play a role in recurrence of a bony deviation and asymmetry of the bony pyramid: (1) incomplete mobilization of the bony vault; (2) incomplete

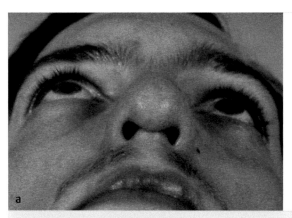
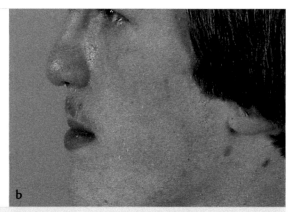

Fig. 9.72 a, b Severe scarring and retraction of the columella due to necrosis following an external approach with closure of the inverted-V incision under tension.

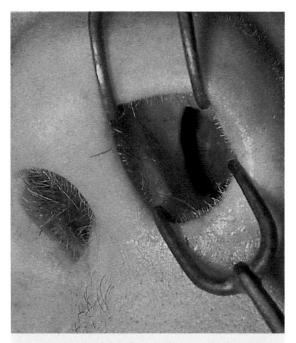

Fig. 9.73 Stenosis of the valve area due to inadequate closure of the IC incision following valve surgery.

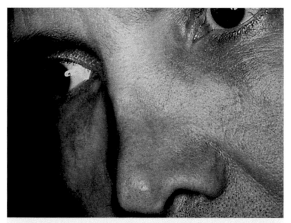

Fig. 9.74 Narrowing of the bony and cartilaginous pyramid due to too much infracture of the lateral nasal walls. (Photograph courtesy Prof. Cottle.)

mobilization of the septum; (3) inadequate undermining of the overlying skin; (4) insufficient repositioning and inadequate fixation of the bony pyramid in its new position; and (5) inadequate postoperative protection (▶ Fig. 9.75).

Treatment: Revision surgery is the only option.

Open Roof

An open roof is a common complication after resection of a bony and cartilaginous hump. The condition may cause a characteristic set of symptoms known as the "open roof syndrome" (▶ Fig. 9.76 and ▶ Fig. 9.77). See also Chapter 2, page 72.

Prevention: Hump resection is avoided if possible; if unavoidable, the roof of the bony pyramid should be closed again. To this end, osteotomies are performed and the ventral margins of the nasal bones are pressed together. Some crushed cartilage or fascia is inserted

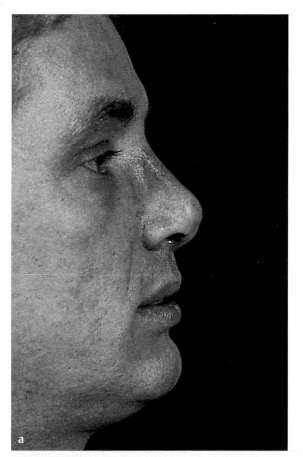
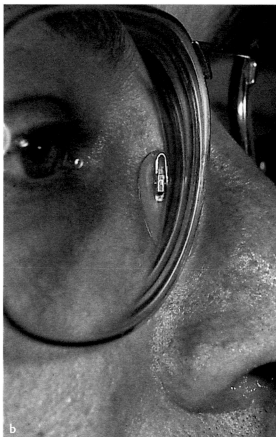

Fig. 9.75 a, b Impression of the bony pyramid due to use of eyeglasses too soon after osteotomies.

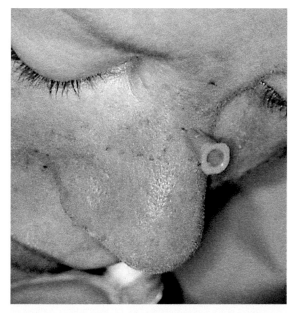

Fig. 9.76 Open roof. Defect of the roof of the bony pyramid caused by resection of a hump without closure and repair of the bony pyramid.

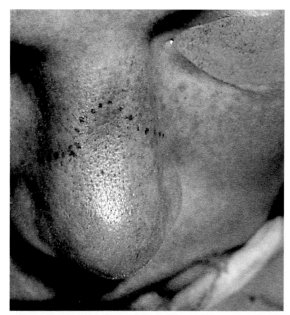

Fig. 9.77 A needle can be pierced through the dorsum.

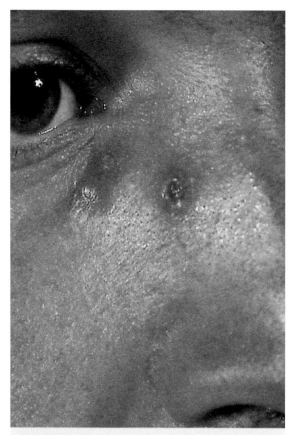

Fig. 9.78 Infected bone sequesters are a complication of a technically incorrect lateral osteotomy.

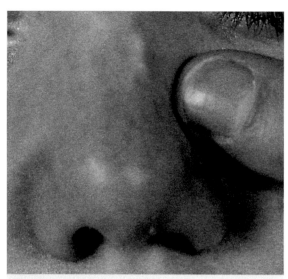

Fig. 9.79 Irregularity of the bony dorsum following osteotomies.

Irregularity of the Bony Dorsum

Irregularities or ridges on the bony dorsum may occur following osteotomies, possibly caused by asymmetrical repositioning of the nasal bones, an open roof, or a bone splinter (▶ Fig. 9.79). They are removed through an IC incision using a narrow rasp and/or chisel. When an open roof is present, new osteotomies are usually required to properly close it (see previous text).

Complications of Lobular Surgery

Complications of lobular surgery are among the most distressing events following nasal surgery. In most instances, they are caused by shortcomings of the surgeon. Modifying the lobule and tip is technically difficult. Failure of lobular and tip surgery is more visible than that of septal and pyramid surgery. Moreover, patients who ask for this type of surgery are often more "nose conscious" and critical than those who want to breathe better. We will confine ourselves here to a discussion of the most common failures.

Too Much (Lateral) Resection of the Cranial Margin of the Lateral Crus

This is a common failure. To narrow the tip, the surgeon decides to resect a strip from the cranial margin of the lateral crus. However, if such a resection is done too laterally or too extensively, it compromises the relationship between the cranial margin of the lateral crus and the lower margin of the triangular cartilage. This produces a depressed and flaccid area that may become sucked in during inspiration, thereby obstructing the vestibule

underneath the skin to smooth the bony dorsum and to keep the skin from adhering to the bone.

Treatment: Revision surgery is the only option to close an open roof.

Bony Sequester

When performing osteotomies, in particular lateral ones, a loose bone splinter may be produced. Beginners in the field usually find it difficult to make just one straight (or curved) cut through the bone. As a result, one or more bone segments devoid of periosteum may come loose and become dislocated. A sequester may be visible and palpable on the lateral bony wall or dorsum. When the inner mucoperiosteum has been lacerated, it may become infected (▶ Fig. 9.78).

Prevention: If a piece of bone breaks off while performing osteotomies, special care is taken to reposition it and fix it in place with internal and external dressings.

Treatment: Dislocated bone splinters are removed by reopening the vestibular or the IC incision. The sequester is grasped and removed using a straight hemostat.

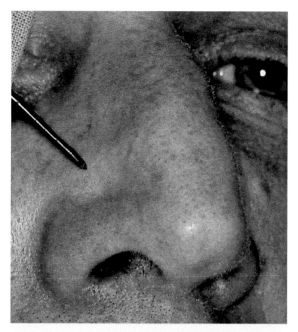

Fig. 9.80 Retraction and weakness of the lateral lobular wall as a result of too much resection from the cranial margin of the lateral crus of the lobular cartilage. The connection of the lateral crus and the triangular cartilage has been lost.

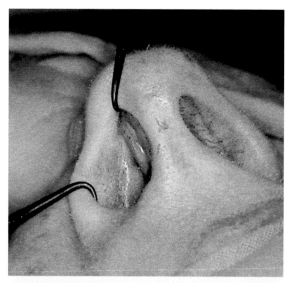

Fig. 9.81 The remaining part of the lateral crus protrudes into the vestibule, causing obstruction and alar collapse on inspiration as a consequence of loss of connection of the lateral crus and the triangular cartilage.

(▶ Fig. 9.80 and ▶ Fig. 9.81). This complication is most often seen in the elderly, in whom the soft tissues are less elastic. The defect is reconstructed by restoring contact between the two cartilages and reinforcing the area by means of a slightly convex graft sculpted from auricular cartilage. This can best be done by the external approach.

Asymmetry of the Domes and/or Lateral Crura

Another common complication of lobular surgery is asymmetry of the tip (domes) and/or the lateral crura. Postoperative asymmetries are usually caused by some surgical failure, though healing may play a role. The risk of asymmetry is greater with the luxation technique than with the open approach. Particularly well known are asymmetries due to incorrect suturing or reconstruction of the domes in an attempt to narrow the tip (▶ Fig. 9.82) The only way to improve the condition is by repairing and repositioning the domes and lateral crura using the open approach.

Cutting through the Domes without Reconstruction

If the domes are vertically cut through and have not been reconstructed, the lateral crus drops in relation to the dome. The skin lateral to the domes may retract, leaving an ugly malformation (▶ Fig. 9.83). This deformity may

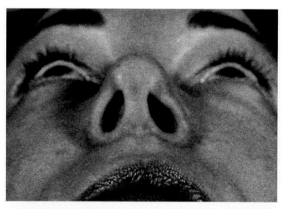

Fig. 9.82 Asymmetry of the alae and nostrils caused by cutting the dome on the left.

be treated by reconstructing the continuity of the domes and by covering the area with a tip graft using the external approach.

Retraction of the Rim of the Nostril

The rim of the nostril may retract after damage with or without infection of the lower margin of the lateral crus (▶ Fig. 9.84). It may also be caused by insufficient repositioning and closure of the infracartilaginous incision (▶ Fig. 9.83).

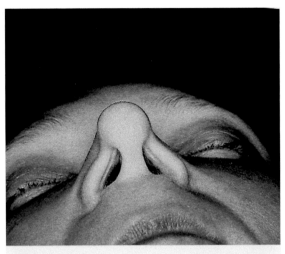

Fig. 9.83 Severe functional and aesthetic deformity of the lobule caused by cutting through the domes without restoring their integrity. Note the scar of the incorrectly placed infracartilaginous incisions. (Photograph courtesy Prof. Cottle.)

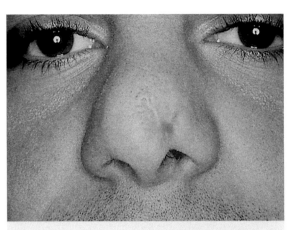

Fig. 9.84 Retraction and scarring of the left ala and caudal lobular notch as a complication of surgery of the caudal margin of the lateral crus. (Photograph courtesy Prof. Cottle.)

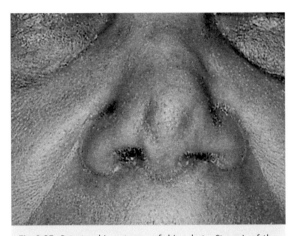

Fig. 9.85 Catastrophic outcome of rhinoplasty. Stenosis of the nostrils and vestibules; retraction and scarring of the tip due to division of the domes without reconstruction; bilateral retraction and scarring of the lateral soft-tissue areas caused by too much resection from the cranial margin of the lateral crus of the lobular cartilages. (Photograph courtesy Prof. Cottle.)

The Catastrophic Outcome

Every experienced nasal surgeon has seen patients in whom nasal surgery has resulted in a disaster. The catastrophic outcome is usually due to a combination of complications. Severe surgical failures, infection, scarring, and extrusion of an implant are the most well-known causes (▶ Fig. 9.85). Based on our experience, we conclude that the basic rules of functional reconstructive nasal surgery must have been broken in these cases.

Complications of Transplants and Implants

Transplants and implants may cause several immediate and late complications. The most common immediate complications are infection, extrusion, and dislocation. The most important long-term problems are extrusion (after trauma or infection), dislocation, bending, resorption, calcification, and growth of the transplant material.

Infection

Infection is one of the most feared complications. Although it occurs more frequently with nonbiological materials, it may also occur with biological transplants of cartilage or bone.

Prevention: The nasal vestibule should be carefully cleaned and disinfected. The transplant must be handled in an aseptic way. The transplant bed should be wide enough to avoid ischemia of the overlying skin or mucosa. Accumulation of blood in the transplant pocket is prevented. Antibiotics are administered systemically starting the day before surgery.

Treatment: Postoperative infection must be suspected in the following situations: when body temperature shows an irregular course; when the patient reports pain; and, in particular, when pain is felt upon touching the external dressing. The stent and tapes should then be removed. If infection appears to have occurred, the IC incision is reopened. Pus is cultured and aspirated. A biological transplant may be left in place. The incision is left partially open for drainage. A slight pressure dressing is applied externally. The infected area is reinspected and cleansed daily. Broad-spectrum antibiotic therapy

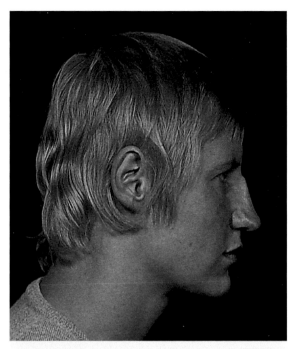

Fig. 9.86 Transplant of rib cartilage that had to be removed as the graft was too long and narrow and had become dislocated.

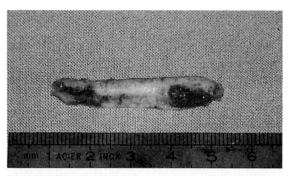

Fig. 9.87 The removed graft.

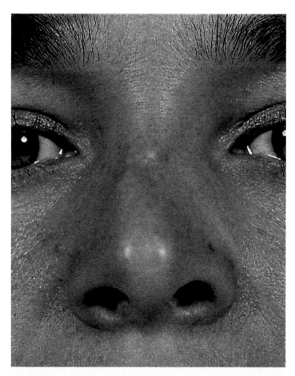

Fig. 9.88 Transplant of rib cartilage that had to be removed due to warping of the graft.

(particularly directed against penicillin-resistant staphylococci) is given both systemically as well as topically in the transplant bed. It may be necessary to adjust the antibiotic treatment depending on the result of the bacteriological tests. If nonbiological material has been implanted, it has to be removed. The chances that the infection will subside with the implant in place are minimal.

Extrusion

If a transplant or implant becomes infected and no immediate action is taken, it will be extruded through necrosis of the skin or mucosa. This should be avoided at all costs, in particular when we are dealing with a dorsal or lobular transplant or implant, as the resulting external scars are ugly and irreparable. Cartilaginous grafts are rarely extruded, although this may occur as an early complication because of infection. If occurring later, it is almost always caused by trauma.

Dislocation

Dislocation, either early or late, is another well-known complication. It may be caused by the shape and dimensions of the transplant, malpositioning, insufficient fixation, or trauma. Transplants should not be too long and too narrow. If too long, they tend to tip. If too narrow, they are often dislocated, which usually necessitates their removal (▶ Fig. 9.86 and ▶ Fig. 9.87).

Bending or Warping

Bending (warping) of a cartilaginous graft may occur if the transplant was not made from the core of the rib (▶ Fig. 9.88 and ▶ Fig. 9.89). See also Chapter 6, page 246.

Resorption

Resorption is the major disadvantage of using cartilage for augmentation, reconstruction, and support. The rate of resorption depends on many factors: the origin of the transplant; the shape and mass of the transplant; the site of transplantation; and the function of the graft. For a more detailed discussion of these factors, we refer to Chapter 9, page 350.

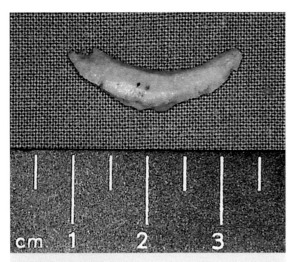

Fig. 9.89 The removed graft.

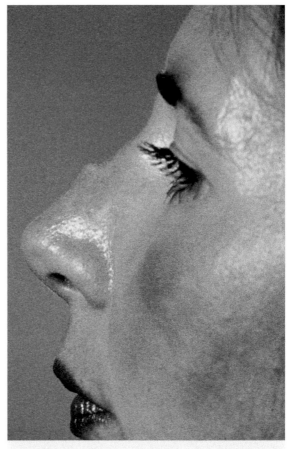

Fig. 9.90 Growth of cartilage reinserted in the dorsum as a skin underlay. The most likely cause is that some perichondrium was still attached. (Photograph courtesy Prof. Pirsig.)

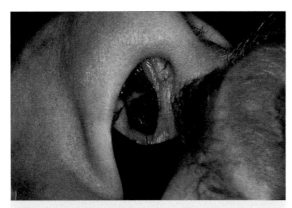

Fig. 9.91 Extrusion of Proplast used to repair a defective anterior septum.

Calcification

After 5 to 10 years, cartilaginous grafts inserted in the nasal dorsum may start to calcify. In general, these calcified areas do not have a negative effect on the result.

Growth of Transplant Material

Though this complication is uncommon, some cases have been reported. Presumably, it could occur in young patients in whom autogeneic cartilage with the perichondrium attached is used (▶ Fig. 9.90).

Nonbiological Implants

Nonbiological implants are bound to become extruded sooner or later, as they do not become integrated in the tissue. A minor trauma or infection may prompt extrusion. This applies first of all to nonbiological implants in the septum and underneath the nasal mucosa. All materials used to date—such as acrylic, Proplast, Silastic, and hydroxyapatite—are usually extruded in weeks or months (▶ Fig. 9.91, ▶ Fig. 9.92, ▶ Fig. 9.93, ▶ Fig. 9.94, and ▶ Fig. 9.95).

This is also a common experience with implants in the dorsum. Extrusion may occur after weeks or months, but also after several years and even decades. The most frequently used materials to augment the nasal dorsum have been: paraffin, ivory, various metals, polyethylene, Silastic, Dacron, polyamide, Supramid, Mersilene, Medpor, and Gore-Tex. Examples of late extrusion of several of these materials are presented in ▶ Fig. 9.96, ▶ Fig. 9.97, ▶ Fig. 9.98, ▶ Fig. 9.99, ▶ Fig. 9.100, ▶ Fig. 9.101, ▶ Fig. 9.102, ▶ Fig. 9.103, ▶ Fig. 9.104, and ▶ Fig. 9.105.

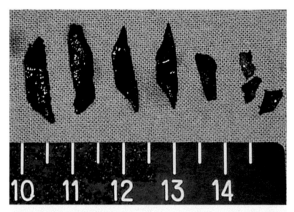

Fig. 9.92 Extrusion of Proplast, implanted submucosally, to narrow a wide nasal cavity.

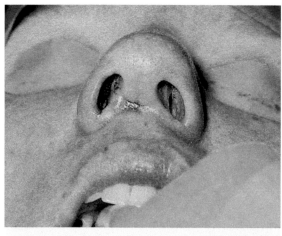

Fig. 9.93 Severe granulomatous reaction with infection caused by a plate of Teflon used to repair a missing anterior septum.

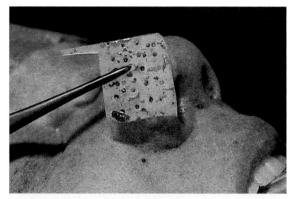

Fig. 9.94 The removed Teflon implant.

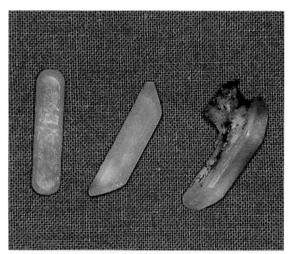

Fig. 9.95 Extruded pieces of acrylic implanted submucosally to narrow a wide nasal cavity in a patient with ozena.

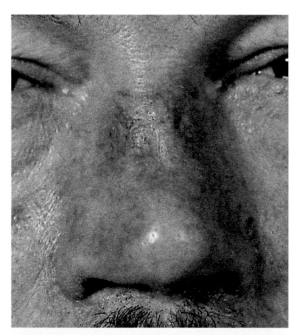

Fig. 9.96 Severe scarring of the bony dorsum after extrusion of paraffin injected to augment the pyramid.

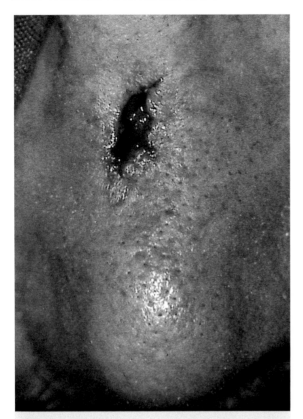

Fig. 9.97 Extrusion of dorsal implant cut from ivory.

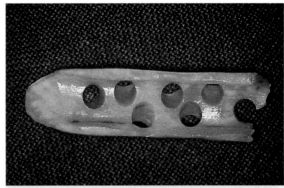

Fig. 9.98 The extruded implant.

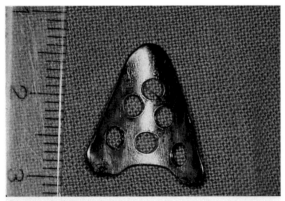

Fig. 9.99 Dorsal implant of steel that had to be removed because of infection and extrusion.

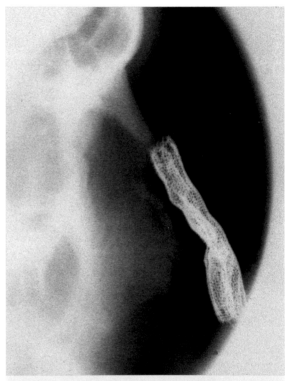

Fig. 9.100 Dorsal implant of tantalum that had to be removed because of infection and extrusion.

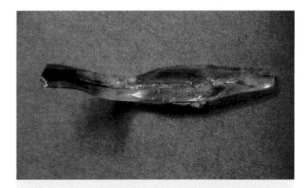

Fig. 9.101 Polyethylene implant that had to be removed because of infection and extrusion 18 years after implantation.

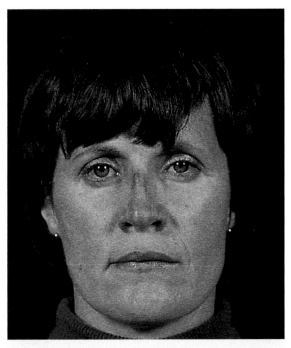

Fig. 9.102 Supramid implant that had to be removed 1 year after implantation

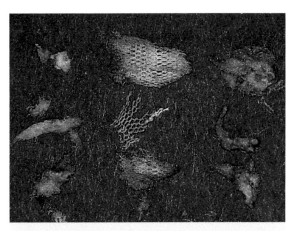

Fig. 9.103 The removed Supramid implant.

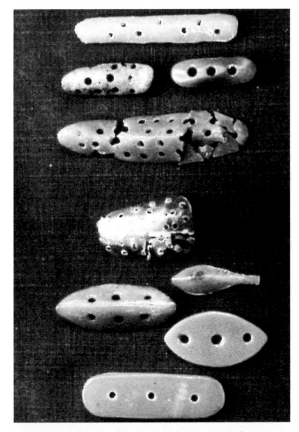

Fig. 9.104 Collection of nonbiological implants, used to augment the nasal dorsum and tip, that had to be removed later. (Photograph courtesy Prof. Hellmich.)

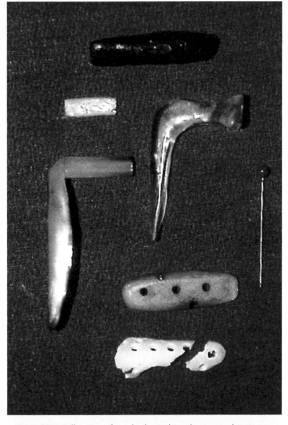

Fig. 9.105 Collection of nonbiological implants, used to augment the nasal dorsum and tip, that had to be removed later. (Photograph courtesy Prof. Hellmich.)

9.10 Patient Complaints and Medicolegal Problems

9.10.1 Dissatisfied Patient

Patients who are dissatisfied with the final result constitute a psychological burden, both to themselves and to the surgeon. If the outcome of the operation is poor according to "objective" criteria, the disappointment of the patient may be understandable. In some instances, however, the patient is unhappy even though the outcome is quite good compared with the preoperative situation. In this event, a discussion based on the preoperative and postoperative photographs may be helpful. We might also consider holding this discussion again in the presence of a relative. If this is not effective, referral to colleague for a second opinion is generally the best option.

It is of utmost importance for the rhinosurgeon to identify the patient with "body dysmorphic disorder" (BDD) preoperatively. These patients represent 1 to 2% of the entire population and, according to some studies, 60 to 70% of them seek cosmetic surgery for minimal or nonexistent "deformities." They are almost always unhappy with their surgical result. Psychiatric care is therefore imperative in these cases.

9.10.2 Claims and Lawsuits

Lawyers and insurance companies often try to have doctors convicted because of a technical failure, such as a septal perforation or a CSF leak. We oppose this tendency. A septal perforation following septal surgery is indeed principally the result of a technical failure. However, this complication can occur even in the hands of the most experienced and careful surgeon. In itself, it is not, therefore, a reason to convict the surgeon. It is the doctor's care in making a diagnosis and giving treatment that should be judged.

Prevention

Some suggestions on reducing the chances of claims and lawsuits have already been presented. Briefly, prevention of medicolegal problems in nasal surgery may be condensed into the following ten questions ("The List of Ten", Huizing 2001):

1. Was the intake history complete?
2. Was the examination performed according to the requirements?
3. Was the diagnosis correct?
4. Was the indication for the conservative or surgical treatment justified?
5. Was the patient duly informed about the diagnosis, the treatment proposal, risks, and alternatives?
6. Was the doctor trained to do the job?
7. Was the treatment state of the art?
8. Were the medical records up to the current standards?
9. Was the complication taken care of immediately and correctly?
10. Was the medical and psychological aftercare sufficient?

Action

In spite of our precautions, a complication may still occur. How are we going to deal with it? The answer is: providing maximum care. This includes:

- *Immediate action*
  Start taking the necessary steps immediately. Do not "run away," no matter how unpleasant the situation may be for yourself.
- *Consultation*
  Immediately consult your (senior) ENT colleague about how to proceed. Also, as soon as possible, consult other specialists when indicated, or (depending on the case) contact a university hospital or other center with special experience in the field.
- *Informing the patient and patient's family*
  Explain to the patient and patient's family what might have happened. Make it clear which steps have to be taken. It is advisable to do this in the presence of a family member and a colleague.
- *Being honest*
  Most patients accept that something may go wrong during their treatment, especially in surgery. They usually do not accept the doctor trying to conceal the truth. If your preoperative information was sufficient, it may now prove of great help.
- *Showing regret*
  It is very important to show regret about what has occurred.
- *Documentation*
  Make a careful and honest documentation of your considerations and steps, preferably handwritten.
- *Remaining in contact with your patient*
  It is of utmost importance to stay in contact with the patient if treatment has been taken over by another colleague or another hospital. Continue to visit him or her. In our experience, patients often do not sue the doctor because of the complication itself but because they are left to deal with it alone.

Questions Asked by Courts

Courts in Western and Northern Europe tend to base their verdict on the answers to the following questions:
- Was the treatment in conflict with the degree of carefulness that might be expected from the average capable ENT doctor?
- Was the treatment state of the art?
- Is the damage due to careless medical treatment?

The terms most frequently used by courts are: "careful," "reproachful," "negligent," "average capable," "standard," and "state of the art."

Chapter 10

Appendix

10

10 Appendix

10.1 Materials

10.1.1 Sutures

In functional reconstructive nasal surgery, incisions are always closed. The only exceptions are minor stab incisions. By closing the incisions, the tissues are adjusted and fixed in their new positions. Postoperative bleeding as well as scarring and stenosis are prevented.

Endonasal mucosal and skin incisions are generally closed with resorbable materials. This applies to the common endonasal skin incisions used for approaches—such as the caudal septal incision (CSI), intercartilaginous (IC) incision, and vestibular incision—as well as all incisions of the septal and buccal mucosa. A great advantage of using resorbable sutures endonasally is that no sutures have to be removed from the inside of the nose during the first postoperative days.

External skin incisions are closed with nonresorbable monofilament synthetic materials. These are also used to close special incisions in the nasal vestibule, such as infracartilaginous incisions.

Fixation of plates or grafts of cartilage to rebuild the septum or other structures is usually done with slowly resorbable materials.

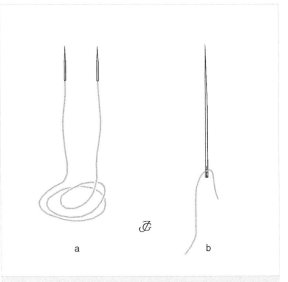

Fig. 10.1 **(a)** Two short straight needles with 4–0 slowly resorbable sutures for transseptal, septocolumellar, and transcolumellar sutures. **(b)** Long straight needle with 3–0 slowly resorbable suture.

> Incisions should be closed at all times. By closing the incisions, the tissues are adjusted and fixed in their new positions, postoperative bleeding is prevented, and scarring and stenosis is avoided.

10.1.2 Needles

Almost all suture material is provided with a more or less curved so-called atraumatic needle. For transseptal, septocolumellar, and transcolumellar sutures we prefer the use of a short straight needle (▶ Fig. 10.1a). For fixation of the caudal end of the septum, we use a long straight needle to temporarily stabilize the septum in its new position, and an atraumatic straight needle with slowly resorbable 3–0 thread to fix it with two or three septocolumellar sutures (▶ Fig. 10.1b). See Chapter 5, ▶ Fig. 5.42 and ▶ Fig. 5.43.

10.1.3 Internal Dressings

There is no consensus on the need for, and type of, internal dressings. In the past, many surgeons, such as ourselves, preferred to apply internal dressings in almost all cases of septal, pyramid, and lobular surgery. Internal dressings serve three purposes: (1) to keep the septum in the midline and prevent septal hematoma; (2) to support the nasal bones, cartilaginous pyramid, and lobular cartilages in their new position; and (3) to limit risk of postoperative bleeding. Currently, the use of internal dressings has diminished, especially in patients in whom no pyramid surgery has been performed.

We used to apply two loosely woven gauze strips either soaked in isotonic saline or with ointment. The first one is applied endonasally to close the septal space and to support the nasal bones and cartilaginous pyramid. The second one is applied in the vestibule after closure of the vestibular incisions.

At present, most surgeons prefer to use preformed strips or "packs" of hydrophilic polyurethane, or polyvinyl acetate (PVA) sponge or foam (see ▶ Fig. 5.36).

> Careful nasal surgery requires a carefully applied internal and external dressing. The internal dressing should not be a "nasal packing" or a "tamponade" as it is commonly called, but an "internal nasal dressing."
> A "nasal packing" or "tamponade" may be the appropriate measure to stop bleeding in cases of epistaxis, not after reconstructive and aesthetic nasal surgery.

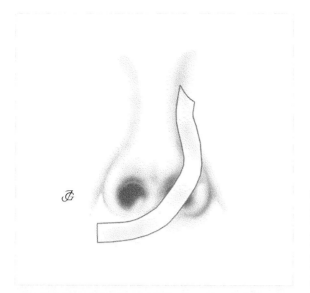

Fig. 10.2 A repositioned pyramid that was preoperatively deviated to the left is kept in the midline by a "unilateral sling."

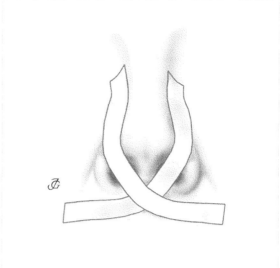

Fig. 10.3 A repositioned pyramid is fixed in the midline by a "bilateral sling."

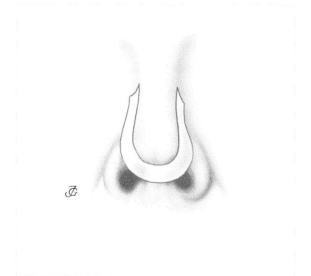

Fig. 10.4 A "tip-narrowing tape" fixes the tissues in their new position after a tip-narrowing procedure.

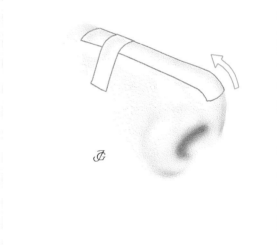

Fig. 10.5 A "tip-lift tape" fixes the tissues in their new position after upward rotation of the tip.

10.1.4 Tapes

Postoperative taping of the external nose is essential in all cases of pyramid and lobular surgery. Tapes are applied (1) to adjust and keep the various soft tissues in their new position and (2) to diminish postoperative edema and the risk of hematomas and ecchymoses.

Depending on our surgical goals, we usually start by applying one or two specific tapes, such as:

- A "unilateral sling" to keep a repositioned pyramid that was preoperatively deviated to the left in the midline (▶ Fig. 10.2)
- A "bilateral sling" to fix a repositioned pyramid in the midline (▶ Fig. 10.3)
- A "tip-narrowing tape" to support a tip-narrowing procedure (▶ Fig. 10.4)
- A "tip-lift tape" to fix an upwardly rotated tip in its new position (▶ Fig. 10.5)

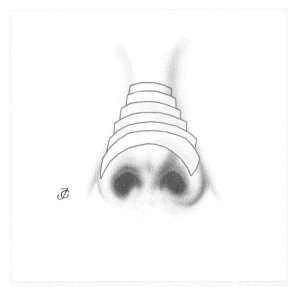

Fig. 10.6 "Pressure tapes" on the dorsum fix a rib graft or other transplant material, and prevent hematoma.

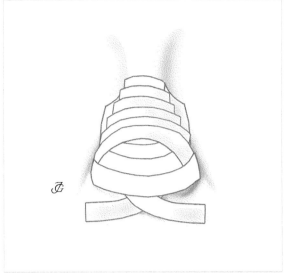

Fig. 10.7 The external nose and the cranial half of the upper lip are completely taped for fixation and protection, and to prevent edema.

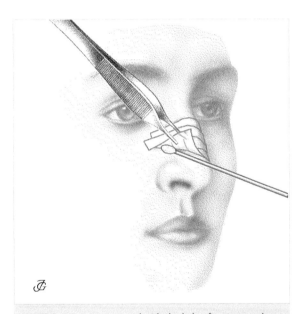

Fig. 10.8 Tapes are removed with the help of cotton wool applicators soaked in benzine. The tapes are "rolled off" the skin by rotating the cotton applicator over the skin while the tape is lifted up by a straight forceps.

We will then apply "pressure tapes" on the whole bony and cartilaginous pyramid, dorsum, lobule, and nasal base to prevent edema and hematoma (▶ Fig. 10.6 and ▶ Fig. 10.7).

Removal and Renewal of Tapes

Tapes should be removed slowly and carefully and preferably by the surgeon himself. He is the only one who knows why and how certain tapes were applied. At the same time, he is the one who can best diagnose complications such as hematomas and infection.

Tapes are removed with the help of cotton wool applicators soaked in benzine. The tapes are "rolled off" the skin by rotating the cotton applicator over the skin while the tape is lifted by a straight forceps (▶ Fig. 10.8).

10.1.5 External Splints (Stents)

External splints or stents are applied postoperatively for fixation, pressure, and protection. Several materials and types of stents are available.

In the past, a plaster of Paris stent was fitted in patients in whom the bony pyramid had been mobilized and repositioned. To provide maximal fixation and protection, such a stent was usually fixed to the forehead (▶ Fig. 10.9 and ▶ Fig. 10.10). In cases where surgery was limited to the cartilaginous pyramid and/or lobule, thermoplastic material may have been chosen (▶ Fig. 10.11).

Plaster of Paris allows a very good fit but also has the disadvantage that making the stent is rather time-consuming and is always a somewhat messy affair. A second drawback is that a stent of plaster cannot be remolded. Thus, if the postoperative swelling subsides after some days and the stent no longer fits, a new one has to be made.

The use of thermoplastic material has the advantages of simplicity and cleanliness, and remolding is easy. There are also soft and moldable metal splints on the market.

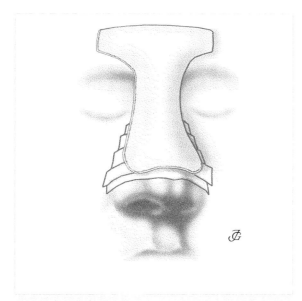

Fig. 10.9 A stent fixed to the forehead provides the best fit and the most protection

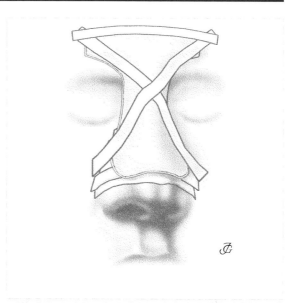

Fig. 10.10 The stent is fixed with tapes to the forehead and cheeks.

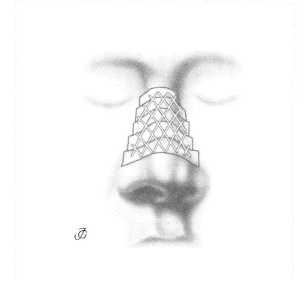

Fig. 10.11 A stent of thermoplastic material offers less protection but can be remolded easily.

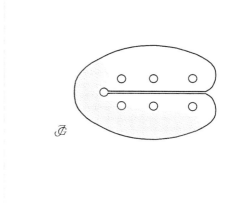

Fig. 10.12 A septal splint may be used to support and fix a reconstructed septum. Splints are fixed with two transseptal, slowly resorbable sutures.

10.1.6 Septal Splints

Bilateral septal splints made from silicone may be of great help in septal reconstruction (▶ Fig. 10.12). Some surgeons use them more or less routinely after septal surgery. Others apply them only when the septum has to be more or less completely rebuilt. Some surgeons prefer to use septal splints with an airway. The advantages of this type of splint are usually less than expected, as these rather massive splints may interfere with the careful application of internal dressings, and are easily blocked.

10.1.7 Intranasal Sheets

Sheets of medical grade silicone or fluoroplastic may be used to prevent synechiae and to keep a reconstructed nasal valve or vestibule open.

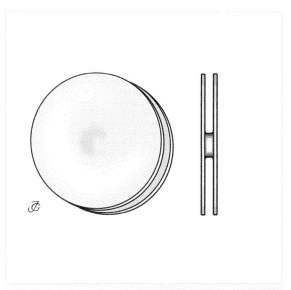

Fig. 10.13 A prosthesis ("septal button") is cut to measure for closing a septal perforation.

10.1.8 Septal Prosthesis (Septal Button)

In patients with a symptomatic septal perforation that cannot be closed surgically, the defect may be obturated with a silicone septal prosthesis or septal button. They are available in different sizes (▶ Fig. 10.13; see also Chapter 5, page 209).

10.1.9 Commercially Available Biological Materials

Nowadays, various biological materials are commercially available, such as fascia, dura cancellous bone (in blocks or granules), and cortical bone. Cancellous chips, small blocks or granules may be implanted submucosally to narrow a nasal cavity which is too wide (see Chapter 8, page 310). Fascia or dura is used for augmentation and repair of defects.

10.2 Instruments

The quality and success of a surgical intervention depend mainly on the following factors: analysis of the pathological condition; surgical concept; skill of the surgeon, anesthesiologist, and surgical assistants; and quality of the instruments.

Since the beginning of modern surgery in the 1880s, hundreds of instruments for nasal surgery have been designed. More than 50 authors have contributed to their development. Often, their names are still linked to the instruments they introduced or popularized. However, most of the tools currently in use are no longer identical to their original designs. Generally, major and minor changes have been made by other surgeons and instrument makers. Nonetheless, in many cases the name of the originator is still linked to the instrument, largely for practical reasons. During surgery, for example, it is simpler to ask for a "Graig" than for a "heavy, biting septum forceps." A side effect of this custom is that younger generations become familiar with the names of some of the pioneers of nasal surgery.

The discussion and illustrations in this chapter only deal with the instruments used in the departments of otorhinolaryngology in Utrecht (The Netherlands) and Ulm (Germany). The authors are fully aware of the fact that many other valuable and effective instruments are available.

> "Tous les moyens sont bons quand ils sont efficacies."
> [All means are fine as long as they are effective.]
> Jean-Paul Sartre

10.2.1 Instruments for Cleansing the Vestibules and Trimming the Vibrissae ("Trim Set")

(▶ Fig. 10.14)
- Alar retractor (Masing type) to expose the vestibule and valve area
- Long (14-cm), slightly curved, blunt scissors to cut the vibrissae
- 14-cm bayonet forceps

Before surgery is started, the vestibules are cleansed and disinfected and the vibrissae are cut and removed. This procedure is carried out at the operating table either before or after induction of anesthesia.

The cut-off vibrissae are removed using cotton wool applicators with some Vaseline. Small strips of gauze are dipped into 80% alcohol to disinfect the vestibules and valve areas.

10.2.2 Instruments and Medications for Anesthesia and Vasoconstriction

(▶ Fig. 10.15)

Local Anesthesia

- Six cotton wool applicators
- Small cup with 200 mg crystalline cocaine
- Small cup with 10 to 15 drops of adrenaline 0.1%
- 10 to 20 mL lidocaine 1% with adrenaline 1:100,000
- 3-mL syringe
- 16-mm/0.5-mm and 40-mm/0.8-mm needles
- Short nasal speculum

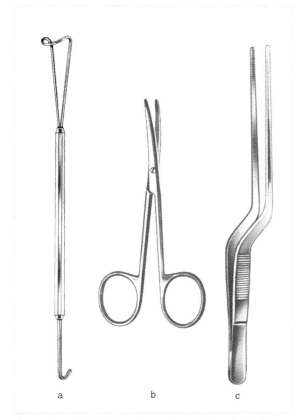

Fig. 10.14 Instruments to cleanse the vestibules and trim the vibrissae ("trimset"). **(a)** Alar retractor (Masing type). **(b)** Long, slightly curved, blunt scissors. **(c)** 14-cm bayonet forceps.

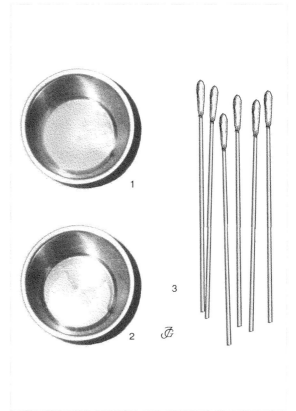

Fig. 10.15 Instruments for local anesthesia and vasoconstriction: small cup with 200 mg crystalline cocaine (1), small cup with 15 drops of adrenaline 0.1% (2), cotton wool applicators (3).

General Anesthesia

- Small cup with 10 mL cocaine 3% with adrenaline 1:20,000
- Small gauzes
- 3-mL syringe
- 16-mm/0.5-mm, 40-mm/0.8-mm, and 50-mm/1.1-mm needles

Regarding the technique of local anesthesia and vaso-constriction, the reader is referred to Chapter 3 (page 132).

10.2.3 Specula

(▶ Fig. 10.16 and ▶ Fig. 10.17)
- *Short, broad speculum (Hartmann–Vienna type):*
  Classic short speculum used for inspection, infiltration anesthesia, and incision of the vestibule
- *Narrow, medium-long speculum (Cottle):*
  Medium-sized speculum with narrow blades used to expose the anterior nasal spine and premaxilla, and to elevate inferior tunnels

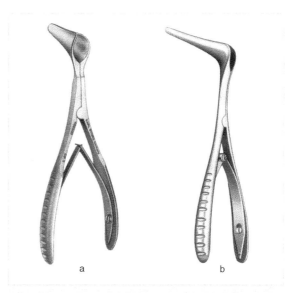

Fig. 10.16 (a) Short, broad speculum (Hartmann–Vienna type). **(b)** Narrow, medium-long speculum (Cottle).

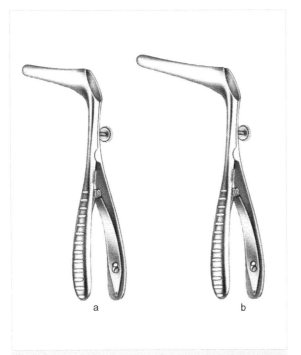

Fig. 10.17 (a) Medium-long speculum (Killian). **(b)** Long speculum (Killian).

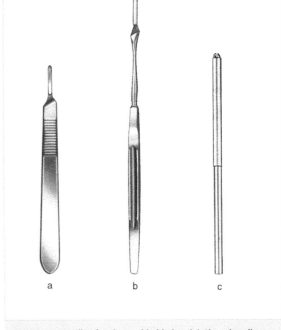

Fig. 10.18 Handles for disposable blades: **(a)** Short handle. **(b)** Long handle. **(c)** Beaver handle.

10.2.4 Knives

Handles

(▶ Fig. 10.18)

- *Short handle and long handle* to mount a disposable No.11, No.15, or No. 20 blade
- *Beaver handle* to mount a No. 64 blade or an angulated No. 66 Beaver blade

Blades

(▶ Fig. 10.19)

- *No. 15 blade (disposable) for:*
  - Making a CSI (hemitransfixion), or vestibular, infra-cartilaginous, columellar, alar-facial, or labiogingival incision; this blade may also be used for IC incisions
  - Modifying the septal, triangular, and lobular cartilage
  - Sculpting grafts
- *No. 11 blade (disposable) for:*
  - Making an IC incision
  - Modifying and cutting cartilage
- *No. 20 blade (disposable) for:*
  - Sculpting large transplants
- *Beaver blade No. 64 (disposable) for:*
  - Cutting scar tissue and synechiae
  - Separating septal mucosal blades
  - Resecting strips and triangles from the septal, triangular, and lobular cartilages
  - Making incisions in the mucosa in turbinate surgery, closing septal perforations, etc.

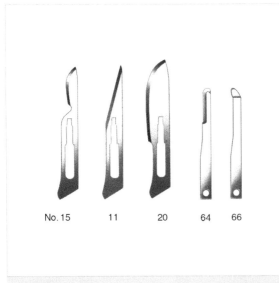

No. 15   11   20   64   66

Fig. 10.19 Disposable blades.

- *Medium-long speculum (Killian):*
  Speculum with medium-long blades used for surgery of the anterior part of the septum, turbinates, and nasal cavity
- *Long speculum (Killian):*
  Speculum with long blades used for surgery of the posterior part of the septum, turbinates, and nasal cavity

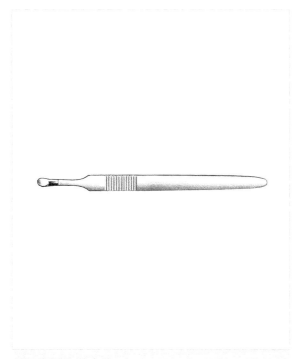

Fig. 10.20 Cottle knife.

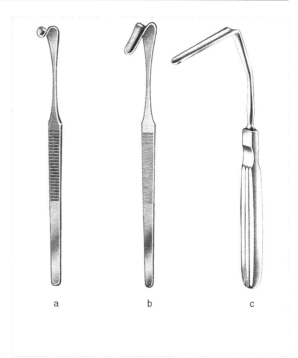

a   b   c

Fig. 10.21 **(a)** Alar retractor (alar protector). **(b)** Short, angulated retractor (Aufricht). **(c)** Long, angulated retractor (Aufricht).

- *Beaver blade angulated No. 66 (disposable) for:*
  - Making incisions in the mucosa when cutting flaps to close septal perforations
  - Resecting strips or triangles of cartilage

Special Knives

- *Cottle knife* (▶ Fig. 10.20):
  Round, sharp knife for dissecting perichondrium from cartilage
  - This knife is especially helpful in exposing the caudal septal end.
  - It should be sharpened frequently.

10.2.5 Retractors

(▶ Fig. 10.21 and ▶ Fig. 10.22)
- *Alar retractor (protector) to:*
  - Retract and protect the ala while making a CSI
  - Inspect the vestibule and valve area
- *Short, angulated retractor ("short Aufricht retractor," "alar protector with lip") to:*
  - Inspect and work on the cartilaginous dorsum through the IC incision
  - Retract the skin while dissecting the lobular cartilages and dorsum in the external approach
  - Open the IC incision when inserting a transplant to augment the dorsum

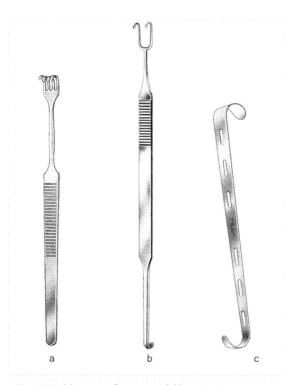

a   b   c

Fig. 10.22 **(a)** Uneven, four-pronged, blunt retractor (Cottle). **(b)** Double retractor (Neivert). **(c)** Double retractor (Aiach).

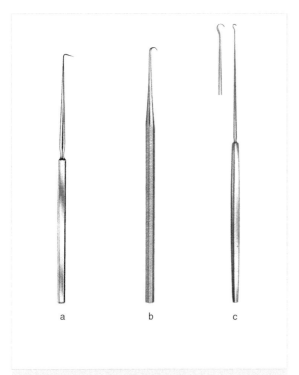

Fig. 10.23 (a) Single straight hook. (b) Single round hook. (c) Small, round (Gillies) hooks.

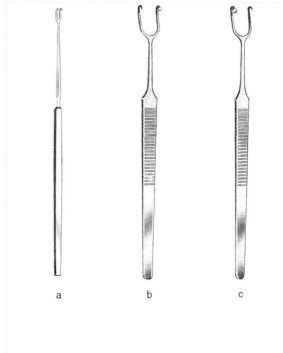

Fig. 10.24 (a) Narrow, two-pronged, sharp hook. (b) Two-pronged hook sharp–dull. (c) Two-pronged hook dull–sharp.

- *Long, angulated retractor (Aufricht) to:*
  ○ Inspect and work on the nasal dorsum through the IC incision
  ○ Push the pyramid and septum in a dorsal direction in the push-down and let-down techniques.
- *Uneven, four-pronged, blunt retractor (Cottle) to:*
  ○ Retract the ala while making an IC incision
  ○ Expose the valve area
- *Double retractor (Neivert) to:*
  ○ Inspect the vestibule and the valve area
  ○ Expose the vestibular base during the maxilla–premaxilla (MP) approach (curved end)
  ○ Expose the lobular cartilage in the luxation technique (flat intermediate part)
- *Double retractor (Aiach):*
  Used to retract the columellar flap while dissecting and modifying the lobular cartilages in the external approach

10.2.6 Hooks

(▶ Fig. 10.23 and ▶ Fig. 10.24)
- *Single straight hook:*
  Used to pull the caudal septal end laterally when dissecting the anterior septum and beginning the superior anterior tunnels
- *Single round hook to:*
  ○ Deliver the dome of the lobular cartilage in the inversion technique

- ○ Deliver the lobular cartilage in the luxation technique
- ○ Retract skin flaps
- *Small, round hooks (Gillies):*
  Used to retract skin and mucosal flaps (e.g., in the external approach or when harvesting auricular cartilage)
- *Narrow, two-pronged, sharp hook (Huizing) to:*
  ○ Retract the columella laterally when dissecting the caudal septal end
  ○ Retract the columellar flap in the external approach
- *Two-pronged hook sharp–dull and two-pronged hook dull–sharp:*
  Used to invert the alar rim and expose the inferior margin of the lateral crus and dome when making an infra-cartilaginous incision
  ○ The sharp end is placed in the part of the incision that has just been made.
  ○ The dull end is placed immediately beneath the lower margin of the cartilage where the next part of the incision is to be made.

10.2.7 Elevators

(▶ Fig. 10.25 and ▶ Fig. 10.26)
- *Double elevator (Cottle):*
  Universal instrument with a slightly curved, blunt end and a slightly curved, semi-sharp end.
  The *blunt end* is used, for instance, to:
  ○ Palpate
  ○ Elevate mucoperichondrial septal tunnels

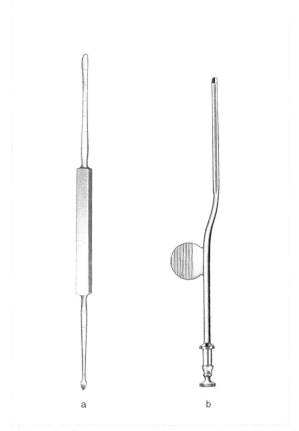

Fig. 10.25 (a) Double elevator (Cottle). **(b)** Suction elevator (Guillen).

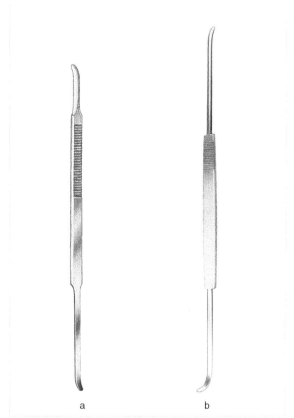

Fig. 10.26 (a) Slightly curved elevator (McKenty type). **(b)** Curved double elevator (McKenty–Cottle type).

- ○ (Re)position mobilized structures
  The semi-sharp end is used, for instance, to:
- ○ Elevate subperiosteal septal tunnels
- ○ Dissect perichondrium from small cartilages (triangular, lobular cartilage)
- ○ Elevate the periosteum from a bony hump
- ○ Separate septal mucosal blades when cartilage and bone is missing
- ○ Reposition the nasal bones after osteotomies
- ○ Mobilize a bony spur or deviation
- ○ Perform submucosal surgery of the turbinates (dissecting the turbinate bone, opening a bulla)
- • *Suction elevator (Guillen):*
  Used to elevate the septal mucoperichondrium and mucoperiosteum and aspirate blood at the same time
  - ○ It is a valuable instrument when bleeding impedes the view, though it should be kept in mind that suction may cause bleeding to persist or increase.
- • *Slightly curved elevator (McKenty) to:*
  - ○ Make subperiosteal paranasal tunnels for lateral and transverse osteotomies
  - ○ Create an inferior septal tunnel

- ○ Elevate the mucoperiosteum of the lateral nasal wall in ozena surgery, and cut a pedicled flap for closure of a septal perforation
- ○ Elevate the periosteum from a bony hump
- • *Curved double elevator (McKenty–Cottle type):*
  Used to elevate the periosteum over the crest of the piriform aperture in the MP approach (especially in Caucasians)
  - ○ The strongly curved end is used to elevate the periosteum over the crest, the slightly curved end is used to begin an inferior septal tunnel.

10.2.8 Forceps

(▶ Fig. 10.27, ▶ Fig. 10.28, ▶ Fig. 10.29, ▶ Fig. 10.30, ▶ Fig. 10.31, and ▶ Fig. 10.32)
- • *Columella clamp or forceps (Cottle):*
  Used to pull the columella first in a caudal and then in a lateral direction to expose the caudal end of the septum and stretch the overlying skin before making a CSI
  - ○ It is available in two sizes: one for adults, one for children.

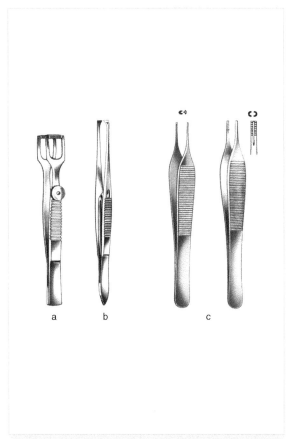

Fig. 10.27 (a) Columellar clamp or forceps (Cottle).
(b) Broad forceps with fine teeth (von Graefe). (c) Narrow
forceps (Adson–Brown) anatomical/surgical.

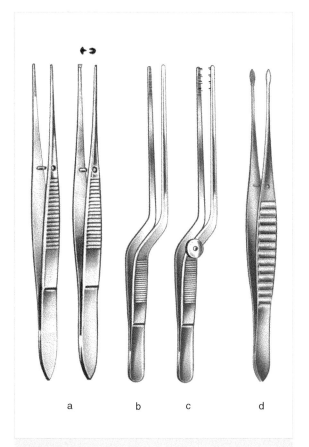

Fig. 10.28 (a) Straight forceps (anatomical/surgical).
(b) Bayonet forceps. (c) Fixation forceps. (d) Cup-forceps
(Cottle).

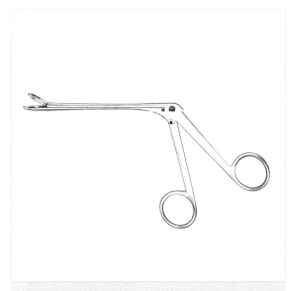

Fig. 10.29 Forceps (Blakesley).

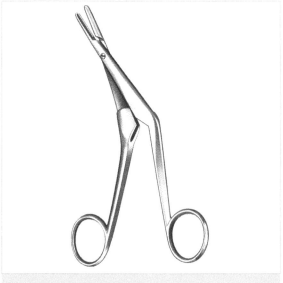

Fig. 10.30 Biting forceps (Craig).

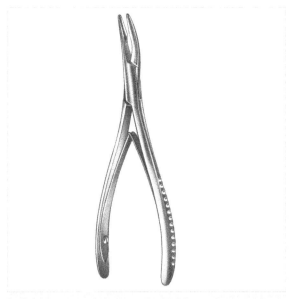

Fig. 10.31 Bone-cutting forceps (Beyer).

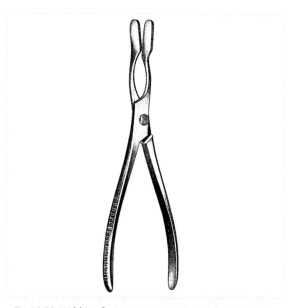

Fig. 10.32 Walsham forceps.

- *Broad forceps with fine teeth (von Graefe, "mouse teeth" forceps) to:*
  - Position (e.g., exorotate) the septal cartilage and fix it in the desired position with septocolumellar sutures
  - Grasp and hold soft tissue flaps
- *Narrow forceps (Adson-Brown):*
  Available as an anatomical and a surgical forceps
  - The anatomical forceps (no teeth) is used to grasp and hold the lobular or triangular cartilages
  - The surgical forceps (small teeth) is used to grasp and hold skin and mucosal flaps.
- *Straight forceps short (12 cm) anatomical/surgical and long (13 cm) anatomical/surgical*
  - The short straight forceps is generally used in the vestibule, the long forceps is mostly used outside the nose (e.g. in preparing grafts).
- *Bayonet forceps short (14 cm) and long (16 cm) to:*
  - Insert plates of bone or cartilage into the septal space for septal repair (16 cm)
  - Apply gauzes for local anesthesia and vaso-constriction (16 cm)
  - Apply internal dressings in the nasal cavity (16 cm) and the vestibule (14 cm)
- *Fixation forceps:*
  Bayonet forceps with wheel to temporarily fix the septal mucosal blades and the transplants inserted for septal reconstruction while applying transseptal sutures and/or splints for final fixation

- *Cup-forceps (Cottle):*
  Slender forceps with ovaloid cup to insert pieces of crushed cartilage or small transplants under the dorsal and lobular skin and to remove small particles
- *Forceps (Blakesley), narrow (No. 1) and middle (No. 2):*
  Long slender forceps to remove loose pieces of cartilage, bone, and soft tissue and to resect polyps and granulation tissue
  - The Blakesley forceps is not designed to fracture bone.
- *Biting forceps (Craig):*
  Strong cutting forceps to resect parts of the cartilaginous or bony septum and to fracture and reposition parts of the bony septum
- *Bone-cutting forceps (Beyer):*
  Strong, slightly curved biting forceps are used to resect the anterior part of a pronounced anterior nasal spine, a protruding wing of the premaxilla, or a bony irregularity at the nasal dorsum
  - The more slender bone-cutting forceps, as used by Lempert (developed for the fenestration operation in otosclerosis), is a good alternative.
- *Nasal bone repositioning forceps (Walsham)*
  Used to reposition an infractured lateral bony nasal wall in patients with an acute nasal injury
  - One leg is introduced intranasally and placed on the mucosa of the inside of the infractured nasal bone; the other leg is placed on the skin.

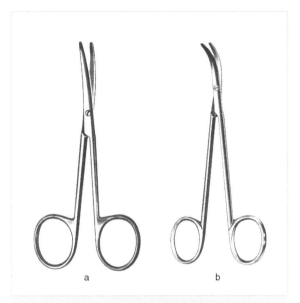

Fig. 10.33 (a) Slightly curved, blunt scissors (Knapp). (b) Strongly curved, blunt scissors (Fomon).

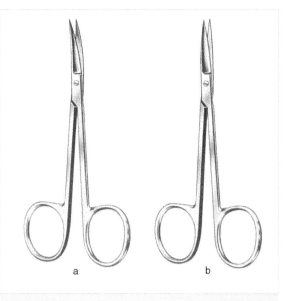

Fig. 10.34 (a) Slightly curved, pointed scissors. (b) Straight, pointed scissors.

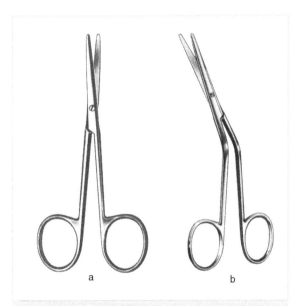

Fig. 10.35 (a) Straight, blunt scissors. (b) Angulated septum scissors (Fomon).

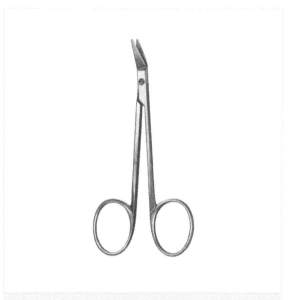

Fig. 10.36 Small, angulated scissors (Walter).

10.2.9 Scissors

(▶ Fig. 10.33, ▶ Fig. 10.34, ▶ Fig. 10.35, ▶ Fig. 10.36, ▶ Fig. 10.37, ▶ Fig. 10.38, and ▶ Fig. 10.39)

- *Slightly curved, blunt scissors (Knapp)—long (13.5 cm) and short (12 cm):*
  Universal scissors used to dissect and cut soft tissues and cartilage, in particular to:
  ○ Undermine the skin of the dorsum and the lobule
  ○ Create a columellar pocket
  ○ Expose the anterior nasal spine
  ○ Cut intranasal sutures and internal dressings
- *Strongly curved, blunt scissors (Fomon):*
  Designed to undermine the skin of the lobule in a retrograde direction through an IC incision and to create a columellar pocket

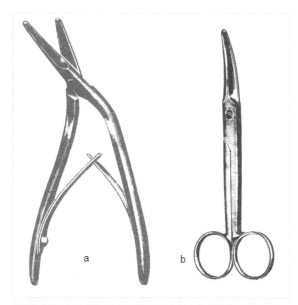

Fig. 10.37 **(a)** Bone scissors (Koffler–Cottle). **(b)** Dressing scissors, slightly curved and blunt (Mayo–Cottle).

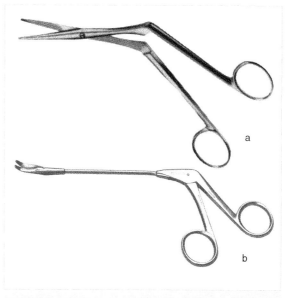

Fig. 10.38 **(a)** Long, narrow, angulated scissors (Heymann). **(b)** Slender, left/right curved scissors (Huizing).

- *Slightly curved, pointed scissors (10.5 cm):*
  Universal scissors for sharp dissection, used in particular to:
  - Dissect the caudal end of the septum
  - Expose and dissect the triangular and lobular cartilage
  - Trim and resect small amounts of cartilage, skin, and mucosa
- *Straight, pointed scissors (10.5 cm)*
- *Straight, blunt scissors (10.5 cm):*
  Small scissors used to:
  - Cut cartilage (e.g., in valve and lobular surgery)
  - Modify cartilaginous grafts
  - Cut mucosa and skin (e.g., in preparing pedicled flaps)
  - Make small resections
- *Angulated septum scissors (Fomon):*
  Used to resect a horizontal (basal) strip from the cartilaginous septum
- *Small, angulated scissors (10 cm) (Walter) to:*
  - Dissect the columellar and lobular skin from the lobular cartilages in the external approach
  - Shorten the caudal septal end
  - Trim the caudal margin of the triangular cartilages
  - Resect a strip from the cranial margin of the lateral crus
- *Bone scissors (Koffler–Cottle):*
  Heavy scissors with small teeth used for cutting bone, in particular the bony septum; they may be used, for example, to:
  - Cut the vomer above and below a spur to allow its resection

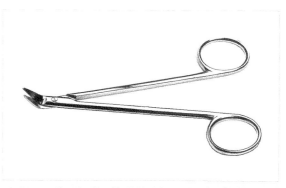

Fig. 10.39 Long angulated, pointed scissors (Huizing).

  - Resect a horizontal bony strip from the bony septum to allow a let-down of the pyramid after bilateral wedge resections
  - Resect a bony plate from the perpendicular plate and/or vomer to be used for reconstruction of the anterior septum
- *Dressing scissors, slightly curved and blunt (Mayo–Cottle):*
  Used to cut gauzes and tapes
  - The scissors are curved in such a way that tape does not stick to the blades.

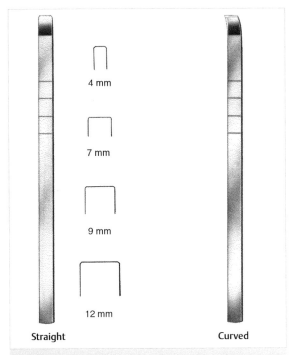

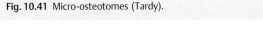

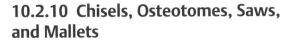

Fig. 10.40 Cottle chisels: straight 4-mm, 7-mm, 9-mm, and 12-mm; curved 6-mm.

Fig. 10.41 Micro-osteotomes (Tardy).

Scissors for Turbinoplasty

(▶ Fig. 10.38 and ▶ Fig. 10.39)

- *Long, narrow, angulated scissors (Heymann)* with small teeth to trim the lower margin of the inferior and middle turbinate and to resect tissue from the turbinate tail
- *Slender, left/right curved scissors (Huizing)* to resect soft tissue in reducing the posterior part of the middle turbinate
- *Angulated (45°) pointed scissors (Huizing)*, 13 cm, to resect and modify the head of the inferior and middle turbinate

10.2.10 Chisels, Osteotomes, Saws, and Mallets

There is a wide variety of different types of chisel and osteotome for nasal surgery on the market. The most important types are discussed in Chapter 6 (page 218).

Our first choice is the set of Cottle chisels, as they are universal. They can be used for all osteotomies, for hump resection, and in septal surgery. Originally, they were designed as a combination of a chisel and an osteotome. The bevel of the chisel enables straight as well as curved osteotomies (see ▶ Fig. 6.14).

Cottle Chisels (or Chisel-Osteotomes)

(▶ Fig. 10.40)

- *4-mm straight chisel*:
  Used to resect small bony crests or a protruding premaxillary wing in septal surgery
- *7-mm straight chisel* used for:
  - Medial and lateral osteotomies
  - Resection of septal spurs and spines
  - Removal of a bony irregularity from the dorsum
- *9-mm and 12-mm straight chisels*:
  Used mainly to resect a bony hump
- *6-mm curved chisel*:
  Used for transverse osteotomies and vertical osteotomies of the bony septum to harvest a plate for repairing a defective anterior septum

Note: Cottle chisels should be sharpened from time to time. It is advisable to slightly smooth the sharp edges to diminish the chances of laceration of the mucosa and skin.

Osteotomes

(▶ Fig. 10.41 and ▶ Fig. 10.42)

- *Micro-osteotomes 2 mm, 4 mm (Tardy)*:
  Used for endonasal (transperiosteal) lateral osteotomies and external transcutaneous transversal osteotomies (see ▶ Fig. 6.33 ▶ Fig. 6.34)
- *Guided osteotomes, curved (left and right)*:
  Used by some surgeons to perform lateral osteotomies
- *Guided osteotomes, straight (different widths)*:
  Used by some surgeons for hump resection

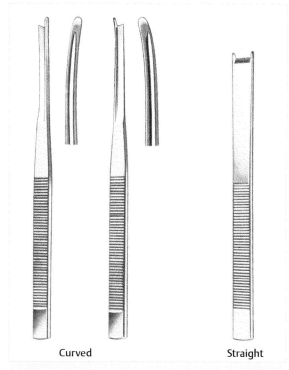

Fig. 10.42 Guided osteotomes: curved (right/left) and straight.

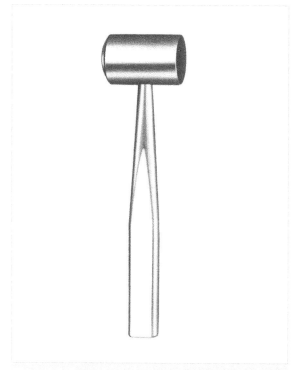

Fig. 10.43 Mallet with flat and round face (Cottle type).

Saws

In the past, saws were used to perform lateral osteotomies and, in some cases, to resect a bony hump. The advantage of using a saw to make a lateral osteotomy was that a straight cut was made that could be completed by a chisel to avoid unnecessary lacerations of the inner mucosa. The great disadvantages of the saw were the production of bone dust, and laceration of the inner mucosa. In the 1980s, the saw was replaced by the chisel. The chisel is a more versatile instrument that allows a curved osteotomy. In the first half of the 20th century, the Joseph saw was the commonly used instrument. It was later succeeded by the Cottle saw with a disposable band saw blade.

Mallets

- *Cottle-type mallet* (▶ Fig. 10.43):
  Heavy mallet with a flat and a rounded face
  - The flat side is used to drive a chisel with the "double-tap" technique. The movements are made in the wrist (see ▶ Fig. 6.18).
  - The rounded side (more force per square centimeter) is used to crush cartilage or bone (see following text).

10.2.11 Rasps and Files

(▶ Fig. 10.44)
- *Double rasp:*
  Used to lower a small bony hump or an irregularity and to smooth the nasal dorsum after hump resection
- *Double file:*
  Used to smooth the bony dorsum after using a rasp

Note: A rasp is only effective when the instrument is pulled. A file is effective in both directions (moving to and fro).

10.2.12 Various

- *Angulated suction tubes (Frazier type;* ▶ Fig. 10.45):
  Diameter 2 mm, 3 mm, and 4 mm
- *Needle holder 13 cm (Neivert):*
  With diamond-covered jaws and offset bow (▶ Fig. 10.46)
- *Cartilage and bone crusher (Cottle;* ▶ Fig. 10.47):
  Used to crush cartilage, bone, and soft tissues before being (re)inserted in the septal space (for septal reconstruction), submucosally, or subcutaneously (as a filler, underlay, or masker)
- *Turbinate crusher (Kressner;* ▶ Fig. 10.48):
  Long, angulated, blunt forceps with flat, hollow jaws to crush and thereby reduce the volume of the inferior turbinate

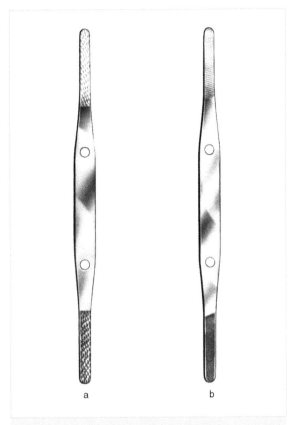

Fig. 10.44 (a) Double rasp. **(b)** Double file.

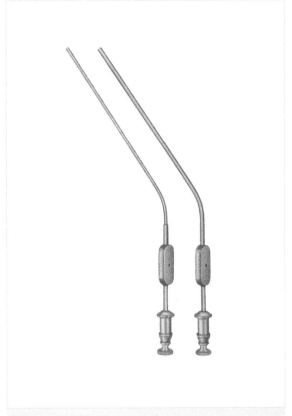

Fig. 10.45 Angulated suction tubes with various diameters (Frazier type).

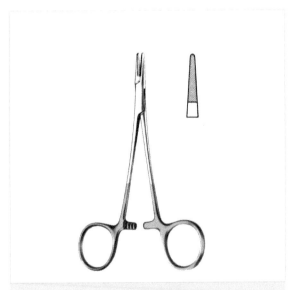

Fig. 10.46 Needle holder with diamond-covered jaws and offset bow.

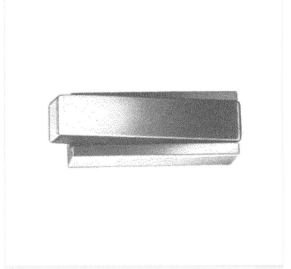

Fig. 10.47 Cartilage and bone crusher (Cottle).

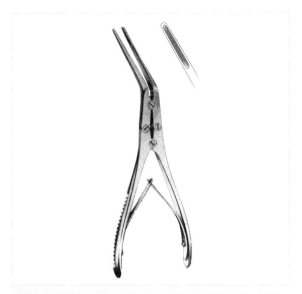

Fig. 10.48 Turbinate crusher (Kressner).

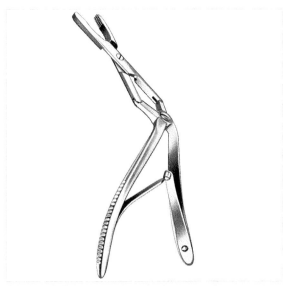

Fig. 10.49 Cartilage morcellizer.

- *Cartilage morcellizer* (▶ Fig. 10.49):
  Forceps used to break the spring of a cartilaginous convexity of the septum or of the lateral crus of the lobular cartilage
- *Measuring stick and caliper* (▶ Fig. 10.50):
  Used to determine the nasal indices, to measure the length, width, and prominence of the various parts of the pyramid, and to plan the size of transplants and implants
- *Bone punch (Hajek;* ▶ Fig. 10.51)
  ○ Small: to enlarge the opening in the anterior sphenoidal wall in transsphenoidal hypophysectomy
  ○ Large: to resect the anterior wall of the antrum (Caldwell–Luc procedure), and the frontal process of the maxilla in external ethmoidectomy
- *Working plate*:
  Used for cutting cartilage and other tissues to the required dimensions before transplantation
- *Whetting stone*:
  Plate of Arkansas stone used to sharpen chisels and the Cottle knife
- *Drawing pen (Devon skin marker regular tip: Devon Industries)* used to:
  ○ Mark the most important points (nasion, K area, tip, subnasale) and lines (nasal base line [NBL])
  ○ Outline the margins of the surgically most relevant nasal structures (bony pyramid, triangular cartilage, lobular cartilage)
  ○ Outline osteotomies, wedge resections, and resections of the domes and lateral crura

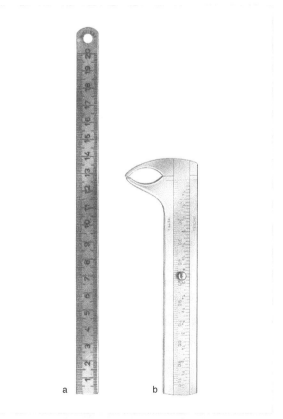

Fig. 10.50 (a) Measuring stick. (b) Caliper.

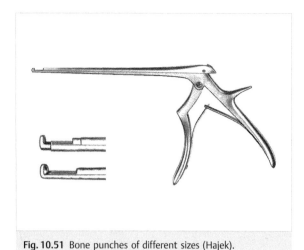

Fig. 10.51 Bone punches of different sizes (Hajek).

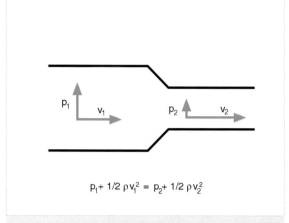

$$p_1 + 1/2\,\rho v_1^2 = p_2 + 1/2\,\rho v_2^2$$

Fig. 10.52 When air flows from a wider into a narrower part of a tube, the velocity (v) of the airstream increases, whereas its pressure (p) falls (Bernoulli's law, 1738).

10.2.13 List of Basic Instruments

For surgeons just getting started in the field of functional corrective nasal surgery who have not had the opportunity to buy a full set of instruments, a list of basic instruments is shown below:

- Cotton wool applicators
- Cups for local anesthetic and vasoconstriction
- Short, broad speculum (Hartmann–Vienna)
- Narrow, medium-long speculum (Cottle)
- Medium-long speculum (Killian)
- Long speculum (Killian)
- Knife handle with No. 15, No. 11, and No. 20 blades
- Beaver handle with No. 64 and No. 66 blade
- Alar retractor (alar protector)
- Short, angulated retractor
- Uneven, four-pronged, blunt retractor (Cottle)
- Single straight hook
- Single round hook
- Two-pronged, sharp–dull hook
- Two-pronged, dull–sharp hook
- Double elevator (Cottle)
- Slightly curved elevator (McKenty)
- Columella forceps
- Narrow forceps (Adson–Brown; surgical, anatomical)
- Straight forceps
- Bayonet forceps
- Blakesley forceps
- Biting forceps (Craig)
- Slightly curved, blunt scissors (Knapp)
- Strongly curved, blunt scissors (Fomon)
- Slightly curved, pointed scissors
- Small, angulated scissors
- Cottle chisels (4-mm, 7-mm, 9-mm)
- Mallet (Cottle)
- Double rasp

- Crusher (Cottle)
- Needle holder (12.5 cm)
- Suction tubes (Frazier)
- Whetting stone
- Drawing pen

10.3 Physical Laws Governing Airstreams

10.3.1 Bernoulli's Law

When air flows without friction through a tube of a constant diameter, pressure is the same at every point along the tube (Bernoulli's law). When air flows from a wider into a narrower part of the tube, the velocity of the airstream increases, whereas its pressure decreases (▶ Fig. 10.52).

When applied to nasal breathing, this implies that the velocity of inspired air increases at areas of narrowing such as the valve area, the head of the turbinates, and pathological obstructions. This may produce a change from a laminar into a turbulent flow, as we discuss in the following text.

Bernoulli's law (1738):

$$p + \frac{1}{2}\rho v^2 = \text{Constant} \tag{10.1}$$

In this formula, ρ is the static pressure; $\tfrac{1}{2}\,\rho v^2$ is the aerodynamical pressure; ρ is the coefficient of density of air (kg/m^3); and v is the velocity of the airflow (m/s).

10.3.2 Hagen–Poiseuille's Equation

In reality, there will be friction from the wall of the tube (the walls of the internal nose) and the viscosity of the air. Consequently, there will be a pressure fall along the

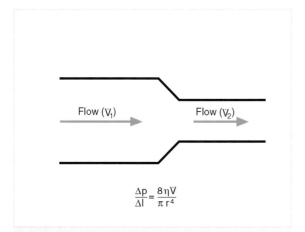

Fig. 10.53 The volume of air ($\dot{V}$) flowing through a tube varies as the second power of the cross-sectional surface (πr^2) of the tube (Hagen–Poiseuille's equation).
Abbreviations: Δp, pressure fall; Δl, distance along the tube; V, volume of air per second; η, coefficient of viscosity of air (Pa.s); r, radius of tube

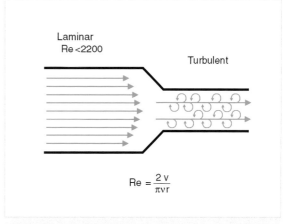

Fig. 10.54 The velocity of the airstream increases where the passage narrows. When the velocity of the molecules exceeds a certain value, the outer layers of air become turbulent and whirls occur. In a tube, the air stream becomes turbulent when Reynolds number exceeds 2200.
Abbreviations: Re, Reynolds number; r, radius of the tube; V, volume of air; v, kinematical viscosity (m²/s)

tube. According to Hagen–Poiseuille's equation, the volume of air flowing through the tube varies as the second power of the cross-sectional surface (πr^2) of the tube (▶ Fig. 10.53).

Applied to the nose, this implies that any narrowing and widening will have a great impact on nasal airflow. A well-known clinical example is the serious impairment of breathing that is caused by a minor obstruction at the nasal valve area.

Hagen–Poiseuille's equation (Hagen 1797–1884, Poiseuille 1799–1869):

$$\frac{\Delta p}{\Delta l} = \frac{8\eta V}{\pi r^4} \tag{10.2}$$

In this equation, Δp is the pressure fall; Δl is the distance along the tube; V is the volume of air per second; η is the coefficient of viscosity of air (Pa.s); and r is the radius of the tube.

10.3.3 Reynolds Number

When the velocity of the air is low, the flow will be laminar. That is, the molecules will follow a straight course. When there is friction by the wall, as in the nose, the velocity of the air will decrease from the axis to the periphery of the airstream.

When the velocity of the air is increased, for instance due to a narrowing, the airstream may become turbulent. This means that the velocity of the molecules of the outer layers of air and their direction are no longer constant, and whirls occur (▶ Fig. 10.54).

Whether a laminar airstream becomes turbulent depends on Reynolds number (Reynolds, 1883). That indicator is determined by the volume of air, the radius of

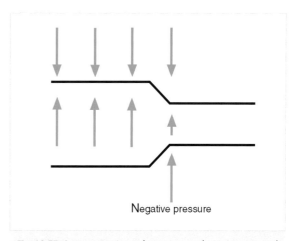

Fig. 10.55 A narrowing in a tube causes a velocity increase and a pressure drop. Air pressure falls in relation to ambient air, creating a relative negative pressure (Venturi effect).

the tube, and the kinematic viscosity of air, according to the formula:

$$Re = \frac{2V}{\pi vr} \tag{10.3}$$

10.3.4 The Venturi Effect

As discussed under 10.3.1 Bernoulli's Law, a narrowing in a tube causes the velocity of air to increase and the pressure to drop. When applied to the nose, this means that air pressure falls in relation to the ambient air (▶ Fig. 10.55), creating a relative negative pressure. Although already mentioned by Bernoulli in 1738, it is generally called the Venturi effect (Venturi 1746–1822).

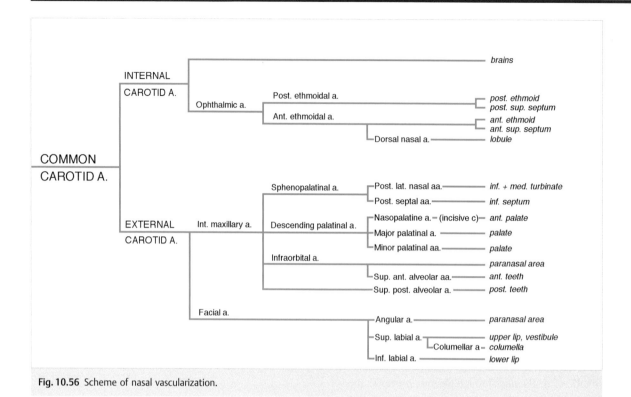

Fig. 10.56 Scheme of nasal vascularization.

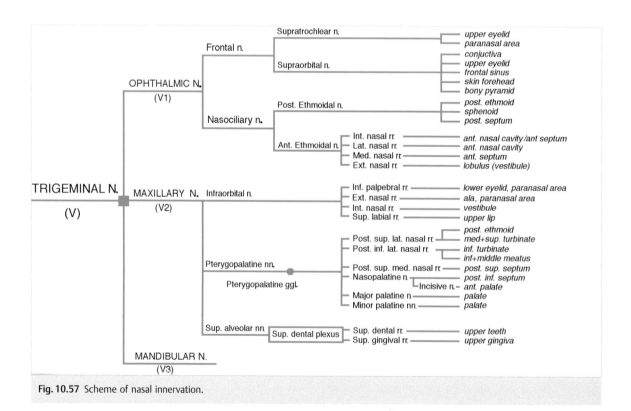

Fig. 10.57 Scheme of nasal innervation.

In the nose, the Venturi effect may produce inspiratory collapse of the lateral nasal wall. Because of the pressure drop, a transmural pressure difference occurs, leading to inward movement of the lateral nasal wall. In patients with a narrow valve area or a loss of rigidity of the lateral nasal wall, alar collapse may result.

10.3.5 Starling Valve

A Starling valve is a semirigid tube with a collapsible segment. This model was introduced by Starling (1866–1927), who stated that the output of the heart per beat is directly proportional to its diastolic filling. Bridger and Proctor (1977) introduced this concept to explain the specific behavior of the anterior nasal segment during inspiratory breathing.

10.3.6 Rohrer's Equation

In 1915, Rohrer postulated the equation

$$V = K_1 V_1 + K_2 V_2 \tag{10.4}$$

to describe the measured data of turbulence. His formula is still quoted but is no longer considered valuable.

10.4 Schemes of Vascularization and Nerve Supply

(▶ Fig. 10.56 and ▶ Fig. 10.57)

10.5 Historical Development of Functional Reconstructive Nasal Surgery

10.5.1 "What's Past is Prologue"

In this chapter, an attempt is made to present an overview of the most important steps in the development of functional reconstructive nasal surgery.

Over centuries, many anatomists, physiologists, and surgeons have contributed to the wealth of knowledge in this specialty. Some of them are still known because their names are attached to certain surgical techniques, diagnostic procedures, or special instruments; others are more or less forgotten.

Killian and Freer, for example, are two names that are associated with submucosal septal surgery. They were preceded, however, by several pioneers, such as Ingals in the United States and Krieg in Germany. The same applies to reconstructive septal surgery as taught by Cottle. He too had important predecessors, such as Metzenbaum and Fomon. In the historical notes presented below, attention is therefore also paid to the scientists and surgeons who pioneered new methods of examination and surgery. In many respects, their contributions to the development of functional reconstructive nasal surgery are just as important as those of the scientists and surgeons that we still know today.

Reconstruction of the Defective Nose

The first step in the development of nasal surgery, or rhinoplasty, was the reconstruction of the defective external nose. Sushruta, an Indian, is reported to have reconstructed a cut-off external nose with pedicled cheek and forehead flaps around 1000 BC. In his time, the loss of the nose because of war injuries or as punishment for adultery was a common deformity. Surgical techniques to repair bodily defects were performed by members of the Koomas caste of tile and brickmakers, and kept secret.

Some of the early Indian methods were adopted by Arabic medicine, and later spread to Sicily, where the technique of the forehead flap was reintroduced by the Branca family around 1442. Later, this technique was also used in southern and northern Italy.

In 1597, Gaspare Tagliacozzi (1545–1599) of Bologna published his classic book *De Curtorum Chirurgia per Insitionem* in three parts. In the third part, he described various techniques for the reconstruction of defective body parts using skin grafts. He restored a defective nose with a pedicled skin flap from the upper arm. One year later, a third publication appeared in Frankfurt under the title *Chirurgia nova*. It was translated into English in 1687. During his time, Tagliacozzi received a lot of criticism, especially from the Church, which considered modeling the body the work of God.

Widespread interest in reconstructive nasal surgery arose again around the turn of the 18th century, mainly because of the many war injuries during the Napoleonic wars. In 1794, B Lucas, an English surgeon working in India, reported to have witnessed the reconstruction of a cut-off nose with a pedicled forehead flap in a prisoner of war. The "curious operation," as he called it in his letter to *The Gentleman's Magazine*, was carried out by a man from the caste of the tile and brickmakers in Poona. Some 20 years later, in 1816, Joseph Carpue of Chelsea, having practiced the operation on cadavers, described how he had successfully restored "a lost nose from the integuments of the forehead in the cases of two officers."

In 1818, Carl von Graefe of Berlin published his book *Rhinoplastik oder die Kunst den Verlust der Nase organisch zu ersetzen*. He introduced the term *rhinoplastik* and compared the Italian with the Indian and German methods. From then on, this surgical technique spread rapidly and the term *rhinoplastik* was adopted by other surgeons, for example, by Busch and von Langenbeck (1864) in Germany, by Labat (1834) and Nelaton (1868) in France (*rhinoplastie*), and by Hardy (1875) in England (*rhinoplasty*).

The Early Publications on Septal and Pyramid Deformities

The first milestones in septal surgery are the early publications on various types of deformity of the septum and the external nose. A monograph on septal deformities by Samuel Quelmaltz, published in 1750, stands out as the very first publication on the nasal septum. Only a few years later, in 1761, Giovanni Morgagni, Professor of Anatomy at Padua, described exostoses and deviations of the septum and their possible origins, such as difficult labor, falls in infancy, and infections. He also discussed the effects of differences in rates of growth between the septum and the upper jaw.

However, it took several decades before nasal pathology was studied again. In 1804, Jacques Deschamps of Paris published the first textbook on the nose and sinuses, while Bernhard von Langenbeck, Professor of Surgery at Berlin, wrote on the irregularities of the septum, such as crests and spurs, in 1843. He was followed by Friedrich Theile of Weimar, who published his study on the prevalence of septal pathology in 1855, and later by Hermann Welcker of Halle, who reported on asymmetries of the nose and the relation between septal deviations and deformities of the maxillary bones in 1882.

Septal Surgery—The First Attempts

Resection of Parts of the Septum

The earliest attempts to correct septal deformities consisted of partial septal resection, which left a defect. The operation was carried out either endonasally (Blandin, Paris, 1835) or through the nasal dorsum. In 1841 and 1845, Johann Friedrich Dieffenbach, Professor of Surgery at Berlin, described in detail how he addressed a septal deviation. In his first publication, he described an external approach through the nasal dorsum, while in his famous book *Die Operative Chirurgie* (1845), he reported on an endonasal method in which the deviated part of the septum was resected and a perforation was left. Because of the development of the head mirror (Hofmann 1845) and the introduction of anterior and posterior rhinoscopy, physicians became increasingly aware of the importance of septal deformities.

Transmucosal Resection of Crests and Spurs

In 1843, Bernhard von Langenbeck described his technique of shaving down a septal spur and crest, while 8 years later, Charles Chassaignac, who worked in Paris, described his method of shaving off a septal deviation after unilateral elevation of the mucosa. In the 1880s, the electrocoagulator, burr, saw (Bosworth 1887), special knife (Moure), and chisel were introduced for the removal of septal spurs and crests.

Septal Medialization Using a Forceps

In 1875, William Adams of London suggested fracturing a deviated septum using a special forceps and supporting it in its new midline position with internal splints. Variations of this technique were later reported by various authors, such as Jurasz (Heidelberg, 1882), Bayer (Brussels, 1882), Jarvis (New York, 1882), and Glasgow (St Louis, 1882). In 1890, Morris Asch of New York described how to forcibly reposition a deviated septum with a special forceps and a stellate punch; the so-called Asch forceps is still in use today.

Walsham of London published a book on nasal obstruction and surgery of the septum in 1897, introducing his forceps (the still well-known Walsham forceps) to medialize the septum and reposition the nasal bones.

Submucosal Septal Surgery

Pioneers

As early as 1847, P Heylen described in the *Gazette médicale de Paris* a technique of resecting the deviated part of the septal cartilage after bilateral elevation of the mucosa. Yet it was Ephraim Ingals of Chicago who fully described the basic principles of submucosal septal surgery in 1882. In the same year, Arthur Hartmann of Berlin also reported on submucosal partial resection of the septum. They were soon followed by Ferdinand Pedersen (Kiel, 1883), Burkhardt (1885), and Robert Krieg (Stuttgart, 1886), who all reported cases in which septal surgery was performed submucosally. In 1889, Robert Krieg was the first to use the term *window resection* (*Fensterresektion*). He is therefore often considered the father of submucosal septal resection.

The operation popularized by Killian and Freer is usually called SMR or "submucous resection." This is incorrect terminology. It should be "submucosal septal surgery," as the surgery is performed under the nasal mucosa, not under the nasal mucus.

Submucosal Septal Resection Becomes a Standard Procedure

In 1899, a technique of submucosal septal resection that preserves a dorsal and a caudal strut of the cartilaginous septum to prevent sagging and retraction was described by Gustav Killian. He reported on 220 cases in which this technique was used in 1904, and one year later his work was translated into English. Killian eventually became Professor of Otorhinolaryngology at Berlin.

Influenced by the work of Ingals, Otto Tiger Freer of Chicago explained his method of submucosal surgery in a series of publications (1902–1905). He advocated a more radical removal of the septal cartilage than Killian. According to Freer, the cartilaginous septum does not contribute to the support of the dorsum, and he claimed that postoperative dorsal sagging is caused by damage to the upper lateral cartilages. Freer introduced a mucosal elevator, which is still used. Between 1903 and 1910, he published eleven articles on the topic.

In the first decade of the 20th century, a vast number of publications on submucosal septal surgery appeared, such as those by Freer, Ballenger, Gleason, and Yankauer in America. In Germany, the most important contributions were those by Killian, Hajek, Bönninghaus, Kretschmann, and Zarniko, while in France, they were those by Moure, Escat, and Bérard.

In 1905, William Ballenger of Chicago introduced his swivel knife, which remained highly popular until the introduction of more conservative techniques of septal surgery in the 1960s, to remove the central part of the septal cartilage. To reduce the complications of dorsal sagging and columellar retraction, most surgeons adopted Killian's method of leaving a dorsal and a caudal strut of cartilage. Nonetheless, dorsal sagging and columellar retraction occurred in a high percentage of cases, as did septal perforations. In 1910, Halle suggested approaching the septum orally.

Septal Reconstruction

Early Attempts

Myron Metzenbaum of Cleveland seems to have been the first to reposition deviated parts of the septum. In 1929, he reported his method of repositioning a deflected anterior septum instead of resecting it. One year later, he described how to reconstruct the septum with bone and cartilage present "within the old traumatized nose."

Peer reported his technique of resection and reinsertion of a deviated caudal end in 1937: when the cartilage was of poor quality, he reconstructed the defect with a graft taken from the dorsal part of the septum. He was therefore the first to use the "exchange" or "transposition" technique.

In 1946, Galloway went one step further. He removed the cartilaginous septum and reconstructed it with a plate shaped from the removed material. This transplant was secured in place with three temporary traction sutures, and then fixed with mattress sutures.

Conservative Reconstructive Septal Surgery

By using smaller transplants, Samuel Fomon of New York (1948) improved the Galloway procedure. He organized numerous instructional courses, and has to be considered one of the pioneers of conservative reconstructive nasal surgery, popularizing hemitransfixion as a universal approach to the septum and stressing the importance of preserving and restoring nasal function.

Maurice H Cottle of Chicago continued Fomon's work during the 1950s and 1960s, and developed new techniques of conservative reconstructive nasal surgery. To repair or reconstruct a severely deformed or missing septum, he introduced the MP approach in 1958. His other noteworthy contributions include reintroducing nasal surgery in children (1951), the push-down technique for hump removal, and nasal roof repair (1954). He also reintroduced manometric recording of nasal breathing. In his instructional courses, he stressed that nasal surgery should in the first place aim to improve nasal function. His many courses, which he gave in the United States, Mexico (1958), Israel (1961), and The Netherlands (1963, 1964, 1965, 1970), prompted a worldwide revival of nasal surgery.

Many other scientists and surgeons have since made important contributions to this area of surgery, among them several of the contributors to this textbook. However, it is beyond the scope of this historical overview to name them all.

Osteotomies

In 1885, Friedrich Trendelenburg of Bonn introduced endonasal lateral osteotomy and transcutaneous transverse osteotomy to redress a deviated nose. Jacques Joseph of Berlin further explored and improved the technique of mobilizing and repositioning the bony pyramid. He developed better instruments, among them a saw (the "Joseph saw") and chisels. Over time, his instruments were modified by other surgeons. After World War II, the saw and chisel-osteotomes designed by Maurice Cottle of Chicago became popular. In the 1970s, Helmut Masing from Erlangen propagated guided chisels, and in the 1980s Eugene Tardy (Chicago) introduced micro-osteotomes to minimize tissue damage when performing bone cuts.

In the 1960s, Cottle described "push-down" of the bony pyramid as a method to correct a bony and cartilaginous hump and, at the same time, keep the dorsum intact. This method was later improved by Huizing (1975), who introduced bilateral wedge resection and the "let-down" of the external pyramid in patients with a prominent nose.

Turbinate Surgery

Surgery of the turbinates has a similar long history to septal surgery, starting in the 19th century. Unfortunately, the techniques that were introduced mostly denied the functional importance of the turbinates. Turbinectomy was introduced in 1882 and, unfortunately, is still in use, despite the irreversible damage that total turbinectomy causes to nasal function. In the early years of the 20th century, Killian and others described the more conservative, but usually insufficiently effective, technique of lateralization. Later, various methods of crushing and partial turbinectomy, commonly named *turbinotomy*, were developed to avoid the disastrous effects of total turbinectomy on nasal function. Some of them are still commonly used despite the fact that by the 1980s, effective function-preserving methods of turbinate reduction had been described and propagated. Names that should be mentioned in this respect are those of Mabry and Pirsig. This book presents a similar technique of "submucosal turbinoplasty" (see page 301).

Rhinoplasty

In 1845, Johann Friedrich Dieffenbach, Professor of Surgery at Berlin, published *Die Operative Chirurgie*, which was the first book that devoted an entire chapter to nasal surgery. Dieffenbach used an external incision on the nasal dorsum to approach the septum. He undermined the dorsal skin, separated the cartilaginous nose from the bony nose, repositioned the lower part, and fixed it in place by taping.

Robert Weir of New York described a (transcutaneous) lateral osteotomy for the first time in 1880: "the operator then made an oblique linear incision through the skin at the side of the nose, introduced a fine bone-chisel and easily cut through the bone, then tilted it into its place."

The endonasal approach in rhinoplasty was first described by John Orlando Roe of Rochester (New York) in 1887. Roe reported his technique of approaching the pathology through an endonasal (IC) incision in his publications on the correction of "pug and hump noses." He named his surgery "corrective rhinoplasty," and also discussed the psychological factors involved in nasal surgery.

Two years later, Friedrich Trendelenburg of Bonn introduced endonasal lateral osteotomy and transcutaneous transverse osteotomy to redress a deviated nose.

Influential publications in the 1890s were those by Robert Weir (1892), who described subcutaneous reduction of a prominent nose, and Goodale (Boston, 1899), who explained a method to reduce a prominent nose that involved resection of a part of the septum underneath the hump, mobilization of the nasal bones, and push-down of the dorsum.

Major Advances in Rhinoplasty

Over a period of more than 30 years, Jacques Joseph of Berlin contributed many world famous publications to the field of plastic surgery of the nose on topics such as nasal reduction (1898, 1905), reduction of a cartilaginous hump or "potato nose" (1902), intranasal hump removal (1904), shortening of the nose (1905), correction of the deviated nose (including the first description of unilateral wedge resection; 1907), "total rhinoplasty" (1914), and reconstruction of nasal and lip defects caused by war injuries (1916–1918). His work culminated in his opus magnum, *Nasenplastik und sonstige Gesichtsplastik*, which was published in 1931. Joseph was visited by hundreds of surgeons who wanted to learn his methods, among them the later famous Gustave Aufricht (New York), Ferris Smyth (Grand Rapids), and Joseph Safian (New York).

The External Approach

In the 1920s, the external approach to the nasal pyramid, the dorsum, and lobule was reintroduced. Sir Harold Gillies (1920), the famous plastic surgeon of London, reported in 1920 on the use of a U-shaped incision at the nasolabial angle in combination with bilateral incisions along the medial crura (the "elephant-trunk incision"), by which he created a columellar flap and obtained access to all nasal structures. Sheehan in 1925 used a vertical columellar incision ("columellar splitting incision") to approach the external nasal pyramid. In 1929 (and again in 1934), Aurel Réthi of Budapest introduced a high horizontal transcolumellar incision as an approach to the nasal dorsum for hump removal and augmentation. This approach was called "external exposure" by EC Padget in 1938.

Réthi's approach was modified by Ante Šerçer of Zagreb in 1957 (and again in 1962), who introduced a midcolumellar incision in combination with bilateral marginal incisions, which allowed him to elevate the lobular skin. He therefore called the technique "decortication." His method was adopted by his pupil and successor Ivo Padovan (1960), who demonstrated it in North America in 1970. There, the technique was further explored and spread by the work of Jack Anderson (New Orleans, 1971), Wilfred Goodman (Toronto, 1973), and later by Peter Adamson (Toronto), Jugo (New York), and Ewout Baarsma (Leiden), among others.

"Tip Surgery"

In recent decades, the cosmetic aspects of nasal surgery have become more and more important. In many countries, nasal surgeons have devoted themselves specifically to aesthetics. Giving in to the demands of our present society, surgery for beauty has gained importance. In particular, the aesthetics of the "nasal tip" have grown in interest, especially in the United States, and more recently also in South America and Europe. It has become accepted to speak of "tip surgery," although we are actually dealing with surgery of the lobule, since the various techniques that have been developed not only remodel the nasal tip, but also the nasal alae, the columella, and the nasal vestibule.

10.6 Bibliography

10.6.1 References

This list contains the majority of publications that are mentioned in the text and have influenced the thinking behind the concepts and the methods described in this book.

Adamson PA. Open rhinoplasty. Otolaryngol Clin North Am 1987; 20: 837–852

American Academy of Sleep Medicine. The International Classification of Sleep Disorders, Revised. Westchester, Illinois: American Academy of Sleep Medicine; 2010: 52–58

Anderson JR. A new approach to rhinoplasty. Trans Am Acad Ophthalmol Otolaryngol 1966; 70: 183–192

Anderson JR. New approach to rhinoplasty: a five year appraisal. Arch Otolaryngol Head Neck Surg 1971; 93: 284–291

Anderson JR. The dynamics of rhinoplasty. In: Proceedings of the Ninth International Congress in Otolaryngology. Amsterdam: Excerpta Medica; 1969: 708–710

Armijo BS, Brown M, Guyuron B. Defining the ideal nasolabial angle. Plast Reconstr Surg 2012; 129: 759–764

Arredondo de Arreola G, López Serna N, de Hoyos Parra R, Arreola Salinas MA. Morphogenesis of the lateral nasal wall from 6 to 36 weeks. Otolaryngol Head Neck Surg 1996; 114: 54–60

Baarsma EA. External septorhinoplasty. Arch Otorhinolaryngol 1979; 224: 169–176

Bachmann W. Die Funktionsdiagnostik der behinderten Nasenatmung. Berlin: Springer; 1982

Bachmann W, Legler U. Studies on the structure and function of the anterior section of the nose by means of luminal impressions. Acta Otolaryngol 1972; 73: 433–442

Barelli PA. Long term evaluation of "push down" procedures. Rhinology 1975; 13: 25–32

Bert P. De la greffe animale [Thesis]. Paris, 1863

Bewarder F, Pirsig W. Spätergebnisse nach submuköser Septumresektion. Laryngol Rhinol 1978; 57: 922–931

Biller JA, Kim DW. A contemporary assessment of facial aesthetic preferences. Arch Facial Plast Surg 2009; 11: 91–97

Binder KH. Dysostosis maxillo-nasalis, ein anrhinencephaler Missbindungskomplex. Dtsch Zahnarztliche Zschr 1962; 17: 438

Bleys RLAW, Popko M, De Groot JW, Huizing EH. Histological structure of the nasal cartilages and their perichondrial envelope. II. The perichondrial envelope of the septal and lobular cartilage. Rhinology 2007; 45: 153–157

Van Bolhuis AH. On the use of processed cancellous bone for narrowing the nasal cavity. Pr Oto Rhino Laryngol 1967; 29: 340–344

Bridger GP, Proctor DF. Maximum nasal inspiratory flow and nasal resistance. Ann Otol Rhinol Laryngol 1970; 79: 481–488

Bridger GP. Physiology of the nasal valve. Arch Otolaryngol 1970; 92: 543–553

Broms P. Rhinomanometry. Lund; 1980

Bruintjes TD, van Olphen AF, Hillen B, Huizing EH. A functional anatomic study of the relationship of the nasal cartilages and muscles to the nasal valve area. Laryngoscope 1998; 108: 1025–1032

Bruintjes TD, van Olphen AF, Hillen B. Review of the functional anatomy of the cartilages and muscles of the nose. Rhinology 1996; 34: 66–74

Bruintjes TjD. On the functional anatomy of the nasal valve and lobule [Thesis]. Utrecht, 1996

Buiter C. Endoscopy of the upper airways. Amsterdam: Excerpta Medica; 1976

Buiter CT. Nasal antrostomy. Rhinology 1988; 26: 5–18

Caplan AI. Cartilage. Sci Am 1984; 251: 84–87

Charlin C. Symptomenkomplex bei Läsionen des N. nasalis. Arch Oftalmol B Aires 1930; 5: 132

Clement PA, Gordts F. Standardisation Committee on Objective Assessment of the Nasal Airway, IRS, and ERS Consensus report on acoustic rhinometry and rhinomanometry. Rhinology 2005; 43: 169–179

Clement PA. Committee report on standardization of rhinomanometry. Rhinology 1984; 22: 151–155

Cole P, Haight JSJ. Posture and the nasal cycle. Ann Otol Rhinol Laryngol 1986; 95: 233–237

Cole P. Acoustic rhinometry and rhinomanometry. Rhinol Suppl 2000; 16: 29–34

Cole P. The four components of the nasal valve. Am J Rhinol 2003; 17: 107–110

Cole P. Upper respiratory airflow. In: Proctor DF, Anderson I, editors. The Nose: Upper Airway Physiology and the Atmospheric Environment. Amsterdam: Elsevier Science; 1982

Collie WR, Pagon RA, Hall JG, Shokeir MH. ACHOO syndrome (autosomal dominant compelling helio-ophthalmic outburst syndrome). Birth Defects Orig Artic Ser 1978; 14 6B: 361–363

Cottle MH, Loring RM, Cohen MH, Kirschman R. Cancellous bone grafts in nasal repair. Ann Otol Rhinol Laryngol 1949; 58: 135–146

Cottle MH, Loring RM, Fischer GG, Gaynon IE. The maxilla-premaxilla approach to extensive nasal septum surgery. AMA Arch Otolaryngol 1958; 68: 301–313

Cottle MH, Loring RM. Surgery of the nasal septum; new operative procedures and indications. Ann Otol Rhinol Laryngol 1948; 57: 705–713

Cottle MH, Loring RM. The expanding scope of nasal surgery. Arch Otolaryngol 1963; 77: 437–441

Cottle MH, Quilty TJ, Buckingham RA. Nasal implants in children and in adults; with preliminary note on the use of ox cartilage. Ann Otol Rhinol Laryngol 1953; 62: 169–175

Cottle MH. An introduction to conservative septum-pyramid surgery. Int Rhinol 1964; 2: 11–24

Cottle MH. Concepts of nasal physiology as related to corrective nasal surgery. Arch Otolaryngol 1960; 72: 11–20

Cottle MH. Corrective Surgery: Nasal Septum and External Pyramid. Chicago: American Rhinologic Society; 1960

Cottle MH. Nasal roof repair and hump removal. AMA Arch Otolaryngol 1954; 60: 408–414

Cottle MH. Nasal surgery in children. Eye Ear Nose Throat Mon 1951; 30: 32–38

Cottle MH. Personal communication. Second International Course in Septum-Pyramid Surgery, 1961

Cottle MH. Rhinology: The Collected Writings of Maurice H Cottle. Barelli PA, Loch WEE, Kern GB, Steiner A, eds. Chicago: American Rhinologic Society; 1987

Cottle MH. Rhino-sphygmomanometry: an aid in physical diagnosis. Int Rhinol 1968; 6: 7–26

Cottle MH. The role of the rhinologist in rhinoplasty. Laryngoscope 1953; 63: 608–618

Cottle MH. The structure and function of the nasal vestibule. AMA Arch Otolaryngol 1955; 62: 173–181

Courtade A. Etude clinique et physiologique de l'obstruction nasale. Arch Int Laryngol Otol Rhinol 1904; 12: 320

Dangouloff M. Des Opérations Conservatrices de la Cloison Nasale. Bordeaux: Imprimeries Gounouilhou; 1925.

Diewert VM. A morphometric analysis of craniofacial growth and changes in spatial relations during secondary palatal development in human embryos and fetuses. Am J Anat 1983; 167: 495–522

Dion MC, Jafek BW, Tobin CE. The anatomy of the nose. External support. Arch Otolaryngol 1978; 104: 145–150

Van Dishoeck HAE. Die Bedeutung der äusseren Nase fur die respiratorische Luftströmung. Acta Otolaryngol 1936; 24: 494–505

Van Dishoeck HAE. Elektromanometer der Nasenfluegelmuskeln und Nasenwiderstandskurve. Acta Otolaryngol 1937; 25: 285–295

Van Dishoeck HAE. Inspiratory nasal resistance. Acta Otolaryngol 1942; 30: 431–439

Van Dishoeck HAE. The part of the valve and the turbinates in total nasal resistance. Int Rhinol 1965; 3: 19–26

Djupesland P, Pedersen OF. Acoustic rhinometry in infants and children. Rhinol Suppl 2000; 16: 52–58

Dorn M, Pirsig W, Verse T. Postoperative management following rhinosurgery interventions in severe obstructive sleep apnea. A pilot study. HNO 2001; 49: 642–645

Døsen LK, Haye R. Surgical closure of nasal septal perforation. Early and long term observations. Rhinology 2011; 49: 486–491

Draf W. Endoskopie der Nasennebenhöhlen. Berlin: Springer; 1978

Eccles R. A guide to practical aspects of measurement of human nasal airflow by rhinomanometry. Rhinology 2011; 49: 2–10

Eckert-Möbius A. Implantation von macerierten spongiösen Rinderknochen zur Behandlung der Ozaena, Rhinitis atrophicans. Z Hals Nasen Ohren Hlk 1923; 7: 108–124

Egyedi P. Degloving the nose. J Maxillofac Surg 1974; 2: 101–103

Eitschberger E, Merklein C, Masing H. [Deviations of septum cartilage after unilateral separation of mucoperichondrium in rabbits]. Arch Otorhinolaryngol 1980; 228: 135–148

Eschelman LT, Schleuning AJ, Brummett RE. Prophylactic antibiotics in otolaryngologic surgery: a double-blind study. Trans Am Acad Ophthalmol Otolaryngol 1971; 75: 387–394

Escher F, Roth F. [Paranasal transethmoid-sphenoidal hypophysectomy in metastatic breast cancer.] Acta Otolaryngol 1957; 48: 44–58

Facer GW, Kern EB. Nonsurgical closure of nasal septal perforations. Arch Otolaryngol 1979; 105: 6–8

Farkas LG. Craniofacial norms. In: Farkas LG, editor. Anthropometry of the head and face, 2nd ed. Appendix A, B, C. New York: Raven; 1994

Federative Committee on Anatomical Terminology. Terminologia Anatomica: International Anatomical Terminology. Stuttgart-New York: Thieme; 1998

Fokkens W, Lund V, Mullol J European Position Paper on Rhinosinusitis and Nasal Polyps group. European position paper on rhinosinusitis and nasal polyps 2007. Rhinol Suppl 2007; 20: 1–136

Fomon S, Bell JW, Berger EL et al. A new approach to ventral deflections of nasal septum. Arch Otolaryngol 1951; 54: 356–366

Fomon S, Gilbert JG, Silver AG, Syracuse VR. Plastic repair of the obstructing nasal septum. Arch Otolaryngol 1948; 47: 7–20

Fomon S, Syracuse VR, Bolotow N, Pullen M. Plastic repair of the deflected nasal septum. Arch Otolaryngol 1946; 44: 141–156

Fomon S. The treatment of old unreduced nasal fractures. Ann Surg 1936; 104: 107–117

Freer OT. Deflection of the nasal septum. A critical review of the methods of their correction by the window resection with a report of 116 operations. Ann Otol Rhinol Laryngol 1905; 14: 213–266

Freer OT. The correction of deflection of the nasal septum with a minimum of traumatism. JAMA 1902; 38: 636–642

Fry HJ. Interlocked stresses in human nasal septal cartilage. Br J Plast Surg 1966; 19: 276–278

Fujita S, Conway W, Zorick F, Roth T. Surgical correction of anatomic abnormalities in obstructive sleep apnea syndrome: uvulopalatopharyngoplasty. Otolaryngol Head Neck Surg 1981; 89: 923–934

Georgiou I, Farber N, Mendes D, Winkler E. The role of antibiotics in rhinoplasty and septoplasty: a literature review. Rhinology 2008; 46: 267–270

Gibson T, Davis WB. The distortion of autogenous cartilage grafts: its cause and prevention. Br J Plast Surg 1957; 10: 257–274

Goldman RB. New technique for corrective surgery of nasal tip. AMA Arch Otolaryngol 1953; 58: 183–187

Goodman WS. External approach to rhinoplasty. Can J Otolaryngol 1973; 2: 207–210

Gray LP. Deviated nasal septum. Incidence and etiology. Ann Otol Rhinol Laryngol 1978; 87: 3–20

Gray VD. Physiologic returning of the upper lateral cartilage. Int Rhinol 1970; 8: 56–59

Grützenmacher S, Lang C, Mlynski R, Mlynski B, Mlynski G. Long-term rhinoflowmetry: a new method for functional rhinologic diagnostics. Am J Rhinol 2005; 19: 53–57

Grymer LF, Hilberg O, Elbrønd O, Pedersen OF. Acoustic rhinometry: evaluation of the nasal cavity with septal deviations, before and after septoplasty. Laryngoscope 1989; 99: 1180–1187

Grymer LF, Illum P, Hilberg O. Septoplasty and compensatory inferior turbinate hypertrophy: a randomized study evaluated by acoustic rhinometry. J Laryngol Otol 1993; 107: 413–417

Grymer LF, Melsen B. The morphology of the nasal septum in identical twins. Laryngoscope 1989; 99: 642–646

Grymer LF, Pallisgaard C, Melsen B. The nasal septum in relation to the development of the nasomaxillary complex: a study in identical twins. Laryngoscope 1991; 101: 863–868

Grymer LF, Bosch C. The nasal septum and the development of the midface. A longitudinal study of a pair of monozygotic twins. Rhinology 1997; 35: 6–10

Gubisch W. The extracorporeal septum plasty: a technique to correct difficult nasal deformities. Plast Reconstr Surg 1995; 95: 672–682

Guiot G, Thibaut B, Borreau M. [Extirpation of hypophyseal adenomas by trans-septal and trans-sphenoidal approaches]. Ann Otolaryngol 1959; 76: 1017–1031

Gunter JP. Anatomical observations of the lower lateral cartilages. Arch Otolaryngol 1969; 89: 599–601

Gunter JP. Tip rhinoplasty: a personal approach. Facial Plast Surg 1987; 4: 263–275

Haavisto LE, Vahlberg TJ, Sipilä JI. Reference values for acoustic rhinometry in children at baseline and after decongestion. Rhinology 2011; 49: 243–247

Hafkamp HC, Bruintjes TD, Huizing EH. Functional anatomy of the premaxillary area. Rhinology 1999; 37: 21–24

Hage J. Collapsed alae strengthened by conchal cartilage (the butterfly cartilage graft). Br J Plast Surg 1965; 18: 92–96

Haight JSJ, Cole P. The site and function of the nasal valve. Laryngoscope 1983; 93: 49–55

Hasegawa M, Kern EB. Variations in nasal resistance (nasal cycle): does it influence the indications for surgery? Facial Plast Surg 1990; 7: 298–306

Hasegawa M, Kern EB. Variations in nasal resistance in man: a rhinomanometric study of the nasal cycle in 50 human subjects. Rhinology 1978; 16: 19–29

Heetderks DR. Observations on the reaction of the normal nasal mucous membrane. Am J Med Sci 1927; 174: 231–244

Heinberg CE, Kern EB. "Midcycle rest" and myocardial infarction. Rhinology 1974; 12: 39–42

Heinberg CE, Kern EB. The Cottle sign: an aid in the physical diagnosis of nasal airflow disturbances. Rhinology 1973; 11: 89–94

Helder AH, Huizing EH. Transplantation terminology in nasal surgery. Rhinology 1986; 24: 235–236

Hellings PW, Prokopakis EP. Global airway disease beyond allergy. Curr Allergy Asthma Rep 2010; 10: 143–149

Hellmich S, Hellmich J. [The intermaxillary bone and Goethe's Mephistopheles]. Laryngol Rhinol Otol (Stuttg) 1982; 61: 552–556

Hellmich S. Cartilage implants in rhinoplasty—problems and prospects. Rhinology 1972; 10: 1–8

Hellmich S. Die Therapie des frischen Septumabszesses. HNO 1974; 22: 278–281

Hellmich S. [Tolerance of preserved homoplastic cartilage implantations in the nose]. Z Laryngol Rhinol Otol 1970; 49: 742–749

Hellmich S. Die Verwendung von Kunstoff bei Nasenplastiken. Laryngol Rhinol Otol 1983; 62: 331–333

Hellmich S. Reconstruction of the destroyed septal infrastructure. Otolaryngol Head Neck Surg 1989; 100: 92–94

Hilberg O, Jackson AC, Swift DL, Pedersen OF. Acoustic rhinometry: evaluation of nasal cavity geometry by acoustic reflection. J Appl Physiol (1985) 1989; 66: 295–303

Hinderer KH. Surgery of the nasal valve. Int Rhinol 1970; 8: 60–67

Hinderer KH. Surgery of the retracted columella. Int Rhinol 1967; 5: 168

Hirsch O. Ueber Methoden der operativen Behandlung von Hypophysistumoren auf endonasalem Wege. Arch Laryngol Rhinol 1910; 24: 129–177

Hoffmann DF, Cook TA, Quatela VC, Wang TD, Brownrigg PJ, Brummett RE. Steroids and rhinoplasty. A double-blind study. Arch Otolaryngol Head Neck Surg 1991; 117: 990–993, discussion 994

Hol MK, Huizing EH. Treatment of inferior turbinate pathology: a review and critical evaluation of the different techniques. Rhinology 2000; 38: 157–166

Hörmann K, Verse T. Surgery for Sleep Disordered Breathing (2nd edition). Heidelberg: Springer; 2010

Howard DJ, Lund VJ. The role of midfacial degloving in modern rhinological practice. J Laryngol Otol 1999; 113: 885–887

Huffman WC, Lierle DM. The deviated nose. Ann Otol Rhinol Laryngol 1954; 63: 62–68

Huizing EH, Mackay IS, Rettinger G. Reconstruction of the nasal septum and dorsum by cartilage transplants—autogeneic or allogeneic? Rhinology 1989; 27: 5–10

Huizing EH, Pirsig W, Wentges R et al. Unanimity and diversity in nasal surgery. Rhinol Suppl 1989; 9: 15–23

Huizing EH. Clinical aspects of implants in functional corrective nasal surgery. In: Veldman JE, editors. Immunobiology, auto-immunity and transplantation in otorhinolaryngology. Amsterdam: Kugler; 1985

Huizing EH. Differential diagnosis of rhinopathy. Outlining of the subject. Acta Otorhinolaryngol Belg 1979; 33: 556–560

Huizing EH. Experience on the use of homologous cartilage in nasal surgery. Acta Otorhinolaryngol Belg 1970; 24: 194–197

Ingels KJ, Kortmann MJ, Nijziel MR, Graamans K, Huizing EH. Factors influencing ciliary beat measurements. Rhinology 1991; 29: 17–26

Huizing EH. Functional surgery in inflammation of the nose and paranasal sinuses. Rhinol Suppl 1988; 5: 5–15

Huizing EH. Implantation and transplantation in reconstructive nasal surgery. Rhinology 1974; 12: 93–106

Huizing EH. Incorrect terminology in nasal anatomy and surgery, suggestions for improvement. Rhinology 2003; 41: 129–133

Huizing EH. Long term results of reconstruction of the septum in the acute phase of a septal abscess in children. Rhinology 1984; 22: 55–63

Huizing EH. Medicolegal problems in otorhinolaryngology: how to prevent, how to deal with medicolegal aspects of euthanasia in the Netherlands. Sven ÖNH Tidskr 2001; 8: 14–17

Huizing EH. [Nose destruction following septum abscess: surgical prevention]. Ned Tijdschr Geneeskd 1985; 129: 577–579

Huizing EH. Nose and society. Rhinol Suppl 1988; 7: 9–38

Huizing EH. Pathophysiology of the ciliary epithelium. Int Rhinol 1967; 5: 73–78

Huizing EH. Push-down of the external nasal pyramid by resection of wedges. Rhinology 1975; 13: 185–190

Huizing EH. Rhinolalia aperta after adenotonsillectomy; treatment by nasopharyngeal implantation of Boplant (Squibb). Pr Oto Rhino Laryngol 1967; 29: 325–334

Huizing EH. Septal reconstruction in relation to function, form and growth of the nose. In: Myers E, editor. New Dimensions in Otorhinolaryngology—Head and Neck Surgery I. Amsterdam: Elsevier Science; 1985: 626–631

Huizing EH. Septum surgery in children; indications, surgical technique and long-term results. Rhinology 1979; 17: 91–100

Huizing EH. [Septum surgery in children]. Ned Tijdschr Geneeskd 1966; 110: 1293–1296

Huizing EH. Some conclusions from our experience with the surgical treatment of ozena. Int Rhinol 1969; 7: 81–87

Huizing EH. Surgery of the lateral nasal wall in atrophic rhinitis and ozena. Rhinology 1976; 14: 79–81

Huizing EH. Surgical drainage of the maxillary sinus. Rhinology 1981; 19: 3–5

Huizing EH. The first descriptions of cilia and ciliary movement by van Leeuwenhoek and de Heide. Rhinology 1973; 11: 128–135

Huizing EH. The management of septal abscess. Facial Plast Surg 1986; 3: 243–254

Hummel T, Sekinger B, Wolf SR, Pauli E, Kobal G. 'Sniffin' sticks': olfactory performance assessed by the combined testing of odor identification, odor discrimination and olfactory threshold. Chem Senses 1997; 22: 39–52

Ikematsu T. [Study of snoring. 4th report: Therapy]. J Jpn Otol Rhinol Laryngol Soc 1964; 64: 434–435

Ingels KJAO, Meeuwsen F, Graamans K, Huizing EH. Influence of sympathetic and parasympathetic substances in clinical concentrations on human nasal ciliary beat. Rhinology 1992; 30: 149–159

Ingels KJAO, Meeuwsen F, van Strien HLCJ, Graamans K, Huizing EH. Ciliary beat frequency and the nasal cycle. Eur Arch Otorhinolaryngol 1990; 248: 123–126

Ingels KJAO, Nijziel MR, Graamans K, Huizing EH. Influence of cocaine and lidocaine on human nasal cilia. Beat frequency and harmony in vitro. Arch Otolaryngol Head Neck Surg 1994; 120: 197–201

Ingels KJAO, van Strien HLCJ, Graamans K, Smoorenburg GF, Huizing EH. A study of the photoelectrical signal from human nasal cilia under several conditions. Acta Otolaryngol 1992; 112: 831–838

Janeke JB, Wright WK. Studies on the support of the nasal tip. Arch Otolaryngol 1971; 93: 458–464

Joseph J. Beitrage zur Rhinoplastik. Berl Klin Wochenschr 1907; 44: 470–472

Joseph J. Die Korrektur der Schiefnase. Dtsch Med Wochenschr 1907; 33: 2033–2040

Joseph J. Intranasale Nasenhöckerabtragung. Berl Klin Wochenschr 1904; 41: 650

Joseph J. Nasenverkleinerungen. Dtsch Med Wochenschr 1904; 30: 1095–1098

Joseph J. Über einige weitere operative Nasenverkleinerungen. Berl Klin Wochenschr 1902; 39: 851–853

Joseph J. Weiteres über Nasenverkleinerung. Münch Med Wochenschr 1905; 52: 1489–1490

Jost G, Levet Y. Parotid fascia and face lifting: a critical evaluation of the SMAS concept. Plast Reconstr Surg 1984; 74: 42–51

Jost G. Mode de suture au cours des rhinoplasties suivant la technique extramuqueuse. Ann Chir Plast 1973; 18: 271

Kamer FM, Churukian MM. Shield graft for the nasal tip. Arch Otolaryngol 1984; 110: 608–610

Kasperbauer JL, Kern EB. Nasal valve physiology. Implications in nasal surgery. Otolaryngol Clin North Am 1987; 20: 699–719

Kayser R. Die exakte Messung der Luftdurchgängigkeit der Nase. Arch Laryngol Rhinol 1895; 3: 101–120

Keck T, Leiacker R, Klotz M, Lindemann J, Riechelmann H, Rettinger G. Detection of particles within the nasal airways during respiration. Eur Arch Otorhinolaryngol 2000; 257: 493–497

Keck T, Leiacker R, Kühnemann S, Rettinger G, Lindemann J. Detection of particles within the nasal airways before and after nasal decongestion. Clin Otolaryngol Allied Sci 2001; 26: 324–328

Keck T, Leiacker R, Lindemann J, Rettinger G, Kühnemann S. [Endonasal temperature and humidity profile after exposure to various climate-controlled inspiratory air] HNO 2001; 49: 372–377

Keck T, Leiacker R, Riechelmann H, Rettinger G. Temperature profile in the nasal cavity. Laryngoscope 2000; 110: 651–654

Keck T, Lindemann J. [Simulation and air-conditioning in the nose] Laryngorhinootologie 2010; 89 Suppl 1: S1–S14

Kennedy DW. Functional endoscopic sinus surgery. Technique. Arch Otolaryngol 1985; 111: 643–649

Kern EB, Laws ER. The transseptal approach to the pituitary gland. Rhinology 1978; 16: 59–78

Kern EB. Rhinomanometry. Otolaryngol Clin North Am 1973; 6: 863–874

Kern EB. Standardization of rhinomanometry. Rhinology 1977; 15: 115–119

Kern EB. Surgical approaches to abnormalities of the nasal valve. Rhinology 1978; 16: 165–189

Keuning J. On the nasal cycle. Int Rhinol 1968; 6: 99–136

Kiesselbach W. Ueber Nasenbluten. Wien Med Zt; 1885: 501

Killian G. Die submuköse Fensterresektion der Nasenscheidewand. Arch Laryngol Rhinol 1904; 16: 362–387

Killian G. The submucous window resection of the nasal septum. Ann Otol Rhinol Laryngol 1905; 14: 363–393

Kittel H, Masing H. Corticosteroid therapy in rhinoplasty. Rhinology 1976; 14: 163–166

Klaff DD. The surgical anatomy of the antero-caudal portion of the nasal septum: a study of the area of the premaxilla. Laryngoscope 1956; 66: 995–1020

Kobal G, Hummel T, Sekinger B, Barz S, Roscher S, Wolf S. "Sniffin' sticks": screening of olfactory performance. Rhinology 1996; 34: 222–226

Knussmann R. Anthropologie. Stuttgart: Gustav Fischer Verlag; 1988

Kuhlo WE, Doll E, Franck MC. [Successful management of Pickwickian syndrome using long-term tracheostomy]. Dtsch Med Wochenschr 1969; 94: 1286–1290

Lang J. Klinische Anatomie der Nase, Nasenhöhle und Nebenhöhlen. Stuttgart: Thieme; 1988.

Lautenschläger A. Die Heilung der Ozaena auf operativem Wege. Klin Wochenschr 1926; 5: 322–325

Lenders H, Pirsig W. Diagnostic value of acoustic rhinometry: patients with allergic and vasomotor rhinitis compared with normal controls. Rhinology 1990; 28: 5–16

Leong SC, Farmer SEJ, Eccles R. Coblation® inferior turbinate reduction: a long-term follow-up with subjective and objective assessment. Rhinology 2010; 48: 108–112

Letourneau A, Daniel RK. The superficial musculoaponeurotic system of the nose. Plast Reconstr Surg 1988; 82: 48–57

Lilja M, Mäkitie AA, Anttila VJ, Kuusela P, Pietola M, Hytönen M. Cefuroxime as a prophylactic preoperative antibiotic in septoplasty. A double blind randomized placebo controlled study. Rhinology 2011; 49: 58–63

Lindemann J, Keck T, Wiesmiller KM et al. Nasal air temperature and airflow during respiration in numerical simulation based on multislice computed tomography scan. Am J Rhinol 2006; 20: 219–223

Lindemann J, Keck T, Wiesmiller K, Rettinger G, Brambs HJ, Pless D. Numerical simulation of intranasal air flow and temperature after resection of the turbinates. Rhinology 2005; 43: 24–28

Lindemann J, Leiacker R, Rettinger G, Keck T. Nasal mucosal temperature during respiration. Clin Otolaryngol Allied Sci 2002; 27: 135–139

Lindemann J, Tsakiropoulou E, Keck T, Leiacker R, Wiesmiller KM. Nasal air conditioning in relation to acoustic rhinometry values. Am J Rhinol Allergy 2009; 23: 575–577

Lindemann J, Tsakiropoulou E, Scheithauer MO, Konstantinidis I, Wiesmiller KM. Impact of menthol inhalation on nasal mucosal temperature and nasal patency. Am J Rhinol 2008; 22: 402–405

Lohuis PJFM, Watts SJ, Vuyk HD. Augmentation of the nasal dorsum using Gore-Tex: intermediate results of a retrospective analysis of experience in 66 patients. Clin Otolaryngol Allied Sci 2001; 26: 214–217

Van Loosen J, Van Zanten GA, Howard CV, Verwoerd-Verhoef HL, Van Velzen D, Verwoerd CD. Growth characteristics of the human nasal septum. Rhinology 1996; 34: 78–82

Lund VJ. Fundamental considerations of the design and function of intranasal antrostomies. Rhinology 1985; 23: 231–236

Mabry RL. "How I do it" — plastic surgery. Practical suggestions on facial plastic surgery. Inferior turbinoplasty. Laryngoscope 1982; 92: 459–461

Malm L, Gerth van Wijk R, Bachert C. Guidelines for nasal provocations with aspects on nasal patency, airflow, and airflow resistance. International Committee on Objective Assessment of the Nasal Airways, International Rhinologic Society. Rhinology 2000; 38: 1–6

Malm L. Resistance and capacitance vessels in the nasal mucosa. Rhinology 1975; 13: 85–89

Masing H, Hellmich S. [Experience with preserved cartilage in nasal reconstruction]. Z Laryngol Rhinol Otol 1968; 47: 904–914

Masing H. Eingriffe an der Nasenscheidewand. In: Naumann HH, editor. Kopf- und Hals- Chirurgie. Stuttgart: Thieme; 1974

Masing H. [Experimental studies on the flow in a nose model]. Arch Klin Exp Ohren Nasen Kehlkopfheilkd 1967; 189: 371–381

Masing H. [On plastic surgery of hematomas and abscesses of the septum]. HNO 1965; 13: 235–238

Mc Caffrey TV, Kern EB. Rhinomanometry. Facial Plast Surg 1986; 3: 217–223

Mendelsohn M, Farrell M. The aesthetic nose: do we agree? J Otolaryngol 1995; 24: 358–361

Messerklinger W. [The ethmoidal infundibulum and its inflammatory illnesses]. Arch Otorhinolaryngol 1979; 222: 11–22

Messerklinger W. Endoscopy of the nose. Baltimore-München: Urban & Schwarzenberg; 1978

Messerklinger W. [Technics and possibilities of nasal endoscopy] HNO 1972; 20: 133–135

Metzenbaum M. Nasal reconstruction by means of the bone and cartilage existing within the old traumatized nose. The Laryngoscope 1930; 40: 488–494

Metzenbaum M. Replacement of the lower end of the dislocated septal cartilage versus submucous resection of the dislocated end of the septal cartilage. Arch Otolaryngol 1929; 9: 282–296

Mink PJ. De neus als luchtweg. Geneeskd Bl 1902; 9: 75–115

Mink PJ. Le nez comme voie respiratoire. Presse Otolaryng Belg 1903; 21: 481–496

Mink PJ. Physiologie der obern? Of obere Luftwege. Würzburg: Verlag F Vogel; 1920

Mladina R. The role of maxillar morphology in the development of pathological septal deformities. Rhinology 1987; 25: 199–205

Mlynski G, Grützenmacher S, Plontke S, Mlynski B, Lang C. Correlation of nasal morphology and respiratory function. Rhinology 2001; 39: 197–201

Mlynski G, Beule A. [Diagnostic methods of nasal respiratory function]. HNO 2008; 56: 81–99

Mueller C, Renner B. A new procedure for the short screening of olfactory function using five items from the "Sniffin' Sticks" identification test kit. Am J Rhinol 2006; 20: 113–116

Nolst Trenité GJ, Verwoerd CDA, Verwoerd-Verhoef HL. Reimplantation of autologous septal cartilage in the growing nasal septum. I. The influence of resection and reimplantation of septal cartilage upon nasal growth: an experimental study in rabbits. Rhinology 1987; 25: 225–236

Nolst Trenité GJ, Verwoerd CD, Verwoerd-Verhoef HL. Reimplantation of autologous septal cartilage in the growing nasal septum. II. The influence of reimplantation of rotated or crushed autologous septal cartilage on nasal growth: an experimental study in growing rabbits. Rhinology 1988; 26: 25–32

Nolst Trenité GJ. Trauma reduction in rhinoplastic surgery. Rhinology 1991; 29: 111–116

Ombrédanne M. Les déviations traumatiques de la cloison chez l'enfant avec obstruction nasale Traitement chirugical et resultants eloignés. Arch Fr Pediatr 1942; 1: 20–26

Padovan IF. External approach in rhinoplasty (decortication). In: Conley J, Dickinson JT, editors. Plastic Reconstructive Surgery of the Face and Neck. Vol 1. Stuttgart: Thieme; 1972: 143–146

Padovan IF. External approach in rhinoplasty (decortication). Symp Otol Rhinol Laryngol Jug 1960; 3/4: 354–360

Pallanch JF, Facer GW, Kern EB, Westwood WB. Prosthetic closure of nasal septum perforations. Otolaryngol Head Neck Surg 1982; 90: 448–452

Papel ID, Ed. Facial Plastic and Reconstructive Surgery 3rd Edition. New York: Thieme; 2009: 127–128

Passàli D, Lauriello M, Anselmi M, Bellussi L. Treatment of hypertrophy of the inferior turbinate: long-term results in 382 patients randomly assigned to therapy. Ann Otol Rhinol Laryngol 1999; 108: 569–575

Peck GC. The onlay graft for nasal tip projection. Plast Reconstr Surg 1983; 71: 27–39

Pedersen OF, Hilberg O. Acoustic rhinometry – standardisation and use. Rhinol Suppl 2000; 16: 1–64

Peer LA. An operation to repair lateral displacement of the lower border of the septal cartilage. Arch Otolaryngol 1937; 25: 475–477

Pentz S, Pirsig W, Lenders H. Long-term results of neonates with nasal deviation: a prospective study over 12 years. Int J Pediatr Otorhinolaryngol 1994; 28: 183–191

Peter K. Atlas der Entwicklung der Nase und des Gaumens beim Menschen mit Einschluss der Entwicklungsstörungen. Jena: Gustav Fisher; 1913

Petruson B. Improvement of the nasal airflow by the nasal dilator Nozovent. Rhinology 1988; 26: 289–292

Philippou M, Stenger GM, Goumas PD, Hillen B, Huizing EH. Cross-sectional anatomy of the nose and paranasal sinuses. A correlative study of computer tomographic images and cryosections. Rhinology 1990; 28: 221–230

Picavet VA, Prokopakis EP, Gabriëls L, Jorissen M, Hellings PW. High prevalence of body dysmorphic disorder symptoms in patients seeking rhinoplasty. Plast Reconstr Surg 2011; 128: 509–517

Pirsig W, Bean JK, Lenders H, Verwoerd CDA, Verwoerd-Verhoef HL. Cartilage transformation in a composite graft of demineralized bovine bone matrix and ear perichondrium used in a child for the reconstruction of the nasal septum. Int J Pediatr Otorhinolaryngol 1995; 32: 171–181

Pirsig W, Haase St. [Phases of postnatal nasal growth. A critical review]. Laryngol Rhinol Otol (Stuttg) 1986; 65: 243–249

Pirsig W, Kern EB, Verse T. Reconstruction of anterior nasal septum: back-to-back autogenous ear cartilage graft. Laryngoscope 2004; 114: 627–638

Pirsig W, Knahl R. [Rhinoplasty in children: a follow-up study in 92 cases]. Laryngol Rhinol Otol (Stuttg) 1974; 53: 250–265

Pirsig W, Königs D. Wedge resection in rhinosurgery: a review of the literature and long-term results in a hundred cases. Rhinology 1988; 26: 77–88

Pirsig W, Lehmann I. The influence of trauma on the growing septal cartilage. Rhinology 1975; 13: 39–46

Pirsig W, Schäfer J. The importance of antibiotic treatment in functional and aesthetic rhinosurgery. Rhinol Suppl 1988; 4: 3–11

Pirsig W. Clinical aspects of the fractured growing nose. Rhinology 1983; 21: 107–110

Pirsig W. [Nasal deformities in the newborn]. HNO 1974; 22: 1–5

Pirsig W. [Regeneration of septal cartilage in children after septoplasty. A histological study]. Acta Otolaryngol 1975; 79: 451–459

Pirsig W. Growth of the deviated septum and its influence on midfacial development. Facial Plast Surg 1992; 8: 224–232

Pirsig W. Historical notes and actual observations on the nasal septal abscess especially in children. Int J Pediatr Otorhinolaryngol 1984; 8: 43–54

Pirsig W. Morphologic aspects of the injured nasal septum in children. Rhinology 1979; 17: 65–75

Pirsig W. Open questions in nasal surgery in children. Rhinology 1986; 24: 37–40

Pirsig W. Operative Eingriffe an der kindlichen Nase. In: Berendes J, Link R, Zöllner F, editors. Hals- Nasen- Ohrenheilkunde im Praxis und Klinik. Vol 2. Stuttgart: Thieme; 1977: 28–39

Pirsig W. Reduction of the middle turbinate. Rhinology 1972; 10: 103–108

Pirsig W. Septal plasty in children: influence on nasal growth. Rhinology 1977; 15: 193–204

Pirsig W. [Septum deviation 1882: beginning of systematic submucous septum surgery] Laryngol Rhinol Otol (Stuttg) 1982; 61: 547–551

Pirsig W. Zur Chirurgie der Nase im Kindesalter: Wachstum und Spätergebnisse [Surgery of the nose in childhood: growth and late results.]. Laryngol Rhinol Otol (Stuttg) 1984; 63: 170–180

Ponikau JU, Sherris DA, Kern EB et al. The diagnosis and incidence of allergic fungal sinusitis. Mayo Clin Proc 1999; 74: 877–884

Popko M, Bleys RLAW, De Groot JW, Huizing EH. Histological structure of the nasal cartilages and their perichondrial envelope. I. The septal and lobular cartilage. Rhinology 2007; 45: 148–152

Poublon RML, Verwoerd CDA, Verwoerd-Verhoef HL. Anatomy of the upper lateral cartilages in the human newborn. Rhinology 1990; 28: 41–45

Powell NB, Zonato AI, Weaver EM et al. Radiofrequency treatment of turbinate hypertrophy in subjects using continuous positive airway pressure: a randomized, double-blind, placebo-controlled clinical pilot trial. Laryngoscope 2001; 111: 1783–1790

Proctor DF, Hardy JB. Studies of respiratory air flow; significance of the normal pneumotachogram. Bull Johns Hopkins Hosp 1949; 85: 253–280

Proetz AW. Air currents in the upper respiratory tract and their clinical importance. Ann Otol Rhinol Laryngol. 1951; 60: 439–467

Proetz AW. Applied Physiology of the Nose 2nd Edition. St Louis: Annals Publishing Company; 1941

Rappai M, Collop N, Kemp S, deShazo R. The nose and sleep-disordered breathing: what we know and what we do not know. Chest 2003; 124: 2309–2323

Rethi A. Operation to shorten an excessively long nose. Rev Chir Plast 1934; 2: 85–87

Rethi A. Ueber die korrektiven Operationen der Nasendeformitäten. Chirurg 1929; 1: 1103–1113

Rettinger G, Engelbrecht-Schnür S. [Sensory impairment of palatine mucosa following septoplasty]. Laryngol Rhinol Otol 1995; 74: 282–285

Rettinger G, Masing H. Rotation of the alar cartilage in collapsed alae. Rhinol 1981; 19: 81–86

Rettinger G, O'Connell M. The nasal base in cleft lip rhinoplasty. Facial Plast Surg 2002; 18: 165–178

Rettinger G. Three-step reconstruction of saddle nose deformities. In: Nolst Trenité GJ, editor. Rhinoplasty. A Practical Guide to Functional and Aesthetic Surgery of the Nose. Amsterdam: Kugler; 1993: 139–148

Evans PH, Brain DJ. The influence of nasal osteotomies and septum surgery on the growth of the rabbit snout. J Laryngol Otol 1981; 95: 1109–1119

Riechelmann H, Karow E, DiDio D, Kral F. External nasal valve collapse – a case-control and interventional study employing a novel internal nasal dilator (Nasanita). Rhinology 2010; 48: 183–188

Robin JL. [Controlled extra-mucosal rhinoplasty with pre-operative measurement of profile modification]. Ann Chir Plast 1973; 18: 119–131

Roe JO. The correction of nasal deformities. Laryngoscope 1908; 18: 782

Roe JO. The deformity termed "pug nose" and its correction by a simple operation. Med Rec 1887; 31: 621. [Reprinted in Aesth Plast Surg 1986; 10: 89–91.]

Rombaux P, Liistro G, Hamoir M et al. Nasal obstruction and its impact on sleep-related breathing disorders. Rhinology 2005; 43: 242–250

Sailer HF. Transplantation of Lyophilized Cartilage in Maxillofacial Surgery. Experimental Foundations and Clinical Success. New York: Kargel; 1983

Sarnat BG, Wexler MR. Growth of the face and jaws after resection of the septal cartilage in the rabbit. Am J Anat 1966; 118: 755–767

Sarnat BG, Wexler MR. Rabbit snout growth after resection of central linear segments of nasal septal cartilage. Acta Otolaryngol 1967; 63: 467–478

Scadding G, Hellings P, Alobid I et al. Diagnostic tools in Rhinology EAACI position paper. Clin Transl Allergy 2011; 1: 2

Schäfer J, Pirsig W. [Preventive antibiotic administration in complicated rhinosurgical interventions—a double-blind study]. Laryngol Rhinol Otol (Stuttg) 1988; 67: 150–155

Schendel SA. Cephalometric analyses. In: Bell WH, editor. Modern Practice in Orthognathic and Reconstructive Surgery. Philadelphia, Pa.: Saunders; 1992

Schuil PJ. Effects of Mediators and Neuropeptides on Human Upper Respiratory Cilia [Thesis]. Utrecht; 1994

Schultz-Coulon HJ. Three-layer repair of nasoseptal defects. Otolaryngol Head Neck Surg 2005; 132: 213–218

Schwab JA, Pirsig W. Complications of septal surgery. Facial Plast Surg 1997; 13: 3–14

Scott JH. The cartilage of the nasal septum: A contribution to the study of facial growth. Br Dent J 1953; 95: 37–43

Šercer A. Dekortikation der Nase. Chir Maxillofac Plast (Zagreb) 1958; 1: 149–152

Šercer A. Die Dekortikation der Nase. In: Sercer A, Mündnich K, editors. Plastische Operationen an der Nase und an der Ohrmuschel. Stuttgart: Thieme; 1962

Shaida AM, Kenyon GS. The nasal valves: changes in anatomy and physiology in normal subjects. Rhinology 2000; 38: 7–12

Sheen JH. Spreader graft: a method of reconstructing the roof of the middle nasal vault following rhinoplasty. Plast Reconstr Surg 1984; 73: 230–239

Sherris DA, Kern EB. The versatile autogenous rib graft in septorhinoplasty. Am J Rhinol 1998; 12: 221–227

Sluder G. Etiology, diagnosis, prognosis and the treatment of sphenopalatine ganglion neuralgia. JAMA 1913; 61: 1201–1206

Sluder G. The role of the sphenopalatine (or Meckel's) ganglion in nasal headaches. N Y Med J 1908; 87: 989–990

Spoor A. A new method for measuring nasal conductivity. Int Rhinol 1965; 3: 27–35

Stammberger H. Endoscopic endonasal surgery—concepts in treatment of recurring rhinosinusitis. Part I. Anatomic and pathophysiologic considerations. Otolaryngol Head Neck Surg 1986; 94: 143–147

Stammberger H. [Personal endoscopic operative technic for the lateral nasal wall—an endoscopic surgery concept in the treatment of inflammatory diseases of the paranasal sinuses]. Laryngol Rhinol Otol (Stuttg) 1985; 64: 559–566

Stoksted P. The physiologic cycle of the nose under normal and pathologic conditions. Acta Otolaryngol 1952; 42: 175–179

Straatman NJA, Buiter CT. Endoscopic surgery of the nasal fontanel. A new approach to recurrent sinusitis. Arch Otolaryngol 1981; 107: 290–293

Sugiura T, Noda A, Nakata S et al. Influence of nasal resistance on initial acceptance of continuous positive airway pressure in treatment for obstructive sleep apnea syndrome. Respiration 2007; 74: 56–60

Sullivan CE, Issa FG, Berthon-Jones M, Eves L. Reversal of obstructive sleep apnoea by continuous positive airway pressure applied through the nares. Lancet 1981; 1: 862–865

Sulsenti G, Palma P. A new technique for functional surgery of the nasal valve area. Rhinol Suppl 1989; 10: 1–19

Sulsenti G. Chirurgia Funzionale ed Estetica del Naso. 1st ed. Bologna: Officine Grafiche Arsitalia; 1972

Tanner JM, Davies PSW. Clinical longitudinal standards for height and height velocity for North American children. J Pediatr 1985; 107: 317–329

Tardy ME, Denneny JC. Micro-osteotomies in rhinoplasty. Facial Plast Surg 1984; 1: 137–145

Tardy ME. Transdomal suture refinement of the nasal tip. Facial Plast Surg 1987; 4: 317

Tasman AJ, Lohuis PJ. Control of tip rotation. Facial Plast Surg 2012; 28: 243–250

Tomkinson A, Eccles R. Acoustic rhinometry: an explanation of some common artefacts associated with nasal decongestion. Clin Otolaryngol Allied Sci 1998; 23: 20–26

Tonndorf J. Der Weg der Atemluft in der menschlichen Nase. Arch Ohr Nas Kehlk Heilk 1939; 146: 41–63

Tos M. Goblet cells and glands in the nose and paranasal sinuses. In: Proctor DF, Anderson I, editors. The Nose—Upper Airway Physiology and the Atmospheric Environment. Amsterdam: Elsevier Science; 1982

Tos M. Mucous elements in the airways. Acta Otolaryngol 1976; 82: 249–251

Trendelenburg F. Ueber die operative Behandlung schiefer Nasen. Verhandl Dtsch Gesell Chir 1889; 19: 82

Uddströmer M. L'importance des cornets pour la résistance dans le nez normal. Acta Otolaryngol 1940; 28: 364–375

Uddströmer M. Nasal respiration: critical survey of some of the current physiological and clinical aspects of respiratory mechanism with description of new methods of diagnosis. Acta Otolaryngol Suppl 1940; 42: 1–46

Unterberger S. Ozaena und gewöhnliche Schrumpfnase Behandlung mit Spongiosa uberplantzung aus dem Darmbeinkamm. Z Hals Nas Ohrenhlk 1929; 23: 346–359

Van Gerven L, Boeckxstaens G, Hellings PW. Up-date on neuro-immune mechanisms involved in allergic and non-allergic rhinitis. Rhinology 2012; 50: 227–235

van Spronsen E, Ebbens FA, Fokkens WJ. Normal peak nasal inspiratory flow rate values in healthy children aged 6 to 11 years in the Netherlands. Rhinology 2012; 50: 22–25

Vase P, Johannessen J. Homograft cartilage in the treatment of an abscess in the nasal septum. J Laryngol Otol 1981; 95: 357–359

Verse T, Maurer JT, Pirsig W. Effect of nasal surgery on sleep-related breathing disorders. Laryngoscope 2002; 112: 64–68

Verse T, Pirsig W. Nasal surgery. In: Hörmann K, Verse T, eds. Surgery for Sleep Disordered Breathing, 2nd ed. Berlin, Heidelberg: Springer; 2010: 25–31

Verse T, Pirsig W. Impact of impaired nasal breathing on sleep-disordered breathing. Sleep Breath 2003; 7: 63–76

Verwoerd CDA, Urbanus NAM, Mastenbroek GJ. The influence of partial resections of the nasal septal cartilage on the growth of the upper jaw and the nose: an experimental study in rabbits. Clin Otolaryngol Allied Sci 1980; 5: 291–302

Verwoerd CDA, Urbanus NAM, Nijdam DC. The effects of septal surgery on the growth of nose and maxilla. Rhinology 1979; 17: 53–63

Verwoerd CDA, Verwoerd-Verhoef HL, Meeuwis CA, vd Heul RO. Wound healing of the nasal septal perichondrium in young rabbits. ORL J Otorhinolaryngol Relat Spec 1990; 52: 180–186

Verwoerd CDA, Verwoerd-Verhoef HL, Meeuwis CA, van der Heul RO. Wound healing of autologous implants in the nasal septal cartilage. ORL J Otorhinolaryngol Relat Spec 1991; 53: 310–314

Verwoerd CDA, Verwoerd-Verhoef HL. Developmental aspects of the deviated nose. Facial Plast Surg 1989; 6: 95–100

Verwoerd CDA, Verwoerd-Verhoef HL. Rhinochirugie bei Kindern: Entwicklungsphysiologische und chirurgische Aspekte der wachsenden Nase. Rhinosurgery in children: developmental and surgical aspects of the growing nose. Laryngo-Rhino-Otol 2010; 89 Suppl 1: S46–S71

Verwoerd CDA, Verwoerd-Verhoef HL. Rhinosurgery in children: surgical and developmental aspects. In: Nolst Trenité GJ, editor. Rhinoplasty. Amsterdam: Kugler; 1993: 149–156

Vuyk HD, Adamson PA. Biomaterials in rhinoplasty. Clin Otolaryngol Allied Sci 1998; 23: 209–217

Vuyk HD. Augmentation mentoplasty with solid silicone. Clin Otolaryngol Allied Sci 1996; 21: 106–118

Walter CD. Composite grafts in nasal surgery. Arch Otolaryngol 1969; 90: 622–630

Ward BB, Feinberg SE, Friedman CD. Tissue matrices for soft tissue and mucosal augmentation and replacement. Facial Plast Surg 2002; 18: 3–11

Weimert TA, Yoder MG. Antibiotics and nasal surgery. Laryngoscope 1980; 90: 667–672

Weir R. Operations for deformities of the nose. N Y Med J 1880; 31: 203–204

Wexler DB, Davidson TM. The nasal valve: a review of the anatomy, imaging, and physiology. Am J Rhinol 2004; 18: 143–150

Wigand ME, Steiner W. [Endonasal antrostomy with endoscopical control for chronic maxillary sinusitis]. Laryngol Rhinol Otol (Stuttg) 1977; 56: 421–425

Wigand ME. Endoskopische Chirurgie der Nasennebenhöhlen und der vorderen Schädelbasis. Stuttgart: Thieme; 1989

Wigand ME. Transnasal ethmoidectomy under endoscopical control. Rhinology 1981; 19: 7–15

Williams HL. The nose as form and function. Ann Otol Rhinol Laryngol 1969; 78: 725–740

De Wit G, Kapteyn TS, van Bochove W. Some remarks on the physiology, the anatomy and the radiology of the vestibulum and the isthmus nasi. Int Rhinol 1965; 3: 37–42

Wustrow F. Schwellkörper am Septum Nasi. Z Anat Entwickl Gesch 1951; 116: 139–142

Zeng B, Ng AT, Qian J, Petocz P, Darendeliler MA, Cistulli PA. Influence of nasal resistance on oral appliance treatment outcome in obstructive sleep apnea. Sleep 2008; 31: 543–547

Zhai L, Bruintjes TD, Hofstee MWA, Huizing EH. Anatomical observations on the attachments of the medial crura. Am J Rhinology 1996; 10: 327–330

Zhai LJ, Bruintjes TD, Boschma T, Huizing EH. The interdomal ligament does not exist. Rhinology 1995; 33: 135–137

Zuckerkandl E. Normale und pathologische Anatomie der Nasenhöhle und ihrer pneumatische Anhänge. Vol I. 2nd ed. Vienna: Braumüller; 1882

Zuckerkandl E. Normale und pathologische Anatomie der Nasenhöhle und ihrer pneumatische Anhänge. Vol II. Vienna: Braumüller; 1892

Zwaardemaker H. Athembeschlag als Hilfsmittel zur Diagnose der nasalen Stenose. Arch Laryngol Rhinol 1894; 2: 174–177

10.6.2 Textbooks and Major Chapters on Nasal Surgery in Chronologic Order

This list presents an overview of textbooks and major chapters on nasal surgery known to the authors. They are here presented in chronological order to illustrate the development of the specialty.

1800–1850

von Graefe CF. Rhinoplastik oder die Kunst den Verlust der Nase organisch zu ersetzen. Berlin: Realschulbuch; 1818

Delpech JM. Chirurgie clinique de Montpellier. Vols 1 and 2. Paris: Gabon; 1823

Dieffenbach JF. Surgical Observations on the restoration of the nose. [Translation from the German by John Stevenson Bushnan]. London: S Highly; 1833

Fritze HE, Reich OFG. Die Plastische Chirurgie in ihrem weitesten Umfang dargestellt. Berlin: A. Hirschwald; 1845.

Dieffenbach JF. Die Operative Chirurgie. Leipzig: Brockhaus; 1845

1850–1900

Mackenzie M. A Manual of Diseases of the Throat and Nose. Vol 2. Berlin: August Hirschwald; 1880

1900–1920

von Bergmann E. Verletzungen der Nase, Frakturen und Dislokationen. In: Heymann P, editor. Handbuch der Laryngologie und Rhinologie. Vol 3. Vienna: Alfred Hölder; 1900: 507

Lange V. Die Erkrankungen der Nasescheidewand. In: Heymann P, editor. Handbuch der Laryngologie und Rhinologie. Vol 3. Vienna: Alfred Hölder; 1900: 439

Nelaton C, Ombrédanne L. La Rhinoplastie. Paris: G. Steinheil; 1904

Joseph J. Korrektive Nasen- und Ohrenplastik. In: Katz L, Preysing H, Blumenfeld F, editors. Handbuch der speziellen Chirurgie des Ohres und der oberen Luftwege. Vol I. Leipzig: Curt Kabitsch; 1912: 124–176

1920–1940

Gillies H. Plastic Surgery of the Face. London: Frowde, Hodder & Stoughton; 1920

Passow A. Die Erkrankungen der Nasenscheidewand mit Anhang das Ansaugen der Nasenflügel von A Brüggemann. In: Denker A, Kahler O, editors. Handbuch der Hals-Nasen-Ohren-Heilkunde. Vol 2. Berlin: Springer; 1926: 444–522

Joseph J. Nasenplastik und sonstige Gesichtsplastik nebst ein Anhang über Mammaplastik. Leipzig: Curt Kabitsch; 1931

Safian J. Corrective Rhinoplastic Surgery. New York: Hoeber; 1935

Seiffert A. Die Operationen am Nase, Mund und Hals. Leipzig: Curt Kabitsch; 1936

Fomon S. Surgery of Injury and Plastic Repair. Baltimore, Md.: Williams & Wilkins; 1939

1940–1960

Aubry M, Freidel C. Chirurgie de la face et de la région maxillo-faciale. Paris: Masson ed.; 1942

Padget EC. Plastic and Reconstructive Surgery. Oxford: Blackwell Science; 1948.

Seltzer AP. Plastic Surgery of the Nose. Lippincott Cie; 1949

Ferris Smyth J. Plastic and Reconstructive Surgery. Philadelphia, Pa.: Saunders; 1950

Brown JB, McDowell F. Plastic Surgery of the Nose. St. Louis: Mosby; 1951

Aubry M, et al. Chirurgie Fonctionelle et Restauratrice du Nez. Paris: Arnette; 1957

Dufourmentel C, Mouly R. Chirurgie Plastique. Paris: Flammarion; 1959

1960–1980

Cottle MH. Corrective Surgery: Nasal Septum and External Pyramid. Chicago: Am Rhinol Soc; 1960

Šerçer A, Mündnich K. Plastische Operationen an der Nase und an der Ohrmuschel. Stuttgart: Thieme; 1962

Converse JM. Reconstructive Plastic Surgery. Vol 1. Philadelphia, Pa.: Saunders; 1964

Denecke HJ, Mayer R. Plastische Operationen am Kopf und Hals. Korrigierende und Rekonstruktive Nasenplastik. Berlin: Springer; 1964

Fomon S, Bell J. Rhinoplasty: New Concepts. Evaluation and Application. Springfield, Ill.: Thomas; 1970

Hinderer KH. Fundamentals of Anatomy and Surgery of the Nose. Birmingham, Ala.: Aesculapius Pub Co; 1971

Masing H. Die Chirurgie der äusseren Nase und der Nasenscheidewand. In: Theissing G, editor. Kurze HNO-Operationslehre. Stuttgart: Thieme; 1971

Sulsenti G. Chirurgia Funzionale ed Estetica del Naso. 1st ed. Bologna: Officine Grafiche Arsitalia; 1972. 2nd ed. Milano: Ghedini Editore; 1992

Huizing EH, Sedee GA, Wentges RThR. Correctieve Neuschirurgie. Report of the Netherlands Society of ORL. ORL 1973: 1–147

Rees TD, Woodsmith D. Cosmetic Plastic Surgery. Philadelphia, Pa.: WB Saunders; 1973

Kazanjian VH, Converse JM. Surgical Treatment of Facial Injuries. 3rd ed. Baltimore, Md.: Williams & Wilkins; 1974

Masing H. Eingriffe an der Nasenscheidewand. In: Naumann HH, editor. Kopf- und Hals Chirurgie. Stuttgart: Thieme; 1974

Skoog T. Plastic Surgery. Philadelphia, Pa.: WB Saunders; 1974

Pirsig W. Operative Eingriffe an der kindlichen Nase. In: Berendes J, Link R, Zöllner F, editors. Hals- Nasen- Ohrenheilkunde im Praxis und Klinik. Vol 2. Stuttgart: Thieme; 1977: 28–39

1980–1990

Rees TD. Aesthetic Plastic Surgery. Philadelphia, Pa.: WB Saunders; 1980

Fritz K. Funktionelle Methoden der Aesthetischen Gesichtschirurgie. Leipzig: Barth; 1981

Denecke HJ, Ey W. Die Operationen an der Nase und im Nasopharynx. Berlin: Springer; 1984

Meyer R. Aesthetic Plastic Surgery. Boston: Little, Brown; 1984

Micheli Pellegrini V. Il Naso Torto. Padua: Ed. Garigliano; 1985

Anderson JR, Ries WR. Rhinoplasty: Emphasing the External Approach. New York: Thieme-Stratton; 1986

Jeppesen F. Septo- and Rhinoplasty. Copenhagen: Munksgaard; 1986

Sheen JH, Sheen AP. Aesthetic Rhinoplasty. 2nd ed. St. Louis: Mosby; 1987

Jost G. Atlas de Chirurgie Esthétique Plastique. 2nd ed. Paris: Masson; 1988

Masing H, Rettinger G. Eingriffe an der Nase. In: Theissing J, editor. Mund-, Hals- und Nasenoperationen. 2nd ed. Stuttgart: Thieme; 1988.

Meyer R. Secondary and Functional Rhinoplasty: The Difficult Nose. Orlando: Grune & Stratton; 1988

Berman WE, editor. Rhinoplastic Surgery. St. Louis: Mosby; 1989

McKinney P, Cunningham BL. Rhinoplasty. New York: Churchill Livingstone; 1989

1990–2000

Johnson CM, Toriumi DM. Open Structure Rhinoplasty. Philadelphia (Pa.): WB Saunders; 1990

Peck GC. Techniques in Aesthetic Rhinoplasty. 2nd ed. New York: Gower Medical; 1990

Tardy ME, Brown RJ Surgical Anatomy of the Nose. New York: Raven Press; 1990

Aiach G, Levignac J. Aesthetic Rhinoplasty. Churchill Livingstone: London; 1991

Krause CJ, Pastorek N, Mangat DS, editors. Aesthetic Facial Surgery. Philadelphia (Pa.): Lippincott, Williams & Wilkins; 1991

Daniel RK, Regnault P. Rhinoplasty. Boston: Little & Brown; 1993

Nolst Trenité GJ, editor. Rhinoplasty. A Practical Guide to Functional and Aesthetic Surgery of the Nose. Amsterdam: Kugler; 1993 (1st ed), 1998 (2nd ed), 2005 (3rd ed), 2011 (4th ed)

Burget GC, Mennick FJ. Aesthetic Reconstruction of the Nose. St Louis, Mo.: Mosby; 1994

McCollough EG, Rousso D, Fedok FG. Nasal Plastic Surgery. Philadelphia, Pa.: WB Saunders; 1994

Ortiz-Monasterio F, Ortiz-Monasterio F, Molina F. Rhinoplasty. Philadelphia, Pa.: WB Saunders; 1994

Zaoli G. Aesthetic Rhinoplasty. Padova: Piccin; 1994

Gubisch W. Septumplastik durch extracorporale Korrektur. Stuttgart: Thieme; 1995

Jugo SB. Surgical Atlas of External Rhinoplasty. London: Churchill Livingstone; 1995

Aiach G, Madjiji A, Horn G, Sheen JH. Atlas of Rhinoplasty: Open and Endonasal Approaches. St Louis: Quality Med Pub; 1996

Tardy ME. Rhinoplasty: the Art and Science. Vols 1 and 2. Philadelphia, Pa.: WB Saunders; 1997

Hoefflin SM. Ethnic Rhinoplasty. New York: Springer; 1998

Tebbets JB. Primary Rhinoplasty. St Louis: Mosby; 1998

Toriumi DM, Becker DG. Rhinoplasty Dissection Manual. Philadelphia, Pa.: Lippincott Williams & Wilkins; 1999

2000–2014

Elsahy N. Plastic and Reconstructive Surgery of the Nose. Philadelphia, Pa.: WB Saunders; 2000

Mang WL. Manual of Aesthetic Surgery. Vol I. New York, Berlin: Springer; 2002.

Meyer R. Secondary Rhinoplasty: Including Reconstruction of the Nose. New York, Berlin: Springer; 2002

Huizing EH, De Groot JAM. Functional Corrective Nasal Surgery. Stuttgart, New York: Thieme; 2002 (1st ed), 2015 (2nd ed)

Baker SR, Naficy S, Jewet B. Principles of Nasal Reconstruction. New York, Berlin: Springer; 2002 (1st ed), 2011 (2nd ed)

Daniel RK. Rhinoplasty: An Atlas of Surgical Techniques. New York, Berlin: Springer; 2002 (1st ed), 2010 (2nd ed)

Papel ID, et al. Facial Plastic and Reconstructive Surgery. Stuttgart, New York: Thieme; 2002 (1st ed), 2009 (2nd ed)

Behrbohm H, Tardy ME, editors. Essentials of Septorhinoplasty. Stuttgart, New York: Thieme; 2003

Behrbohm H, Tardy E. Functional-Aesthetic surgery of the Nose – Septorhinoplasty. Stuttgart, New York: Thieme; 2003

Daniel RK. Mastering Rhinoplasty. New York: Springer; 2004 (1st ed), 2010 (2nd ed)

Sachs ME. Mastering Revision Rhinoplasty. New York: Springer; 2006

Theissing RG. Werner JA. HNO-Operationslehre. Stuttgart, New York: Thieme; 2006

Becker DG, Park SS. Revision Rhinoplasty. Stuttgart, New York: Thieme; 2007

Mennick FJ. Nasal Reconstruction: Art and Practice. Elsevier Health Sciences; 2008

Godin MS, editor. Rhinoplasty – Cases and Techniques. Stuttgart, New York: Thieme; 2012

Guyuron B. Rhinoplasty. Elsevier; 2012

Lohuis JFM. Advanced Caucasian and Mediterranean Rhinoplasty. Kugler Publications; 2014

Index

Note: Page numbers set bold or italic indicate headings or figures, respectively.